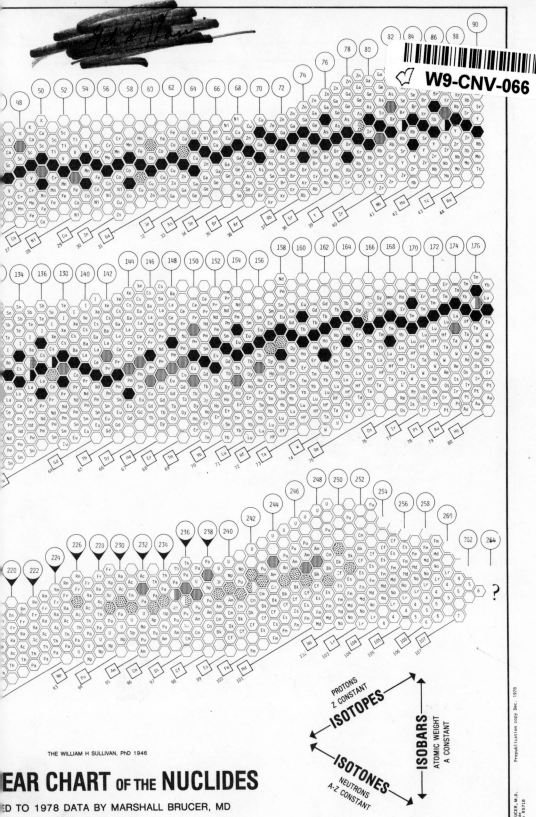

THE WILLIAM H SULLIVAN, PhD 1946

EAR CHART OF THE NUCLIDES

ED TO 1978 DATA BY MARSHALL BRUCER, MD

PROTONS
Z CONSTANT
ISOTOPES

ISOBARS
ATOMIC WEIGHT
A CONSTANT

ISOTONES
NEUTRONS
A-Z CONSTANT

Prepublication copy Dec. 1978

MARSHALL BRUCER, M.D.
5535 Via Celeste
Tucson, Arizona 85718

TEXTBOOK OF NUCLEAR MEDICINE TECHNOLOGY

TEXTBOOK OF
Nuclear medicine technology

PAUL J. EARLY, B.S.

President, Nuclear Medicine Associates, Inc.,
Cleveland, Ohio; Consultant in Nuclear Medicine,
Ohio University, Athens, Ohio

MUHAMMAD ABDEL RAZZAK
M.B.B.Ch., D.M., M.D.(Cairo), F.A.C.P.(U.S.A.)

Professor of Medicine, Medical Unit and Division of Nuclear Medicine,
Faculty of Medicine, Cairo University, Cairo, A.R.E.;
Nuclear Medicine Consultant, Medical Services,
Egyptian Armed Forces

D. BRUCE SODEE, M.D., F.A.C.P.

Director, Nuclear Medicine Institute, Cleveland, Ohio; Director,
Nuclear Medicine Department, Hillcrest Hospital, Cleveland,
Ohio; Formerly Associate Professor of Radiology (Nuclear Medicine),
George Washington University, Washington, D.C.

THIRD EDITION

with **590** illustrations

The C. V. Mosby Company

ST. LOUIS • TORONTO • LONDON   1979

The C. V. Mosby Company
11830 Westline Industrial Drive, St. Louis, Missouri 63141

Library of Congress Cataloging in Publication Data

Early, Paul J
  Textbook of nuclear medicine technology.

  Bibliography: p.
  Includes index.
  1. Nuclear medicine. I. Abdel Razzak,
Muhammad, joint author. II. Sodee, D. Bruce,
1930-   joint author. III. Title.
R895.E18 1978   616.07'57   78-31659
ISBN 0-8016-1488-0

C/VH/VH 9 8 7 6 5 4 3 2 1   02/C/238

Preface

As in the first edition of *Textbook of Nuclear Medicine Technology,* we have attempted to present contents in this text to correspond with the growth of what is now a new specialty of medicine. As our clinical basis grows, it becomes increasingly important for personnel in this field to continuously update their knowledge in instrumentation, radiochemistry, anatomy, and physiology. Some of the more basic information has been removed so as to avoid duplication of basic courses that are usually a prerequisite to a student entering the field of nuclear medicine.

This text is designed to introduce the student to nuclear science and clinical theory, which constitute the two parts of this book. These parts represent the works of a large variety of authors compiled over a long period of time. In discussion of generally accepted theory and practice, no attempt has been made to document statements with precise references.

Additions to Part One of this edition draw attention to dosimetry, expanding the MIRD concept of dosimetry to include S factors. A special section on film and film characteristics, written by David T. Williams, has been included in this edition. Computers and instrumentation receive special attention in an effort to present some of the advances since the last edition. Also, sections on radiation health, radiation biology, and radiation safety have been expanded in this edition. The ALARA philosophy has been included in the latter.

Additions to Part Two draw attention to recent advances in clinical procedures and techniques. Some of the older radiopharmaceuticals have been deleted from this edition because of their limited use in state-of-the-art nuclear medicine. These have been replaced with more current radiopharmaceuticals and discussions of their uses.

It should be emphasized that this text is designed to be used in concert with our other book, *Technology and Interpretation of Nuclear Medicine Procedures,* which contains experiments and procedures that will facilitate the learning of the principles discussed in this text. Acknowledgements are extended to all contributors; illustrators Susan Nicolet and David Warnock; and to our secretaries, Georgene Sodee and Ann Canty, who have aided in the production of this manuscript. Special thanks is extended to Roger Cloutier of the Oak Ridge Associated Universities, Oak Ridge, Tennessee, for generating the corrected version of the universal decay table (Appendix B).

Paul J. Early
Muhammad Abdel Razzak
D. Bruce Sodee

Contents

APPENDIXES

PART ONE

NUCLEAR SCIENCE

1 Anatomy of the atom

In any treatise of the basic sciences a detailed discussion of the structure of matter, molecules, and the constituent atoms must first be presented. In any treatise of the basic *nuclear* sciences a discussion of the constituent parts of the atom should be presented, since these parts play such an important role in the understanding of the nuclear sciences. All the parts of the atom that are important to the nuclear sciences, particularly to nuclear medicine, are presented in this chapter.

NATURE OF MATTER

The atom is composed of a central positively charged core known as a *nucleus*. Traveling in a path around the nucleus are one or more smaller negatively charged particles of mass, called *electrons*. Bohr compared this arrangement to a miniature solar system—the nucleus representing the sun and the electrons representing the planets circling the sun.

The electron

Definition and description. The electron is a high-velocity extranuclear particle that has a more or less fixed elliptic path around the nucleus. The electron possesses a known mass that remains constant for electrons of all atoms. The number of electrons that are circling the nucleus is a variable, and that number in an electrically neutral atom is dictated by the constituents of the nucleus. Two criteria may be used to differentiate the electron particle from other particles in the atom: *mass* and *electrical charge* (Table 1-1). With the electron as a reference point, the electron has a relative mass of 1 and a negative charge. This negative charge apparently cannot be separated from the electron. Possessing a negative charge, the electron exhibits forces of attraction or repulsion to other charged particles. These forces were first noticed by Coulomb, and the principle is now an accepted principle of physics. Coulomb's law states in part that *like charges repel; unlike charges attract.*

Mystery of the electron. Because of Coulomb's law and the fact that negative electrons circle the positive nucleus, the question of what effect all this has in the atom may well be asked. A repulsion effect between electrons is exhibited as a distribution in space as they circle the nucleus. The mystery arises from the lack of attraction of the electrons to the nucleus. What prevents the electron from being attracted to the nucleus?

Table 1-1. Mass and charge of particles of the atom

Particle	Charge	Mass
Electron	Negative	1*
Proton	Positive	1,836
Neutron	Neutral	1,840
Neutrino	Neutral	~0

*Reference mass.

The attraction is prevented through the action of two phenomena working simultaneously. (1) Since the electron is a particle circling the nucleus at high velocities, the electron counteracts the attraction by the nucleus to a certain degree by centrifugal force, the force of inertia that tends to make rotating bodies move away from the center of rotation. (2) A certain amount of energy from the atom known as *binding energy* is expended for no other reason than to retain the electron in its preordained orbit.

The nucleus

On learning of the existence of the nucleus, scientists became intrigued with the fact that the nucleus contained almost all of the weight attributed to the atom. The nucleus therefore became a primary target of research. The effort to discover the composition and function of the nucleus still continues. Many aspects of the nucleus are known; others are unknown, but theories have been formulated about them. One fact that is considered indisputable is that the nucleus itself is made up of small particles. The two particles most important to students of nuclear medicine are the *proton* and the *neutron*. These particles are normal constituents of the nucleus and are commonly referred to as *nucleons*. This positively charged core of every atom contains almost the entire mass of the atom but only a small part of its volume. It has been calculated that the nucleus is only 1/100,000 the size of the entire atom, but it is so dense that a child's marble of the same density would weigh approximately 36,400,000 tons. The nucleus is very stable and is impervious to chemical or physical changes; however, radiation can cause changes within it.

The proton. The proton (p) possesses a known mass, which remains constant. It has a positive charge associated with it that cannot be separated from it. The charge is equal in magnitude to the negative charge of the electron. It is because of the presence of these protons within the nucleus that the nucleus possesses a positive charge. In fact, in the hydrogen atom, the proton *is* the positive nucleus. In all other atoms the proton is one of the constituents. The mass of the proton is much greater than that of the electron. It has a mass 1,836 times that of the electron (Table 1-1). The number of protons within the nucleus determines the type of atom; for example, all carbon atoms have 6 protons, and all atoms containing 6 protons are carbon atoms.

The neutron. The neutron (n) also possesses a known mass that remains constant. This mass is just slightly greater than the mass of a proton (1,840). This particle, as the name implies, has no electric charge. Because of the neutral charge it cannot attract or repel charged particles. In fact, it is this very property that makes the neutron important. With a lack of charge, the neutron cannot be affected by the charged particles in the atom and can penetrate right into the heart of the atom. Under proper conditions the neutron can actually be incorporated into the nucleus or disrupt it. The former is referred to as neutron activation; the latter is referred to as fission. Both of these phenomena will be discussed later.

Mystery of the nucleus. The nucleus can be considered to be an aggregate of positive charges because of its proton constituents. According to Coulomb's law, the protons should repel one another, and the repulsive effects of the positive charges should cause the nucleus to fragment. However, this does not seem to be the case. An explanation is that the protons — and therefore the nucleus — are contained through binding energy. The nucleus expends a large amount of energy to keep the nucleons bound to one another.

The neutrino. The neutrino cannot be considered a normal constituent of the nucleus, but it results from interactions within the nucleus. This particle plays a more or less important role in nuclear medicine, since it is emitted during several methods of atomic decay. At the present time, only a description of the particle is warranted. The neutrino (v) is, as the name would indicate, a particle possessing a neutral charge. The mass of the neutrino approaches zero mass.

The mass and charge of all these particles are summarized in Table 1-1.

Energy shells

The atom has been defined as the smallest unit of matter that exhibits the chemical properties of an element. It is composed of a nucleus containing protons and neutrons of varying numbers and is surrounded by one or more negatively charged electrons circling in rather well-defined orbits, or *energy shells*. The number of electrons in each energy shell varies according to the chemical element. Each shell can contain only a certain number of electrons. That number is defined by the *$2n^2$ formula*, in which *n* is the number of the energy shell. The energy shells are numbered beginning with that shell closest to the nucleus and proceeding outward numerically. According to the $2n^2$ formula, the first energy shell can contain no more than 2 electrons. The second energy shell can contain no more than 8 electrons, the third energy shell can contain no more than 18 electrons, the fourth energy shell can contain no more than 32 electrons, and so on. Rather than being designated by numbers, the shells are labeled alphabetically beginning with K and proceeding outward. Therefore the K shell can have no more than 2, the L shell no more than 8, and the M shell no more than 18 electrons. A more lengthy discussion of energy levels, both orbital as well as nuclear, will be found at the end of Chapter 2.

NUCLEAR SHORTHAND

In every phase of business and professional life, there is a need to express one-self in concise, definitive terminology. Nuclear physics is no different. For this reason, a shorthand system has been devised to specify every atom and every form of that atom. This identification process is carried out with the aid of the *chemical symbol,* the *atomic number,* and the *mass number* in accordance with the following format:

$$\ _Z^A X$$

X represents the chemical symbol
A represents the mass number
Z represents the atomic number

The *mass number* (A) has the superscript position immediately preceding the chemical symbol and indicates the number of protons and neutrons in the nucleus. (In the past, this number held the superscript position immediately following the chemical symbol.) The *atomic number* (Z) has the subscript position immediately preceding the chemical symbol and indicates the number of protons in the nucleus just as it does on the periodic chart of the atoms. Since the proton number of any element is synonymous with the element itself, this shorthand method has been shortened even further by indicating only the element and the mass number. These two terms are sufficient to identify the atom. The *neutron number* (N) can be found by subtracting the atomic number from the mass number:

$$N = A - Z$$

THREE SIMPLEST ATOMS

In a detailed study of the three simplest atoms—hydrogen, helium, and lithium—some basic principles can be learned of the nature of the more complex atoms that occur in nature (Fig. 1-1). These principles will be delineated after the discussion of each of these atoms.

Hydrogen

The simplest of all atoms is the hydrogen atom (H). This element is a colorless, odorless gas that occurs throughout all living material. It represents 10% of the body weight of the biochemical standard man. Hydrogen, the simplest atom in the periodic chart of the atoms, possesses the atomic number 1, indicating 1 proton and therefore 1 electron. The number of neutrons in the nucleus of any atom can be learned by rounding off the atomic weight and subtracting the atomic number. The rounding off of the atomic weight of hydrogen, 1.0079, would result in the number 1. Since the atomic number is 1, there are no neutrons in the most abundant form of the hydrogen atom. The symbol for this form is $_1^1$H.

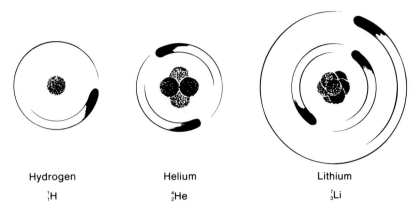

| Hydrogen | Helium | Lithium |
| ^1_1H | ^4_2He | ^7_3Li |

Fig. 1-1. Nuclear components and electron configurations of the three simplest atoms—hydrogen, helium, and lithium. It should be noted, however, that these atoms have not been drawn proportionally. If the constituents of the hydrogen atom, for example, were depicted correctly, it would be impossible to display the atom on the page. It has been calculated that if the nucleus of the hydrogen atom were the size of a baseball, the electron would be circling in an orbit wide enough to encompass New York City. It should also be remembered that atoms are three-dimensional. The electrons do not circle the nucleus in a flat field relationship as depicted here, but can circle the nucleus from an infinite number of angles.

Helium

Helium (He), occupying the next position on the periodic chart, is also a colorless and odorless gas. It has an atomic number of 2 and an atomic weight of 4.0026. The helium nucleus consists of 2 protons and 2 neutrons, accounting for the symbol ^4_2He.

In order that the helium atom be electrically neutral, 2 orbiting electrons are required because there are 2 protons in the nucleus. This same pattern is followed throughout all the atoms.

Lithium

Lithium (Li) is a metal considered not essential for biologic materials. Lithium occupies the next position in the order of complexity, having an atomic number of 3 and an atomic weight, when rounded off, of 7. This would indicate that the lithium atom has 3 protons, 4 neutrons, and, in an electrically neutral atom, 3 orbiting electrons, as shown in the symbol ^7_3Li.

Principles

In studying these three simplest atoms, four important principles are demonstrated:

1. To maintain electrical neutrality, the number of orbiting electrons must equal the number of protons within the nucleus. Hydrogen has 1 proton and there-

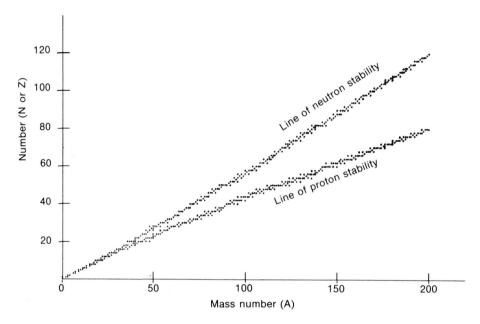

Fig. 1-2. Graph showing the number of neutrons to the number of protons for all known stable forms of an element and plotted against their mass number. The graph displays neutron and proton lines of stability. The graph also illustrates the fact that as atoms become more complex, more neutrons are required to maintain stability.

fore 1 electron. Helium has 2 protons and therefore 2 electrons. Lithium has 3 protons and therefore 3 electrons.

2. The mass of the electron lends very little to the total mass of the atom under study. In the hydrogen atom the nucleus consists of 1 proton. Since the proton is 1,836 times greater than the electron in mass, the nucleus is of the same order of magnitude. In the helium atom the nucleus is 7,350 times greater in weight than the electron. The mass of any atom is very closely equal to the sum of the masses of the protons and the neutrons comprising its nucleus. The mass of the orbital electrons can in general be disregarded.

3. The electron configuration of each atom has a certain order. In hydrogen the electron is added to the K shell. In helium the second electron is added to the K shell, thereby completing that shell's full complement of electrons according to the $2n^2$ formula. In the lithium atom the third electron must be added to the L shell, since the K shell has received its full complement of electrons. A somewhat similar orderly progression continues throughout the entire chart of the atoms, although many irregularities exist, especially beyond potassium (K).

4. The number of neutrons within the nucleus varies with respect to the number of protons that exist within the nucleus. In the case of hydrogen there are no neutrons. Helium contains an equal number of protons and neutrons. Lithium has

a larger number of neutrons than protons. In fact, proceeding from lithium in complexity, the number of neutrons must increase at a faster rate than the number of protons to maintain nuclear stability, that is, to maintain a nonradioactive status (Fig. 1-2). This relationship begins to express itself as early as the third atom in the order of complexity. It continues until an atom such as polonium 210 is reached, which contains 84 protons and 126 neutrons. Even with this obvious abundance of neutrons, the nucleus cannot maintain stability, and the atom is subject to radioactive decay.

BIBLIOGRAPHY

Blahd, W. H.: Nuclear medicine, New York, 1965, McGraw-Hill Book Co.

Bogardus, C. R., Jr: Clinical applications of physics of radiology and nuclear medicine, St. Louis, 1969, Warren H. Green, Inc.

Boyd, C. M., and Dalrymple, G. V.: Basic science principles of nuclear medicine, St. Louis, 1974, The C. V. Mosby Co.

Chandra, R.: Introductory physics of nuclear medicine, Philadelphia, 1976, Lea & Febiger.

Chase, G. D., and Rabinowitz, J. L.: Principles of radioisotope methodology, ed. 3, Minneapolis, 1967, Burgess Publishing Co.

Goodwin, P. N., and Rao, D. V.: The physics of nuclear medicine, Springfield, Ill., 1977, Charles C Thomas, Publisher.

Gottschalk, A., and Potchen, E. J.: Diagnostic nuclear medicine, Baltimore, 1976, The Williams & Wilkins Co.

Hendee, W. R.: Medical radiation physics, Chicago, 1970, Year Book Medical Publishers, Inc.

Johns, H. E.: The physics of radiology, ed. 2, revised edition, Springfield, Ill., 1964, Charles C Thomas, Publisher.

King, E. R., and Mitchell, T. G.: A manual for nuclear medicine, Springfield, Ill., 1961, Charles C Thomas, Publisher.

Pizzarello, D. J., and Witcofski, R. L.: Medical radiation biology, Philadelphia, 1972, Lea & Febiger.

Prasad, K. N.: Human radiation biology, New York, 1974, Harper & Row, Publishers.

Quimby, E. H., and Feitelberg, S.: Radioactive isotopes in medicine and biology, ed. 2, Philadelphia, 1963, Lea & Febiger.

Rollo, F. D.: Nuclear medicine physics, instrumentation, and agents, St. Louis, 1977, The C. V. Mosby Co.

Shilling, C. W.: Atomic energy encyclopedia in the life sciences, Philadelphia, 1964, W. B. Saunders Co.

United States Department of Health, Education and Welfare: Radiological health handbook, revised edition, Washington, D.C., September 1960, United States Department of Commerce Clearinghouse for Federal Scientific and Technical Information.

Wagner, H. N.: Principles of nuclear medicine, Philadelphia, 1968, W. B. Saunders Co.

Wang, C. H., and Willis, D. L.: Radiotracer methodology in biological science, Englewood Cliffs, N.J., 1965, Prentice-Hall, Inc.

2 Nuclides and radionuclides

In recent years the terms *isotope* and *radioisotope* have fallen into disfavor. These two terms had been used for many years to describe all forms of all elements. Since this is not entirely correct usage of the two terms, they have been replaced by the terms *nuclide* and *radionuclide,* respectively. The term nuclide was proposed as a more precise term than isotope because the meaning of nuclide is any nucleus plus its orbital electrons. The term isotope refers to two or more forms of the same element. It would be incorrect to say iodine 127 is the only stable isotope of iodine, since there is only one stable form, not two or more. It would be more meaningful to describe iodine 127 as the only stable nuclide of iodine. Furthermore, it would be improper to refer to ^{197}Hg and ^{131}I as radioactive isotopes (radioisotopes). They are actually radioactive nuclides (radionuclides) because they are two different elements. A correct usage of the term radioisotopes would be that ^{197}Hg and ^{203}Hg are radioisotopes because they are two forms of the same element.

ISOTOPES

An isotope may be defined as one of two or more forms of the same element having the same atomic number (Z), differing mass numbers (A), and the same chemical properties. These different forms of an element may be stable or unstable (radioactive). However, since they are forms of the same element, they possess identical chemical properties. These chemical properties remain the same even though, if unstable, their radioactive properties differ. Another way of defining isotopes is that they are forms of the same element, but each form has a different weight because of the varying number of neutrons in the nucleus (Fig. 2-1).

There are over 270 known nuclidic forms of stable elements; 40 of these exist in nature and are termed *naturally occurring* nuclides. In addition to these, more than 900 radionuclides have been produced artificially.

Three isotopes of hydrogen. The periodic chart lists atomic numbers (chemical numbers) as whole numbers and atomic weights as decimal fractions. It would seem that if the nucleus consists of protons and neutrons and each nucleon represented one unit of atomic weight (the electrons not adding significantly to the weight of the atom), then all atoms should have an atomic weight that would be a multiple of one. However, this is not the case. For example, hydrogen has an atomic weight of 1.008. This must have caused great concern to early investigators,

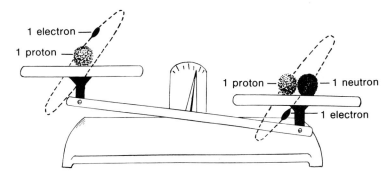

Fig. 2-1. Diagram illustrating that the difference between two isotopes can be expressed as a weight differential caused by an increased or decreased number of neutrons in their nuclear configurations.

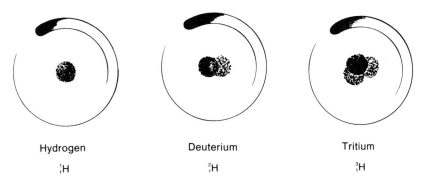

Hydrogen

^1_1H

Deuterium

^2_1H

Tritium

^3_1H

Fig. 2-2. Three isotopes of hydrogen — ordinary hydrogen, deuterium, and tritium. The number of protons and electrons remains the same for all three forms, but the neutron number increases.

since the earliest known form of hydrogen had only 1 proton and should have had an atomic weight of 1.000. This not being the case, early investigators found it necessary to hypothesize the existence of some other form of the element that reacted identically to hydrogen but was heavier. This would cause the resultant weight to be something greater than 1.000, the degree being dependent on the abundance of this heavier form. The existence of isotopes was postulated as one of the possible factors in this obvious discrepancy. Hydrogen was found to occur in nature in two different forms, ordinary hydrogen and deuterium, thus proving the hypothesis.

Hydrogen. Ordinary hydrogen, ^1_1H (sometimes called *protium*), is the most abundant form of the element hydrogen. Its nucleus has only 1 proton ($Z = 1$) and no neutrons ($A = 1$) (Fig. 2-2). It is naturally occurring and stable.

Deuterium. Another isotope of hydrogen is deuterium. Deuterium, ^2_1H, consists of 1 proton ($Z = 1$) and 1 neutron ($A = 2$) and is the least abundant form. It occurs in a ratio of 8 parts to every 1,000 parts of ordinary hydrogen. Deuterium is naturally occurring and stable. It has also been called *heavy hydrogen*. Since ordinary hydrogen has 1 proton and deuterium has 1 proton plus 1 neutron, deuterium is twice the weight of the most abundant form.

It is interesting to note that deuterium occurs at a ratio of 8:1,000 parts of all hydrogen atoms in nature. This ratio of abundance would justify the atomic weight differential of the hydrogen atom as 1.008. The atomic (chemical) weight of an element is derived from all the *stable* forms of the element, considering the atomic weight of each form of the element and its percent abundance in nature. For example, if both forms occurred in nature at a rate of 50:50, and since ^{2}H is twice the weight of ^{1}H, the atomic weight would be 1.500.

Tritium. There is a third isotope of hydrogen, but it does not occur naturally. It is the artificially produced tritium, $^3_1$H. Tritium is sometimes symbolized as ^{3}T. This isotope contains 1 proton (Z = 1) and 2 neutrons (A = 3) and is therefore three times the mass of the most abundant form. It is sometimes referred to as *extra-heavy hydrogen*. Since hydrogen is an intimate part of body chemistry, the use of tritium plays an important role in medical and agricultural research. It is also used as one of the nuclides measured in the Nuclear Regulatory Commission's stratospheric sampling program. It is formed by neutron bombardment of nitrogen 14 after the detonation of an atomic device, yielding carbon 12 and tritium.

·   ·   ·

All three forms have only 1 proton in their nuclei and only 1 electron in their orbits (Fig. 2-2). Since the electrons determine the chemical characteristics and their number is the same on all three forms, these isotopes, whether stable or unstable, react identically in a chemical situation. The difference in mass is caused solely by the number of neutrons within the nucleus.

Neutron to proton ratio. From studying these isotopes of hydrogen, the principle of neutron to proton ratio and nuclear stability can be observed. In the cases of ordinary hydrogen and deuterium the presence or absence of 1 neutron does not alter the stability of the nucleus. In both cases the nucleus is nonradioactive. However, the incorporation of 1 more neutron into the nucleus, as in the case of tritium, exceeds the bounds of nuclear stability. Why the nucleus becomes unstable at that point is not clearly understood, but tritium becomes an unstable or radioactive nuclide of hydrogen because there are too many neutrons.

This principle is also true with all other nuclides. Each element has its own unique ratio or combination of neutrons and protons. Any deviation from this, either too few neutrons and too many protons or too many neutrons and too few protons, results in nuclear instability.

The method by which a nuclide decays (changes into another nuclide) is that method that will result in the nucleus becoming stable or closer to stability. If the decay process contains only one step, then the resultant new nuclide is stable. If the decay process contains many steps, then the nuclide formed after the first step will be unstable and more than one step is necessary before a stable form of an element is reached.

OTHER "ISOS"

Isobar. By definition, isobars are 2 atoms that have the same mass number but different atomic numbers and therefore different chemical properties. To state it another way, the nucleus of each of these atoms contains the same sum of protons and neutrons, but the division between protons and neutrons is different. An example of isobars would be lithium 7($_3^7$Li) and beryllium 7($_4^7$Be). Both nuclides have a total of 7 nucleons. Lithium has 3 protons and 4 neutrons, and beryllium has 4 protons and 3 neutrons. Isobars in nuclear medicine are of no particular importance per se.

Isotone. Isotones are nuclides having the same number of neutrons. In no other way are 2 isotones similar. They differ in atomic number, mass number, and chemical properties. They are mentioned primarily because the trilinear chart of the nuclides has been formulated on the basis of isotopes, isobars, and isotones. An example of isotones would be $_{53}^{131}$I and $_{54}^{132}$Xe. In each case N = 78.

Table 2-1 summarizes the differences between isotopes, isobars, and isotones.

Isomer. An isomer is one of two or more nuclides that has the same mass number and atomic number as the others but exists for measurable times in the excited state. When a nucleus is in an excited state and decays by gamma emission, the transition from the higher to the lower energy usually takes less than 10^{-13} seconds. Nuclei that take longer than 10^{-9} seconds are called isomers. Two examples of isomers are technetium 99m and strontium 87m.

ATOMIC ENERGY LEVELS

Both x rays and gamma rays represent energy releases as a result of changes in energy levels either within the nucleus or in the extranuclear structure. X rays are releases of energy as a result of changes within the orbital pattern of the electrons. Gamma rays are releases of energy as a result of changes occurring within the nucleus itself. To understand these energy releases an explanation of both the orbital energy levels and the nuclear energy levels is warranted.

Table 2-1. Summary of the differences between isotopes, isobars, and isotones

	Atomic number (Z)	Mass number (A)	Neutron number (N)	Chemical properties
Isotopes	Same	Different	Different	Same
Isobars	Different	Same	Different	Different
Isotones	Different	Different	Same	Different

ORBITAL ENERGY LEVELS

Although it has been said that an electron is more or less assigned to a definite orbit, the analogy of an atom to a miniature solar system is to some degree an over-simplification. Unlike the planets circling the sun, the electron can actually exist anywhere, although it is most often found in its regularly assigned orbit. Unlike the usual illustrations of the atom, it has been suggested that the electron does not follow a circular path around the nucleus but more nearly an elliptical path. In fact, some scientists subscribe to the theory that the K shell electron(s) has such an elliptical pattern that the orbit of the K shell electron actually passes through the nucleus. Furthermore, since like charges repel one another, the electrons repel each other in their respective orbits so that these electrons are actually arranged in space symmetry. There are two types of energies involved in the course of an electron, and each plays a definite role in the action and subsequent reaction of electron disturbance. These energies are the binding energy and the energy state of the electron itself.

Binding energy. The binding energy of the electron is the energy required to remove the particle from its orbit. If the binding energy of a K shell electron of a particular atom was 70,000 electron volts (70 kev), as in Fig. 2-3, that electron must be supplied with an energy equal to or greater than 70 kev to remove it from its energy shell. This energy could be supplied to that electron by a high-energy particle or photon radiation, at which time the energy of the interacting particle or ray would be decreased in energy by an amount equal to the binding energy. The same principle is true for an L shell electron except that less energy is required to

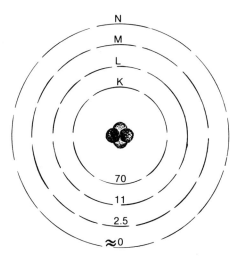

Fig. 2-3. Representative electron binding energies of a hypothetical atom. The binding energy is larger for those electrons circling closer to the nucleus. To remove an electron from its orbit, the removing force must possess an energy equal to or greater than the binding energy.

remove it, since the binding energy becomes less as the electron is positioned farther away from the nucleus. In a typical atom, in which the K shell electron would have a binding energy of 70 kev, the binding energy of the L shell electron may be reduced to as little as 11 kev, the M shell electron to 2.5 kev, and the N shell electron ≈0, the latter being the case with all outer shell electrons. In each of these cases, energy equal to or greater than that of the binding energy of the electron must be supplied to remove that electron from its orbit.

Energy state of the electron. The energy state of an orbital electron can, perhaps, best be described by comparing it, through a crude analogy, to a racetrack (Fig. 2-4). For each car to stay abreast with the others it must possess a different speed (energy). According to the illustration, the car on the outside track (the M track) must travel at 75 mph to keep abreast with the car on the inner track (the K track) traveling at 65 mph. Therefore the 75 mph car has a greater energy state than does the car on the inner track. Should the car on the inside track drop from the race, either the car in the middle track or the car on the outside track would have the ability to take its place. To do so, each car must decrease its speed, that is, decrease its energy state to maintain its position in the race.

Such is also the case of the orbiting electrons. Should the K shell electron be

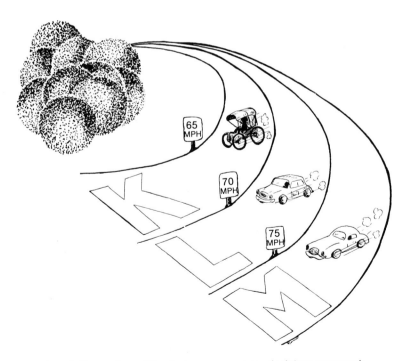

Fig. 2-4. Comparison of the electron energy state principle to a racetrack.

removed from its orbit for some reason, the L or the M shell electron would take its place. To do so, there would necessarily have to be a decrease in the energy state of that orbiting electron. At the same time there would be an increase in the binding energy, since the electron is assuming the role of the K shell electron that possesses more binding energy. Should a K shell electron be removed, the probability that that space would be filled by the L electron and the L space filled by the M electron would be greater than of the M falling down into the K shell electron. In any case, just as nature abhors a vacuum, an electron shell abhors a vacancy. By depicting the energy states of the electrons as analogous to a racetrack, the intention is to simplify the phenomena of *optical radiation* and *characteristic radiation.*

Optical radiation. The ability of atoms under certain conditions to emit radiations that fall into the visible spectrum allowed scientists a means of identifying the atom by identifying the color of the light. This type of radiation is termed *optical radiation.* It results from the fact that when an atom is given a certain amount of energy (termed *excited state*), the electron will move to a certain corresponding path (subshell) farther from the nucleus. This move would not be enough to move it into another orbit. (In the case of the racing car, the car would not move into the 80 mph racetrack, but would move into a suborbit that might correspond to the outer portion of the 75 mph track, thereby necessitating the car to go 77 mph to keep aligned.) To go to this subshell, the electron would have to assume additional energy, just as would the racing car. As soon as the source of energy is removed, the electron drops back to the original orbit and emits a photon of an energy corresponding to the energy loss by the electron. The photon would be of a frequency and wavelength equal to some form of the visible light spectrum, thereby serving as a means of color identification.

This same principle applies to *excitation* of an atom by a passing particle (α or β) or electromagnetic radiation (γ- or x-radiation). An orbital electron is raised in energy state with the subsequent release of that energy when the electron drops into its normally occupied energy shell.

Characteristic radiation. The same principle holds true for electrons falling into an energy shell closer to the nucleus. In the event that a K shell electron would be removed, the vacancy would be filled by either the L shell electron or the M shell electron. Since the L shell electron would have to decrease in energy state by assuming the role of a K shell electron, the energy differential must be released in the form of x-radiation. This is known as characteristic radiation, or *fluorescent radiation.* It is important to note that these emissions are not known as gamma radiations. The only difference between gamma and x radiation is their *source,* or origin. X rays originate from the orbital structure of the atom, and gamma rays always originate from the nucleus. At no time could these characteristic radiations be referred to as gamma rays. The term *characteristic radiation* has been applied because the energy of the resultant x ray is characteristic of the energy loss by an electron falling from an orbit distant from the nucleus to an orbit closer to the nucleus. All electrons falling into the K shell, regardless of their origin, would emit x rays, called *characteristic K-radiation;* all electrons falling into the L shell would emit characteristic L-radiation and so on.

The actual situation is considerably more complex than that described previously. Electrons are capable of rotating about and moving back and forth with respect to their position with the nucleus. The energy pathways in which these electrons travel and still stay within their primary energy shells are called *subshells.* The total subshells for each primary energy shell are known, as well as is the number of electrons to be found on each subshell. (Fig. 2-5 and Table 2-2).

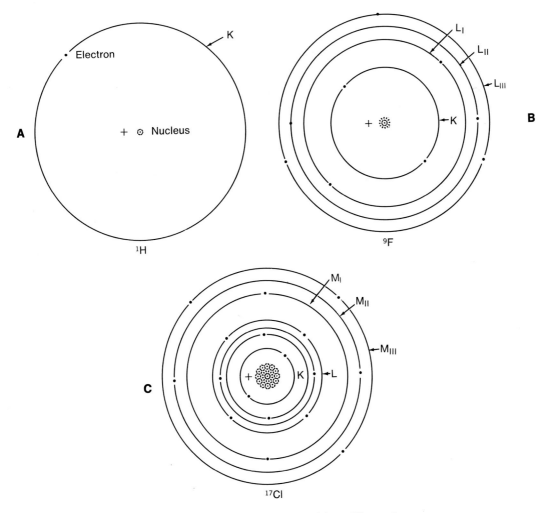

Fig. 2-5. Subshell arrangements of three different size atoms.

Table 2-2. The occupation capacities of the electron shells of the atom

n	*Primary shell letter designation*	*Subshell designation*							*Total capacity*
		I	*II*	*III*	*IV*	*V*	*VI*	*VII*	
1	K	2	–	–	–	–	–	–	2
2	L	2	2	4	–	–	–	–	8
3	M	2	2	4	4	6	–	–	18
4	N	2	2	4	4	6	6	8	32
5	O	2	2	4	4	6	6	8	32

Changes between subshells (within the same primary energy shell) occur constantly, so that physicists avoid trying to predict the exact location of any electron at any time. They attempt to predict only the probability that an electron is at a given energy level. For each change, a discrete amount of energy is released. Changes between primary energy shells can also occur; however, it requires an electron vacancy in a lower level or a degree of excitation sufficient to overcome the binding energy of that electron. Whenever changes in electron position of this magnitude occur, the resultant release of energy falls usually in the x-ray portion of the electromagnetic spectrum (Chapter 3).

The laws of physics forbid the movement of some electrons of one energy shell to another shell. It is not felt that a discussion of these rules are within the scope of this textbook. Suffice it to say that the changes that are permitted result in energy emissions bearing names such as "$K\alpha1$ x-ray". A $K\alpha1$ x-ray is the energy released as a result of the L_{III} electron dropping into the K shell, called a K-L_{III} transition. Other transitions worthy of note because they yield energies that could require consideration in radiation dosimetry are as follows: $K\alpha2$ x-ray = K-L_{II} transition, $K\beta1$ x-ray = K-M_{III} transition, $K\beta2$ x-ray = K-N_{II} transition, and L x-rays = x-rays arising because of any vacancy in the L shell.

NUCLEAR ENERGY LEVELS

The concept of energy states as discussed regarding the orbital structure is also applicable to the nucleus, except that releases of energy resulting from changes within the nucleus are of much greater magnitude than those of the electrons. There are two possible results should an elevation in energy state (excited state) be experienced by the nucleus. There may be particle emission caused by conditions involving binding energy or photon (gamma) emission caused by conditions involving the energy state of the nucleus.

Binding energy. Just as there is a binding energy involved with the orbiting electrons, so also is there a binding energy involved with the nucleus. The binding energy in the nucleus is the energy required to remove a single proton, neutron, or alpha particle from the nucleus. The existence of binding energy can be demonstrated by comparing the mass relationship of an intact helium 4 nucleus (2 pro-

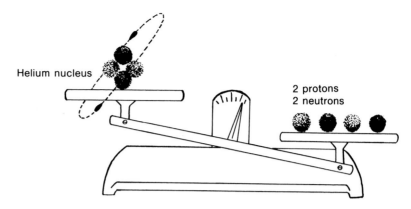

Helium nucleus

2 protons
2 neutrons

Fig. 2-6. Proof of nuclear binding energy. The intact helium 4 nucleus weighs less than the individual components weighed separately. This suggests that some of the nuclear mass has been converted to binding energy.

tons, 2 neutrons) to the weight of 2 protons and 2 neutrons weighed separately (Fig. 2-6). The intact helium 4 atom actually weighs less than the sum of its constituent parts because some of the actual mass of the helium 4 nucleus has been converted to energy (binding energy). The nuclear binding energy is the equivalent energy difference between the sum of the masses of the protons and neutrons as they would exist separately and the equivalent energy of the mass of the nucleus itself. This difference is also called *mass defect* (Chapter 3).

It is believed that the protons and neutrons are in a constant state of motion. When energy is supplied to an atom, the degree of motion increases. This condition can be caused by the absorption of a photon, collisions with other particles or systems, or the natural radioactivity of the nucleus.

Since the nucleons are in motion, there are many chances for collisions between nuclear particles. When energy is added to the nucleus, the number of collisions increases. When a collision occurs, some or all of the energy of the colliding particle is transferred to the particle into which it collides. By this transfer of energy, the particle receives and retains an inordinate amount of energy until such time as it would lose that energy by a subsequent collision. If the energy that the particle receives exceeds the binding energy of that particle in the nucleus, the particle will be subject to ejection from the nucleus if no subsequent collision occurs. This would then constitute *particle emission.*

This phenomenon could be compared to a pool table. A dormant cue ball can be supplied with energy through the action of striking it with a cue stick. As the cue ball is propelled over some distance of the pool table, it collides with other balls on the table. Through this collision the cue ball transfers some or possibly all of its energy to other balls on the table. Should the energy transferred to another ball on the table be sufficient, the ball could possibly exceed the limits of the rebound cushions and be ejected from the pool table. This would be analogous to particle emission. Energies transferred to the nucleons that exceed their binding energy result in the loss of a particle from the nucleus, just as energy transferred to the pool balls, sufficient to overcome the containing effect of the table cushions, results in the loss of a pool ball from the table. This analogy typifies one mode of decay exactly. The analogy must be altered somewhat for other modes of decay that result in the production of particles other than protons and neutrons. These "foreign" particles, then, receive high energies with their subsequent emission from the nucleus.

Energy state of the nucleons. The concept of energy state of the electron is also applicable to that of the nucleus. When energy is added to the nucleus, but not enough to cause particle emission, the nucleus may merely be raised to another energy state. The most frequent cause for this is particle emission. The particle does not require all the energy given to the nucleus to bring about its ejection. Therefore energy remains in the nucleus, raising it to an excited state. Actually, both the protons and the neutrons have their own set of discrete energy levels to which either nucleon can be raised if sufficient energy is supplied to the nucleus. A nucleus is in its *ground state* when all of its lower energy levels are filled. This can be compared to stepladders with several missing rungs (Fig. 2-7). Only the intact rungs in the ladder would be representative of energy levels to which the nucleons could be raised. If each rung of the ladder represented 100 kev, the nucleons could be raised only to an energy level of 200, 400, 500, or 800 kev. In Fig. 2-7, *A*, the nucleus is in its ground state because all the nucleons occupy the lowest rungs (or energy levels). In Fig. 2-7, *B*, an excited state of the nucleus is represented in which a nucleon has been raised to an excited level of 500 kev. When this occurs, the nucleus instantaneously returns to ground state and releases energy corresponding to the energy differential. This energy release is known as gamma radiation. The return to ground state could occur as a one-step, one-gamma affair (monoenergetic), as in Fig. 2-7, *B*, or as a series of jumps with more than one gamma being released, as in Fig. 2-7, *C*. It is not likely that in exciting the nucleus the nucleus would not receive sufficient energy to raise the excitation state of the neutron to 500 kev but may only raise it to 400 kev. The reverse could also be true; the nucleus may have received a greater amount of energy, thereby raising the nucleus to 800 kev. It is impossible to predict which particular atom in a given sample of atoms would receive more energy or less energy so that these variations in neutron and proton excitation levels would be known. It is possible, however, to predict the percentages of nuclei receiving these varying energies. It is also possible to predict the percentages of gamma emissions having specific energies. The gamma energy that occurs the most times is referred to as the *primary energy peak,* that is, iodine 131 = 364 kev. This does not mean that iodine 131 has gamma emissions of only one energy. It means simply that the gamma emission of 364 kev occurs the greatest number of times for any given number of iodine 131 atoms undergoing the "de-excitation" process.

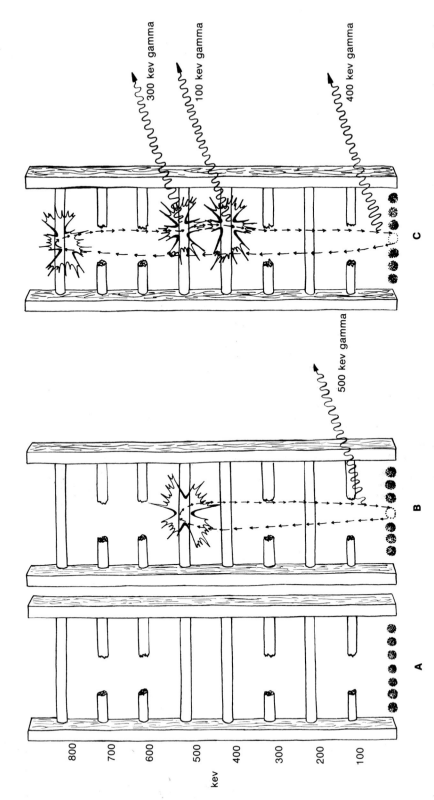

Fig. 2-7. Comparison of the nuclear energy state principle to a ladder. **A,** A nucleus at ground state. **B,** The emission of a monoenergetic gamma. **C,** A more complex decay scheme.

The concept of atomic energy levels is extremely difficult. The analogies of racetracks, pool tables, and ladders can, without hesitation, be considered over-simplifications. There is no such thing as a perfect analogy, and these are certainly no exceptions. They are included to assist the student of nuclear medicine in the understanding of extremely difficult principles. Any one of them could be subject to criticism should the analogy be extended beyond its intended purpose.

ELECTRON VOLT

In all exposures to the fundamentals of physics and electricity, terms that have become commonplace are words such as *volt, ampere,* and *erg.* In nuclear medicine the unit of definition seems to center on the term *electron volt* (ev). As the name implies, an electron volt has a relationship to an electron and to the volt. In physics the fundamental unit of work is the erg, or the *joule.* A more useful energy unit for nuclear medicine purposes is the electron volt, with its multiples, thousand electron volts (kev) and million electron volts (mev). The electron volt is defined as the amount of kinetic energy acquired when an electron falls through a potential difference of 1 volt (Fig. 2-8). In some instances, kev is similar to kv (used on x-ray equipment). If 1 electron falls through a potential difference of 1 v, it is equivalent to 1 ev; therefore, if 1 electron falls through a potential difference of 1,000 v, it is equivalent to 1,000 ev (1 kev). In this instance both kv and kev relate to 1,000 v potential difference. In other instances kev is totally different from kv; if 1,000 electrons fall through a potential difference of 1 v, it is also equivalent to 1,000 ev (1 kev). In this example the potential difference is 1 v and quite unlike kv.

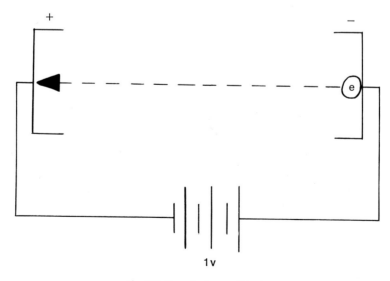

Fig. 2-8. One electron volt (ev).

The amount of work performed by 1 ev, expressed in joules, is found to be the product of the charge of the electron (in coulombs) and the potential difference through which it falls. The charge of 1 electron is known to be 1.60×10^{-19} coulombs. Therefore:

$$1 \text{ ev} = 1.00 \times 1.60 \times 10^{-19} \text{ coulombs} = 1.60 \times 10^{-19} \text{ joules} \qquad (2\text{-}1)$$

Thus 1 ev has the capacity to do the work of 1.60×10^{-19} joules. Through the use of this formula the electron volt has been converted to the joule, a fundamental unit of work. This conversion figure will be used in the following chapters.

BIBLIOGRAPHY

Blahd, W. H.: Nuclear medicine, New York, 1965, McGraw-Hill Book Co.

Bogardus, C. R., Jr: Clinical applications of physics of radiology and nuclear medicine, St. Louis, 1969, Warren H. Green, Inc.

Boyd, C. M., and Dalrymple, G. V.: Basic science principles of nuclear medicine, St. Louis, 1974, The C. V. Mosby Co.

Chandra, R.: Introductory physics of nuclear medicine, Philadelphia, 1976, Lea & Febiger.

Chase, G. D., and Rabinowitz, J. L.: Principles of radioisotope methodology, ed. 3, Minneapolis, 1967, Burgess Publishing Co.

Goodwin, P. N., and Rao, D. V.: The physics of nuclear medicine, Springfield, Ill., 1977, Charles C Thomas, Publisher.

Gottschalk, A., and Potchen, E. J.: Diagnostic nuclear medicine, Baltimore, 1976, The Williams & Wilkins Co.

Hendee, W. R.: Medical radiation physics, Chicago, 1970, Year Book Medical Publishers, Inc.

Johns, H. E.: The physics of radiology, ed. 2, revised edition Springfield, Ill., 1964, Charles C Thomas, Publisher.

King, E. R., and Mitchell, T. G.: A manual for nuclear medicine, Springfield, Ill., 1961, Charles C Thomas, Publisher.

Prasad, K. N.: Human radiation biology, New York, 1974, Harper & Row, Publishers.

Quimby, E. H., and Feitelberg, S.: Radioactive isotopes in medicine and biology, ed. 2, Philadelphia, 1963, Lea & Febiger.

Rollo, F. D.: Nuclear medicine physics, instrumentation, and agents, St. Louis, 1977, The C. V. Mosby Co.

Shilling, C. W.: Atomic energy encyclopedia in the life sciences, Philadelphia, 1964, W. B. Saunders Co.

United States Department of Health, Education and Welfare: Radiological health handbook, revised edition, Washington, D.C., September 1960, United States Department of Commerce Clearinghouse for Federal Scientific and Technical Information.

Wagner, H. N.: Principles of nuclear medicine, Philadelphia, 1968, W. B. Saunders Co.

Wang, C. H., and Willis, D. L.: Radiotracer methodology in biological science, Englewood Cliffs, N.J., 1965, Prentice-Hall, Inc.

3 Nature of radiation

Every human being is exposed daily to a variety of radiations whether he recognizes it or not. The popular concept of radiation, however, is somehow synonymous only with radiations emanating from an x-ray tube, from radioactive materials, or from fallout. In addition to these, there are several other types of radiations, all of which manifest themselves in different ways. Some of these radiations can be felt, such as the radiant energy whereby heat is transferred. Other radiations are audible, or at least the devices that receive these radiations, such as the radio, translate them to audible sound. Other radiations can be seen, such as light, which, when focused through a prism, can be further subdivided into all the colors of the spectrum.

There are other radiations that can neither be heard, seen, felt, nor otherwise perceived by the human senses. Examples of these are x rays and gamma rays. All of these radiations are among the members of the electromagnetic spectrum and are spoken of in terms of waves of energy. [Note that none of these radiations are affected by electrical or magnetic properties of matter; hence the name *electromagnetic.*] *

*Ignore

ENERGY WAVES AND THEIR CHARACTERISTICS

A wave in the electromagnetic spectrum is not unlike a wave resulting from a disturbance within a body of water. Throwing a rock into a large body of water would result in the familiar ripples, beginning at the point where the rock touched the water and progressing outward in a circular fashion. Close inspection of these waves would reveal that each wave is an entity in itself, each having a definite length. Those waves occurring near the point of impact occur more frequently than those at a distance from the point of impact, and they travel away from the point of impact. The *wavelength* is defined as the distance from a point on one wave to the same point on the subsequent wave. It could be said that the wavelength of those waves at the point of impact is shorter than those at a distance. The *frequency* is defined as the number of wave formations per unit time. It could be said that the frequency of waves would be greater near the point of impact than distant to the point of impact. The *velocity* is defined as the speed at which these waves travel.

All electromagnetic waves possess these same three characteristics of wavelength, frequency, and velocity. The velocity (c) of an electromagnetic wave is a constant. All waves travel at the same velocity regardless of their position on the

24

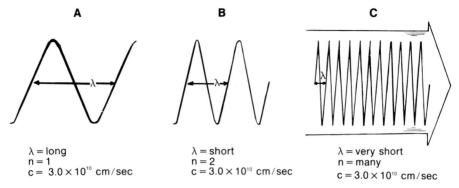

A

λ = long
n = 1
c = 3.0 × 10¹⁰ cm/sec

B

λ = short
n = 2
c = 3.0 × 10¹⁰ cm/sec

C

λ = very short
n = many
c = 3.0 × 10¹⁰ cm/sec

Fig. 3-1. Characteristics of electromagnetic waves. **A,** The wavelength, frequency, and velocity of a wave. **B,** As the wavelength decreases, the frequency increases and velocity remains unchanged. **C,** The quantum nature of radiation; the wave behaves like a bundle of energy, having direction and traveling at the speed of light.

electromagnetic spectrum. The speed of light waves is 186,000 miles per second (3.0×10^{10} cm/sec), and all members of the electromagnetic spectrum travel at this velocity. Wavelength (λ) and frequency (n) are variables and are *inversely proportional* to one another. This is readily apparent in Fig. 3-1. If the wavelength is decreased, the frequency with which that wave would occur per unit time would necessarily increase (Fig. 3-1, *B*).

The following formula shows a very important relationship between wavelength, frequency, and velocity for electromagnetic waves:

$$c = n \times \lambda$$

c = Velocity in cm/sec
n = Frequency in waves (vibrations)/sec
λ = Wavelength in cm

Since $c = 3 \times 10^{10}$ cm/sec, that value can be substituted immediately. If the frequency is known, the wavelength can be calculated, or, conversely, if the wavelength is known, the frequency can be calculated. Since the wavelength of radiations of interest to nuclear medicine personnel is extremely small, the angstrom unit (Å) has been devised as an expression of length, rather than the centimeter. The angstrom unit has a value of 10^{-8} cm.

ELECTROMAGNETIC SPECTRUM

The electromagnetic spectrum is usually displayed on the basis of wavelength in angstrom units. It could also be displayed in terms of frequency or energy. Fig. 3-2 attempts to incorporate all three variables in its display of the electromagnetic spectrum.

The spectrum may best be discussed by imagining ourselves to be in a room

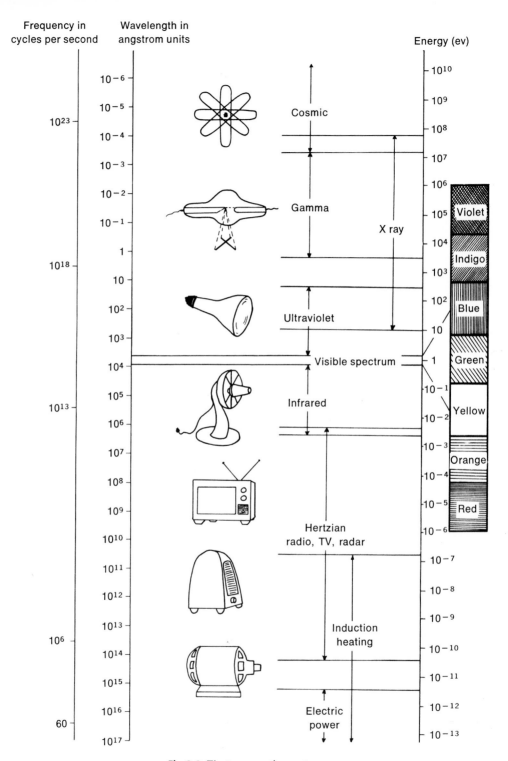

Frequency in cycles per second

Wavelength in angstrom units

Energy (ev)

	10^{-6}	10^{10}
	10^{-5}	10^{9}
10^{23}	10^{-4}	10^{8}
	10^{-3}	10^{7}
	10^{-2}	10^{6}
	10^{-1}	10^{5}
	1	10^{4}
10^{18}	10	10^{3}
	10^{2}	10^{2}
	10^{3}	10
	10^{4}	1
	10^{5}	10^{-1}
10^{13}	10^{6}	10^{-2}
	10^{7}	10^{-3}
	10^{8}	10^{-4}
	10^{9}	10^{-5}
	10^{10}	10^{-6}
	10^{11}	10^{-7}
	10^{12}	10^{-8}
10^{6}	10^{13}	10^{-9}
	10^{14}	10^{-10}
	10^{15}	10^{-11}
	10^{16}	10^{-12}
60	10^{17}	10^{-13}

Cosmic

Gamma

X ray

Ultraviolet

Visible spectrum

Infrared

Hertzian radio, TV, radar

Induction heating

Electric power

Violet

Indigo

Blue

Green

Yellow

Orange

Red

Fig. 3-2. Electromagnetic spectrum.

containing a variety of electrical and electronic instrumentation, seated before an instrument that has a capacity of dialing in wavelengths ranging from 10^{17} Å to 10^{-5} Å. By setting the dial of the instrument at 10^{17}Å, the operator would feel heat, since heat waves occur at this wavelength. If the dial were turned slightly, to decrease the wavelength, the radio would begin to play. A further turn of the dial would allow reception by the television set. When the dial is turned even further to allow reception of even shorter wavelengths, the radar monitoring scope would begin to indicate reception of information. With another turn of the dial an intense and deeply penetrating heat in the form of infrared radiation from a heat lamp would be experienced. As the dial is turned further, the room would become illuminated by a deep red light. Subsequent turns of the dial would change the color of the light from red to orange, orange to yellow, yellow to green, green to blue, blue to indigo, and indigo to violet. Eventually the sunlamp will glow, allowing exposure to ultraviolet radiation. Up to this point, changes in wavelengths have demonstrated phenomena that, with appropriate aids, could be felt, seen, or heard. Further changes in wavelength, indicating reception of even shorter waves, cannot be perceived by the human senses. The first of these that would be encountered would be x-rays, next would be gamma rays, and finally, at the shortest wavelength setting possible, would be cosmic radiation. In this hypothetical situation a variety of waves of energy would be experienced, all of which differ from one another in wavelength, frequency, and energy.

It is important to note that although emissions from radioactive materials are spoken of in terms of alpha particles, beta particles, and gamma rays, alpha and beta particles do not appear on the electromagnetic spectrum. Only gamma rays exist as electromagnetic waves. Alpha particles and beta particles are particulate matter and therefore possess mass. They are not waves of energy and for this reason are not seen on the spectrum, even though these particles sometimes behave as waves of energy and waves of energy sometimes behave as particles.

Relationship of wavelength to frequency

Since the electromagnetic spectrum is based on wavelength, it is apparent that the wavelengths of the various entities must be known. Red light, which has the longest wavelength of the visible light spectrum, has a value of 0.00007 cm or 7,000 Å. Green light is known to have a wavelength of 5,000 Å, and blue light has a wavelength of 4,000 Å. If the wavelength of the radiation is greater than 7,000 Å or shorter than 4,000 Å, the radiations are no longer visible to the human eye and fall into the infrared and ultraviolet ranges respectively. The frequency of radiation from blue light (4,000 Å) can be calculated as shown in formula 3-1:

$$n \times \lambda = c \tag{3-1}$$

$$n = \frac{c}{\lambda} = \frac{3.0 \times 10^{10}}{0.00004} = 7.5 \times 10^{14} \text{ waves/sec}$$

Proceeding further up the electromagnetic spectrum, the wavelength begins to become very short and the corresponding frequency begins to become very great. At this point the quantum nature of radiation must be considered.

Quantum nature of radiation. Sometimes electromagnetic waves produce results that cannot be explained by the action of waves of energy. A question arises as to whether these waves can actually be regarded as waves at all, or whether they should be regarded as mass. This is especially true with such waves as x rays, gamma rays, and cosmic rays, which have very short wavelengths. These waves can assume properties, not of waves, but of particles, as is seen in Fig. 3-1, *C.* They can be likened to bullets possessing great energy and traveling in a given direction. This bundle of energy is called a *quantum* or a *photon,* and the amount of energy carried by the photon depends on the frequency of the radiation. The frequency, in turn, is an inverse function of wavelength. The *energy of the photon is directly proportional to frequency* as indicated by formula 3-2:

$$E = h \times n \tag{3-2}$$

E = Energy in joules
h = Planck's constant in joule sec = 6.61×10^{-34} joule sec
n = Frequency in seconds

Since the energy of the photon is directly proportional to frequency and frequency is inversely proportional to wavelength, then *energy is inversely proportional to wavelength* also. As the wavelength decreases, the energy of the photon increases, and vice versa.

Relationship of wavelength to energy

It has already been demonstrated in formula 2-1 that 1 ev is equal to 1.6×10^{-19} joules. With this value and formulas 3-1 and 3-2 it is possible to calculate the energy of any photon of radiation, given the wavelength. To express a photon with a wavelength of 1.0 Å in terms of energy, three steps are required:

1. Convert wavelength to frequency (formula 3-1)*

$$c = n \times \lambda$$

$$n = \frac{c}{\lambda} = \frac{3 \times 10^{10}}{10^{-8}} = 3 \times 10^{18} \text{ waves/sec (equivalent to 1 Å)}$$

2. Convert frequency to energy in joules (formula 3-2)*

$$E = h \times n$$
$$E = 6.61 \times 10^{-34} \times 3 \times 10^{18}$$
$$E = 19.83 \times 10^{-16} \text{ joules (equivalent to 1 Å)}$$

---

*Since formula 3-1 is $n = \dfrac{c}{\lambda}$ and formula 3-2 is $E = hn$, formula 3-1 can be substituted into formula 3-2 to read $E = \dfrac{hc}{\lambda}$

3. Convert joules to electron volts by comparing it to the value of 1 ev, that value being 1.6×10^{-19} joules

$$1 \text{ Å} = \frac{19.83 \times 10^{-16}}{1.6 \times 10^{-19}} = 12.4 \times 10^3 \text{ ev (or 12.4 kev)}$$

With these formulas, given the wavelength of any type of radiation, it is possible to convert wavelength to energy in electron volts or, conversely, energy in electron volts to wavelength. Since energies of the various radionuclides are known, it is possible to place them in their proper positions on the electromagnetic spectrum.

If a photon with a wavelength of 1.0 Å has an energy of 12.4 kev as just determined, then a photon with a wavelength of 0.01 Å has an energy of 1,240 kev, or 1.24 mev, and this relationship holds true for any wavelength. Since this is the case, another relationship can be formulated whereby wavelength can immediately be converted to energy in electron volts without going through the three steps just discussed.

$$E = \frac{12,400}{\lambda} \quad = \quad \frac{12.4}{\lambda} \quad \text{for keV units}$$

E = Energy in electron volts
λ = Wavelength in angstrom units

MASS-ENERGY EQUIVALENCE

For centuries it was believed by all that mass was mass and energy was energy; no thought was given to the possibility that the two were interconvertible. It was not until the present century that the possibility was advanced and proved. Einstein's contribution to nuclear science was an extremely important one and helped explain some of the phenomena of nuclear disintegration. He explained that mass is really a form of energy and that mass and energy could be converted from one to the other with formula 3-4:

$$E = mc^2 \tag{3-4}$$

E = Energy in joules
m = Mass weight in kg
c = Velocity of light in m/sec

By this equation it is possible to calculate the amount of energy released if 1 gram of matter were completely destroyed and converted to energy:

$$E = 10^{-3} \times (3 \times 10^8)^2$$
$$= 10^{-3} \times 9 \times 10^{16}$$
$$= 9 \times 10^{13} \text{ joules}$$

The conversion of joules to the more useful electron volt would yield an immense number, not of particular importance at this time.

More important, just as one can convert 1 kg of mass to energy, so also one can calculate the energy released should an atom become annihilated or, even more appropriate, should a subatomic particle (a proton, neutron, or electron) be converted to energy. This is accomplished by the use of the *atomic mass unit* (amu). The atomic mass unit is defined as one twelfth of the arbitrary mass assigned to carbon 12 ($^{12}_{6}C$). It is known that 1 amu is equal to 1.49×10^{-10} joules. According to formula 2-1, 1 ev is equal to 1.6×10^{-19} joules, and 1 mev is equal to 1.6×10^{-13} joules; therefore:

$$1 \text{ amu} = \frac{1.49 \times 10^{-10}}{1.6 \times 10^{-13}} = 0.9312 \text{ g } 10^3 \text{ mev, or } 931.2 \text{ mev*} \tag{3-5}$$

This figure (931.2) becomes of value as a conversion factor to convert mass to an equivalent amount of energy whenever a loss of mass has been observed after any nuclear reaction or interaction. Examples of its use in a nuclear reaction will be shown in Chapter 4. An example other than a nuclear reaction is that of a helium atom. It has previously been discussed that the intact helium atom actually weighs less than the sum of its constituent parts weighed separately because some of the mass has been converted to binding energy. The actual energy realized by such a loss of mass can be calculated by the use of this relationship between atomic mass units and energy. Helium 4 is composed of 2 protons, 2 neutrons, and 2 electrons. It has an amu value of 4.003874. The sum of its component particles, however, is indicated in the following:

$$\begin{aligned}
\text{amu of protons} &= 1.007277 \times 2 = 2.014554 \\
\text{amu of neutrons} &= 1.008665 \times 2 = 2.017330 \\
\text{amu of electrons} &= 0.000549 \times 2 = \underline{0.001098} \\
\text{sum of components} &= 4.032982
\end{aligned}$$

Based on these values, the component particles of helium 4 weighed separately are heavier than the intact helium 4 atom by 0.030379 amu (4.032982 − 4.002603 = 0.030379 amu). Since 1 amu has been determined to be equal to 931.2 mev (formula 3-5), the binding energy within the atom of helium 4 is equal to 28.2898 mev according to the following calculation:

$$E = 0.030379 \times 931.2 \text{ mev} = 28.2898 \text{ mev}$$

What has actually occurred is that the atom, to keep itself intact, must convert 0.03 units of atomic mass into 28.3 mev of energy. The atom uses a small fraction of this energy as binding energy to keep the electrons in their energy shells. The major part of this energy is used by the nucleus to keep its nucleons (primarily the protons carrying the positive charges) from repelling one another to the point of disrupting it.

The fact that the nucleus possesses the ability to convert units of mass to pure energy tends to place the entire phenomenon in the realm of sheer fantasy. The

---

*A proportion:

$$\frac{1 \text{ mev}}{1.6 \times 10^{-13} \text{ joules}} = \frac{x}{1.49 \times 10^{-10} \text{ joules}}$$

$$1.6 \times 10^{-13} x = 1.49 \times 10^{-10}$$

$$x = 931.2 \text{ mev}$$

possibility of having a piece of matter in one instance converted to invisible energy in another instance is a fact that sometimes seems difficult to understand. However, this same type of phenomenon occurs almost every time a reaction or interaction occurs in a nucleus.

A better example of the conversion of mass to energy is that of the reaction between a positron and an electron. It is known that when these 2 units of mass collide, they completely annihilate one another, and all of their mass is converted to energy according to the following calculations:

$$\text{amu of electron} = 0.000549$$
$$\text{amu of positron} = \underline{0.000549}$$
$$0.001098$$
$$0.001098 \times 931.2 = 1.02 \text{ mev}$$

The resultant energy of the annihilation reaction between a positron and an electron is 1.02 mev. Actually the energy is not represented as 1 photon of 1.02 mev but as 2 photons of 0.51 mev emitted in exactly opposite directions from one another (p. 47).

GENERAL CLASSIFICATIONS OF RADIOACTIVITY

In general, there are two classifications of radioactivity and of radioisotopes: natural and artificial. Naturally occurring radionuclides are those nuclides that emit radiation spontaneously. No additional energy is necessary to place them in an unstable state. Artificial radioactivity is that radioactivity resulting from man-made unstable nuclides. Such nuclides are made unstable by bombarding stable nuclides with high-energy particles. Both types of radioactivity play an important role in nuclear medicine.

Natural radioactivity

It has been suggested that particles within the atom are in a constant state of motion. This motion within the nucleus results in collisions between nucleons whereby energy is transferred to other nucleons. This transfer of energy sometimes results in a nucleon achieving energy greater than the binding energy, in which case the particle is allowed to escape the nucleus. This particle escape is termed a *disintegration*. The process of *decay* and the act of particle escape allow the nucleus to reduce the number of protons or neutrons or both to a point at which the binding energy can contain the remainder of the nucleons. In this way, stability is eventually achieved.

All nuclides with the atomic number (Z) greater than 82 are radioactive because they possess an unstable number of protons or neutrons. Many of these are naturally occurring. There are also instances of naturally occurring radionuclides of lesser atomic number, such as potassium 40 and carbon 14.

These naturally occurring radionuclides are found in all parts of the world; therefore, all the peoples of the world are subjected to their radiation effects. The amount of radiation caused by these nuclides would vary from place to place based on local geographic conditions. Some genetic mutations are attributable in part to such exposures to naturally occurring radioactivity. These radiations could also have contributed to some of the phases of the evolutionary process. The source of these radiations is both extraterrestrial and terrestrial. Cosmic rays arising from outside the earth's atmosphere constitute the radiations of extraterrestrial origins. Those of terrestrial origin are found in the earth's crust, and radioactive materials having gaseous form are found in the air.

Generally, only a few steps are necessary in the process of decay before a stable ratio of neutrons to protons is reached. Occasionally, however, the process of achieving stability will require as many as 18 different steps. Such as sequence of events is called a *radioactive series*. There are currently 4 such series in existence: the thorium series, decaying to stable lead 208; the actinium series, decaying to stable lead 207; the uranium series, decaying to lead 206; and the neptunium series, decaying to bismuth 209. It has been suggested by some scientists that there may have been more radioactive series that existed at some point in time, but they have all since attained stability.

Artificial radioactivity

Artificial radioactivity is the same as natural radioactivity, except that the radionuclides are man made. It is possible to subject stable nuclides to high-energy particles to produce instability. This instability can be effected by subjecting a stable nuclide to such devices as a cyclotron or a nuclear reactor (pile), wherein the stable nuclides are bombarded with neutrons, protons, deuterons, or alpha particles. In such bombardment, some of these bombarding particles will be absorbed by the nucleus of the target material. In each case an alteration has occurred in the proton to neutron relationship. By such changes in the nucleus the number of particles within the nucleus is altered to a point where the binding energy can no longer contain them. Accordingly, a particle is ejected from a nucleus and a new nuclide is formed, which may be either radioactive or stable. If it is a stable nuclide, the reaction ends. The manner in which these artificial radionuclides are produced will be discussed in Chapter 5.

BIBLIOGRAPHY

Casarett, A. P.: Radiation biology, Englewood Cliffs, N.J., 1968, Prentice-Hall, Inc.

Chandra, R.: Introductory physics of nuclear medicine, Philadelphia, 1976, Lea & Febiger.

Johns, H. E.: The physics of radiology, ed. 2, revised edition, Springfield, Ill., 1964, Charles C Thomas, Publisher.

Rollo, F. D.: Nuclear medicine physics, instrumentation, and agents, St. Louis, 1977, The C. V. Mosby, Co.

Shilling, C. W.: Atomic energy encyclopedia in the life sciences, Philadelphia, 1964, W. B. Saunders Co.

Wagner, H. N.: Principles of nuclear medicine, Philadelphia, 1968, W. B. Saunders Co.

4 Methods of radioactive decay

IDENTIFICATION OF EMISSIONS

There are basically three emissions from radionuclides — alpha and beta particles and gamma rays. A means of identifying these radiations had to be devised, and this problem became the doctoral thesis of Mme. Marie Curie around the turn of the century. To carry out the experiment of identification, Mme. Curie devised a simple technique. She took a large block of lead with a hole in its center into which she placed a source of radium. In this manner, since the radiations emanate at an infinite number of angles from the source, those that did not radiate upward through the hole would be absorbed by the surrounding lead. A piece of photographic film was placed above the lead block. In this way, radiations emanating from the radium source and going through the hole in the lead block would be detected by an area of darkening on the film. In an effort to learn if these radiations had electrical charges, Mme. Curie included a magnetic field in a direction perpendicular to the direction of the emissions (Fig. 4-1). She reasoned that, if charged, the positively charged emissions would be deflected to the right according to the rules of physics for positive charges in a magnetic field, and the negatively charged emissions would be deviated to the left. Those with no charge would remain unaffected by the magnetic field. Furthermore, in the presence of the magnetic field, if all three types of emissions were present, three areas of darkening would be seen on the photographic plate. Since Mme. Curie did detect three areas of darkening, she arbitrarily labeled the emissions after the first three letters of the Greek alphabet. Those that were deflected to the right and had a positive charge were called *alpha* emissions, those that were deflected to the left and negatively charged were called *beta* emissions, and those that remained undeflected with no charge were called *gamma* emissions.

CHARACTERISTICS OF EMISSIONS

Many experiments have been performed to learn more about radioactivity. In addition to the conclusions of Mme. Curie's experiment, many other characteristics are now known.

It is an accepted fact that a radioactive nuclide will emit one, two, or all three of these basic radiations. There are comparatively few radionuclides that possess the ability to decay by both alpha and beta emission with the subsequent release of a gamma ray. Most radionuclides decay by either alpha emission or beta emis-

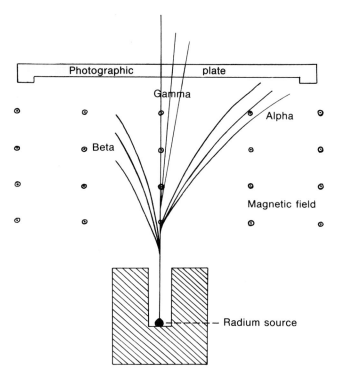

Fig. 4-1. Electrical properties of radioactive emissions. An illustration of Mme. Curie's experiment to prove that alpha emissions are positively charged, beta emissions are negatively charged, and gamma emissions are neutrally charged.

sion. In either case, gamma emission could be a subsequent reaction. Those radionuclides that decay by alpha emission only or beta emission only are termed *pure alpha emitters* and *pure beta emitters,* respectively.

It is also known that the process of decay creates other nuclides that may be either radioactive or stable. (Note the word *nuclides,* not isotopes.) ^{203}Hg, for instance, does not eventually decay to ^{197}Hg (an isotope); it decays by beta-gamma emission to ^{203}Tl (another nuclide). This is called *transmutation,* the conversion of one element into another.

Another indisputable fact is that the process of decay is a series of random events. It is impossible to predict exactly which atom is going to undergo disintegration at any given time. However, it is possible to predict, on the average, how many atoms will disintegrate during any interval of time. Because of this predictability, the rate of disintegration can be used as a method of quantitative analysis. These disintegrations can be detected, those detected can be counted, and the results can be expressed as counts per unit time.

It has also been demonstrated that temperature, pressure, or chemical combination have absolutely no effect on the rate of decay. Radioactive materials can be placed in a freezer without any demonstrable change in the half-life. The same is true should a source of radioactivity be subjected to heat and pressure, as in an autoclave for sterilization purposes.

The fact that chemical combination does not alter the radioactive characteristics is the rationale responsible for labeling or "tagging" chemicals, by replacing stable atoms of a compound with radioactive atoms. ^{197}Hg-labeled chlormerodrin, a mercurial diuretic, is an example. In labeling this compound the stable form of mercury is replaced by the unstable form. In this way, neither the mercurial diuretic nor the ^{197}Hg is altered in any way, and the body reacts to either form similarly.

METHODS OF DECAY

The original radionuclide in any method of decay is called a *parent;* the nuclide to which it decays is called a *daughter*, which may be stable or unstable. If a daughter nuclide is stable, the decay process is terminated. If the daughter is unstable, a new decay process begins that may differ entirely from its predecessor.

Alpha emission

Definition and origin. The alpha particle (α, $^4_2\alpha$, or $^4_2$He) is a helium nucleus consisting of 2 protons and 2 neutrons. This particle is the same as the helium atom with the exception that there are no orbital electrons. Because there are no negative charges to neutralize the positively charged nucleus, the alpha particle possesses an electric charge of $+2$ on emission. Since the particle is without electrons, it will not be satisfied until it acquires 2 electrons, making it an electrically neutral helium atom.

Alpha particles originate in the nuclei of heavier atoms. For the most part, these atoms occupy the upper one third of the chart of the nuclides. It is obvious that if alpha emissions occurred as a result of nuclear changes in the lighter nuclides, the nuclide would be discarding a major portion of its nucleus. Alpha decay is a fast and efficient means of bringing the neutron to proton ratio closer to a stable ratio. Since an alpha particle removes 2 protons and 2 neutrons from the parent nuclide, the new nuclide contains 2 fewer protons and 2 fewer neutrons. In effect, the atomic number (Z) would be decreased by 2, the neutron number (N) would be decreased by 2, and the mass number (A) would be decreased by 4.

Ionization and penetration. Since an alpha particle has an electrical charge of $+2$, its immediate purpose is to acquire 2 electrons to become electrically neutral. As the alpha particle passes through matter, it attracts electrons from nearby atoms (Fig. 4-2). Because of the strong electrical attraction of the alpha particle ($+2$), its huge mass (7,400 times the size of the electron), and the almost nonexistent binding energy of outer shell electrons, the alpha particle can actually overcome the binding forces of the electron's parent atom, causing the electron to be released in space. As a result the electron is free to ionize other atoms in the sur-

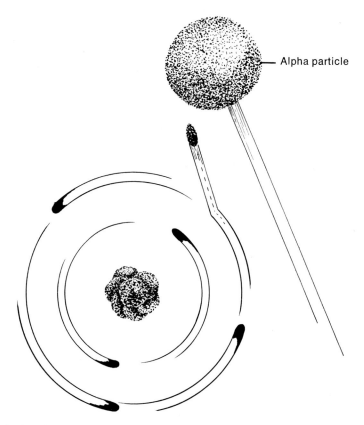

Alpha particle

Fig. 4-2. Ionization of matter by a passing alpha particle. NOTE: Artist's concept is misleading because alpha particles are approximately 7,400 times larger than the mass of the electron.

rounding media (provided it has enough energy to do so), to combine with positive ions in the vicinity, or to become one of the free electrons that occur in all matter. This process of removal of an electron from an atom is called *ionization*. The result of this ionization process is the creation of an *ion pair* consisting of a negative ion (the electron) and a positive ion (the atom from which the electron was removed). *Primary ionization* is that produced by the originally charged particle; *secondary ionization* is that subsequently produced by the ions that resulted from the primary event (electrons, primarily).

This process of attracting the electron by the alpha particle causes a slowing down and loss of kinetic energy of the particle itself because the alpha particle uses some of its energy to remove the electron. This process of ionization will continue many, many times with subsequent atoms in the path of the alpha particle. The particle will create more ion pairs until it loses all its kinetic energy and comes to *rest mass*. The particle picks up the 2 electrons necessary for electrical neutrality and comes to rest as a helium atom, a chemically inert gas. At this point it ceases to be of radiobiologic significance.

An alpha particle loses an average of 34 ev per ionization event in air. If energy loss by the alpha particle were the only consideration, this would mean that an alpha particle with 3,400,000 ev of energy (3.4 mev) would undergo 100,000 ionization events (100,000 ion pairs) before expending all of its energy and coming to rest mass. It would require less than 2 cm of air to expend all the energy of such an alpha particle. As matter increases in density, less distance is required to expend the energy of the alpha particle; therefore, penetration decreases.

The *range* of an alpha particle, that is, the distance the charged particle travels from its point of origin to the place where it no longer acts as a destructive radiation particle, is about 4 cm in air. This value changes considerably in tissue, in which the range is reduced to a few thousandths of a centimeter. For this reason, an alpha particle is unable to penetrate the epidermis of the skin. It is not to be assumed, however, that an alpha particle is without injurious radiation effects because it cannot penetrate the skin. The most common methods of alpha contamination are inhalation or ingestion of alpha-laden materials. This is not of particular importance in the usual nuclear medicine laboratory, since alpha emitters are not used in routine nuclear medicine procedures.

Ionization is often spoken of in terms of *specific ionization,* that is, the number of ion pairs formed per unit of path traveled by a moving charged particle through matter. For particles of the same energy the specific ionization increases with mass and charge. For this reason, alpha particles have a higher specific ionization than other particles because they have more mass and 2 positive charges. Furthermore, specific ionization is inversely proportional to velocity, since the slower moving particle spends more time in the vicinity of the atom and therefore has a greater chance to ionize it. The specific ionization in air for a 1 mev alpha particle is about 60,000 ion pairs per centimeter of path traveled.

An alpha particle is also capable of *excitation* of an atom as it approaches or passes through it. To excite an atom is to increase the energy state of an orbital electron by the transfer of some of the energy of the alpha particle to the electron. By increasing the energy state the electron assumes a new suborbit distant to the nucleus. The electron cannot stay in this excited state, so it immediately releases the excess energy and returns to its original orbit.

Example. Since an alpha particle consists of 2 protons and 2 neutrons, there would necessarily be 2 fewer protons and 2 fewer neutrons in the parent atom. A typical alpha emitter is $^{226}_{88}$Ra. Following is the reaction of alpha emission:

$$^{226}_{88}\text{Ra} \rightarrow {}^{222}_{86}\text{Rn} + {}^{4}_{2}\text{He}$$
$$(\text{radium}) \rightarrow (\text{radon}) + (\text{alpha})$$

Accordingly, the new nuclide, radon 222, has a mass number reduced by 4 and an atomic number reduced by 2.

Beta emission

A beta particle (β) is a high-velocity electron ejected from a disintegrating nucleus. The particle may be either a negatively charged electron, termed a *negatron* (β^-), or a positively charged electron, termed a *positron* (β^+). Both types of beta particles have the same mass, regardless of their charge. Although the precise definition of "beta emission" refers to both β^- and β^+ particles, the common usage of the term refers only to the β^- particle, as distinguished from positron emission, which refers to the β^+ particle. The remainder of this text will treat β^- and β^+ particles as betas and positrons, respectively.

Beta decay

Definition and origin. The beta particle (β^-) is a high-velocity, negatively charged electron emitted from a nucleus of an atom undergoing disintegration. The beta particle is identical to the orbital electron in mass and electrical charge. Both possess a charge of -1 and a mass $1/_{1,836}$ that of a proton and equivalent to 0.000548 amu.

Since a β^- particle is defined as being ejected from the nucleus, the question arises of how an electron can be emitted from the nucleus when there is no electron in the nucleus. What actually happens is that a neutron is converted into a proton, an electron (β^-), and a neutrino as shown below:

$$\text{Neutron} \rightarrow \begin{array}{c} \text{Proton} \\ + \\ \text{Electron}\ (\beta^-) \\ + \\ \text{Neutrino}\ (\nu) \end{array}$$

The immediate result of the neutron breakdown is that the electron (β^-) and the neutrino are ejected from the nucleus, whereas the proton remains. The parent atom is increased in atomic number by 1, with no change in mass number. (Mass number is protons plus neutrons, and one has been converted to the other, so there is no change in the total number.)

Examples. An example of a beta emitter is phosphorus 32. It decays to sulfur 32 with the emission of a beta particle and a neutrino according to the following:

$$^{32}_{15}\text{P} \rightarrow {}^{32}_{16}\text{S} + \beta^- + \nu$$

In this reaction no gamma is released; therefore ^{32}P is a pure beta emitter. Others are carbon 14 ($^{14}_{6}$C), cesium 137 ($^{137}_{55}$Cs), and strontium 90 ($^{90}_{38}$Sr).

An example of a beta-gamma emitter is iodine 131. ^{131}I decays by beta emission to xenon 131 according to the following:

$$^{131}_{53}\text{I} \rightarrow {}^{131}_{54}\text{Xe} + \beta^- + \nu + \gamma$$

Other beta-gamma emitters are mercury 203 ($^{203}_{80}$Hg), gold 198 ($^{198}_{79}$Au), iron 59 ($^{59}_{26}$Fe), molybdenum 99 ($^{99}_{42}$Mo), and sodium 24 ($^{24}_{11}$Na).

Debit mass and credit energy. It is important to realize that whenever the disintegration of a nucleus occurs, regardless of the method of decay, there is a release of energy. The source of this excess energy is the nucleus itself because of a disparity in the mass of the new nuclide. This unaccounted mass is expressed in atomic mass units (amu) in the calculations of the ^{32}P reaction that follow (amu values taken from Appendix C):

$$
\begin{array}{r r}
\text{amu } ^{32}_{15}\text{P} & 31.973910 \\
\text{less amu 15 electrons} = 0.000549 \times 15 = & \underline{0.008235} \\
\text{amu of } ^{32}_{15}\text{P nucleus} & 31.965675 \,(A) \\[4pt]
\text{amu } ^{32}_{16}\text{S} & 31.972074 \\
\text{less amu 16 electrons} = 0.000549 \times 16 = & \underline{0.008784} \\
\text{amu of } ^{32}_{16}\text{S nucleus} & 31.963290 \,(B) \\[4pt]
\text{amu of } ^{32}_{15}\text{P nucleus} & 31.965675 \,(A) \\
\text{less amu of } ^{32}_{16}\text{S nucleus} & \underline{31.963290} \,(B) \\
\text{mass difference} & 0.002385 \\
\text{less } \beta^- \text{ mass} & 0.000549 \\
\text{less neutrino mass} & \underline{0.000000} \\
\text{unaccounted mass} & 0.001836
\end{array}
$$

It was not until Einstein that this question of what happened to the rest of the mass could be answered. He said that mass or energy could not be destroyed but that each could be converted into the other. In these reactions some mass is always lost, but an equivalent amount of energy is always gained. It has already been shown (formula 3-5) that 931.2 is the conversion factor to convert mass (amu) to energy expressed as mev. Therefore the energy released from decay of ^{32}P to ^{32}S is as follows:

$$\text{Energy released in mev} = 0.00183 \times 931.2 = 1.70 \text{ mev}$$

The energy resulting from this neutron breakdown is expended in three different ways: (1) Some of the energy goes to the electron so that it may be ejected from the nucleus. (2) Some of the energy goes to the neutrino so that it may be ejected from the nucleus. (3) In any radionuclide other than a pure beta emitter, some of the energy is retained by the nucleus. The latter elevates a nucleon to a new energy level. The consequence of this elevated energy level or excited state is that, with the exception of isomeric transition (p. 49), the excess energy is instantaneously released in the form of gamma radiation. The energy levels to which the excited nucleus is elevated are discrete energy levels and are well known. Therefore the energy released in the form of gamma radiation is also well known. This is not the case with the β^- particle and the neutrino. The amount of energy that is expended on the beta particle or the neutrino is unpredictable from one atom to another, but the energy distribution is known based on percentages.

Energy distribution of a pure beta emitter. In the pure beta emitter all the energy resulting from a neutron breakdown is expended on the beta particle and neutrino to eject it from the nucleus. There is no elevated energy state of the nucleus and therefore no subsequent gamma emission. Fig. 4-3 shows the distribution of energy to the ^{32}P beta particle as a function of energy plotted on the abscissa (horizontal axis) versus frequency of occurrence on the ordinate (vertical axis). As indicated, the maximum energy (E_{max}) of any beta particle from this radionuclide is that of 1.7 mev. The number of atoms in a given sample producing a beta particle of 1.7 mev is very, very low. Conversely, the number of atoms in the given sample producing a beta particle of 0.6 mev is much higher. E_{max} indicates that the maximum energy resulting from the neutron breakdown is 1.7 mev. Since all the energy in a pure beta emitter is expended on either the beta particle or the neutrino, whatever portion of the energy that the beta particle does not receive, the neutrino receives. Therefore an atom that supplies the beta particle with all the energy resulting from the neutron breakdown would have a neutrino that has just enough energy to be ejected from the nucleus. However, one of its sister atoms in the same sample that gives only 0.6 mev of energy to the beta particle would have a neutrino possessing the energy difference of 1.1 mev. According to Fig. 4-3, the situation in which a beta particle receives 0.6 mev and the neutrino receives 1.1 mev of energy occurs much more frequently than that in which the beta particle receives the total energy and the neutrino very little or vice versa. This whole concept of energy distribution can be crudely summed up as whatever energy the

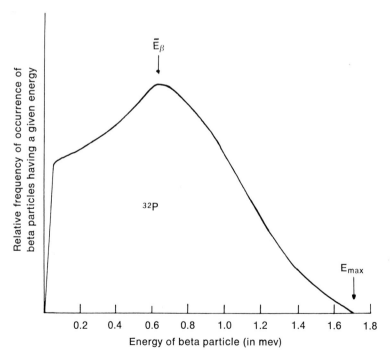

Fig. 4-3. Distribution of resultant energy to ^{32}P beta particles following the conversion of a neutron to a proton with the expulsion of an electron and a neutrino from the nucleus.

beta particle does not use, the neutrino receives. If this were actually the case, the beta particle must be considered as most charitable. However, most of the beta particles need only approximately one third of the available energy, leaving the other two thirds for the neutrino. This energy value is generally considered to be its average energy represented by the symbol $\overline{E}_\beta$ (E bar beta). Since it is approximately equivalent to one third of all the available energy, $\overline{E}_\beta \approx \frac{1}{3}E_{max}$. In any nuclide that is not a pure beta emitter the nucleus would contribute some of its energy to the nucleus itself. Energy distribution between the beta particle and the neutrino would remain similar.

Purpose. When a nucleus undergoes beta disintegration, the daughter nuclide possesses a nucleus with an atomic number increased by 1 and the mass number remains the same. A neutron has been changed into a proton; therefore the proton number is increased by 1. However, the mass number has not been changed because what has been lost in neutrons has been gained in protons. This type of decay would occur in any nuclide having too many neutrons or too few protons or both. Beta decay is the only method available to such an unstable nucleus. The neutron number is decreased, and the proton number is increased in an attempt to achieve stability. It may be, however, that the new nuclide may also be unstable for the same reason, and it may subsequently disintegrate by the same method. This process will continue until a stable proportion of neutrons and protons exists. (Disintegration of a nucleus means only that it changes in composition, not that it no longer exists.)

This situation exemplifies the conditions that exist in every atom of tin 127 ($^{127}_{50}$Sn) (Fig. 4-4). ^{127}Sn contains 77 neutrons and 50 protons. For some reason not completely understood, this neutron to proton ratio is unstable because there are too many neutrons and too few protons. Its only course of action is beta decay. In decaying by beta emission, ^{127}Sn becomes antimony 127 ($^{127}_{51}$Sb); this nucleus with 76 neutrons and 51 protons is still unstable. Consequently, it decays by beta emission to tellurium 127 ($^{127}_{52}$Te), and this nucleus with 75 neutrons and 52 protons is unstable also. Finally, it decays by beta emission to iodine 127 ($^{127}_{53}$I), which has a stable ratio of 74 neutrons to 53 protons, and the decay series ends. ^{127}I happens to be the only stable isotope of iodine and is the form of the element that is found in iodized salt, fish, and so on.

Since the unstable parent atom decays by beta emission to a daughter atom that has the same mass number but a different atomic number and therefore different chemical properties, it can be said that beta decay gives rise to an isobar. The process is termed *isobaric transition*.

Ionization and penetration. Beta particles also possess the ability to excite or ionize atoms or both. The method of ionization, however, is somewhat different from the ionization of alpha particles. An alpha particle attracts an orbital electron and thus creates an ion pair. The beta particle repels the orbital electron from its energy shell to create an ion pair (Fig. 4-5). Each ion pair produced by the β^- par-

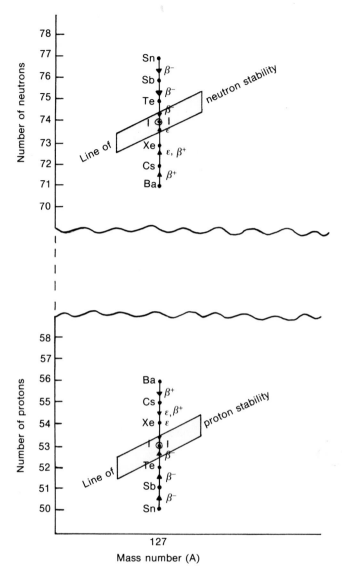

Fig. 4-4. Magnification of Fig. 1-2 at the level of A = 127 demonstrating that unstable atoms decay to stability by whatever method is required to achieve a stable ratio of neutrons to protons.

ticle represents a loss of energy by the beta particle. These processes of excitation and ionization continue until the beta particle loses all its kinetic energy. At this point the beta particle is said to have attained rest mass. It can now combine with some positively charged ion to make it a neutral atom once again. This process is termed *deionization*. It can also become a free electron, in which capacity it does not combine with anything. The specific ionization of a 1 mev beta particle in air is about 45 ion pairs per centimeter of path traveled. Compared to an alpha particle,

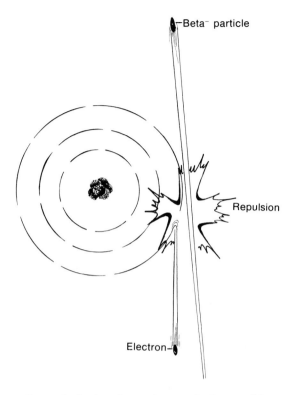

Fig. 4-5. Ionization of matter by a passing beta particle.

the specific ionization of a beta particle is greatly reduced. This is largely because the charge of an alpha particle is twice and its mass 7,400 times that of a beta particle. Furthermore, an alpha particle has a lower velocity than a beta particle and is in the area of any one atom for a longer period of time, which increases its probability of attracting an orbital electron to it.

As with alpha particles, beta particles lose an average energy of 34 ev per ionization event. Similarly, considering only the loss of particle energy, a 3.4 mev beta particle would undergo 100,000 ionization events before losing its radiobiologic significance. It differs from the alpha particle, however, in its penetration. As the specific ionization values indicate, a beta particle incurs fewer ionization events per unit of path traveled, so it travels farther than an alpha particle of equal energy. The penetrating power of beta particles is approximately 100 times as great as that of alpha particles. However, the penetration power of beta particles is only a small fraction of that of gamma rays. Alpha particles are completely absorbed by a thin sheet of paper, whereas an inch of wood or 1/25 inch of aluminum is required to stop a beta particle. In tissue a 1 mev beta particle has a range of 0.42 cm. However, this particle is not harmless from a radiobiologic standpoint. It is well to remember that phosphorus 32, a pure beta emitter, is used as a therapeutic agent for such clinical states as leukemia, polycythemia, and ascites. In each case the epidermis is bypassed either by intravenous or intracavitary administration.

Bremsstrahlung. *Bremsstrahlung* is the German word for braking radiation. Bremsstrahlung is the production of electromagnetic radiation by the deceleration (actually, negative acceleration) that a fast, charged particle undergoes when it is deflected by another charged particle. The charged particles in the case of Bremsstrahlung are the beta particle and the nucleus of an atom near which the beta particle passes. When a beta particle passes near an atomic nucleus, its path of travel will be changed somewhat in the direction of the nucleus because of the attraction of unlike charges. This change in direction is spoken of as acceleration, but it is a negative acceleration. The beta particle slows down and loses energy. In these instances the energy lost is released in the form of x rays (Fig. 4-6). These x rays are equal in energy to that energy lost by the beta particle. This is one of the phenomena that occur in x-ray tubes and their subsequent x-ray production. In the case of x-ray machines, however, electrons are used rather than beta particles.

Bremsstrahlung is also the reason that high Z material, such as lead, is not always the answer to radiation protection. With beta emitters, the amount of Bremsstrahlung increases with the density of the material through which it passes.

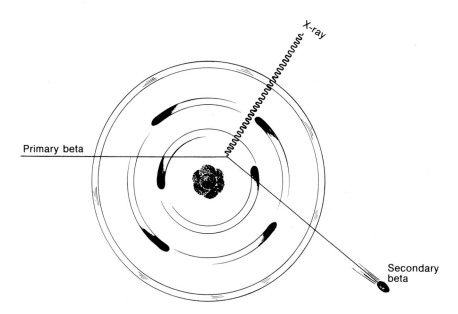

Fig. 4-6. Bremsstrahlung. A beta particle passes near the nucleus of an atom and is attracted to it. This results in a loss of energy and change in direction. That loss of energy is expressed as x ray, or Bremsstrahlung.

Therefore, since Bremsstrahlung is x ray, it is not as easily shielded as is the beta particle. It is considered a better practice during the administration of these pure beta emitters to use some low Z material, such as plastic or lucite, as an adequate barrier for the beta particle and to reduce the amount of Bremsstrahlung produced in the shielding material. In fact, the plastic syringe, used in the administration of the material is usually adequate shielding.

Positron decay

Definition and origin. The positron (β^+) is a high-velocity, positively charged electron emitted from the nucleus of an atom undergoing disintegration. The positron differs from the electron and the beta particle only in that it has an opposite electrical charge. It has the mass of an electron but the electrical charge of a proton. The nuclear origin of the positron is the proton. A proton, under the influence of all the nucleons in its nucleus, is converted into a neutron, an electron with a positive charge (positron), and a neutrino, as shown below:

$$\text{Proton} \rightarrow
\begin{array}{c}
\text{Neutron} \\
+ \\
\text{Electron } (\beta^+) \\
+ \\
\text{Neutrino}
\end{array}$$

The immediate result of the proton breakdown is that the positive electron (β^+) and the neutrino are ejected from the nucleus while a neutron remains. The parent atom is reduced in atomic number by 1, with no change in mass number. (Similar to beta decay, one of the units comprising the mass number is converted to the other so that there is no change. In positron decay, however, it is the opposite of beta decay; a proton becomes a neutron.)

Examples. An example of a positron emitter is nitrogen 12. It decays to carbon 12 with the emission of a β^+ particle and a neutrino according to the following:

$$^{12}_{7}\text{N} \rightarrow {}^{12}_{6}\text{C} + \beta^+ + \nu$$

In this reaction no gamma is released; therefore, ^{12}N is a pure positron emitter. ^{18}F is another.

A further example of a positron emitter and one more pertinent to nuclear medicine is gallium 68. It decays to zinc 68 with the emission of a positron, a neutrino, and energy (γ) according to the following:

$$^{68}_{31}\text{Ga} \rightarrow {}^{68}_{30}\text{Zn} + \beta^+ + \nu + \gamma$$

Another important positron emitter is sodium 22 $(^{22}_{11}\text{Na})$.

Debits and credits. Just as with beta decay, the disintegration of a nucleus with the subsequent emission of a positron yields energy as a result of loss through conversion of mass. The mass-energy equivalence can be calculated because amu values are known. A calculation of the ^{12}N reaction follows:

$$
\begin{array}{rl}
\text{amu } ^{12}_{7}\text{N} & 12.018641 \\
\text{less amu 7 electrons} = 0.000549 \times 7 = & \underline{0.003843} \\
\text{amu of } ^{12}_{7}\text{N nucleus} & 12.014798 \text{ (A)}
\end{array}
$$

$$
\begin{array}{rl}
\text{amu } ^{12}_{6}\text{C} & 12.000000 \\
\text{less amu 6 electrons} = 0.000549 \times 6 = & \underline{0.003294} \\
\text{amu of } ^{12}_{6}\text{C nucleus} & 11.996706 \text{ (B)}
\end{array}
$$

$$
\begin{array}{rl}
\text{amu of } ^{12}_{7}\text{N nucleus} & 12.014798 \text{ (A)} \\
\text{less amu of } ^{12}_{6}\text{C nucleus} & \underline{11.996706} \text{ (B)} \\
\text{mass difference} & 0.018092 \\
\text{less } \beta^{+} \text{ mass} & 0.000549 \\
\text{less } \nu \text{ mass} & \underline{0.000000} \\
\text{unaccounted mass} & 0.017543
\end{array}
$$

Having determined the mass difference, the mass-energy equivalence can be determined as follows:

$$\text{Energy released (mev)} = 0.017543 \times 931.2 = 16.33 \text{ mev}$$

Purpose. By undergoing positron decay the proton number is decreased by 1, and the neutron number is increased by 1. This would result in a daughter product having 1 less atomic number and the same mass number, another example of isobaric transition. This type of decay is exactly opposite to beta decay. This type might occur in an unstable nucleus in which there are too many protons and/or too few neutrons to bring the number of neutrons and protons to a stable ratio. In many instances positron emission is in competition with electron capture (p. 70), since both methods of decay have identical results.

It may be, however, that positron emission will only bring the neutron to proton ratio closer to stability. This is the case with barium 127 ($^{127}_{56}$Ba) (Fig. 4-4). ^{127}Ba contains 71 neutrons and 56 protons. This ratio of neutrons to protons is not stable, so it decays by β^{+} emission to cesium 127 ($^{127}_{55}$Cs). ^{127}Cs is still unstable, so it decays by β^{+} emission or electron capture (primarily the latter) to xenon 127 ($^{127}_{54}$Xe). ^{127}Xe still contains an unstable ratio of neutrons and protons, and it decays entirely by electron capture to iodine 127 ($^{127}_{53}$I). The series has finally reached stability at this point because iodine 127 has 74 neutrons and 53 protons, and these are the numbers necessary for stability.

It is of particular importance to learn what happens to the positron once it is ejected from the nucleus. Three reactions are of importance: ionization, Bremsstrahlung, and the annihilation reaction.

Ionization and penetration. The degree of ionization and Bremsstrahlung is similar to that which occurs with the beta particle for as long as the positron survives. The methods, however, are different because of an opposite electrical charge. Ionization occurs when the positron attracts the negatively charged orbital electron from its orbit; the beta particle repels it from its orbital path.

Bremsstrahlung. Bremsstrahlung differs also, since the nucleus has a preponderance of positive charges and the positron is also positive. The negative acceleration seen in the Bremsstrahlung phenomenon would be that of a repulsion away from the nucleus rather than an attraction toward it. This negative acceleration is, as in the beta particle, a loss of energy to that positron, and this energy is released in the form of an x ray. The x ray is equal in energy to the energy lost by the positron particle.

Annihilation reaction. The most important reaction of the positron after ejection is the annihilation reaction. It is for this reason that the positron is short lived; the average life is approximately 10^{-9} seconds. The annihilation reaction is the result of a collision between the positively charged positron that has lost all its kinetic energy and an always present negatively charged electron. The masses of both particles are completely annihilated. Accordingly, energy must be released equivalent to the masses of 1 electron and 1 positron. That mass energy equivalence is 1.02 mev of energy as indicated below:

$$\text{amu of electron} = 0.000549$$
$$\text{amu of positron} = \frac{0.000549}{0.001098}$$
$$0.001098 \times 931.2 \text{ mev} = 1.02 \text{ mev}$$

The energy that results is not 1 photon with an energy of 1.02 mev but 2 photons of 0.511 mev radiating in exactly opposite directions of one another. The available energy is equally divided between the 2 photons. This reaction is seen in Fig. 4-7.

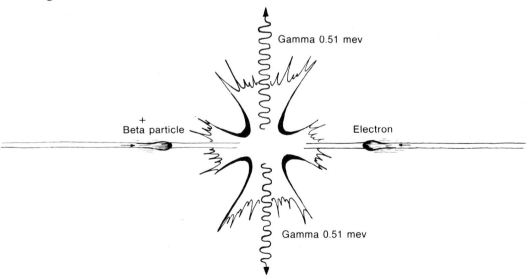

Fig. 4-7. Annihilation reaction. A positron is attracted to an electron, whereupon both particles are annihilated and converted to energy (2 gamma photons each with an energy of 0.511 mev).

Electron capture

Another mode of radioactive decay used by unstable nuclei having too few neutrons and too many protons is that of electron capture (ϵ). Electron capture is similar to positron decay in that the end results are similar, but the methods used to achieve these ends differ. As stated previously, it is generally believed that energy shells are not perfectly circular around the nucleus but are elliptic in shape. It is even thought that possibly the K shell electron passes through the nucleus during one of its orbits and is captured by the nucleus. Whatever the case, it is known that one of the orbiting K shell electrons is captured by the nucleus. When this electron is captured, the nucleus transforms a proton into a neutron and a neutrino is ejected (Fig. 4-8). It is usually the K shell electron that is captured by the nucleus (K capture). This method of decay is known to exist with electrons from the L energy shells as well. In these cases the phenomenon is known as L capture. Capture of unbound (free) electrons by nuclei has not been observed to date. Whatever electron is captured, a vacancy will exist in that shell that must be filled. Electrons fall down into the vacancy, and characteristic x-radiation results, as described in Chapter 2.

By the decay process of electron capture the parent nucleus produces a daughter nucleus with a neutron number increased by 1 and a proton number decreased

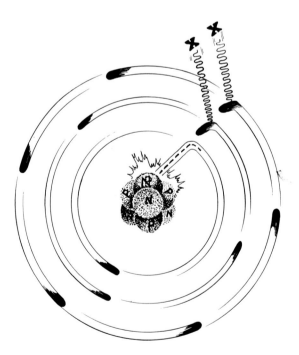

Fig. 4-8. Electron capture. The nucleus attracts an orbital electron, which combines with a proton to form a neutron. The secondary process of filling the orbital vacancy results in emission of characteristic x-radiation.

by 1. In so doing, the daughter product becomes an isobar of the parent. This is the third method of isobaric transition. Chromium 51 ($^{51}_{24}$Cr) is an example of electron capture; its decay scheme is shown at the end of this chapter (p. 72). Other pertinent radionuclides that decay by electron capture are iodine 123 ($^{123}_{53}$I), iodine 125 ($^{125}_{53}$I), mercury 197 ($^{197}_{80}$Hg), cobalt 57 ($^{57}_{27}$Co), strontium 85 ($^{85}_{38}$Sr), selenium 75 ($^{75}_{34}$Se), and germanium 68 ($^{68}_{32}$Ge).

Isomeric transition. An isomer, in nuclear terms, is one of 2 nuclides having the same mass number and the same atomic number, which can exist for measurable times in the excited state. This differs from the chemical meaning of the term. It has been stated before that in most cases this state of excitation must be instantaneously relieved by the emission of a gamma ray. In some radionuclides, however, this does not occur instantaneously. Isomeric transition is the radioactive transition from one nuclear isomer to another of lower energy. It is part of the decay process of certain radionuclides. An example of this would be molybdenum 99 ($^{99}_{42}$Mo). Molybdenum 99 decays by beta-gamma emission to technetium 99 ($^{99}_{42}$Tc). In the process of decay a point is reached at which the nucleus is able to retain its excited level (142 kev) for a half-life period of 6 hours. Since the molybdenum nucleus has ejected the beta particle and the neutrino, it has already lost 1 neutron and gained 1 proton. It is no longer molybdenum 99, but technetium 99. Furthermore, it can only be technetium 99 when the nucleus is at ground state, which it is not. It acts as though it were another radionuclide, a semistable technetium 99 atom. For this reason, the atom that can exist in this increased energy state of the nucleus is referred to as being in a *metastable* state. This state is signified by *m* after the mass number (technetium 99m). Not until the nucleus loses that energy is it known as a true technetium 99 atom. Isomeric transition is regarded as a form of decay because of the emission of the gamma ray. Sometimes, however, it only represents a change in energy state, not a change in nuclear composition. Other pertinent radionuclides that decay by isomeric transition include strontium 87m (^{87m}Sr) and barium 137m (^{137m}Ba).

Gamma emission

Radioactive decay by alpha emission, beta emission, positron emission, or electron capture usually leaves some of the energy resulting from these changes in the nucleus. As a result, the nucleus is raised to an excited level. None of these excited nuclei (with the exception of isomeric transition) can remain in this high-energy state. They must instantaneously release this energy so that the nucleus can return to ground state or its lowest possible energy state. This energy is released in the form of gamma radiation and the gamma has an energy equal to the change in energy state of the nucleon. These photons are members of the electromagnetic spectrum and have a wavelength corresponding to very short x rays. As stated previously, a gamma ray differs from an x ray only in its origin; gamma rays originate in the nucleus; x rays originate in the orbital electron structure. Although of different origin, gamma rays and x rays have precisely the same characteristics. Their powers of excitation, ionization, and penetration are exactly the same. For this reason they are used interchangeably in medical diagnosis and treatment.

Gamma rays carry no electrical charge; therefore they are not subject to forces of attraction or repulsion as are alpha, beta, and positron particles. Unlike these particles, gamma rays are the only emissions from an unstable nucleus that fall into the electromagnetic spectrum. Since they are not particles, the postemission product differs from the preemission form of the element only in a decreased energy state. There is no change in atomic number, neutron number, or mass number. Furthermore, some nuclear reaction or interaction must have preceded the gamma emission for the nucleus to be in an excited state. Reactions include neutron bombardment and charged particle bombardment. Interactions include alpha decay, beta decay, and positron decay.

Ionization and penetration. Gamma rays are also capable of producing ionization. It is referred to as *indirect* ionization, however. Gamma photons are capable of striking orbital electrons, thereby ejecting them from their orbits at very high velocities. These rapidly moving secondary electrons ionize the atoms in the surrounding media. The same is true of x rays.

The degree of penetration by a gamma ray is much greater than that of the other nuclear emissions. Penetration is such that, theoretically, enough shielding could never be provided to entirely stop all gamma rays. Even with a mile of lead there would be some gamma rays not totally absorbed but passing its full length. The degree of absorption or degree of attenuation can be predicted (p. 117).

Interactions with matter. There are three ways that gamma photons can interact with matter that have importance to nuclear medicine. These are the Compton effect, the photoelectric effect, and pair production. All three methods result in the loss of energy by the gamma ray and its eventual absorption.

Compton effect. The Compton effect (Fig. 4-9) (also called incoherent scattering) occurs when an incident gamma ray (primarily of medium energy) interacts with a free or loosely bound (outer shell) electron. In this interaction with matter a portion of the energy of the incident gamma ray is transferred to the electron. The energy expended depends on the angle at which the incident gamma ray hits the electron. If the electron is hit head-on, then a major portion of the energy is given to the electron. If the hit is one of a glancing nature, very little of the energy is transferred to the electron. As a result, the electron (Compton electron) is ejected from the orbital structure, and a gamma ray of reduced energy *(secondary, Compton,* or *scatter)* emerges from the atom with a change in direction. The incident gamma ray has been reduced in energy by two factors. First, it has had to use some of its energy to overcome the binding energy of the electron that was removed. Second, it has transferred some of its energy to that electron. Therefore the energy of the secondary gamma ray is equal to the energy of the incident

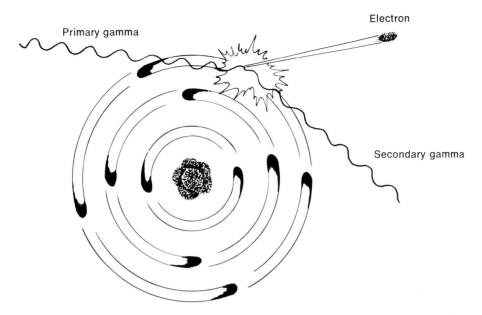

Fig. 4-9. Compton effect. A gamma photon of medium energy strikes an outer orbital electron and releases it from its orbit. This results in the production of a secondary gamma of reduced energy.

gamma ray, less the binding energy of the electron released, less the energy given to that electron. Inasmuch as this secondary gamma is changed in direction and is of reduced energy, it becomes of extreme importance to nuclear medicine. (Without knowledge of instrumentation — spectrometry — and Compton scatter, results from scanning techniques and function studies could be misinterpreted. This will be discussed in greater detail under spectrometry, Chapter 9.)

Photoelectric effect. The photoelectric effect (Fig. 4-10) occurs when an incident gamma ray (primarily of low energy) interacts with an inner-orbital electron. When this reaction occurs, the entire energy of the gamma ray is transferred to the electron, and the gamma is totally absorbed. The electron, called a *photoelectron,* is released from its energy shell and the atom. Since the electron had a binding energy to contain it within its orbit, energy had to be used by the incident gamma ray to overcome that binding energy. Therefore the electron would have the energy of the gamma ray less the amount of energy required to overcome the binding energy. Since a vacancy exists within that inner orbit, other orbital electrons will fall into that vacancy with a subsequent emission of characteristic x rays.

In the process of absorption of gamma rays, the gamma ray usually goes through a series of Compton collisions, progressively reducing it in energy until it can finally be totally absorbed by the photoelectric process.

Pair production. Pair production is the third way in which gamma rays interact

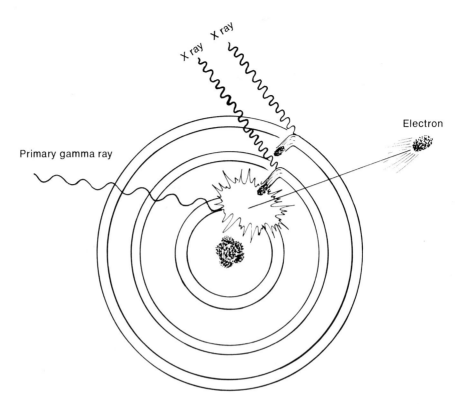

Fig. 4-10. Photoelectric effect. A low-energy gamma photon strikes an inner orbital electron and releases it from its orbit, which effects total absorption of the gamma photon. Characteristic x-radiation results from the filling phenomenon.

with matter. This phenomenon occurs when high-energy gamma rays interact in the vicinity of the nucleus. In pair production the energy of the gamma ray is completely absorbed in the vicinity of the strong electrical field of the nucleus with a subsequent production of a negatron and a positron (Fig. 4-11). For this to occur the incident gamma ray must have a minimum energy of 1.02 mev. If these conditions are met, the positron and the negatron are ejected from the atom. The beta particle acts as other beta particles in that it passes through matter, creating ion pairs along its path, until such time as it is incorporated into an atom or becomes a free electron. The positron, however, almost instantaneously collides with an electron. This results in the subsequent annihilation of both particles and the emission of 2 gamma rays of 0.511 mev. Since the conversion of the mass of 2 beta particles is equal to 1.02 mev and since the amount of energy is equally divided between the 2 annihilation gamma photons regardless of the energy of the incident gamma ray (provided it is greater than 1.02 mev), the energy of the annihilation gamma rays would always be equal to the 0.511 mev. If the incident gamma ray is greater in energy than 1.02 mev, the excess energy is given to the β^+

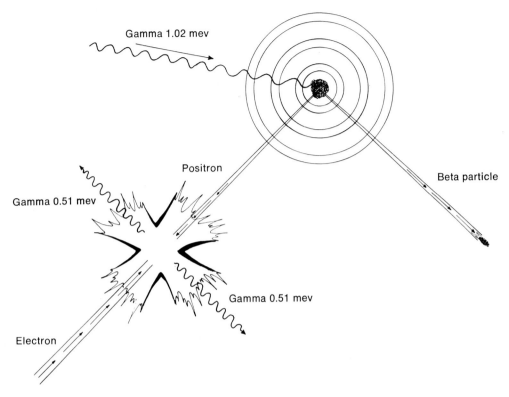

Fig. 4-11. Pair production. A high-energy gamma ray interacts near the nucleus, producing two particles, a beta particle (negatron) and a positron. The positron annihilates almost immediately.

and β^- as kinetic energy that must be lost before the β^+ can undergo annihilation. Regardless of the energy of the incident gamma ray (provided it is 1.02 mev or greater), the energy of the annihilation gamma ray is always 0.511 mev. This gamma interaction represents an energy-to-mass-to-energy relationship. The reaction was begun with energy (gamma) and was converted to mass ($\beta^- + \beta^+$), which in turn was converted to energy (2 gammas of 0.511 mev).

Internal conversion. After almost all nuclear interactions the nucleus is left in an excited state. This elevated energy state is usually decreased to ground state immediately by the emission of a gamma ray equal to the change in energy level. In some cases, however, when this gamma ray emerges from the nucleus, the gamma ray can be naively regarded as transferring all its energy to one of its own orbital electrons, usually the K shell electron. The electron is then ejected from the atom and possesses an energy equal to that of the gamma ray less the binding energy (Fig. 4-12). The gamma ray has internally converted its own atom, hence the name internal conversion. The electron that is ejected from the atom is called the *conversion electron.* Since these electrons have energy and are capable of ion-

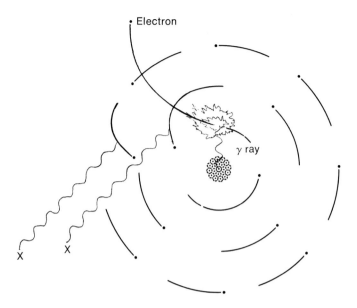

Fig. 4-12. Internal conversion. A gamma ray being released from the nucleus strikes and ejects a K shell electron. The characteristic x-ray emissions are a result of the loss of energy by other orbital electrons falling into the vacancy created by the ejected electron.

izing other atoms, it must be a consideration in the calculations of radiation dose from internal emitting radionuclides. This reaction occurs most with high Z materials.

Auger electrons. Another process resulting from changes in energy state and changes in electron configuration in the orbital shells is the release of Auger electrons. It can occur when a vacancy is created in an inner shell. Fluorescent (characteristic) radiation is then emitted as an electron assumes the lower energy state necessary to fill that vacancy. If this energy release (in the form of an x ray) possesses the capability of interacting with and removing electrons from neighboring atoms (that is, photoelectric and Compton interactions), then it also possesses the capability of removing its own electron from orbit. This electron, given energy from the fluorescent radiation and removed from its orbit, is called an *Auger electron* (Fig. 4-13). As with internal conversion electrons, these electrons have energy and are capable of ionizing other atoms; therefore, they must be a consideration when calculating internal radiation dosimetry. This interaction occurs with low Z materials.

Auger electrons are known as to their frequency and average energy for all of the radionuclides. Further, they can be identified not only as to the energy shell from which they are ejected, but by the change of electron position that caused the characteristic radiation as well. For instance, an Auger electron can be identified

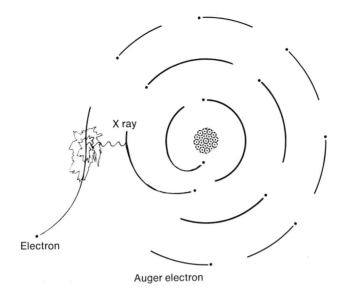

Fig. 4-13. Auger electron. Characteristic x ray emitted from one of the orbital electrons as it assumes a lower energy state strikes another orbital electron and removes it from orbit.

as a KLL Auger e, which means that it is an Auger electron emitted from the L shell as a result of the transition of another L shell electron to a vacancy in the K shell. Other appellations are as follows: KLX Auger e = an Auger electron emitted from the X shell, when X stands for any shell higher than the L shell, as a result of the transition of an L shell electron to a vacancy in the K shell; KXY Auger e = an Auger electron emitted from the Y shell as a result of the transition of an X shell electron to a vacancy in the K shell, when X and Y each stand for any shell higher than the L shell; LMM Auger e = an Auger electron emitted from the M shell as a result of the transition of another M shell electron to a vacancy in the L shell; MXY Auger e = an Auger electron emitted from the Y shell as a result of the transition of an X shell electron to a vacancy in the M shell, when X and Y each stand for any shell higher than the M shell.

Triple production. This is another photon interaction with matter not important to nuclear medicine but included in the interest of completeness. Triple production is similar to pair production except that it requires a photon of very high energy (greater than 2.04 mev) to interact in the field of an orbital electron causing three changes: (1) creation of a negatron, (2) creation of a positron, and (3) the removal of the electron from orbit. Since radionuclides with such high energies are not routinely used in nuclear medicine, this interaction phenomenon has little importance to this text.

Coherent scattering (Thomson scattering). This is an interaction with matter not necessarily important to nuclear medicine but included here in the interest of completeness. Coherent scattering occurs when the photon of very weak energy is absorbed by an orbital electron. In the process of absorption, the electron begins to vibrate, thereby releasing electromagnetic waves of the same energy as the incident photon. The resultant photon is no different than the incident photon with respect to wavelength, frequency or energy, except that it differs in direction. This is the only interaction with matter in which the photon is "scattered" without losing any energy. This phenomenon is not important to nuclear medicine because it occurs only with photons of very low energy.

The neutron. Since the neutron has no charge and is a comparatively large particle, it is unaffected by other particles containing electrical charges. The neutron can penetrate through the orbital structure directly into the nucleus where it is either absorbed, as in the case of neutron capture and transmutation (Chapter 5), or possibly disrupts the nucleus, as in the case of fission. Another special consideration of neutrons is that they are produced in enormous quantities in the fission process, either controlled as in the case of a nuclear reactor, or uncontrolled as in the detonation of a nuclear bomb. Neutrons can have energies from as low as 0.025 ev (thermal neutrons) to higher than 1 million ev (fast neutrons).

The ionizing effects of neutrons are greater than those of gamma or x rays. They also have one special feature regarding their ability to ionize hydrogen, which is a major constituent of all biologic materials. Ordinary hydrogen has a nucleus composed of only 1 proton, which is less in mass than the neutron. On subjecting biologic materials to neutron bombardment, the neutron possesses the unique quality of ionizing its hydrogen atoms by removing the nucleus, rather than the usual orbital electron.

PRINCIPLES OF RADIOACTIVE DECAY

When radiopharmaceuticals are introduced into a biologic system, two processes are usually taking place to reduce the amount of radioactivity in the body. One that is always present is the reduction of radioactivity because of the physical decay of the radionuclide. There is no way to stop, slow, or speed up this process. The other, which may or may not be present, is the biologic elimination of the material. Most materials introduced into the body will at some time be eliminated. Some materials, however (such as colloidal gold 198 and technetium 99m – labeled sulfur colloid), are removed from circulation by the reticuloendothelial system and are never excreted by any elimination system. The units of measurement by which these radioactivity reduction times are defined as physical half-life, biologic half-life, and effective half-life. Physical half-life is specifically defined by the use of the term *curie.*

The curie. When a radioactive nucleus changes to another nucleus, the change is called *decay,* or *disintegration.* The rate of decay is spoken of in terms of disintegrations per unit of time, usually in seconds or minutes. The curie (Ci) is defined as a unit of radioactivity in which the number of disintegrations per second is 3.7 $\times$ 10^{10}. By multiplying this unit by 60 the definition can be expressed as disintegrations per minute (dpm), 2.2 $\times$ 10^{12} dpm. Multiples and submultiples of the curie unit can be expressed similarly in disintegrations per second and disintegrations per minute according to Table 4-1.

At the meeting of the International Commission on Radiation Units and Measurements (ICRU) in July 1974, it was recommended that within a period of not less than about 10 years, the curie be replaced with the new SI unit,* the reciprocal second (sec^{-1}). This new unit is to be used to express the unit of activity as a function of the rate of spontaneous nuclear transformations of radionuclides, as one per second (dps, as we are used to thinking of it). Further, it was suggested that this new unit of activity be given the name *becquerel,* bearing the symbol *Bq.* The becquerel, therefore, would be equal to one distintegration per second or approximately 2.703 $\times$ 10^{-11} Ci. A 15 mCi dose of technetium 99m would then be referred to as 555 megabecquerels (555 MBq). (Refer to Appendix G for other conversions.)

Physical half-life

The physical half-life (T$_{1/2}$ or T$_p$) is often called the *radioactive half-life.* It is defined as the length of time required for one half of the original number of atoms in a given radioactive sample to disintegrate. This reduction of the number of atoms through disintegration of their nuclei is known as radioactive decay and is inherent to all radioactive materials. The rate of decay of a given isotope remains constant. It cannot be influenced by temperature, pressure, or chemical combination. Furthermore, every atom in a radioactive sample has the same probability of disintegrating.

---

*An abbreviation for Système International d'Unités, an international system of units designed to end the confusion of various units of length and weight used by various countries.

Table 4-1. Multiples and submultiples of the curie

Units	Disintegrations per second (dps)	Disintegrations per minute (dpm)
Megacurie	3.7 $\times$ 10^{16}	2.2 $\times$ 10^{18}
Kilocurie	3.7 $\times$ 10^{13}	2.2 $\times$ 10^{15}
Curie (Ci)	3.7 $\times$ 10^{10}	2.2 $\times$ 10^{12}
Millicurie (mCi)	3.7 $\times$ 10^{7}	2.2 $\times$ 10^{9}
Microcurie (μCi)	3.7 $\times$ 10^{4}	2.2 $\times$ 10^{6}
Millimicrocurie (mμCi) also called nanocurie	3.7 $\times$ 10 or 37	2.2 $\times$ 10^{3} or 2,200
Micromicrocurie ($\mu\mu$Ci) also called picocurie	3.7 $\times$ 10^{-2}	2.2

Because of decay, all radioactivity decreases with time, since fewer atoms are left as some atoms decay. Since the fraction of nuclei disintegrating per unit time is always the same and since progressively fewer atoms are left, the fraction of remaining atoms represents fewer and fewer atoms with the passage of time. This fraction of the remaining number of atoms that decay per unit of time is called the *decay constant* (λ). The larger the fraction, the faster the process of decay. Stated another way, the larger the decay constant, the shorter the half-life. Therefore $T_{1/2}$ is inversely proportional to λ. If one were to plot on linear paper the number of atoms present in a given radioactive sample versus time, the curve shown in Fig. 4-14, *A*, would be obtained. It is apparent that the same length of time is required for 100 atoms to decay to 50 atoms as is required for 50 atoms to decay to 25 at-

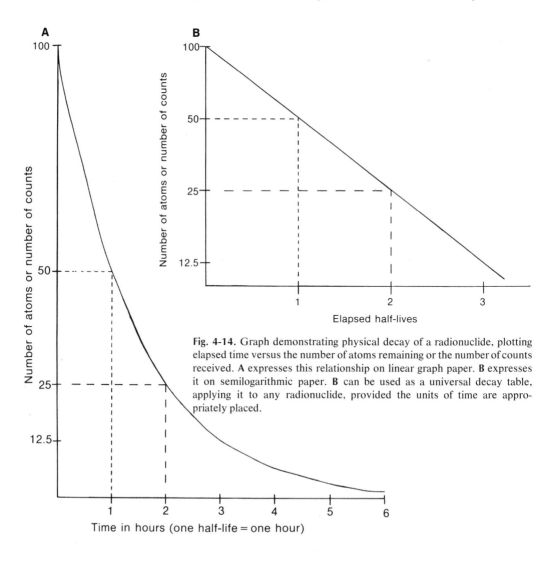

Fig. 4-14. Graph demonstrating physical decay of a radionuclide, plotting elapsed time versus the number of atoms remaining or the number of counts received. A expresses this relationship on linear graph paper. B expresses it on semilogarithmic paper. B can be used as a universal decay table, applying it to any radionuclide, provided the units of time are appropriately placed.

oms. The length of time during which the number of atoms diminish to one half is referred to as the half-life. Half-lives range in value from thousandths of a second to millions of years. Notice that the curve approaches the abscissa asymptotically, which would imply that some atoms live forever in their excited state. This is not true. If an atom is excited, it must relieve that excitation with the emission of a gamma ray at some point in time. This decay curve is only applicable to large numbers of atoms. If the same curve was plotted on semilogarithmic paper with the number of atoms on the logarithmic scale and time on the linear scale, then a straight line would be obtained (Fig. 4-14, *B*). The rate of decay can therefore be said to have an exponential function.

Fig. 4-15 also exemplifies the concept of decay constant. It shows that one half

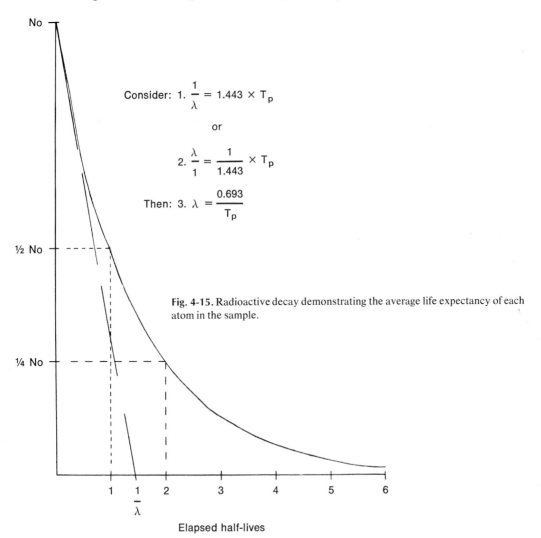

Consider: 1. $\dfrac{1}{\lambda} = 1.443 \times T_p$

or

2. $\dfrac{\lambda}{1} = \dfrac{1}{1.443} \times T_p$

Then: 3. $\lambda = \dfrac{0.693}{T_p}$

Fig. 4-15. Radioactive decay demonstrating the average life expectancy of each atom in the sample.

Elapsed half-lives

of the atoms decay per unit time (in this case the unit of time is one half-life). In the first unit of time 100 atoms decay to 50 atoms; in the second unit of time the 50 atoms remaining decay to 25 atoms. In each unit time the fraction of the number of atoms remaining in the sample is constant at one half (decay constant).

Average life expectancy (mean life). The active life of any particular radioactive atom can have any value between zero and infinity. However, the *mean life* of a large number of atoms is a definite quantity. It is related to the decay constant, being equal numerically to its reciprocal $(\frac{1}{\lambda})$. It can be described as the period of time that it would take for all the atoms of a radionuclide to decay provided that they decayed at the initial rate of decay until all the atoms were gone. Although one half of all nuclei decay in one half-life, the average life becomes longer because in the subsequent half-lives, nuclei live longer. The average life expectancy is always equal to 1.443 times the physical half-life (Fig. 4-15).

In Fig. 4-15, the number of nuclei originally in the sample (N_0) is plotted against time in half-lives. Accordingly, after one half-life has elapsed, only one half of the original radioactive nuclei are still present in the sample. After two half-lives, only one fourth of the original radioactive nuclei are present in the sample. If one were to extend the slope of the curve received at 0 half-life until it intercepted the abscissa, this extension would intercept at 1.443 half-lives. This is the life expectancy of each radioactive atom and is the reciprocal of the decay constant $(\frac{1}{\lambda})$.

Decay formula. The curve for radioactive decay can be expressed by the following equation:

$$N_t = N_o e^{-\lambda t}$$

N_t = Number of atoms at some point in time
N_o = Number of atoms originally present
e = Base of the natural logarithm, 2.718
λ = Decay constant
t = Time elapsed
Minus sign indicates that the number of atoms are decreasing

λ can be proved mathematically to be equal to $\dfrac{0.693}{T_{1/2}}$ (Fig. 4-13)

Substituting:

$$N_t = N_o e^{-\frac{0.693t}{T_{1/2}}}$$

This formula can be expressed similarly in terms of activity as follows:

$$A_t = A_o e^{-\frac{0.693t}{T_{1/2}}}$$

A_t = Activity after a period of elapsed time
A_o = Activity in the original sample

The use of the last formula is seen in the following problem:

A sample of iodine 131 was known to have an activity of 10 mCi on January 14 at 12 noon CST. What would the activity be on January 16 at 3 PM EST? (Note: Calculations of elapsed time must also include variations in time zones. Elapsed time in this case is exactly 50 hours.)

$$A_o = 10 \text{ mCi}$$
$$t = 50 \text{ hr}$$
$$T_{1/2} = 8.1 \text{ days or } 194 \text{ hr} - \text{both time units (t and } T_{1/2}) \text{ must be the same}$$

Solve for A_t

$$
\begin{aligned}
A_t &= A_o e^{-\frac{0.693t}{T_{1/2}}} \\
&= 10 \text{ mCi} \times e^{-0.693 \times \frac{50 \text{ hr}}{194 \text{ hr}}} \\
&= 10 \times e^{-\frac{34.65}{194}} \\
&= 10 \times e^{-0.18*} \\
&= 10 \times .84 \\
&= 8.4 \text{ mCi}
\end{aligned}
$$

Accordingly, the activity of the sample on January 16 at 3PM EST is 8.4 mCi.

Decay tables. The factor found on any decay table for iodine 131 with an elapsed time of 2 days plus 2 hours (50 hours) is 0.84, or it may be listed at 84% remaining, the result of $e^{-0.693t/T_{1/2}}$. In either case, the original activity is multiplied by 0.84 to find the present activity. All decay tables for the various radionuclides are nothing more than the compilation of these values for various periods of elapsed time. Appendix B shows a universal decay table.

Since decay tables are more convenient to use, most nuclear medicine personnel prefer them to the use of the decay formula. Two practical problems involving their use should be mentioned: (1) how is the decay table used when an aliquot of the radioactive solution is needed *prior* to the calibration date and (2) how is the decay table used when the decay factors do not cover a sufficient period of time?

The first problem could present itself when an order of radioactive material is received from a supplier prior to its calibration date. If the new source is to be used, it becomes necessary to first calculate the amount of activity on hand (this will be larger than that indicated on the label); then the volume that will represent the desired dose must be calculated. (Some tables include these factors.) The following problem will demonstrate the correct use of decay tables.

Problem. A 10 mCi source of ^{198}Au in a volume of 10 ml, calibrated for June 10 at 12 noon EST was received on June 9. What would be the activity on June 9 at 12 noon EST?

Solution (using decay table). Decay factor for ^{198}Au after one day of elapsed time = 0.77. This factor may be used, but instead of multiplying the activity by the decay factor, divide by the decay factor:

---

*The value for e^{-x} can be found in Appendix E.

$$\frac{10\,\text{mCi}}{0.77} = 13\,\text{mCi}$$

Similarly, using concentration:

$$\frac{1\,\text{mCi/ml}}{0.77} = 1.3\,\text{mCi/ml}$$

Expressing it another way:

To determine activity on hand *before* calibration date:

$$A_t = A_o \div DF$$

A_t = Activity on hand
A_o = Activity indicated on the vial
DF = Decay factor

Problem. The second problem involving decay tables presents itself when the decay factors given do not cover a sufficient period of time.

A 10 mCi source of ^{198}Au has an elapsed time of 85 hours from date of calibration, and the decay table has values only to 70 hours. What is the activity on hand?

Solution. The easiest approach is to correct for one half-life, knowing that ^{198}Au has a 65-hour half-life. Then using the decay factor representative of the time differential from one half-life (65 hours) to the remaining period of elapsed time (85 hours), that is, 20 hours (85 hours − 65 hours), multiply by one half of the original activity:

1. Activity at time zero (A_o) = 10 mCi
2. Activity at 65 hours or 1 half-life ($A_{T_{1/2}}$) = 5 mCi
3. Elapsed time = 85 hr
4. Elapsed time − $T_{1/2}$ (in this case) = 20 hours remaining time
5. Decay factor for remaining time = 0.81
6. Using $A_{T_{1/2}}$: 5 mCi $\times$ 0.81 = 4.05 mCi activity on hand

Accordingly, the original vial of 10 mCi ^{198}Au would contain 4.05 mCi 85 hours later.

Expressing it another way:

$$A_t = A_{T_{1/2}} \times DF \text{ (for remaining time)}$$

A_t = Activity on hand
$A_{T_{1/2}}$ = Activity after one half-life*
DF = Decay factor for total elapsed time (one half-life*)

This would also apply to concentrations, if this was the desired method of record keeping.

Biologic half-life

Biologic half-life (T_b) is the time required for the body to eliminate one half of the dose of any substance by the regular processes of elimination. This time is the

---

*This could also be the value after 2 or more half-lives, depending on the circumstances.

same for both stable and radioactive isotopes of any given element. The principal methods of elimination are by way of the urine, feces, exhalation, and perspiration. Biologic half-life is an important consideration when attempting to predict radiation damage to the human body from internal emitters. Any radionuclide that is retained by the body for only a short period of time will have a relatively small radiobiologic effect, regardless of whether it has a long physical half-life or a short physical half-life.

Effective half-life

Because both the physical and biologic half-lives must be taken into consideration when predicting the amount of radiation that is absorbed per unit mass of tissue, a third term is used to express the difference between the two. This is called the *effective half-life*.

The effective half-life is defined as the time required for the radioactivity from a given amount of a radioactive element deposited in the tissues or organs to diminish by 50% as a result of the combined action of radioactive decay and loss of the material by biologic elimination. The effective half-life (T_e) is usually experimentally determined.

A relatively simple example of experimentally determining effective half-life is that of iodine 131 in the thyroid gland. Iodine 131, labeled sodium iodide, is administered to the patient, and an uptake is determined at 24 hours after administration by a standard thyroid uptake counter. Uptakes are continued every subsequent 24-hour period. By plotting the count on day 1 and comparing subsequent daily counts, one may find the activity in the thyroid reaches 50% at 6 days, even though the physical half-life of iodine 131 is approximately 8 days. Obviously, biologic elimination has acted on the iodine 131 in the thyroid gland so that the 50% rate is reached before the physical half-life. The effective half-life in this case is something less than the physical half-life. The biologic half-life always decreases the effective half-life to a value less than that of the physical half-life. The only time that this would not be the case is in the event of no biologic elimination, as with colloidal gold in the liver. In this case the effective half-life is equal to the physical half-life. In no case is the effective half-life larger than the physical half-life. If the biologic half-life is known, the effective half-life can be mathematically calculated by the following expression:

$$T_e = \frac{T_p \times T_b}{T_p + T_b}$$

The usual case, however, is that both the effective half-life (experimentally determined) and the physical half-life are known. Using these two values the biologic half-life can be determined by the following formula:

$$T_b = \frac{T_p \times T_e}{T_p - T_e}$$

DECAY SCHEMES
Principles

A decay scheme provides a ready reference for a variety of data. Quick identification is possible of such information as mode of decay, energy states of the nuclei and their subsequent gamma emissions, and the nuclide to which the radionuclide decays. These decay schemes have a wide variation in complexity. Those that decay directly to the daughter product without emitting electromagnetic radiation are the simplest forms. These would include the pure alpha emitters and pure beta emitters. Those decay schemes with resultant electromagnetic radiation vary greatly in complexity. Some, such as cobalt 60, have a very simple decay scheme. Others, such as iodine 131 and molybdenum 99, have extremely complex decay schemes.

Decay schemes are patterned by placing the parent nucleus at the top of the decay scheme. Diagonal lines extending from the right or the left of the parent indicate the mode of decay. Those diagonal lines that angle to the right represent the mode of decay whereby the daughter nuclide is of higher atomic number than the parent. Those diagonal lines that angle to the left represent the modes of decay whereby the daughter nuclide is of lower atomic number than the parent. Alpha decay, positron decay, and electron capture all result in the daughter nuclide being of lower atomic number than the parent. Beta decay is the only method resulting in a daughter nuclide of higher atomic number than the parent.

A pure beta emitter is an example of the simplest form of decay. ^{32}P is repre-

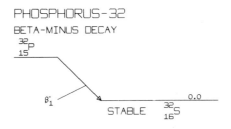

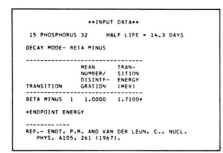

Courtesy Dillman, L. T., and Von der Lage, F. C.: MIRD pamphlet #10, New York, 1975, Society of Nuclear Medicine.

sentative of such a scheme. The "Input Data" box* indicates that the parent radionuclide, phosphorus 32, has a 14.3-day half-life and decays by β^- directly to sulfur 32, which is stable. One hundred percent (mean number/disintegration = 1.0000) of all ^{32}P nuclei decay by this method; the maximum energy is 1.7100 mev. All the energy is distributed to the beta particle and the neutrino. The nucleus does not receive any energy from this reaction; therefore, neither is the nucleus raised to an excited level nor is there a subsequent gamma emission. Note that in this mode of decay the diagonal line is angled to the right, indicating an increase in atomic number by the daughter. The atomic number of phosphorus 32 is 15 decaying to sulfur 32 with an atomic number of 16. Simple decay schemes can also be represented by pure alpha emitters, by pure positron emitters, or in nuclides that undergo 100% electron capture. In these cases all diagonal lines would be angled to the left because in all cases the daughter has a lower atomic number than the parent.

In general, the scintillation crystals used in routine diagnostic nuclear medicine procedures detect only gamma emissions. For the nuclide to be of importance to diagnostic nuclear medicine, gamma emission must be a part of its decay scheme. There are exceptions to this, such as beta emitters used with liquid scintillation detectors and positron emitters. For gamma rays to be emitted, the radionuclide must decay in such a way that only part of the energy involved in the transition from parent to daughter is distributed in the ejection particles. When this occurs, the nucleus is raised to an excited energy state, and in returning to ground state this energy is emitted in the form of gamma rays. These increases in energy state are represented by horizontal lines drawn between the parent and daughter nuclide and are representative of the various energy levels to which the nucleus can be raised. These horizontal lines would be analogous to the rungs on the stepladder used previously to describe the nuclear energy levels. A relatively simple example of such a decay scheme involving gamma emission would be that of cobalt 60. Cobalt 60 is an unstable nucleus with a half-life of 5.26 years, and it decays by beta decay to the stable nickel 60. In this transition, however, only a portion of the energy resulting from the change within the nucleus is distributed to the beta particle and the neutrino. The remainder of the energy is retained by the nucleus, and the nucleus is raised to an excited state. The energy state to which the nucleus is raised varies depending on whether the nucleus of the particular cobalt 60 atom decays by β^-_1 or β^-_2. As the "Input Data" box indicates, 99.8% of all cobalt 60 atoms decay by β^-_1, which itself has an emission energy (transition energy) of 0.313 mev. The rest of the atoms of cobalt 60 (1.2%) decay by β^-_2, which has an emission energy of 1.486 mev. The energy state to which the nucleus of cobalt 60 is raised after the emission of β^-_1 is 2.5057 mev. Rather than decaying from this elevated energy state with one release of energy to achieve

---

*"Output Data" box will be explained in chapter 7, Dosimetry.

ground state, it releases 2 gamma quanta to achieve ground state. In jumping from 2.5057-mev to 1.3325-mev energy state, there is a release of a gamma photon (γ_1) of 1.1732 mev in energy, the energy difference between the two energy states. Note that this occurs in 99.8% of all atoms, which is to be expected since only 99.8% of all cobalt 60 atoms decay by β^-_1, and therefore reach this level of excitation. This release of energy is followed immediately by another release of energy of 1.3324 mev (γ_2) representative of the change in energy state from the 1.3324-mev level to ground state. Note that this transition energy occurs 100% of the time. The reason is that all atoms of cobalt 60, whether they decay by β^-_1 or β^-_2, have their nuclei excited to an energy state of 1.3324 mev at sometime during their decay. The total energy involved in the transition of cobalt 60 to nickel 60 is 2.818 mev regardless of whether it decays by β^-_1 or β^-_2.

Decay schemes are simplified methods to describe the mode of decay and subsequent energy release in the form of gamma radiation produced by changes in an unstable nucleus. The directions of the arrows that represent the modes of decay, although not intended, assume a similarity to the Madame Curie experiment discussed at the beginning of this chapter. The negatively charged particle, representing the beta decay, is angled in one direction; the positively charged particles, representing alpha decay and positron decay (also electron capture), are angled in the opposite direction; the gamma ray with no charge is drawn perpendicular to the parent nucleus.

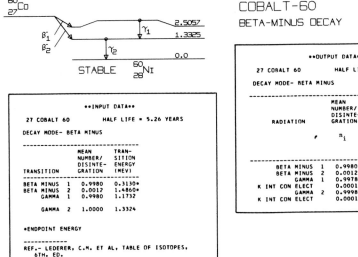

Courtesy Dillman, L. T., and Von der Lage, F. C.: MIRD pamphlet #10, New York, 1975, Society of Nuclear Medicine.

Alpha decay

Alpha decay can be represented by the decay of radium 224 as follows. Ninety-four and eight-tenths percent of the atoms of radium 224 (Z = 88) decay by an alpha particle of 5.7837 mev to radon 220 (Z = 86). Since an alpha particle is a helium nucleus, the parent atom loses 2 protons and 2 neutrons (an atomic number of 2 and a mass number of 4) to become radon 220. Five and two-tenths percent of all atoms of radium 224 decay by an alpha particle that leaves the nucleus in an excited state with a new energy level of 0.2410 mev. The atom instantaneously emits a gamma ray of 0.2410 mev to become radon 220. The daughter product has a decreased atomic number, so the angle of the schematic is to the left. Radon 220 itself is an unstable nucleus and an inert gas. Being unstable, it will continue to decay and does so by alpha emission. This is a portion of the series that will eventually decay to stable lead 214. This chain of decay can be easily followed by referring to Brucer's trilinear chart of the nuclides, a portion of which appears on p. 94. Radium 224 is a very simple alpha decay scheme. There are others much more complex in nature.

Beta (beta-minus) decay

The decay scheme of a pure beta emitter, phosphorus 32, has already been discussed on p. 64. This is a simple decay scheme in which no electromagnetic radiation is emitted. As energies to the beta particles vary and as energy states of the nucleus vary, the decay scheme becomes more and more complex.

Gold 198. A more complex decay scheme involving 3 beta particles of different energies and 3 gamma photons of different energies is that of gold 198. Gold 198 (Z = 79) decays by beta decay to stable mercury 198 (Z = 80). The percentage of all gold 198 atoms that decay with a beta particle having a maximum energy of 0.9612 mev (β_2) is 98.6%. This leaves the nucleus in an excited energy state of 0.4117 mev. This state of excitation is instantaneously relieved by the emission of a gamma ray of 0.4117 mev (γ_1). This path of decay represents an energy differential between parent and daughter nuclei of 1.37 mev; the beta particle has a maximum energy of 0.9612 mev, and the gamma has an energy of 0.4117 mev.

The percentage of all gold 198 atoms that emit a beta particle with a maximum energy of 0.29 mev (β_1) is 1.3%. The energy state of the nucleus is raised to 1.0876 mev. There are two ways to relieve this excited state. The nuclei may reach ground state immediately by the emission of a gamma ray of 1.0876 mev (γ_3), or they may do it in a two-step fashion by the emission of a gamma ray of 0.6758 mev (γ_2) plus a gamma ray of 0.4117 mev (γ_1). Both paths represent an energy differential between parent and daughter of 1.37 mev just as the β_2-γ_1 route does.

There is also a possibility that 0.02% of all gold 198 atoms would distribute all their energy to the beta particle and the neutrino, in which case the atom decays directly by beta decay (β_3) to stable mercury 198 with no emission of electromag-

RADIUM-224
ALPHA DECAY

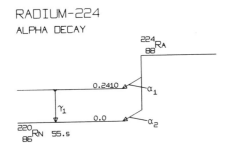

GOLD-198
BETA-MINUS DECAY

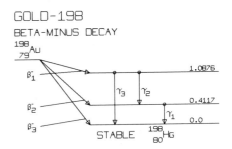

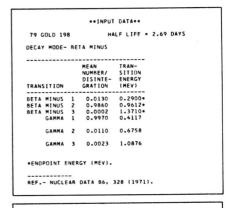

```
            ••INPUT DATA••

  88 RADIUM 224       HALF LIFE = 3.64 DAYS

  DECAY MODE- ALPHA

  --------------------------------------
                    MEAN      TRAN-
                    NUMBER/   SITION
                    DISINTE-  ENERGY
  TRANSITION        GRATION   (MEV)
  --------------------------------------
      ALPHA   1     0.0520    5.5427
      ALPHA   2     0.9480    5.7837
      GAMMA   1     0.0520    0.2410



  ------------
  REF.- LEDERER, C.M. ET AL, TABLE OF ISOTOPES,
  6TH. ED.
```

```
               ••INPUT DATA••

    79 GOLD 198         HALF LIFE = 2.69 DAYS

  DECAY MODE- BETA MINUS

  --------------------------------------
                     MEAN      TRAN-
                     NUMBER/   SITION
                     DISINTE-  ENERGY
  TRANSITION         GRATION   (MEV)
  --------------------------------------
  BETA MINUS  1      0.0130    0.2900•
  BETA MINUS  2      0.9860    0.9612•
  BETA MINUS  3      0.0002    1.3710•
     GAMMA    1      0.9970    0.4117

     GAMMA    2      0.0110    0.6758

     GAMMA    3      0.0023    1.0876


  •ENDPOINT ENERGY (MEV).

  ------------
  REF.- NUCLEAR DATA B6, 328 (1971).
```

```
            ••OUTPUT DATA••

  88 RADIUM 224       HALF LIFE = 3.64 DAYS

  DECAY MODE- ALPHA

  ----------------------------------------------
                    MEAN      MEAN     EQUI-
                    NUMBER/   ENERGY/  LIBRIUM
                    DISINTE-  PAR-     DOSE
   RADIATION        GRATION   TICLE    CONSTANT

                     n_i       Ē_i      Δ_i
                              (MeV)    (g-rad/
                                       μCi-h)
  ----------------------------------------------
       ALPHA   1    0.0520    5.4472   0.6033
  RECOIL ATOM       0.0520    0.0990   0.0109
       ALPHA   2    0.9480    5.6840   11.4773
  RECOIL ATOM       0.9480    0.1033   0.2086
       GAMMA   1    0.0400    0.2410   0.0205
  K INT CON ELECT   0.0044    0.1425   0.0013
  L INT CON ELECT   0.0056    0.2242   0.0026
  M INT CON ELECT   0.0018    0.2374   0.0009
  K ALPHA-1 X-RAY   0.0020    0.0837   0.0003
  K ALPHA-2 X-RAY   0.0011    0.0810   0.0002
  K BETA-1 X-RAY    0.0007    0.0948   0.0001
  LMM AUGER ELECT   0.0052    0.0097   0.0001
  MXY AUGER ELECT   0.0170    0.0035   0.0001

  ------------
  DAUGHTER NUCLIDE, RADON 220  IS RADIOACTIVE
  AND MAY CONTRIBUTE TO THE DOSE.
```

```
            ••OUTPUT DATA••

    79 GOLD 198         HALF LIFE = 2.69 DAYS

  DECAY MODE- BETA MINUS

  -----------------------------------------------
                    MEAN      MEAN     EQUI-
                    NUMBER/   ENERGY/  LIBRIUM
                    DISINTE-  PAR-     DOSE
   RADIATION        GRATION   TICLE    CONSTANT

                     n_i       Ē_i      Δ_i
                              (MeV)    (g-rad/
                                       μCi-h)
  -----------------------------------------------
  BETA MINUS   1     0.0130    0.0811   0.0022
  BETA MINUS   2     0.9860    0.3163   0.6643
  BETA MINUS   3     0.0002    0.4648   0.0002
      GAMMA    1     0.9555    0.4117   0.8380
  K INT CON ELECT    0.0287    0.3286   0.0201
  L INT CON ELECT    0.0095    0.3979   0.0081
  M INT CON ELECT    0.0031    0.4089   0.0027
      GAMMA    2     0.0107    0.6758   0.0154
  K INT CON ELECT    0.0002    0.5927   0.0003
      GAMMA    3     0.0022    1.0876   0.0053
  K ALPHA-1 X-RAY    0.0139    0.0708   0.0021
  K ALPHA-2 X-RAY    0.0076    0.0688   0.0011
  K BETA-1 X-RAY     0.0048    0.0802   0.0008
  K BETA-2 X-RAY     0.0013    0.0831   0.0002
  L ALPHA X-RAYS     0.0060    0.0099   0.0001
  L BETA X-RAYS      0.0056    0.0118   0.0001
  LMM AUGER ELECT    0.0206    0.0081   0.0003
  MXY AUGER ELECT    0.0622    0.0028   0.0003
```

Courtesy Dillman, L. T., and Von der Lage, F. C.: MIRD pamphlet #10, New York, 1975, Society of Nuclear Medicine.

Courtesy Dillman, L. T., and Von der Lage, F. C.: MIRD pamphlet #10, New York, 1975, Society of Nuclear Medicine.

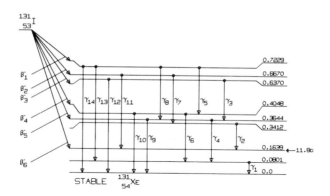

Courtesy Dillman, L. T., and Von der Lage, F. C.: MIRD pamphlet #10, New York, 1975, Society of Nuclear Medicine.

••INPUT DATA••

53 IODINE 131   HALF LIFE = 8.06 DAYS

DECAY MODE- BETA MINUS

TRANSITION	MEAN NUMBER/ DISINTE- GRATION	TRAN- SITION ENERGY (MEV)
BETA MINUS 1	0.0200	0.2470*
BETA MINUS 2	0.0067	0.3030*
BETA MINUS 3	0.0664	0.3330*
BETA MINUS 4	0.0000	0.5650*
BETA MINUS 5	0.8980	0.6060*
BETA MINUS 6	0.0080	0.8060*
GAMMA 1	0.0660	0.0801
GAMMA 2	0.0035	0.1772
GAMMA 3	0.0006	0.2723
GAMMA 4	0.0607	0.2843
GAMMA 5	0.0011	0.3180
GAMMA 6	0.0003	0.3250
GAMMA 7	0.0037	0.3257
GAMMA 8	0.0001	0.3585
GAMMA 9	0.8380	0.3644
GAMMA 10	0.0006	0.4048
GAMMA 11	0.0029	0.5029
GAMMA 12	0.0657	0.6367
GAMMA 13	0.0014	0.6430
GAMMA 14	0.0174	0.7228

*ENDPOINT ENERGY (MEV).

REF.- GRAEFFE, G. AND WALTERS, W.R., PHYS. REV. 153, 1321 (1967).
LEDERER, C.M. ET AL, TABLE OF ISOTOPES, 6TH. ED.

••OUTPUT DATA••

53 IODINE 131   HALF LIFE = 8.06 DAYS

DECAY MODE- BETA MINUS

RADIATION	MEAN NUMBER/ DISINTE- GRATION n_i	MEAN ENERGY/ PAR- TICLE $\bar{E}_i$ (MeV)	EQUI- LIBRIUM DOSE CONSTANT Δ_i (g-rad/ uCi-h)
BETA MINUS 1	0.0200	0.0691	0.0029
BETA MINUS 2	0.0067	0.0867	0.0012
BETA MINUS 3	0.0664	0.0964	0.0136
BETA MINUS 5	0.8980	0.1916	0.3666
BETA MINUS 6	0.0080	0.2839	0.0048
GAMMA 1	0.0258	0.0801	0.0044
K INT CON ELECT	0.0343	0.0456	0.0033
L INT CON ELECT	0.0043	0.0751	0.0007
M INT CON ELECT	0.0014	0.0792	0.0002
GAMMA 2	0.0029	0.1772	0.0011
K INT CON ELECT	0.0004	0.1426	0.0001
GAMMA 3	0.0006	0.2723	0.0003
GAMMA 4	0.0578	0.2843	0.0350
K INT CON ELECT	0.0023	0.2497	0.0012
L INT CON ELECT	0.0004	0.2792	0.0002
GAMMA 5	0.0010	0.3180	0.0007
GAMMA 6	0.0003	0.3250	0.0002
GAMMA 7	0.0036	0.3257	0.0025
GAMMA 8	0.0001	0.3585	0.0001
GAMMA 9	0.8201	0.3644	0.6366
K INT CON ELECT	0.0147	0.3299	0.0103
L INT CON ELECT	0.0023	0.3594	0.0017
M INT CON ELECT	0.0007	0.3635	0.0006
GAMMA 10	0.0006	0.4048	0.0005
GAMMA 11	0.0029	0.5029	0.0031
GAMMA 12	0.0653	0.6367	0.0886
K INT CON ELECT	0.0002	0.6021	0.0003
GAMMA 13	0.0014	0.6430	0.0020
GAMMA 14	0.0173	0.7228	0.0267
K ALPHA-1 X-RAY	0.0249	0.0297	0.0015
K ALPHA-2 X-RAY	0.0128	0.0294	0.0008
K BETA-1 X-RAY	0.0068	0.0336	0.0004
K BETA-2 X-RAY	0.0014	0.0345	0.0001
KLL AUGER ELECT	0.0041	0.0244	0.0002
KLX AUGER ELECT	0.0018	0.0285	0.0001
LMM AUGER ELECT	0.0477	0.0031	0.0003
MXY AUGER ELECT	0.1147	0.0009	0.0002

DAUGHTER NUCLIDE, XENON 131M IS RADIOACTIVE AND MAY CONTRIBUTE TO THE DOSE.
BRANCHING TO 0.1639 MEV, 11.8 DAY HALF LIFE, ISOMERIC LEVEL IN XENON-131 IS 0.0144 PER DISINTEGRATION OF IODINE-131.

netic radiation. The maximum energy of such a beta particle would be 1.37 mev, the energy differential between parent and daughter.

The largest number of beta particles (98.6%) decay in such a manner as to elevate the nucleus to an energy state of 0.412 mev. This being the case, the energy used in detecting gold 198 with radiation detection devices is 0.412 mev. In addition to the 98.6%, contributions are received from β^-_1, since one of its paths in relieving its excited state is by the 0.412 mev route, which further increases the percentage of atoms decaying by that energy emission to 99.7%. In looking at a gamma spectrum of gold 198, if the detection device was sensitive enough, three gamma peaks would be displayed: a very large peak at 0.412 mev and two much smaller peaks at 0.676 mev and 1.088 mev. The peak of choice in any study using gold 198 would be the peak of 0.412 mev.

Iodine 131. An even more complex beta-gamma spectrum is that of iodine 131. Iodine 131 decays by beta decay to stable xenon 131 by way of a metastable state of xenon 131 at 0.1639 mev energy state. The nuclei of iodine 131 can decay by six different methods represented by six different beta particles all varying in energy. The differential between parent and daughter is 0.970 mev, regardless of which beta-gamma pathway is calculated. Since 89.8% of all nuclei of iodine 131 decay by the β^-_5-γ_9 pathway and γ_9 has an energy of 0.364 mev, the energy used to detect iodine 131 is 0.364 mev. With iodine 131 there are no contributors from other beta pathways to increase the percentage of 0.364-mev gammas, as was the case of gold 198. In fact, the opposite is true. The β^-_5 pathway results in two different gammas (γ_4 and γ_9), each having different energies. In effect, this would actually reduce the percentage of nuclei giving the 0.364 gamma. This is realized by the study of gamma percentages of the 89.8% of iodine 131 atoms that decay by the β^-_5 route; only 83.8% continue the decay process by the γ_9 route (0.364 mev); the remaining 6% decay by the γ_4 route.

Electron capture

Iodine 125. A simple decay scheme representing the electron capture phenomenon is that of iodine 125 (Z = 53). Iodine 125 decays by electron capture to an excited state of tellurium 125. One-hundred percent of all atoms of iodine 125 achieve this excited state in the process of their transition, which is relieved by the emission of a gamma photon of 35 kev (0.0354 mev), an energy that represents the change in energy state from excited to ground. The daughter, tellurium 125, has an atomic number that is less than the parent, so the diagonal line is angled to the left.

An interesting phenomenon regarding this particular radionuclide is shown in the examination of the "Output Data." As previously noted, electron capture necessarily involves the production of x rays because of the "filling" phenomenon; it can also result in the production of x rays as a result of *internal conversion*. While this is a phenomenon common to many radionuclides, it is of particular interest with iodine 125, since the energies of all of these x rays (see mean energies $\bar{E}_i$ of K alpha and K beta x rays in "Output Data") are very close to the transition energy of the gamma photon (see Gamma-1 in "Input Data") and, therefore, indistinguishable with the use of routine nuclear medicine laboratory counting equipment. Further, since many of these events occur, for all practical purposes, at the same time, a second energy peak can be found around 55 to 60 kev, representing a coincident counting of these simultaneous events. Since these simultaneous counting events occur as a constant percentage of the number of disintegrating atoms, it is considered proper to include these counts in the windows used for in vitro counting. This relationship could be destroyed, of course, if the amount of radioactivity in the sample was greater than the counting capacity of the instrument. See Chapter 11, "Considerations of Counting and Imaging," for a discussion of this matter.

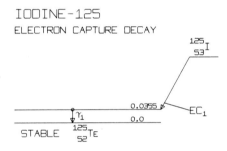

Courtesy Dillman, L. T., and Von der Lage, F. C.: MIRD pamphlet #10, New York, 1975, Society of Nuclear Medicine.

Chromium 51. Another radionuclide used in nuclear medicine procedures that involves electron capture is chromium 51. Chromium 51 decays to vanadium 51 by two methods of electron capture. Eighty-nine and eight-tenths percent of all atoms of chromium 51 decay by electron capture to the ground state of vanadium 51, whereas 10.2% leave the nuclei in an excited energy state. The 10.2% that decay by way of the excited nucleus do so by raising its nuclear energy state to 0.320 mev. That energy state is instantaneously relieved by the release of a gamma photon equivalent to the change in energy state (0.320 mev). Vanadium 51 is a stable form of the element vanadium. As with the decay of iodine 125 to tellurium 125, chromium 51 produces a daughter nuclide that is reduced in atomic number; therefore, the diagonal of the decay scheme is angled to the left. It is interesting to

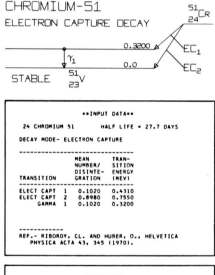

Courtesy Dillman, L. T., and Von der Lage, F. C.: MIRD pamphlet #10, New York, 1975, Society of Nuclear Medicine.

note that this gamma peak of 320 kev represents only 10.2% of all the available atoms of chromium in any sample. The other 89.8% go undetected by standard detection methods. This also explains the unusual readings on dose calibrator constancy checks when chromium 51 is measured using a constancy source.

Positron (beta-plus) decay

Oxygen 15. Oxygen 15 is an example of a positron emitter. Oxygen 15 (Z = 8) decays to nitrogen 15 (Z = 7), which is stable. One-hundred percent of all atoms of oxygen 15 decay directly to their ground state, with no energy remaining to excite the nucleus and, consequently, no gamma photon emission. The energy differential between the daughter and parent is 1.7000 mev, which is seen in the "Input Data" box as the transition energy of the positron particle. This energy is shared with the neutrino as they are both ejected from the nucleus, much the same as in beta decay. The daughter product has a decrease in atomic number so that the diagonals are angled to the left. Since this radionuclide is a pure positron emitter, the only way that it is useful to photon-sensitive (gamma or x rays) counting equipment, such as that found in routine nuclear medicine departments, is through the eventual annihilation of the positron and the subsequent release of two gamma photons.

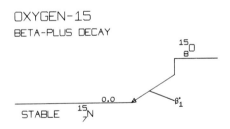

OXYGEN-15
BETA-PLUS DECAY

$^{15}_{8}$O

0.0

STABLE $^{15}_{7}$N

β^+_1

```
            ••INPUT DATA••

   8 OXYGEN 15          HALF LIFE = 124. SECONDS

   DECAY MODE- BETA PLUS

   ------------------------------------
                  MEAN      TRAN-
                  NUMBER/   SITION
                  DISINTE-  ENERGY
   TRANSITION     GRATION   (MEV)
   ------------------------------------
   BETA PLUS   1  1.0000    1.7000•

   •ENDPOINT ENERGY

   ------------
   REF.- LEDERER, C.M. ET AL, TABLE OF ISOTOPES,
     6TH. ED.
```

```
            ••OUTPUT DATA••

   8 OXYGEN 15          HALF LIFE = 124. SECONDS

   DECAY MODE- BETA PLUS

   -----------------------------------------
                         MEAN     MEAN    EQUI-
                         NUMBER/  ENERGY/ LIBRIUM
                         DISINTE- PAR-    DOSE
   RADIATION             GRATION  TICLE   CONSTANT
   -----------------------------------------
                         n_i      Ē_i     Δ_i
                                  (MeV)   (g-rad/
                                          µCi-h)
   -----------------------------------------
   BETA PLUS     1        1.0000   0.7206  1.5349
   ANNIH. RADIATION       2.0000   0.5110  2.1768
```

Courtesy Dillman, L. T., and Von der Lage, F. C.: MIRD pamphlet #10, New York, 1975, Society of Nuclear Medicine.

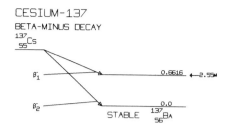

CESIUM-137

BETA-MINUS DECAY

$^{137}_{55}$Cs

β^-_1 ——————————— 0.6616 ←—2.55M

β^-_2 ——————————— 0.0

STABLE $^{137}_{56}$BA

```
              ••INPUT DATA••

    55 CESIUM 137        HALF LIFE = 30.0 YEARS

  DECAY MODE- BETA MINUS

  ---------------------------------
                 MEAN      TRAN-
                 NUMBER/   SITION
                 DISINTE-  ENERGY
  TRANSITION     GRATION   (MEV)
  ---------------------------------
  BETA MINUS  1  0.9460    0.5140•
  BETA MINUS  2  0.0540    1.1760•

  •ENDPOINT ENERGY (MEV).

  ------------

  REF.- HANSEN, M.M. ET AL, Z. PHYSIK 218,425
    (1969).
    KARTASHOV, V.M. ET AL, SOV. J. NUCL. PHYS. 6,
    656 (1968).
```

```
              ••OUTPUT DATA••

    55 CESIUM 137        HALF LIFE = 30.0 YEARS

  DECAY MODE- BETA MINUS

  ---------------------------------
                 MEAN      MEAN     EQUI-
                 NUMBER/   ENERGY/  LIBRIUM
                 DISINTE-  PAR-     DOSE
  RADIATION      GRATION   TICLE    CONSTANT
  ---------------------------------
                 $n_i$      $\bar{E}_i$    $\Delta_i$
                           (MeV)    (g-rad/
                                    μCi-h)
  ---------------------------------
  BETA MINUS  1  0.9460    0.1747   0.3520
  BETA MINUS  2  0.0540    0.4269   0.0491

  ------------

  DAUGHTER NUCLIDE, BARIUM 137M IS RADIOACTIVE
  AND MAY CONTRIBUTE TO THE DOSE.
  BRANCHING TO 0.6616 MEV, 2.55 MINUTE HALF LIFE,
  ISOMERIC LEVEL IN BARIUM-137 IS 0.946 PER
  DISINTEGRATION OF CESIUM-137.
```

Courtesy Dillman, L. T., and Von der Lage, F. C.: MIRD pamphlet #10, New York, 1975, Society of Nuclear Medicine.

Isomeric transition

Cesium 137. A simple example of a decay scheme representing isomeric transition is cesium 137. Cesium 137 (Z = 55) decays by 2 beta particles of 0.514 mev and 1.1760 mev. The beta particle having a maximum energy of 0.514 mev (β^-_1) represents 94.6% of all cesium 137 atoms; the 1.1760 mev beta particle (β^-_2) represents only 5.4% of all the atoms of cesium 137. β^-_2 decays directly to ground state barium 137 (Z = 56), which is stable. β^-_1 decays to an excited state of the nucleus. Unlike other forms of decay in which there is an excited state of the nucleus, this excitation state can be held for a half-life of 2.55 minutes. This isomeric state is known to be barium 137m (Z = 56). The isomer decays to ground state, barium 137, releasing a gamma photon of 0.662 mev. The transition from parent to daughter represents an energy differential of 1.176 mev. The daughter product has an increased atomic number, so the diagonals are angled to the right.

Molybdenum 99. A more complex decay scheme representing isomeric transition and pertinent to nuclear medicine is molybdenum 99. All atoms of molybdenum 99 (Z = 42) have a 66.7-hour half-life and decay by 1 of 8 beta particles to technetium 99 (Z = 43) through the isomeric state of technetium 99m. This isomeric state has a half-life of 6.03 hours and is the form of the radionuclide that is

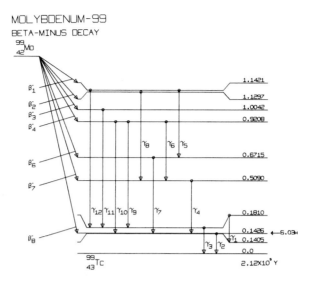

MOLYBDENUM-99
BETA-MINUS DECAY

Courtesy Dillman, L. T., and Von der Lage, F. C.: MIRD pamphlet #10, New York, 1975, Society of Nuclear Medicine.

Continued.

••INPUT DATA••

42 MOLYBDENUM 99   HALF LIFE = 66.7 HOURS

DECAY MODE- BETA MINUS

TRANSITION		MEAN NUMBER/ DISINTE- GRATION	TRAN- SITION ENERGY (MEV)
BETA MINUS	1	0.0012	0.2340*
BETA MINUS	2	0.0001	0.2470*
BETA MINUS	3	0.0014	0.3730*
BETA MINUS	4	0.1850	0.4560*
BETA MINUS	5	0.0001	0.6150*
BETA MINUS	6	0.0004	0.7050*
BETA MINUS	7	0.0143	0.8680*
BETA MINUS	8	0.7970	1.2340*
GAMMA	1	0.0630	0.0405
GAMMA	2	0.0633	0.1405
GAMMA	3	0.0760	0.1810
GAMMA	4	0.0145	0.3664
GAMMA	5	0.0001	0.3807
GAMMA	6	0.0002	0.4115

••INPUT DATA••

42 MOLYBDENUM 99 (CONTINUED)

TRANSITION		MEAN NUMBER/ DISINTE- GRATION	TRAN- SITION ENERGY (MEV)
GAMMA	7	0.0005	0.5289
GAMMA	8	0.0002	0.6207
GAMMA	9	0.1370	0.7397
GAMMA	10	0.0480	0.7782
GAMMA	11	0.0014	0.8231
GAMMA	12	0.0011	0.9610

*ENDPOINT ENERGY (MEV).

REF.- VAN EIJK, C.W. FT AL, NUCL. PHYS. A121, 440 (1968).

```
            ••OUTPUT DATA••

   42 MOLYBDENUM 99      HALF LIFE = 66.7 HOURS

   DECAY MODE- BETA MINUS

   --------------------------------------------------
                         MEAN      MEAN      EQUI-
                         NUMBER/   ENERGY/   LIBRIUM
                         DISINTE-  PAR-      DOSE
              RADIATION  GRATION   TICLE     CONSTANT

                         n_i       E̅_i       Δ_i
                                   (MeV)    (g-rad/
                                            µCi·h)

   --------------------------------------------------
            BETA MINUS  1   0.0012   0.0658   0.0001
            BETA MINUS  3   0.0014   0.1112   0.0003
            BETA MINUS  4   0.1850   0.1401   0.0552
            BETA MINUS  6   0.0004   0.2541   0.0002
            BETA MINUS  7   0.0143   0.2981   0.0090
            BETA MINUS  8   0.7970   0.4519   0.7673
               GAMMA    1   0.0130   0.0405   0.0011
   K INT CON ELECT          0.0428   0.0195   0.0017
   L INT CON ELECT          0.0053   0.0377   0.0004
   M INT CON ELECT          0.0017   0.0401   0.0001
               GAMMA    2   0.0564   0.1405   0.0168
   K INT CON ELECT          0.0058   0.1194   0.0014
   L INT CON ELECT          0.0007   0.1377   0.0002
               GAMMA    3   0.0657   0.1810   0.0253
   K INT CON ELECT          0.0085   0.1600   0.0029
   L INT CON ELECT          0.0012   0.1782   0.0004
   M INT CON ELECT          0.0004   0.1806   0.0001
               GAMMA    4   0.0143   0.3664   0.0112
               GAMMA    5   0.0001   0.3807   0.0000
               GAMMA    6   0.0002   0.4115   0.0002
               GAMMA    7   0.0005   0.5289   0.0005
               GAMMA    8   0.0002   0.6207   0.0003
               GAMMA    9   0.1367   0.7397   0.2154
   K INT CON ELECT          0.0002   0.7186   0.0003
               GAMMA   10   0.0479   0.7782   0.0794
   K INT CON ELECT          0.0000   0.7571   0.0001
               GAMMA   11   0.0014   0.8231   0.0024
               GAMMA   12   0.0011   0.9610   0.0022
   K ALPHA-1 X-RAY          0.0253   0.0183   0.0009
   K ALPHA-2 X-RAY          0.0127   0.0182   0.0004
   K  BETA-1 X-RAY          0.0060   0.0206   0.0002
   KLL AUGER ELECT          0.0087   0.0154   0.0002
   KLX AUGER ELECT          0.0032   0.0178   0.0001
   LMM AUGER ELECT          0.0615   0.0019   0.0002
   MXY AUGER ELECT          0.1403   0.0004   0.0001

   --------------
   DAUGHTER NUCLIDE, TECHNETIUM 99M IS
   RADIOACTIVE AND MAY CONTRIBUTE TO THE DOSE.
   BRANCHING TO 0.1426 MEV, 6.03 HOUR HALF LIFE,
      ISOMERIC LEVEL IN TECHNETIUM-99 IS 0.860 PER
      DISINTEGRATION OF MOLYBDENUM-99.
```

of interest in nuclear medicine procedures. Molybdenum 99 decays primarily (79.7%) by a beta particle (β_8^-) having an energy of 1.234 mev to the metastable form of technetium with an increased nuclear energy state of 0.1405 mev. It relieves that energy state by the emission of a gamma photon (γ_2) of 0.1405 mev. The transition from molybdenum 99 to technetium 99 represents an energy change of 1.376 mev, regardless of which pathway the nucleus decays. Technetium 99 is itself unstable, having a half-life of 2.12×10^5 years, and decays by beta decay, with no electromagnetic radiation, to ruthenium 99, a stable form of that element.

BIBLIOGRAPHY

Blahd, W. H.: Nuclear medicine, New York, 1965, McGraw-Hill Book Co.

Bogardus, C. R., Jr.: Clinical applications of physics of radiology and nuclear medicine, St. Louis, 1969, Warren H. Green, Inc.

Casarett, A. P.: Radiation biology, Englewood Cliffs, N. J., 1968, Prentice-Hall, Inc.

Chandra, R.: Introductory physics of nuclear medicine, Philadelphia, 1976, Lea & Febiger.

Goodwin, P. N., and Rao, D. V.: The physics of nuclear medicine, Springfield, Ill., 1977, Charles C Thomas, Publisher.

Gottschalk, A. and Potchen, E. J.: Diagnostic nuclear medicine, Baltimore, 1976, The Williams & Wilkins Co.

Hendee, W. R.: Medical radiation physics, Chicago, 1970, Year Book Medical Publishers, Inc.

Johns, H. E.: The physics of radiology, ed. 2, revised edition, Springfield, Ill., 1964, Charles C Thomas, Publisher.

King, E. R., and Mitchell, T. G.: A manual for nuclear medicine, Springfield, Ill., 1961, Charles C Thomas, Publisher.

Quimby, E. H., and Feitelberg, S.: Radioactive isotopes in medicine and biology, ed. 2, Philadelphia, 1963, Lea & Febiger.

Rollo, F. D.: Nuclear medicine physics, instrumentation, and agents, St. Louis, 1977, The C. V. Mosby Co.

Shilling, C. W.: Atomic energy encyclopedia in the life sciences, Philadelphia, 1964, W. B. Saunders Co.

Shapiro, J.: Radiation protection, Cambridge, Mass., 1972, Harvard University Press.

Wagner, H. N.: Principles of nuclear medicine, Philadelphia, 1968, W. B. Saunders Co.

5 Origin of nuclides

Following is a discussion of six methods whereby nuclides are produced, not all of which are currently used to obtain the nuclides needed in a nuclear medicine department.

FISSION

Fission, stated simply, is the production of small nuclei from a large nucleus. It may be strictly defined as an exergonic (energy-liberating) process of splitting certain heavy nuclei into two more or less equal fragments. These fragments are known as fission products. Fission may occur spontaneously or may be induced by the capture of bombarding particles, primarily neutrons. In addition to fission fragments, neutrons and energy in the form of gamma rays are usually by-products. The fission products from such reactions are generally from atomic numbers 42 (molybdenum) to 56 (barium) but may range from atomic numbers 30 through 64. Approximately 200 different radioactive nuclides are formed as fission products in the detonation of a nuclear device (atomic bomb). Uranium and plutonium are generally used in a nuclear reactor to produce some of the radioactive materials used in nuclear medicine. There are 40 or more different ways in which the nuclei of uranium and plutonium can split when fission occurs so that 80 or more different fission products can be produced.

Fission is a process that can either be controlled (the energy released does not reach explosive quantities) or made uncontrolled as in an atomic device. The latter results in a nuclear explosion. The controlling of a fission reaction is based primarily on the slowing down of the highly energetic neutrons released from the reaction. Following is a typical example of a fission reaction:

$$\begin{array}{c} \nearrow\ {}^{103}_{42}\text{Mo} \xrightarrow{\beta^-}\ {}^{103}_{43}\text{Tc} \xrightarrow{\beta^-}\ {}^{103}_{44}\text{Ru} \xrightarrow{\beta^-}\ {}^{103}_{45}\text{Rh}\ (\text{stable}) \\ {}^{235}_{92}\text{U} + {}^{1}_{0}\text{n} \longrightarrow {}^{236}_{92}\text{U} \qquad + 2\ {}^{1}_{0}\text{n}\ +\ \text{energy} \\ \searrow\ {}^{131}_{50}\text{Sn} \xrightarrow{\beta^-}\ {}^{131}_{51}\text{Sb} \xrightarrow{\beta^-}\ {}^{131}_{52}\text{Te} \xrightarrow{\beta^-}\ {}^{131}_{53}\text{I} \xrightarrow{\beta^-}\ {}^{131}_{54}\text{Xe}\ (\text{stable}) \end{array}$$

Uranium 235 absorbs a neutron to become uranium 236, liberating 2 neutrons plus energy in the form of gamma photons. Uranium 236 splits into approximately two equal parts to begin two fission chains. One of these chains begins with molybdenum 103 and continues to stable rhenium 103; the other begins with tin 131 and continues to the stable xenon 131. Involved in these two fission chains are several radionuclides, other forms of which are used in nuclear medicine procedures (radioisotopes of molybdenum, tin, iodine, and xenon). Obviously, this could be one method of producing radionuclides for use in nuclear medicine. This is currently one of the methods of producing molybdenum 99 for fission generators. Although molybdenum 103 is shown in the reaction, a different type of split would have yielded molybdenum 99, the parent of the "fission moly" generators.

According to this reaction, each fission process liberates 2 neutrons. Assuming that each neutron generates another fission process, 4 neutrons would be released in the second generation. If each of these neutrons generated a fission process, the third generation would release 8 neutrons; the fourth, 16 neutrons; the fifth, 32 neutrons; and so on. Should this fission process go uncontrolled, the amount of energy and continued production of neutrons would reach the point of explosion. Such is the case of the atomic bomb. It has been calculated that in fewer than 90 generations the neutron yield would be sufficient to cause the fission of every nucleus in 110 pounds of uranium. This would result in the liberation of the same amount of energy as in the explosion of 1 million tons of TNT. If uncontrolled, this ninetieth generation will be attained in less than one-millionth of a second.

Fortunately, with nuclear reactors, fission can be controlled through the use of absorbing media resulting in a self-sustaining reaction. In this way, by-products of fission can be continuously produced and used for peaceful purposes.

FUSION

Fusion can be defined simply as the joining of light nuclei to form a heavier nucleus. When this occurs, neutrons and energy are released. This is also an exergonic process. Following is a typical example of fusion:

$$\mathrm{{}^2_1H + {}^2_1H \longrightarrow {}^3_2He + {}^1_0n + 3.22\,mev}$$

Two deuterium molecules are brought together against extremely large forces of electrostatic repulsion until they actually fuse to produce a new nucleus. This fusion can only be accomplished by the acceleration of these deuterium particles to extremely high velocities. These velocities represent temperatures of millions of degrees. Only at this point will the particles collide with sufficient energy to fuse.

Although this is not a way in which radioactive materials are produced for nuclear medicine uses, it does represent a very interesting and hopefully useful source of energy. Its importance lies in the fact that water could be used as a source of energy because deuterium (^{2}H) occurs in 8 parts per 1,000 of ordinary hydrogen (^{1}H). The present problem is that, unlike the fission reaction, the fusion reaction is not self-sustaining. It requires the constant application of extremely high temperatures to sustain the reaction. For it to be self-sustaining, the energy released from fusion must be fed back into the reaction. To date, only limited progress has been made, although many researchers are working on the problem. Advances are being made with the use of lasers to initiate the fusion reaction. When and if such a method is devised, it has been estimated that a cubic mile of water will provide enough energy for all man's needs forever.

A nonpeaceful use of the fusion reaction is the thermonuclear weapon. The term *thermonuclear weapon* is used because the weapon relates directly to the fusion reaction and can be brought about only in the presence of very high temperatures. This thermonuclear weapon is commonly referred to as the hydrogen bomb as opposed to the fission atomic bomb. The million-degree temperature necessary to bring about a nuclear fusion reaction is provided by the initiation of the reaction with a nuclear fission reaction. A quantity of deuterium is combined with a fission weapon, and, on detonation, a combined fission-fusion reaction takes place with the release of enormous energy. Weight for weight, the fusion of deuterium nuclei provides over three times as much energy as the fission of uranium or plutonium. It has been calculated that 1 pound of uranium produces as much energy as 8,000 tons of TNT, whereas 1 pound of deuterium produces energy equivalent to 26,000 tons of TNT.

NEUTRON ACTIVATION (NEUTRON CAPTURE)

One of the most common production methods of radioactive materials used in nuclear medicine departments is neutron activation (neutron capture). Neutron activation involves the capture of a neutron into a stable nucleus with the subsequent emission of a gamma ray. This process is usually referred to as an (n, γ) process. Production of gold 198 from gold 197 by neutron activation is written as follows:

$$^{197}Au + {}_{0}^{1}n \rightarrow {}^{198}Au + \gamma$$

Following is a shorthand method for indicating this neutron activation phenomenon:

$$^{197}Au\,(n, \gamma)\,{}^{198}Au$$

The product is always an isotope of the target element, but since it has incorporated a neutron into its nucleus, the product has a mass number increased by 1. The process usually involves neutrons of relatively low energy called *slow neutrons,* or *thermal neutrons.* The bombardment of stable forms of an element by neutrons is generally carried out in nuclear reactors.

Neutron activation, in addition to being a means of obtaining radionuclides, has also become a dynamic tool in research and is developing into an exciting new field in medicine. Many areas of utilization have not even been touched yet. Some, however, are well known. Neutron activation is used not only in medicine but also in the field of crime detection. Neutron activation analysis has been used to determine the presence of heavy metal poisons in tissues. This has been extremely valuable in medical-legal problems. It can also be used to quantitate very small quantities of elements in serum and other biologic samples. A human hair can be subjected to neutron activation for purposes of identification, chemical analysis, and so on. A paper chromatograph of a serum sample can be subjected to neutron activation analysis in an effort to determine the constituents of the serum. These are just a few of present-day applications of neutron activation.

Since the product of such a reaction is an isotope of the target element, there is no possible way to separate these on a chemical basis. Furthermore, it is impossible to create a situation in the reactor whereby all atoms of gold 197 incorporate a neutron to become gold 198. The material that is removed from the reactor after bombardment is necessarily a mixture of the two isotopes. For this reason, the gold 198 administered to a patient will also have a certain amount of stable gold 197. The latter is referred to as a *carrier*. To inform the user of the quantity of gold 197 in the gold 198 dose, the term *specific activity* is ordinarily used. Another useful unit is *specific weight*.

Specific weight. It is often the problem of the researcher to determine the specific weight of the material introduced into the human body. Knowing the specific weight becomes valuable from the standpoint of toxicity, in that the researcher does not want to approach the toxic dose of any material to successfully perform the study. Also, the "load" introduced into the human body must not upset the normal physiologic balance of the material. For example, if in any thyroid diagnostic procedure the amount of iodine exceeds the normal daily intake, the normal physiology of the thyroid is altered.

Problem. A dose of 50 μCi is used as an uptake and scanning dose. How much ^{131}I is introduced into the iodine pool? (^{131}I is used as the example because it is carrier-free.)

Solution. The determination of specific weight involves two mathematical procedures: (1) determination of the number of atoms in the sample and (2) determination of the specific weight. These are calculated as follows:

1. Determine the number of atoms by the formula:

$$\lambda N = A$$

A = Activity in disintegrations per minute
(1 μCi = 2.22 $\times$ 10^6 dpm; so 50 μCi = 1.11 $\times$ 10^8 dpm)

$\lambda = \dfrac{0.693}{T_{1/2}}$ (since A is in minute units, so must T$_{1/2}$ be in minute units)

N = Number of atoms

Solving for N:

$$\frac{0.693}{8.1 \text{ days} \times 24 \text{ hr/day} \times 60 \text{ min/hr}} \times N = 1.11 \times 10^8 \text{ dpm}$$

$$\frac{0.693}{11,664} N = 1.11 \times 10^8$$

$$5.94 \times 10^{-5} N = 1.11 \times 10^8$$

$$N = 1.87 \times 10^{12}$$

2. Determine specific weight of the sample by the formula:

$$W = \frac{A \times N}{K}$$

W = Weight of sample (grams)
A = Atomic weight of radionuclide
N = Number of atoms
K = Avogadro's number = 6×10^{23}

Solving for W:

$$W = \frac{131 \times 1.87 \times 10^{12}}{6 \times 10^{23}}$$

$$= \frac{244.97 \times 10^{12}}{6 \times 10^{23}}$$

$$= 40.83 \times 10^{-11} \text{ grams or } 4 \times 10^{-7} \text{ mg or } 4 \times 10^{-4} \mu g$$

It has been determined that a 50 μCi dose introduces 0.0004 μg of iodine 131 into the iodine pool. Since the daily adult intake of iodine is considerably more than this,* the iodine pool remains physiologically unaltered. Furthermore, approximately 20 mCi could be administered without altering the iodine pool.

Specific activity. Another parameter of interest in nuclear medicine and one that relates activity to weight is specific activity. Specific activity is strictly defined as the ratio of activity to the specific weight of the radionuclide. It is usually expressed as millicuries per milligram or curies per gram. Using the information just determined on specific weight and the strict definition of specific activity, the preparation in the problem just given would have a specific activity of:

$$\frac{50 \, \mu Ci}{40 \times 10^{-8} \text{ mg}} = \frac{50 \times 10^{-3} \text{ mCi}}{40 \times 10^{-8} \text{ mg}} = 1.25 \times 10^5 \text{ mCi/mg}$$

The strict definition of specific activity is rarely used with commercial preparations of radionuclides, however. The specific weight used in their formula is sometimes the weight of the stable nuclide or, more commonly, the weight of the chemical compound to which the radionuclide is labeled; for example, in the case of ^{197}Hg-labeled chlormerodrin, the specific activity refers to the microcuries of mercury 197 per milligram of the chlormerodrin molecule (μCi ^{197}Hg/mg chlormerodrin). This information regarding specific activity is found on all radiopharmaceutical labels.

Even though neutron activation is the most common method of obtaining radionuclides, the inability to separate the stable form of the element (carrier) from the unstable increases the problems of chemical toxicity levels. To obtain a de-

---

*In 1969 the average diet in the United States contained approximately 150 μg/day. By 1974 the average was estimated to have increased to 450 μg/day for males and 382 μg/day for females. Data suggest that these levels may eventually reach 1,050 μg/day. (Data from Talbot, J. M., Fisher, D. K., and Carr, C. J.: A review of the effects of dietary iodine on certain thyroid disorders, Fed. Am. Soc. Exp. Biol. 7:11-13, 1976.)

sired level of radioactive material in a patient, it may be necessary to introduce an undesirable level of the element or an undesirable level of the labeled compound. (A compound is said to be labeled when it consists in part of radioactive atoms, such as ^{131}I-labeled iodohippurate sodium [Hippuran].)

The value of specific activity may be illustrated by a hypothetical example. A laboratory has just received a shipment of ^{197}Hg-labeled chlormerodrin. The specific activity as stated on the label is 200 μCi/mg, calibrated for Monday at 8AM. The calibration date informs the user of the radiopharmaceutical that the specific activity is true as stated only at the time of calibration. (This also holds true for two other values found on the label: activity and concentration.) The value would be different before or after the date and time of calibration.

For ease of calculation, it will be assumed that ^{197}Hg has a half-life of 48 hours and that the standard dose for a given study was 2.0 mCi. The following schedule would then prevail:

	Specific activity	Activity injected	Chlormerodrin injected
Monday 8 AM	200 μCi/mg	2,000 μCi	10 mg
Wednesday 8 AM	100 μCi/mg	2,000 μCi	20 mg
Friday 8 AM	50 μCi/mg	2,000 μCi	40 mg

Chlormerodrin is a well-known mercurial diuretic. Assume that 20 mg of chlormerodrin is a standard diuretic dose. By Wednesday morning at 8 AM a medical problem presents itself, and by Friday it worsens. In order to inject the standard dose of radioactivity, the patient must also receive the standard diuretic dose. Perhaps, in the medical management of some patients for whom diuresis is a contraindication the nuclear medicine procedure may have to be delayed or omitted. Although this is a hypothetical situation, it demonstrates the value of specific activity, and it can be related similarly to toxicity levels.

Specific activity is not to be mistaken for concentration. This information is also found on all radiopharmaceutical labels. Concentration is defined as the ratio of activity to volume. It is usually expressed in units of millicuries per milliliter or microcuries per milliliter. A vial containing 10 mCi activity in a volume of 10 ml will be expressed as having a concentration of 1.0 mCi/ml. As with specific activity, this value is only true at the date and time of calibration.

It might be well to point out a practical problem with volume, especially as it applies to the use of a multiple-dose vial. In using a solution of radioactive material whose concentration permits five or more withdrawals, a lack of volume is often encountered on the last withdrawal. The vial must be disposed of because of insufficient volume even though the inventory indicates otherwise. This is usually not an error of calculation on the part of the nuclear medicine personnel or of the radiopharmaceutical supplier. In such instances the lack of volume can be accounted for by the "hang-up" in needles, rubber stopper, and the vial itself. Commercial suppliers of "cold" (nonradioactive) materials in multiple-dose form can in many cases compensate for this by adjusting the volume. However, because the regulations of the Food and Drug Administration are such that volume and concentration must be included on the label of radioactive drugs, such compensatory action may not be taken. Obviously, if 1 ml more of diluent is added to correct for this situation, the volume and the concentration would also have to change. Calculation would then be based on the increased volume, and no purpose would be served.

TRANSMUTATION

Transmutation can be described as a process in which one element is converted into another. More specifically, it is the transformation of a nuclide of one element into a nuclide of a different element by nuclear reaction. Transmutation is often referred to as the answer to the alchemist's dream. Hundreds of years ago a group of "scientists" tried in vain to change common metals into gold. Their object was to bring about transmutation. Now, after years of investigation and accumulated knowledge of the nature of radioactive materials, the process of conversion from one element to another element by decay is well known. However, transmutation applies specifically, in the case of radionuclide production, to converting one stable element into another unstable element. An example of such a reaction is the conversion of stable sulfur 32 into radioactive phosphorus 32. This is accomplished by bombarding sulfur 32 with neutrons in such a manner as to eject a proton from its nucleus. In this manner, an element having one more neutron and one less proton is produced—phosphorus 32. This process is described as an (n, p) reaction according to the following:

$$\,^{32}_{16}\text{S} + \,^{1}_{0}\text{n} \rightarrow \,^{32}_{15}\text{P} + \,^{1}_{1}\text{p}$$

The shorthand method is written as follows:

$$\,^{32}_{16}\text{S}(\text{n, p})\,^{32}_{15}\text{P}$$

Like neutron activation, transmutation also involves neutron bombardment (as well as bombardment with protons, deuterons, and alpha particles). In the case of transmutation, however, rather than being bombarded with a slow neutron, the target element is bombarded with a fast neutron. The incorporation of a fast neutron into the nucleus is immediately followed by the emission of a proton. The advantage of the transmutation process is that the target and the product are no longer isotopes but are nuclides. Being two different elements, they are subject to separation by standard chemical techniques. Phosphorus 32 can easily be separated from the sulfur 32. In this way a pure product of phosphorus 32, referred to as *carrier-free,* is obtained. In a shipment of phosphorus 32 from a radiopharmaceutical supplier the specific activity on the label will indicate *C.F.* for carrier-free. Ideally, this would be the method of producing all radiopharmaceuticals, but methods are not known by which to produce all radiopharmaceuticals in this manner.

LINEAR ACCELERATORS AND CYCLOTRONS

Under the usual conditions that prevail in the atom, charged particles are unable to enter and/or interact with nuclei of other atoms because they have insufficient energy to penetrate the orbital electrons or the nucleus. A negatively charged particle, as it nears an atom, is repelled away from the negatively charged orbital electrons. Likewise, a positively charged particle would be repelled away from a positively charged nucleus. However, if sufficient energy is supplied to these charged particles, they can overcome these repulsion effects and penetrate the nucleus, causing an interaction. Devices that provide the energy necessary to perform this action are called *particle accelerators.* There are two basic types: the type that moves the particle in a straight path, called the *linear accelerator,* and the type that moves the particle in a circular path, such as a *cyclotron, betatron,* and *synchrotron.* Such devices can accelerate particles to the point at which they possess energy from 1 million to 1 billion ev.

The linear accelerator is a high-energy particle accelerator consisting of cylinders of increasing lengths arranged in a straight line. These linear accelerators can be as long as 2 miles in length. The particle acceleration is provided by means of a pulsing electrostatic or magnetic field.

One explanation of the function of linear accelerators is as follows. If a positively charged particle such as an alpha particle, proton, or deuteron (nucleus of deuterium atoms) were used at the beginning of the linear accelerator and the first cylinder was charged negatively, the particle would be attracted by electrostatic attraction through the first cylinder, thereby gaining energy. As the particle nears the second cylinder, which is increased slightly in length, the charge of the cylinder through which it has just passed is reversed to a positive charge and the cylinder toward which it is approaching is charged negatively. The particle is attracted by the unlike charge in the second cylinder and repelled by the like charge in the cylinder through which it has just passed. This process of reversal of charges between cylinders continues throughout the entire length of the linear accelerator; each time it occurs the particle is accelerated further. In this way the particle can achieve tremendous energy levels. By achieving such high energies, the particles can overcome the repulsive effects of the nucleus and actually interact with it. In this way, stable nuclei are made unstable and accelerators become a source of radionuclides.

Another explanation of the internal workings of the linear accelerator is that electrons are fed into one end of the tube down which an electromagnetic wave of radiofrequency is traveling. The electrons are carried forward on this wave not unlike a surfboard being carried by an ocean wave. Linear accelerators of this type are used for radiotherapy. In this way very high energy electrons (4 to 8 mev) may be produced through a distance of 1 to 2 m. It is important that charged particles are used. Higher energies are possible with greater distance. Neutrons, gamma rays, and neutrinos are unacceptable as a bombarding material in this type of unit.

The principle of reversed electromagnetic charges is used in the cyclotron. The cyclotron was first described in 1931 by Lawrence and Livingston as a type of particle accelerator. In the cyclotron the particles are repeatedly accelerated through intermediate voltages to achieve high energy. The cyclotron consists of two hollow semicircular pieces of metal with a short gap between them. These semicircular pieces of metal are called Ds because of their shape. The Ds are mounted between the poles of the large electromagnet with the straight side of the Ds abutting one another. Two Ds arranged in this manner assume the shape of a circle; hence the name cyclotron. The particles are attracted into the first D that has an opposite electrical charge. The particle moves through the semicircular path of the D until it reaches the gap. At this point the electromagnetic fields are reversed. The D through which the particle just passed changes in charge so as to have a repulsive effect, and the D into which it will now move will have an attractive effect. In this way the particle is accelerated. This process continues throughout the extent of the cyclotron until it reaches the target material. The particle now possesses extremely high energies and interacts with the target material to produce an altered nucleus, which is unstable. The source of the particles is arranged in the center of the circle formed by the two Ds and the particles proceed outward in a spiral fashion until they reach the target material.

The cyclotron is generally a more versatile device compared with a reactor or a linear accelerator It has an advantage over the linear accelerator because space does not present the problem for a cyclotron that it does for a linear accelerator. It has more advantages over a nuclear reactor because of the wider variety of nuclear particles it can employ. Another major advantage is that it is capable of producing certain useful radionuclides, primarily short-lived, that are not produced in significant quantities in nuclear reactors. A further advantage over reactors is that radioisotopes may be produced with much higher specific activity; they are often carrier-free. The disadvantage to the cyclotron over the nuclear reactor is that of operating costs. The operating cost for cyclotrons is much greater than that for nuclear reactors.

Protons are commonly used as a bombarding material in the cyclotron. Their source is a small amount of hydrogen placed in the center of the cyclotron. The hydrogen is then bombarded with electrons from tungsten filament, removing the single electron in the orbit of the hydrogen atom and leaving the positive ion in the source. The nucleus of the hydrogen atom is a proton. At the present time, many of the standard nuclear medicine radionuclides are by-products of a nuclear reactor for economic reasons. Cyclotrons are employed for radioisotope production when they offer a significant advantage over reactors. This is occurring more and more.

GENERATORS

Another method of radionuclide production is the generator. The generator has become a very convenient method of obtaining short-lived radionuclides at places distant to large-scale production sites. Short-lived radionuclides have gained wide acceptance in the field of nuclear medicine because, by their use, larger doses of radiopharmaceuticals can be injected with resultant decreased radiation dose to the patient and organs of interest, increased statistics necessary for more meaningful imaging results, and a continuous availability of a short-lived radionuclide in the nuclear medicine laboratory. Examples are molybdenum 99/technetium 99m generators and tin 113/indium 113m generators.

Physical characteristics. All generators are modifications of a basic physical arrangement. The generator consists of a small glass column containing an ion exchange material. The parent nuclide is firmly affixed (adsorbed) onto this material. The column of ion exchange material is held by a porous glass frit at the bottom of the column and a plastic ring at the top. An outer plastic housing is usually provided to guard against breakage during shipment and handling. Both ends of the system should be sealed to preserve sterility and pyrogen-free conditions within the column.

Principle of operation. The basis of operation for a radionuclide generator is that a relatively long-lived parent nuclide continually produces through radioactive decay a shorter-lived daughter nuclide. Separation of the daughter nuclide can be performed easily and repeatedly, usually on the basis of chemical separation techniques. This separation process is referred to as *elution,* or "milking."

The daughter nuclide is eluted from the parent nuclide (which remains on the ion exchange medium) and collected at the bottom of the column. Other elution processes are known, such as distillation, solvent extraction (MEK, methyl ethyl ketone), and precipitation; however, the simplicity of ion exchange media lends itself well to the routine nuclear medicine laboratory. The daughter is eluted by introducing the recommended reagent through the top of the column and collecting the product solution from the bottom of the column. The product is then assayed for concentration of daughter nuclide.

This process of elution can be repeated as many times as is thought necessary; however, the percent yield will vary. After the daughter has been eluted, the daughter activity is low but begins to increase (regenerate) until it eventually approximates the activity of the parent again (Fig 5-1). At this point, if undisturbed, the activity of the daughter nuclide appears to assume the half-life of the parent. The next elution repeats the cycle. (The parent continues to decay also but at a much slower rate than the daughter.) If the column has completely regenerated, the usual yield is approximately 70% of the parent activity. In the case of the ^{99}Mo/^{99m}Tc generator, regeneration requires approximately 24 hours. Any elutions that are performed before that time will result in lower yields per elution; however, a large net yield can be realized if several premature elutions are performed over any period of time. For example, one elution per day (at 8 AM) will yield ^{99m}Tc between 70% and 90% of the activity of the ^{99}Mo, whereas two elutions per day (at 8 AM and 2 PM) will yield 99^mTc at approximately 105% to 120% of the activity of ^{99}Mo. This is due to the exponential buildup of the daughter

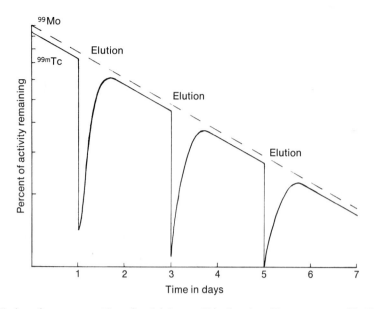

Fig. 5-1. Elution of a generator. Plot of molybdenum 99/technetium 99m generator with [99]Mo decay seen as a dotted line and ^{99m}Tc decay seen as a solid line. Note that the generator is eluted on days one, three, and five, changing in no way the course of the decay of [99]Mo. Following each elution, it requires approximately four physical half-lives to return to equilibrium. Regeneration is an exponential function with approximately 50% regeneration during the first half-life, 25% more during the second half-life, and so on. Daughter activity (^{99m}Tc) never reaches 100% parent activity ([99]Mo) because 7.6% of all [99]Mo atoms decay to ^{99m}Tc, bypassing the metastable state.

product after elution. This increased net yield carries with it a sacrifice of concentration.

The principle of generators becomes almost impossible to believe because the question always arises of how can the generator regenerate when 1 atom of molybdenum 99 with a 67-hour half-life decays to technetium 99m with a 6-hour half-life? The question is best answered not on a one-atom-to-one-atom basis but with many atoms. An analogy may help clarify the situation.

Radioactive decay (Chapter 4) can be compared to a reservoir of water with an outlet at its base (Fig. 5-2). The molecules of water flowing through the outlet represent atoms undergoing the decay process, whereas the molecules in the tank represent radioactive atoms that have not yet decayed. The rate of flow of water molecules in both tanks is controlled only by the height of the column of water (flow rate is proportional to height of column), since the size of their outlets is the same. As the height of the column decreases by one half, the flow rate decreases proportionally. This is also true in a sample of radioactivity; as the number of atoms in the original sample is reduced to one half (half-life), the rate of decay is reduced proportionally.

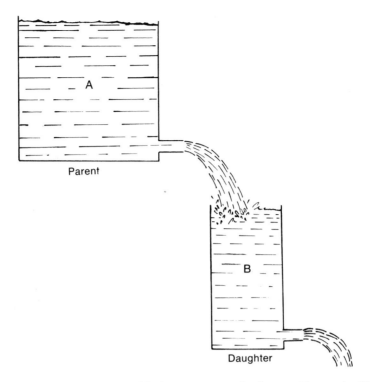

Parent

Daughter

Fig. 5-2. Illustration comparing radionuclide decay to a reservoir of water with an outlet. The number of molecules of water, the rate of flow from the outlet, and the diameter of the outlet are representative of the number of atoms in the radioactive sample, the rate of decay, and the fraction of the remaining number of atoms that decay per unit time (λ), respectively. The two reservoirs of water of varying size with outlets of the same size, in which the larger empties into the smaller, are analogous to a generator whose parent radionuclide has a longer half-life than the daughter radionuclide.

It becomes clear from this analogy that for 2 radionuclides having two different half-lives but the same number of disintegrations per unit time, the radionuclide having the longer half-life must have a larger number of atoms in the sample.* This situation is represented by the two reservoirs of water, tank A and tank B in Fig. 5-2. Since the flow rate (or disintegration rate) is exactly the same in both reservoirs, tank B will reach half height (half-life) is a shorter period of time because it has less water (fewer atoms).

Fig. 5-2 also demonstrates the probability of decay. It is impossible to predict which water molecules flowing from tank A to tank B will, in turn, flow from tank B. Some water molecules will flow immediately to the outlet and out of tank B,

---

*It is as simplistic as this: the difference in the number of atoms is related to the difference in half-life. ^{99}Mo has a half-life that is ten times longer than ^{99m}Tc; therefore, ^{99}Mo has ten times the number of atoms for the same amount of radioactivity. The first formula on p. 82 bears out this relationship. This is also one of the reasons why longer-lived radionuclides deliver a larger radiation dose than do shorter-lived radionuclides.

whereas others will flow inside tank B before being expelled. The overriding principle is that it is possible to predict the number of water molecules that will flow out of tank B per unit time. The same is true with a radioactive series of unstable parent and daughter atoms. The radioactive daughter atom may decay immediately on being transmuted or may exist in its unstable state for a longer period of time. Although it is impossible to predict which atom will decay immediately, it is possible to predict how many atoms will decay from a given radioactive sample per unit time.

The analogy of reservoirs can also be extended to the operation of a generator. Since generators currently in use are those of relatively long-lived parents and relatively short-lived daughter products, the reservoirs of Fig. 5-2 accurately depict the situation. At the time of the initial elution, both reservoirs are full to capacity and the flow rates (decay rates, activity, disintegrations per unit time) are the same. The first elution decreases tank B to ≈ 30% capacity, and tank A remains undisturbed. Because the height of the column of water has been reduced, the flow rate has also been reduced, analogous to decreased activity of the daughter product. As tank A continues to flow at the same rate into tank B, tank B will begin to fill up; at the same time, the outflow continues at an increasingly greater rate because the column of water increases in height. The same is true in the generator. The parent nuclide continues to decay at the same rate, but because tank B has fewer atoms after elution, the rate of decay is decreased. After elution and since the parent nuclide continues to decay to the daughter at the same rate, the number of daughter atoms becomes increasingly greater and therefore the number of disintegrations per unit time (activity) becomes increasingly greater also. Eventually a point is reached at which tank B is filled to the same height as tank A and the flow rates of both reservoirs are again equal. The same point of complete regeneration is reached in the generator when the activity of the daughter nuclide is the same as the parent nuclide. Furthermore, because the transmutation of the parent nuclide to the daughter nuclide is at the same rate as the daughter nuclide is to its successor, the half-life of the daughter appears to be the same as the parent. This is not true, of course, because the removal of the daughter from the parent allows the daughter to display its own characteristic half-life. The point at which the ratio of the two activities remains constant and both appear to decay with the half-life of the parent is called *equilibrium.*

Two terms are used to describe two different types of equilibrium. These are *transient* equilibrium and *secular* equilibrium. Transient equilibrium is a condition that exists when the parent radionuclide has a physical half-life that is not much longer than that of the daughter nuclide. A good example of this type of equilibrium is the molybdenum 99/technetium 99m generator system. Secular equilibrium, on the other hand, is a condition that exists when the parent radionuclide has a physical half-life that is considerably longer than that of the daughter nuclide. An example of this type of equilibrium is the tin 113/indium 113m generator system.

TRILINEAR CHART OF THE NUCLIDES
Marshall Brucer, M.D.

At the beginning of the twentieth century the main problem in chemistry was the periodic table. The table was filling rapidly, but some puzzling inconsistencies occurred among the naturally radioactive elements. Some thorium substances with very different physical properties could not be separated chemically. Uranium was geochemically related to lead, but there seemed to be more than one atomic weight for lead, all with the same chemical properties.

Kasimer Fajans, a German physical chemist, developed a "displacement law" to explain the pattern of radioactive decay. In 1912 he found a way to explain the puzzling inconsistencies, but it demanded more than one "element" in one place on the periodic table. Frederick Soddy, a physical chemist in Glasglow, generalized this solution to the entire periodic table. During the nineteenth century "atomic weight" was not a true "mass" but was a relative "proportional number" of each element balanced against the others in ordinal progression up the periodic table. Atomic weight, thus, could be an average of all the atomic numbers making up a chemical element. Soddy called these the "isotopes" of the element. A few years later (1917) he pointed out that if some substances had equal atomic number (chemical properties) but different atomic weight (a physical property), then there must also be substances with equal weight but different atomic number. Eventually, the latter were called *isobars*.

The number of electrons in an atom had already (in 1913) been related to the number of positive charges (protons) in the nucleus of the atom. This was the atomic number (Z). It was postulated in 1920 that the remainder of the nucleus was made up of uncharged particles much like the proton but neutral in charge (neutrons). Chadwick, in England, discovered these in 1932. The atomic number was the number of protons (iodine has 53, hence $_{53}I$). The atomic weight was the number of protons plus neutrons (one of the iodines has 53 plus 78, hence $^{131}_{53}I$). If there are isotopes with equal proton number and isobars with equal mass, then there should also be substances with an equal number of neutrons. Replace the "p" (for proton) in isotope with an "n" (for neutron) and the word becomes "isotone."

In 1921 Otto Hahn, a German chemist, while trying to straighten out some difficulties in the uranium chain of decay, found two substances with entirely different half-lives but that were the same isotope, isobar, and isotone. By 1935, in the search for new radioisotopes, physicists were finding more of these unusual species. In 1936 Lisa Meitner, the long-time physicist-associate of Hahn, called these *nuclear isomers*.

Discovery of the artificial radioisotopes

Atom smashing to study atomic structure was popular around 1933. Frederick Joliot and Irene Curie in Paris noticed that the aluminum target they were bombarding with polonium alpha particles remained radioactive after the bombardment stopped. After careful investigation, on Feb. 10, 1934, Joliot and his wife (the daughter of Marie Curie) published a note on the production of a new artificial isotope of phosphorous ($^{30}_{15}$P). Thirty-six years after she and her husband had discovered the first naturally radioactive element (polonium), Madame Curie had the pleasure of hearing her daughter and son-in-law announce the discovery of the first artificial radioactive substance made with alpha particles from her first discovery in 1898.

On reading the announcement of the discovery of artificial radioactive isotopes, Enrico Fermi, at the University of Rome, thought that the newly discovered neutron would be a better bombardment projectile than alpha particles. Within 2 months of the production of the first phosphorous 30, he had bombarded many elements and found 33 radioisotopes (and 13 others that were probably also radioactive). Physicists immediately began the search for others.

Terminology

During World War II, Fermi's nuclear reactor and the newer cyclotrons were used to create still different nuclear reactions to produce even more radioactive nuclides. By 1947 there were about 800 known species; it was becoming too complex to talk about an *isotope-isobar-isotone-isomer*. In 1947 Turner, an American physicist, proposed the word *nuclide* to signify any specific arrangement of protons and neutrons. The term was quickly adopted, and this branch of science became nuclear, not isotope, physics; chemistry became nuclear, not isotope, chemistry. However, before World War II the nuclear sciences had revolved around the chemical similarity of reactions of isotopes. The first chemical and then biologic use of a nuclide had been because of its chemical isotopy. The name *isotopes* caught hold with physicians and political administrators who did not know the historical background; newspapers picked up the catchword. By the time medical people began to use radionuclides the improper term "radioisotopes" was embedded in the language.

Yet the medical and tracer people were not using isotopes. Once they had obtained, for example, an isotope of iodine, they measured its decay to xenon; they were using isobar relationships. The nuclear reactor people were using isotone relationships. With the founding of the first medical society of physicians using these nuclear reaction products, the improper use of the term "radioisotopes" was corrected and physicians adopted the name *nuclear medicine*.

Development of the trilinear chart of the nuclides

In 1946 William H Sullivan, one of the chief chemists at Oak Ridge, Tennessee, put all the known radioactive and stable nuclides onto a trilinear chart of many hexagons. Each hexagon represented one nuclide. One axis of the hexagonal array signified isotopes, the second axis signified isobars, and the third axis signified isotones. Production, chemistry, physics, or medical use did not matter to Sullivan. He had plotted the first trilinear chart that showed all the nuclides in their true, structural relationship.

Every physicist who looked at Sullivan's 1946 trilinear chart knew that there were more nuclides to be discovered. There were 800 nuclides known in 1947; by 1968 approximately 1,800 had been found; by December 1978 there were almost 2,452, and a few more seemed necessary to make the chart symmetric. If each hexagon is to be a complete designation of a nuclide, a tremendous amount of data is involved — much too much for a simple chart. Also, the fine details are changing with each increase in accuracy. Summary *Tables of Isotopes* are out of date before they are published, and a special journal, *Nuclear Data,* is published periodically to keep researchers up to date.* Physicists and chemists need the complete tabular data. Clinical physicians need only a small fragment, and this much can be put in chart form. Fig. 5-3 shows 15 of the almost 2,500 nuclides.

The central box in each hexagon gives the proper name of the nuclide. All of the iodines (I) have the same number of protons ($_{53}$I). One nuclide of iodine has 76 neutrons and 53 protons, which equals 129 nucleons ($^{129}_{53}$I); one has 79 neutrons ($^{132}_{53}$I). Iodines 115 to 141 have been demonstrated, and there may be a few more. Six of the 27 known iodine nuclides have isomers of appreciable half-life; hence, there are more than 33 different kinds of iodine. Only one kind is stable ($^{127}_{53}$I). Each hexagon on the trilinear chart shows not only a nuclide (and maybe an isomer) but also its isobaric, isotopic, and isotonic relationship to its neighbors in the periodic table.

Choice of data

By the time Sullivan's chart had gone through a few editions, the data had become so complex that Sullivan had to leave something out. He wanted to make a medical chart; but with the rapid changes in medical demands, he did not know what data was important (and neither did anyone else). However, some items were obviously important to physicians.

Half-life. Half-life is so important in medical use that it was put immediately above the name plate. For example, iodine 141 has a half-life of 0.43 seconds; iodine 129 has a half-life of 15.7 million years. The amount of any nuclide that can be given to a patient is probably the first consideration of a clinician. However, is "amount" the physical dose of radiation or the chemical dose of the nuclide? "Dose" of a radionuclide is usually measured in millicuries (a mCi is the number of atoms that will result in 37 million disintegrations per second). Because the disintegrations of iodine 129 occur over such a long time span, it would take about 62 gm of chemical to produce 1 mCi of radiation; a proper large chemical dose is in the milligram range. But only femtograms of iodine 141 are needed for a millicurie. (A

---

*Nuclear Data, Section B, New York, 1967 to date, Academic Press, Inc.

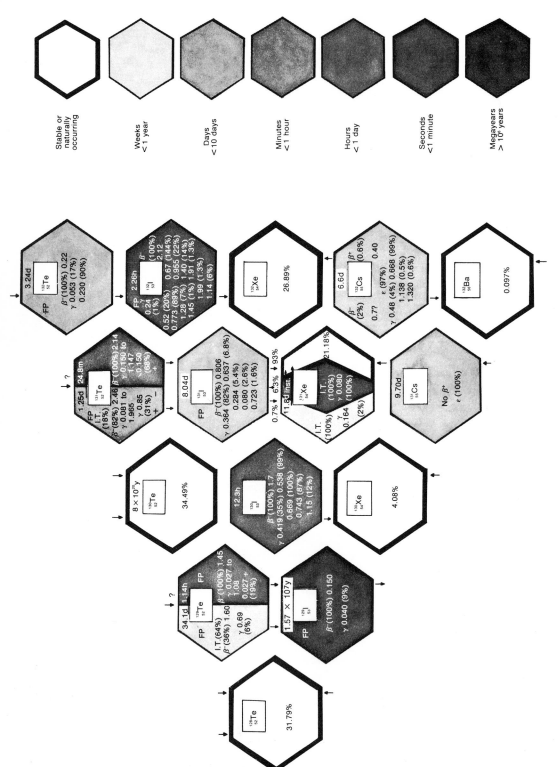

Fig. 5-3. Portion of the trilinear chart of the nuclides demonstrating arrangement and information content of the chart. (Courtesy Mallinckrodt Inc., St. Louis, Mo.)

femtogram is $\frac{1}{1,000}$ of a picogram, which is $\frac{1}{1,000}$ of a nanogram, which is $\frac{1}{1,000}$ of a microgram, which is $\frac{1}{1,000}$ of a milligram, which is $\frac{1}{1,000}$ of a gram.) A true "tracer" chemical dose of the short-lived iodines (hours to weeks) can be given with extremely large physical doses of radiation. Both concepts of "amount" are implied in half-life.

A 24-hour thyroid uptake could be measured with short-lived iodine 132. But, even if a full millicurie were given, at 24 hours there would only be one half of $\frac{1}{2}$ of $\frac{1}{2}$ of $\frac{1}{2}$ . . . (10 half-lives) left, and approximately three fourths of this would have been excreted. To administer the original millicurie, a day's shipping time from the pharmaceutical house would have to be allowed. A curie would be ordered to give a millicurie to measure a fraction of a microcurie—this is feasible and has been done, but it is not practical.

Radiation characteristics. Just as important as half-life is whether the energy of radiation emission is highly penetrating or below the limits of the detecting instruments. The trilinear chart gives the energy of iodine 132 as 773 kev plus many other energies. This is supervoltage radiation that demands tremendous shielding. On a complete table of isotopes, many nuclides are described that have a clinically convenient half-life but emit energies in the multimillion volt range. No matter what their biologic specificity, the tremendous shielding necessary in their use might be totally impractical in a busy clinical laboratory and might be totally unacceptable to clinical instruments.

A high-energy gamma ray has little chance of being stopped by a piece of tissue. If it is stopped, however, it has great effect. A low-energy gamma ray will not cause as much effect, but it is more likely to be stopped. The same is true in a radiation-measuring instrument. Gamma rays much under 0.1 mev or much over 0.5 mev cause problems in the clinical laboratory. This is why most medical nuclides are selected from the medium range, for example, iodine 131 = 0.364 mev and technetium 99m = 0.140 mev. With the recent development of the thin crystal, fast gamma camera, the lower energy nuclides (0.1 mev to 0.2 mev) have a great advantage in detection sensitivity.

Pattern of decay. The concept of milking a short-lived daughter nuclide from a long-lived parent was already in medical use before World War I. Radium 226 with a half-life of 1,600 years decays to 3.8-day radon 222. For many medical uses the shorter-lived (and less expensive) radon is more valuable than the longer-lived radium. Early in the 1920s G. Failla, a New York medical radiation physicist, devised a method to milk (elute) the radon from a large radium source and gave it the very expressive name "radon cow."

Tellurium 132 has a 3.24-day half-life; its daughter nuclide, 2.26-hour iodine 132, can be milked from a well-shielded tellurium source in the laboratory. This first artificial nuclide cow (the euphemism is "generator") was devised in the early 1950s. It was valuable in the development of the concept of dual nuclide studies. Shielding, contamination, cost, transportation, procurement, and many problems connected with half-life can be solved by the use of a cow system. In 1964 the molybdenum 99/technetium 99m generator revolutionized radiopharmaceuticals, and over 200 cow systems are now theoretically available for development.

Iodine 131, the most common radionuclide of early nuclear medicine had a surprisingly complex decay scheme. Only 93% decays to stable xenon 131. Once its beta emission has occurred, the iodine 131 atom becomes xenon 131 in a metastable state. Eight hesitations can occur during the emission of gamma rays before the xenon achieves stability. Seven of these hesitations have nanosecond and picosecond durations and hence are of no medical concern, but 0.42% of the decays are through an 11.9-day isomer of xenon 131; this half-life is longer than that of the original 8-day iodine 131. Although 0.42% is too small to be of any concern in routine clinical work, during a long-term iodine retention study, within a few weeks there may be more xenon 131m than there is iodine 131 in a closed system. To some extent absorption in fat makes the body a closed system for xenon.

The gamma emission of iodine 131 at 364 kev can now easily be distinguished from the gamma emission of xenon 131m at 164 kev. The older iodine 131 literature, before spectroscopy, lists the iodine 131 half-life at 8.08, 8.07, or 8.05 days (now 8.04). Some of the confusion was caused by measurement in an open system (^{131}I only) or in a closed system (^{131}I + ^{131m}Xe).

The 6.6-day cesium 132 nuclide shown in Fig. 5-3 decays with the emission of either a negatron (β^-) or a positron (β^+). The negatron decay yields barium 132; the positron decay yields xenon 132. A double decay pattern is more common at the upper end of the periodic table where decay can be partially alpha and partially beta emission. It is not very serious in routine medical pharmacology, but it can be very serious in precise chemical work.

When multiple daughters are present in a decay system, the succeeding daughters can confuse counting problems in routine work. The same confusion can be caused by multiple nuclides produced by almost every production technique. Even a negligible chemical impurity can be a significant radiation impurity. The first iodine radionuclide used in thyroid therapy (1939) was iodine 130. It was the preferred isotope because of its relative radiochemical purity. Iodine 131 was then made from the cyclotron bombardment of tellurium, and at least ten different isotopes of iodine were produced. It is now impossible to determine which of the isotopes were being measured in some of the early studies of iodine metabolism.

When fission product iodine 131 first became available in 1946, it was the first of the iodine nuclides to have a relative radiochemical purity. But then, when higher specific activity was thought to be desirable, iodine 131 could be made even more cheaply in a nuclear reactor by neutron bombardment of tellurium 130. The pharmaceutical manufacturer bought 1.25-day tellurium 131, which decays to 8-day iodine 131 during shipment. A simple final chemical extraction of iodine yielded a very pure and very high specific activity iodine 131.

Medical trilinear chart

Inside the front cover is the 1979 revision of the trilinear chart of the nuclides.* For ordinary clinical laboratory work, half-life, decay pattern, and proportion and energy of beta and gamma emission are all that can be included on a simplified chart of the nuclides. Some of the details that are essential to physicists and chemists are also essential in pharmaceutical research. Neutron cross sections might be of great importance in diagnostic procedures involving neutron activation analysis. The average beta emission energy is essential in initial radiation dosage estimates. Alternative production methods invariably present the toxicologic problems of contaminating activities. However, there is no room for such data on a simplified chart. The trilinear chart does show the pattern of decay and the great diversity of radionuclides that are theoretically available in the practice of nuclear medicine.

---

*The 1979 revision of Brucer's trilinear chart of the nuclides is available from Mallinckrodt, Inc., St. Louis, Mo. 63147.

BIBLIOGRAPHY

Brucer, M.: Vignettes in nuclear medicine, St. Louis, 1967-1979, Mallinckrodt Inc.

Chandra, R.: Introductory physics of nuclear medicine, Philadelphia, 1976, Lea & Febiger.

Gottschalk, A., and Potchen, E. J.: Diagnostic nuclear medicine, Baltimore, 1976, The Williams & Wilkins Co.

Johns, H. E.: The physics of radiology, ed. 2, revised edition, Springfield, Ill., 1964, Charles C Thomas, Publisher.

Quimby, E. H., and Feitelberg, S.: Radioactive isotopes in medicine and biology, ed. 2, Philadelphia, 1963, Lea & Febiger.

Rollo, F. D.: Nuclear medicine physics, instrumentation, and agents, St. Louis, 1977, The C. V. Mosby Co.

Shilling, C. W.: Atomic energy encyclopedia in the life sciences, Philadelphia, 1964, W. B. Saunders Co.

Wagner, H. N.: Principles of nuclear medicine, Philadelphia, 1968, W. B. Saunders Co.

6 Radiation measurement and protection

The many aspects of radiation measurement and consequent protection should become a primary consideration any time radioactive materials are used. The actual effects of radiation are not completely known, but it can generally be stated that all radioactivity is injurious; therefore, steps must be taken to prevent unnecessary exposure. A number of factors affect the radiation as to its possible injurious effect. These specific factors include type and energy of radiation, penetration power, ionization ability, radioactive half-life, biologic half-life, and effective half-life. In addition, personnel who will use radioactive materials must be introduced to the various units of radiation measurement and must recognize the necessity for certain limitations to radiation exposure.

MEASUREMENT OF RADIATION

Basically, two parameters are used to define the various terms of radiation measurement: the ionization of matter by radiation and the energy absorbed by matter from radiation. From these two basic concepts three kinds of radiation measurement have been derived: (1) the roentgen(r), (2) the radiation absorbed dose (rad), and (3) the roentgen equivalent, man (rem). A fourth unit describes the number of atoms that disintegrate per unit time, the curie and its submultiples. All of these are used or have been used in the past as units of radiation measurement. The curie has been described on p. 57.

The roentgen. The roentgen was originally defined as the amount of x- or gamma radiation that produces 1 electrostatic unit (esu) of charge as a result of interactions in 1 cc of dry air at standard temperature and pressure. It is now defined in equivalent units as 2.58×10^{-4} coulombs/kg air. At the meeting of the International Commission on Radiation Units and Measurements (ICRU) in July 1974, it was recommended that within a period not less than about 10 years this unit of exposure be replaced with a new SI unit—the coulomb per kilogram. This new unit of exposure would then be equal to 3,876 r in the old terminology. No name was recommended for this new unit at that July 1974 meeting.

There are two important items to be emphasized regarding the definition of this exposure unit regardless of its name. First, the exposure unit is a measure of the total exposure and does not involve the time over which exposure is administered. Second, it is a unit only of x rays or gamma rays.

The rad (radiation absorbed dose). The rad is a measure of the amount of energy imparted to matter by ionizing radiation per unit mass of irradiated material at the place of interest. One rad is equal to 100 ergs of absorbed energy per gram of absorbing material. There are two areas that warrant emphasis in this definition. First, a rad includes any ionizing radiation, as distinguished from the roentgen, which applies only to x rays or gamma rays. Second, the rad is only a measure of the energy absorbed by the material of interest and is not directly related to quantity or intensity of the radiation field. The rad also came under scrutiny at the ICRU meeting in July 1974. It was suggested that a new SI unit be assigned to this unit of dose, that it be called the joule per kilogram when used for ionizing radiation, and that it be given the name *gray,* with the symbol *Gy.* This new unit of dose would then be equal to 100 rad, using the old terminology.

The RBE (relative biologic effectiveness). RBE is a term used to indicate that different types of radiation have different effects in biologic materials or biologic systems. More specifically, it is the ratio of an absorbed dose of x rays or gamma rays to the absorbed dose of any radiation required to produce an identical biologic effect. This definition can be written as a formula:

$$\text{RBE} = \frac{\text{Dose in rads to produce some effect with x rays or gamma rays}}{\text{Dose in rads to produce same effect with radiation under investigation}}$$

For example, it is known that an absorbed dose of 0.05 rad of alpha radiation produces the same biologic effect as an absorbed dose of 1 rad of x- or gamma radiation. The RBE for an alpha particle would be determined by the following:

$$\text{RBE} = \frac{1.0 \text{ rad}}{0.05 \text{ rad}} = 20$$

Accordingly, the RBE value for an alpha particle is 20. Although all ionizing radiations are capable of producing similar biologic effects, the effect varies from one type of radiation to another based on the absorbed dose (rad) (Table 6-1). This relative biologic effectiveness of physically different ionizing radiations depends solely on the number of ionization events, commonly referred to as linear energy transfer (LET). Since the LET is a function of the charge and velocity of the ionizing particle, it requires less alpha radiation to produce the same biologic effect as x- or gamma radiation.

Table 6-1. RBE and QF values for various types of radiation

Radiation	RBE	QF
Alpha	20	10
Beta (≤30 kev)	1.7	1.7
Beta (>30 kev)	1	1.0
Gamma	1	1.0
X-	1	1.0

The rem (roentgen equivalent, man). The rem is a unit of human biologic dose as a result of exposure to one or many types of ionizing radiation. It is equal to the absorbed dose in rads times the relative biologic effectiveness of the particular type of radiation being absorbed. Another way of expressing it is as follows:

$$\text{Radiobiologic dose in rem*} \ = \ \text{Dose in rad} \ \times \ \text{RBE}$$

Should the radiation being measured be that of x-, gamma, or beta radiation greater than 30 kev, the rem value would be equal to the rad value, since the RBE value of all three types of emissions is 1.

There is a distinct difference between the three major forms of radiation measurement. The roentgen is considered the unit of exposure dose, the rad is a unit of absorbed radiation dose, and the rem is a unit of biologic dose. All three units are used in various situations in nuclear medicine. The roentgen, or more commonly its submultiple the milliroentgen, is used as a value for most survey meter readings. The rad is used as a unit to describe the amount of exposure received by the organ of interest on injection of a radiopharmaceutical; the rem is the unit used to express exposure values of some personnel monitoring devices (film badges, for example).

Considerable confusion has arisen regarding the use of the RBE and, therefore, the rem. It is obvious from the preceding discussion that different ionizing radiations cause different biologic effects. What is not so obvious (without highly controlled animal experiments) is that, even though Table 6-1 attempts to do it, there is no single RBE value that can be used for all tissue by any one category of radiation. RBE values for the same type of radiation vary from tissue to tissue. A very high RBE has been found for cataracts in mice, whereas a very low RBE has been found for testicular atrophy, all with the same type of radiation.

The concept of RBE or rem dose is a unit now limited to use in radiation biology. This was at the suggestion of the ICRU in their Report No. 11 in 1968. In fact, Jacob Shapiro in his text *Radiation Protection* suggests in a footnote that "the term RBE was originally used as a multiplication factor of 'rads' to give 'rem' but this practice is no longer employed." The term that is similar to the RBE and is currently being used is the *quality factor*, symbolized by the abbreviation *QF*.

The QF (quality factor). QF is another name for expressing the LET dependent response by a biologic system and was initially intended to be used specifically for radiation protection. If the biologic response per rad of two different types of radiation are the same, then the QF is the same. Refer to Table 6-1 for comparisons between RBE and QF values. A distinction may be made between the two terms; the measurement made for determining the relative effectiveness of two different types of radiations is the RBE; the factor expressing this relative effectiveness is the QF. QFs are usually determined by way of animal experiments.

---

*Referred to as RBE dose (rems).

Another problem in attempting to determine biologic effectiveness is one of the distribution of the dose. Internally administered radionuclides are not uniformly distributed within the body. Therefore, the dose delivered to that body, would have a greater or lesser effect depending on that distribution. Therefore, the *DF (dose distribution factor)* is also a consideration. Another way of expressing all these factors is as follows:

$$\text{Radiation protection dose in rem}^* = \text{Dose in rad} \times \text{QF} \times \text{DF}$$

The specific ionization (SI). The SI is the average number of ion pairs (primary or secondary) that are produced per unit of path traveled by the incident radiations. As mentioned in the section of this text on alpha decay, a 1.0 mev alpha particle will cause the formation of approximately 60,000 ion pairs per cm (air), expending an average of 34 ev of energy per ion pair. (Energy is also lost as a result of the excitation of nearby atoms. It is estimated that 2.2 atoms are excited by the ionization of a neighboring atom in air.) With this information, the LET can be computed.

Linear energy transfer (LET). The LET differs from the SI in that it is the average loss in energy per unit of path traveled by the incident radiations. Obviously, the two parameters are very closely related. One deals with the number of events, the other deals with the deposition of energy in each segment of tissue. The LET is simply the product of the SI and the average energy expended on the production of each ion pair. Expressed as a formula:

$$\text{LET} = \text{SI} \times \text{energy expended per ion pair produced}$$

therefore,

the LET of a 1.0 mev alpha = 60,000 ion pairs/cm (air) $\times$ 34 ev energy expended/pair

$$= 2.04 \text{ mev/cm (air)}$$

The distance that any incident radiation can travel (range) can be determined knowing the energy of the incident radiation and LET of the material through which it is passing, according to the following mathematical relationship:

$$\text{Range} = \frac{\text{E}}{\text{LET}}$$

therefore,

the range of a 1.0 mev alpha in air $= \dfrac{1.0 \text{ mev}}{2.04 \text{ mev/cm(air)}}$

$$= 0.49 \text{ cm of air}$$

It is obvious that as the LET increases, or the energy decreases, the range decreases.

Relationships of units

Note that when both the LET and the SI units were discussed, they were expressed as the *average*. These two units are not constant throughout the medium

*Referred to as DE(rems) or dose-equivalent (rems).

through which the incident radiation is passing. An alpha particle passing through tissue will have ionization events spaced farther apart at its entrance into the tissue than at the end of its pathway (Fig. 6-1, *A*). As the alpha particle progresses into the tissue, the speed with which the particle is traveling becomes slower and slower because of the loss of energy through its ionization activities. As the particle nears the end of its pathway, the SI increases tremendously as a result of the very slow speed of the particle and its probable influence on almost each atom that it passes. The same relationship exists for LET and RBE (Fig. 6-1, *B* and *C*).

Conversions between radiation units

Conversions can be made among all of these units but usually only through rather complicated mathematical manipulations; roentgens can be calculated in rads, rads can be calculated in rems, and so on. The Nuclear Regulatory Commission* regulations state that roentgens, rads, and rems are almost identical, and for all practical purposes x-, gamma, and beta radiations are treated as having identical values. Precise conversion methods are not within the scope of this book. There is, however, one conversion that may find practicality in the nuclear medicine laboratory. This is the conversion of units of activity (millicuries) to exposure rate (milliroentgens per hour: mr/hr). This correlation can be used to calibrate survey meters.

If there is a known source of activity, one can calculate the exposure rate from any gamma point source by the following formula:

$$mr/hr = \frac{n \times I_\gamma}{s^2}$$

n = Number of millicuries
I_γ = mr/hr at 1 meter/mCi
s = Distance in meters

Since this formula is for any gamma point source, a point source of cobalt 60 can be used as a calibration source. The formula and the I_γ values can be found in the *Radiological Health Handbook*.† These values are constant for each gamma source. In the case of cobalt 60, I_γ = 1.32. (Other I_γ values: ^{226}Ra = 0.825, ^{131}I = 0.21, ^{99m}Tc = 0.072, and ^{125}I = 0.067.)

The formula just given can be used to find a survey meter reading for a 5 mCi point source of cobalt 60 at a distance of 1 meter:

$$mr/hr = \frac{5 \times 1.32}{1^2}$$

$$mr/hr = 6.60$$

---

*Formerly Atomic Energy Commission.
†Published by the United States Department of Health, Education and Welfare, Division of Radiological Health, Washington, D.C., September 1960.

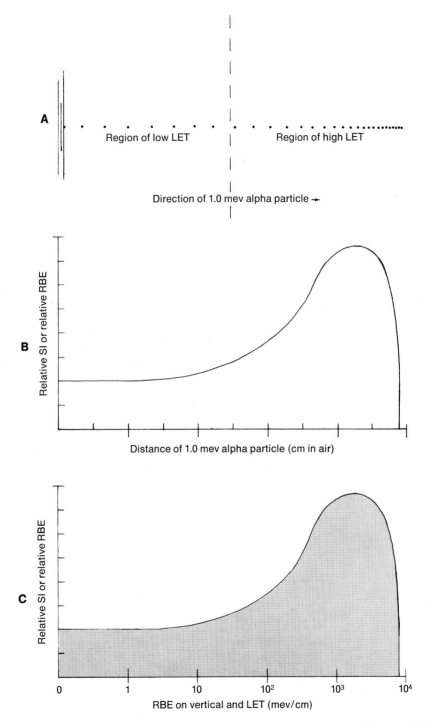

Fig. 6-1. **A,** Relationship of interactions of an alpha particle as it passes through matter (air). **B,** Relationship of the specific ionization (or RBE) of a 1.0 mev alpha particle to distance. The reason that the specific ionization decreases near the termination of the alpha pathway is that the alpha particles have been slowed to the point that they capture electrons, reducing their charge and thus their ionization capabilities. **C,** Relationship of RBE to LET for a 1.0 mev alpha particle in air. The reason that the RBE decreases near the termination of the alpha pathway is that at this point more energy than is necessary has been deposited in the tissue to fulfill some desired response — usually cell death.

A similar calculation is available for radium as the calibration source:

$$mr/hr = \frac{\text{Number of milligrams of radium}}{s^2}$$

s = Distance to the source in yards

The same formula using distances in terms of centimeters is as follows:

$$mr/hr = \frac{8,400 \times \text{Number of milligrams of radium}}{s^2}$$

s = Distance in centimeters

Any of these formulas may prove beneficial to persons working in the nuclear medicine department because continuous calibration of survey meters is necessary. In some cases a calibration check source is provided with the survey meter. Its value should be known and checked at each use. Should the value vary, the survey meter should be recalibrated with an NBS traceable standard. Too often this check source is used solely to check for functional batteries.

MAXIMUM PERMISSIBLE DOSE (MPD)

Since radiation is generally thought to be harmful to human beings, the ideal would be no radiation exposure at all. However, the use of radiation and radioactive materials in many instances has proved to be beneficial to mankind. Since man is therefore going to use these radiation-emitting materials, some methods must be devised to allow their use within safe limits. This establishment of a compromise became the problem of the National Council on Radiation Protection and Measurements (NCRP). The NCRP was to establish the dose of ionizing radiation that in light of present knowledge is not expected to cause appreciable bodily injury to a person at any time during his lifetime. The acceptance of such a dose involves the acceptance of a risk as well because a possibility that the radiation dose will manifest itself during the lifetime of the exposed person or in subsequent generations does exist. The probability, however, is so low that the risk is acceptable to the average individual. Such a dose was termed by the NCRP as a "permissible" dose, and on April 18, 1958, the Council established the Maximum Permissible Dose (MPD). This statute allows the radiation worker to receive a maximum dose to the whole body of 5 rems per year after the age of 18 according to the following formula:

$$MPD = 5 (N - 18) \text{ rem}$$
$$N = \text{Age in years}$$

The Nuclear Regulatory Commission still suggests the use and interpretation of this formula. In 1971, however, the NCRP redefined the acceptable occupational exposure limits. They also added values for which no guidelines had been presented before, such as recommendations for pregnant women and students below the age of 18 years of age. These dose-limiting recommendations can be found in Table 6-2.

The interpretation of the MPD formulation is explained in Title 10 of the *Code*

Table 6-2. National Council on Radiation Protection and Measurements dose-limiting recommendations, 1971*

Maximum permissible dose equivalent for occupational exposure	
Combined whole-body occupational exposure	
Prospective annual limit	5 rems in any one year (1.25/qtr)
Retrospective annual limit	10-15 rems in any one year
Long-term accumulation to age N years	$(N - 18) \times 5$ rems
Skin	15 rems in any one year
Hands	75 rems in any one year (25/qtr)
Forearms	30 rems in any one year (10/qtr)
Other organs, tissues, and organ systems	15 rems in any one year (5/qtr)
Fertile women (with respect to fetus)	0.5 rem in gestation period
Dose limits for the public or occasionally exposed individuals	
Individual or occasional	0.5 rem in any one year
Students < 18	0.1 rem in any one year
Emergency dose limits	
Life saving (>45 years old, if possible)	100 rems
Less urgent	25 rems

*From NCRP Report No. 39, Basic radiation protection criteria, Washington, D.C., 1971, NCRP. Available from NCRP Publications, P.O. Box 30175, Washington, D.C. 20014.

of Federal Regulations, Part 20.101 (10CFR20.101) by stipulating the two methods of recording and calculating the radiation exposure to occupational personnel.

The method used by most routine nuclear medicine departments is to limit the radiation exposure received by occupational personnel to doses per calendar quarter* according to the following schedule:

1. Whole body; head and trunk; active blood-forming organs; lens of the eyes; gonads – 1.25 rems per quarter
2. Hands and forearms; feet and ankles – 18.75 rems per quarter
3. Skin of the whole body – 7.5 rems per quarter

The licensee may not permit any individual to receive a dose in excess of any of these values. With this method the licensee is required to complete or at least be able to supply the information requested on Form NRC-5. Records are not required of the individual's accumulated occupational exposure doses prior to each quarter. A licensee may permit any employee to receive any two or all three of the specified radiation doses concurrently, provided a separate Form NRC-5 is maintained for each type of dose. All such records are preserved for 5 years.

The other method of calculating the radiation exposure to occupational personnel is to use the MPD formula in its strictest sense, a method generally considered consistent with only very hazardous uses of radioactive materials. The MPD formula is applicable to radiation exposure to the whole body, head and trunk, lens of the eye, active blood-forming organs, or gonads. The formula indicates that

*Thirteen complete, consecutive weeks; *or* the period between a date in January of any year to the same date in April, in July, and in October; *or* the quarters may be the first 14 weeks, the next 12 weeks, the next 14 weeks and the last 12 complete, consecutive calendar weeks.

the maximum permissible dose to these organs and sections of the body shall not exceed 5 rems multiplied by the number of years beyond age 18. The Committee also stipulates that the dose in any quarter-year (13 consecutive weeks) could be as large as 3 rems if the total occupational exposure during the lifetime of the individual does not exceed the MPD value calculated by the formula.

The interpretation of this formula implies that one cannot work with radiation before the age of 18. The implication is clarified with statement 5 on p. 107. Furthermore, it places a premium on older personnel because, as one gets older, more radiation can be accumulated per year (provided the person never receives maximum exposure). According to this formula, one could build up a "bank" or reserve of permissible exposure (age-prorated maximum). One application of the use of the bank of permissible exposure is as follows. If a radiation worker had 7 rems in his bank of permissible exposure, he could receive 3 rems per quarter for the entire next year (or 12 rems for that year) before using up his bank of permissible exposure (Table 6-3). Beyond this period of time, radiation exposures would be limited to 1.25 rems per quarter (or 5 rems per year).

Before permitting any individual to use this method in a restricted area so as to receive exposures greater than the quarterly value of the prospective annual limit (Table 6-2), each licensee, according to Title 10CFR20.102, must do the following:

1. Obtain a completed Form NRC-4, signed by the individual, showing each period of time after the individual attained the age of 18 in which the individual received an occupational dose of radiation, and
2. Calculate on Form NRC-4 . . . the previously accumulated occupational dose received by the individual, and the additional dose allowed for that individual . . . . In any case where a licensee is unable to obtain reports of the individual's occupational dose for a previous complete calendar quarter, it shall be assumed that the individual has received the maximum permissible dose.*

In addition to the exposure limits to critical organs shown in Table 6-3, there are several other stipulations regarding radiation exposure:

1. Accumulated dose of external exposure (radiation workers)

---

*The assumed MPD value should be 3.75 rems per calendar quarter before 1/1/61 and 1.25 rems per calendar quarter after 1/1/61.

Table 6-3. Exposure permissible per quarter for a person with a bank of 7 rems

Quarter	Bank at start of quarter (rem)	Suggested MPD per quarter (rem)	Total MPD (rem)	Allowable MPD per quarter (rem)	Bank at end of quarter (rem)
1	7.	1.25	8.25	3	5.25
2	5.25	1.25	6.5	3	3.5
3	3.5	1.25	4.75	3	1.75
4	1.75	1.25	3	3	0

    a. Skin of the whole body: MPD = 10(N − 18), and the dose in any 13 consecutive weeks shall not exceed 6 rems

    b. Hands and forearms; feet and ankles: MPD = 75 rems per year, and the dose in any 13 consecutive weeks shall not exceed 25 rems

2. Emergency dose (radiation workers): An accidental or emergency dose of 25 rems to the whole body or a major portion thereof occurring only once in the lifetime of the person need not be included in the determination of the radiation exposure status of that person.

3. Medical dose (radiation workers): Radiation exposure resulting from necessary medical and dental procedures need not be included in the determination of the radiation exposure status of the person concerned.

4. Dose to persons outside of controlled areas: The radiation or radioactive material outside a controlled area attributable to normal operation within the controlled area shall be such that it is improbable that any individual will receive a dose of more than 0.5 rems in any one year from external radiation.

5. No employer shall permit any employee who is under 18 years of age to receive in any period of one calendar quarter a dose in excess of 10% of the above limits.

All such records will be preserved for the lifetime of the individual. Regardless of the method used to calculate occupational personnel radiation exposure, any excesses are considered overexposures and must be reported to the Commission as specified in Title 10CFR20.403. In addition, any personnel experiencing these overexposures must be removed from all exposure to radiation for the balance of the quarter.

    Regulation G1910.96 (n) of the Occupational Safety and Health Act (OSHA) indicates that "Every employer shall maintain records of the radiation exposure of all employees for whom personnel monitoring is required . . . and advise each of his employees of his individual exposure on at least an annual basis."

SPECIFIC FACTORS INVOLVED IN RADIATION PROTECTION
Type of radiation

    In nuclear medicine three types of emissions are of primary concern: alpha particles, beta particles, and gamma rays. In addition, there are x rays resulting from several phenomena of interaction with matter, but these are generally very weak in nature and of no particular concern as far as radiation protection is concerned. One fact to be considered is that of external emission versus internal emission — whether the radiation comes from outside the body and penetrates the epidermis into the body or whether the emitters are already inside the body after being introduced by way of ingestion, inhalation, or intravenous injection. Gamma rays and x rays are able to penetrate the epidermis of the skin and therefore present the same hazard whether they are external or internal emitters. Such is not the case with alpha and beta emitters. Alpha and beta particles cannot ordinarily penetrate the outer layers of the skin. As external emitters they do not usually constitute a serious problem with radiation protection. If they are used as internal emitters, however, the problem of alpha and beta radiation damage becomes severe.

Penetration power

As just stated, alpha particles and beta particles are not generally regarded as radiation hazards as external emitters. A 1.0 mev alpha particle has a range in tissue of 0.0006 cm and in air of 0.49 cm, while a 5 mev alpha particle has a range of 0.0037 cm in tissue. An alpha particle would require an energy of 7.5 mev to penetrate human skin. Under ordinary circumstances a piece of paper will stop an alpha particle.

The penetration power of beta particles is about 100 times that of alpha particles. An inch of wood or 1/25 inch of aluminum is required to stop a beta particle. The range in tissue for a 1 mev beta particle is 0.42 cm and for a 5 mev beta particle 2.2 cm. Although an external beta emitter is generally considered not to be of consequence as far as radiation protection is concerned, a beta particle can penetrate from a few millimeters to 1 cm beneath the skin. There is a rapid deceleration of the particle as a result of its interaction with tissue. Protective shielding for the pure beta emitter deserves special attention since a high Z material will increase the amount of Bremsstrahlung produced and, therefore, increase the radiation exposure of internal organs. The plastic syringe used for administration of the material is usually adequate shielding for the beta particle, with a minimum of x rays produced because of the low Z nature of the plastic.

Gamma rays have extremely high penetration power and can create radiation hazards as either external or internal emitters. The gamma ray cannot be stopped by paper or small amounts of aluminum or lead. In general, protection is spoken of in terms of inches of lead and feet of concrete. In contrast to total absorption of an alpha or beta particle, only 3% of the gamma ray energy is absorbed in 1 cm of tissue. The rest is either absorbed in a much larger volume of tissue or travels through and completely out of the body.

Ionization

Ionization in tissue, either directly or indirectly, is thought to be the most important biologic interaction of radiation. Almost all the damage to tissue is as a result of this phenomenon. The ability to ionize varies tremendously among alpha, beta, and gamma emissions. A term that is used to describe this phenomenon is *specific ionization,* which has been discussed previously in this chapter.

There is an important correlation between the ionization ability and the penetration power of the various emissions. The alpha particles are very weak in their penetration power, but their ionization ability reaches tremendous proportions. If alpha particles bypass the epidermis, they present a tremendous problem in radiation biology. This is also true of beta emitters. Although beta emitters do not have as great an ionization ability, they have increased penetration power. However, their penetration power is not such that they can penetrate far beyond the skin. Based on their ionization ability, beta emitters can cause tremendous biologic damage provided the protective layer of the skin is bypassed. It is for this reason that phosphorus 32, a pure beta emitter, is used therapeutically in cases of leukemia and polycythemia. The rationale for its use is based solely on its ability for localized destruction of tissue function. Since most radiopharmaceuticals are beta-gamma emitters, the beta component represents the largest contribution of radiation dose as an internal emitter. In some cases 90% to 95% of the dose is from the beta component. Although alpha and beta particles cannot penetrate the skin, there must still be protection against them. Because of their ability to ionize tissue once they have bypassed the skin, they present more of a radiation hazard than gamma photons, although the damage will be localized.

PRACTICAL METHODS OF RADIATION PROTECTION

For personnel involved in the use of radioactive materials, methods of radiation protection should be foremost in their thoughts at all times. The total picture of the actual effects of radiation is not known and may not be known for many centuries to come. However, assuming that all ionizing radiations are potentially harmful, man can cope with the problem by constantly being alert to methods of protection. Practical limitations established by national and international committees to assist the occupational radiation worker have already been discussed. The rationale for these limits is that even peaceful uses of the atom require some exposure to emissions. It is impossible and impractical to shield workers from them completely. There is also a constant bombardment by cosmic radiation from outside the earth's atmosphere. These cosmic rays are highly energetic and, practically speaking, no amount of protection can shield us completely from these rays. Man has learned to live with these omnipresent cosmic radiations. Complete shielding is also impractical because many beneficial uses of atomic energy would be removed from modern medical technology, such as x-ray therapy and diagnosis and nuclear medicine therapy and diagnosis. For precisely this reason, nuclear medicine personnel must be constantly aware of the practical methods of radiation protection. These methods are distance, shielding, and time. With the judicious use of all three of these methods, the amount of radiation to which the radiation worker subjects himself or herself can be kept at a minimum and well within the limitations established by the NCRP.

Distance

Distance constitutes one of the best methods of radiation protection and is one of the routine methods used. It is not only a very effective means of radiation protection, but in many instances it is the least expensive. As one moves away from the source of radiation, one naturally expects to receive less radiation. The novice might think that as the distance is doubled from the source at a given position, the radiation to the person would be reduced by one half; however, the radiation is reduced to one fourth. This is known as the inverse square law, which states that the amount of radiation at a given distance from a source is inversely proportional to the square of the distance. By doubling the distance, the dose is one-fourth the original; by halving the distance, the dose is four times the original.

The name of the law defines the nature of the law itself. By increasing the distance by a factor of 2, the dose is decreased by the inverse square of 2 (namely, $1/4$), according to the following:

Distance factor	*Inverse*	*Inverse square*
2	$1/2$	$(1/2)^2 = 1/4$

Accordingly, by reducing the distance by a factor of $1/2$, the dose is increased by the inverse square of $1/2$ (namely, 4):

Distance factor	*Inverse*	*Inverse square*
$1/2$	$2/1$	$(2/1)^2 = 4/1 = 4$

This relationship is seen in Fig. 6-2.

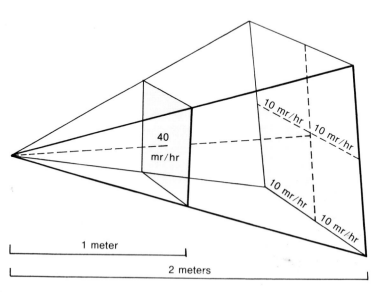

Fig. 6-2. Inverse square law. As radiations are emitted from a point source, an arbitrary area is selected a 1 m, representative of a radiation intensity of 40 mr/hr. At 2 m (twice the distance from the point source) that same radiation field of 40 mr/hr has expanded to an area four times the size of the original area. Consequently, the original area (gray) now receives only one fourth of the entire radiation.

The inverse square law can also be expressed as a formula. By utilization of this formula and knowing the intensity at a given distance, one can mathematically determine the intensity at another known distance or the distance at which one could receive a required intensity. The formula follows:

$$\frac{I}{i} = \frac{d^2}{D^2} \text{ or } ID^2 = id^2$$

I = Intensity at a distance (D) from a point source
i = Intensity at a different distance (d)

The following examples demonstrate the inverse square law:

1. 300 mr/hr is measured at 8 cm. What is the dose rate at 2 cm?

$$\frac{x}{300} = \frac{8^2}{2^2}$$

$$x = \frac{8^2}{2^2} \times 300 = \frac{64}{4} \times 300 = 4,800 \text{ mr/hr}$$

2. 600 mr/hr is measured at 10 cm. What is the distance at which 150 mr/hr is received?

$$\frac{600}{150} = \frac{x^2}{10^2}$$

$$x^2 = \frac{600}{150} \times 10^2$$

$$x = \sqrt{\frac{600 \times 100}{150}} = \sqrt{400} = 20 \text{ cm}$$

Both of these examples could have been calculated without the use of the formula. In example 2 the dose rate desired is one fourth of that measured at 10 cm from the point source. According to the inverse square law, this would require twice the distance, or 20 cm.

The principle of the inverse square law is easily demonstrated by any survey meter and a point source. If the point source is placed at a distance of 0.5 meter from the detector and the reading is recorded by moving the source to a distance of 1 meter, the intensity is reduced to one fourth. The inverse square law applies most accurately with the use of gamma emitting point sources; that is, with sources in which the radioactivity is contained in a very small volume. It does not apply to extended sources or to multiple sources.

The inverse square principle explains the suggested use of long-handled tongs and remote control handling devices with application to large quantities of radiation. It also plays a role in the calculation of visiting time to a recently treated patient. It may be that a patient's family could stay only 10 minutes at the bedside, but by not allowing the visitors within 6 feet, their stay could be prolonged based on inverse square relationships.

Shielding

Shielding is also a very practical method of radiation protection. The use of shielding materials such as lead sheets and lead bricks is nothing new to even the most inexperienced radiation worker. This shield is simply a body of material used to prevent or reduce the passage of radiation. In the case of alpha and beta radiation, very little shielding is required to absorb the emissions completely. An alpha particle is stopped by a sheet of paper, a beta particle is stopped by an inch of wood, but feet of concrete or inches of lead are necessary to absorb gamma radiation. The general practice is to use enough shielding for complete absorption of alpha and beta particles. This is not true, however, with gamma or x-radiation. With these two types of emissions, shielding is used to reduce the amount of radiation.

The shielding aspect of beta particles deserves special consideration. It is known that $1/4$ inch of plastic will stop a beta particle; therefore a syringe will provide adequate shielding in itself. If a syringe containing ^{32}P, for example, is placed near a scintillation detector, a large number of counts will be received. The detector is actually registering the electromagnetic radiation resulting from Bremsstrahlung.

In order that radiation be completely absorbed or reduced in intensity, energy must be lost by the radiations themselves. The energy of charged particles is lost primarily by a series of ionization events or excitation of atoms within the shielding medium. Energy from electromagnetic radiation is lost by three methods: photoelectric effect, Compton effect, or pair production, depending on the energy of the radiation itself. For those gamma rays below 1.02 mev in energy, the process of absorbing is usually a series of Compton collisions whereby the energy gradually diminishes. Eventually the radiations are sufficiently decreased in energy that total absorption occurs through the photoelectric effect. For those gamma rays above 1.02 mev of energy, pair production occurs with the eventual formation of two gamma rays of 0.511 mev. They are eventually absorbed by the Compton and photoelectric interactions.

As far as the shielding material itself is concerned, density and thickness go hand-in-hand in reducing radiation intensity (Fig. 6-3). If a material 1 cm thick with a density of 10 gm/cm³ (grams per cubic centimeter is a standard unit of density) was placed between a source and a detector, it would have the same stopping power as a material 10 cm thick having a density of 1 gm/cm³ placed similarly. For this reason, units of *density thickness* have become accepted in grams per square centimeter according to the following:

$$\frac{gm}{cm^3} \times cm = \frac{gm}{cm^3} \times \frac{1}{cm^{-1}} = gm/cm^2$$

Shielding, however, is considerably more complicated than just these simple concepts in density thickness. It is easy, although hazardous, to suggest a direct

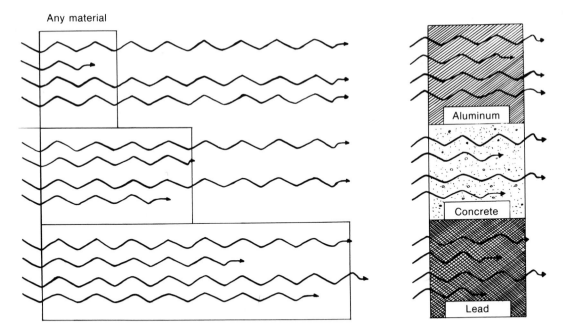

Fig. 6-3. Absorption characteristics of shielding materials. As density and/or thickness of the shielding material increases, the absorption of radioactive emissions by the material also increases.

relationship of density to atomic number (Z). In general, it is true that the higher the atomic number, the higher the material's density and vice versa. However, there are plenty of exceptions to the rule. Gold and lead are good examples. Gold has a Z of 79 with a density of 19.3 gm/cm³; lead has a higher Z of 82 and a lower density of 11.0 gm/cm³. Densities also change when materials assume different physical states, and yet their atomic numbers remain the same. A good example of this is water. It has an effective atomic number of 7.4 but assumes different densities depending on its physical state—whether ice, liquid, or vapor.

Attenuation coefficients. Any discussion of shielding must present some units for measuring the quantity of radiation that is absorbed (attenuated) by some absorber. Two such units are the *linear attenuation coefficient* and the *mass attenuation coefficient*. They differ in that the latter unit considers the density of the attenuating medium.

Linear attenuation coefficient. The linear attenuation coefficient (symbol, μ) is defined as the fraction of the number of photons removed from the radiation field per centimeter of absorber. It is expressed as a constant percentage of photons absorbed, much like the decay constant, λ, in the physical half-life formula. A condition with a μ value of 20% per centimeter (written 0.20 cm^{-1}) would indicate that the remaining number of photons in a photon beam would be reduced in in-

$$\frac{N}{N_0} = e^{-.2x} = e^{-.2} \quad \text{for } 1 \text{ cm}$$
$$= .8187$$

(handwritten marginalia: "? .", "?", "Conceptually wrong!")

tensity by 20% for each centimeter of the absorbing medium (Fig. 6-4). A μ value is specific for the energy of the photons and the type of absorber. If either change, so also does the linear attenuation coefficient. Table 6-4 lists a variety of linear attenuation coefficients for a variety of photon energies in different media.

Mass attenuation coefficient. The mass attenuation coefficient, (symbol, μ/ρ) is another useful unit. It is obtained by dividing the linear attenuation coefficient by the density (ρ) of the absorbing medium. The unit is expressed in terms of cm²/gm. By the same token, the μ value could be determined by multiplying the mass attenuation coefficient (cm²/gm) by the density (gm/cm³).

The relationship between μ and μ/ρ is seen in Fig. 6-5. Since water has a density of unity, μ and μ/ρ are the same. Since density changes with the various physical states of water, the linear attenuation coefficient also changes. The reason is that attenuation by the absorber changes, and this unit reflects only the attenuation by the absorbing medium per centimeter. Contrast that to the mass attenuation coefficient, which remains the same regardless of the change in physical state of the medium. The reason for this is that this unit reflects the density of the entire absorbing medium, not just the thickness. It can also be concluded from this figure, that 1 gm of water, ice, or water vapor will absorb the same amount of photons per gram. This relationship is not important in medicine because sizes of human organs do not allow this type of consideration. Further, since the mass attenuation coefficient remained the same for all physical forms of water regardless of density or volume, the mass attenuation coefficient is not important to medicine either. Therefore, the shielding formula uses the linear attenuation coefficient.

Attenuation in the photoelectric range. Another interesting phenomenon occurs in the attenuation of various energy photon beams. It is easily understood that as the energy of the photon increases, the probability of attenuation decreases. In other words, the mass attenuation coefficient is changing with the energy, and as the absorbing medium becomes less and less effective, the μ/ρ decreases and the percent transmission increases. One would suspect that a curve generated by plotting mass attenuation coefficient versus photon energy would result in a

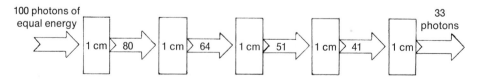

Fig. 6-4. Attenuation of a photon beam through 5 cm of an absorbing medium whose $\mu = 0.20$ cm⁻¹. Each cm of the absorber reduces the remaining number of photons by 20%. Note that energy is monochromatic. Attenuation of polychromatic beams is much less predictable.

Table 6-4. Linear attenuation coefficients for a variety of media and photon energies*

Attenuator with ρ in gm/cm³	Pb 11.34	Al 2.7	H₂O 1.0	NaI 3.67
μ at 20 kev	984.4	9.278	0.711	62.39
μ at 27.4 kev	447.2	3.985	0.434	23.86
μ at 140 kev	27.1	0.386	0.153	2.496
μ at 364 kev	3.164	0.262	0.111	0.459
μ at 511 kev	1.724	0.224	0.096	0.327

*Adapted from Gottschalk, A., and Potchen, E. J.: Diagnostic nuclear medicine, Baltimore, 1976, The Williams & Wilkins Co.

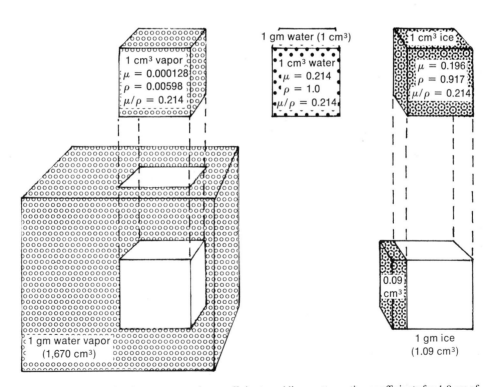

1 gm water (1 cm³)

1 cm³ vapor
$\mu = 0.000128$
$\rho = 0.00598$
$\mu/\rho = 0.214$

1 cm³ water
$\mu = 0.214$
$\rho = 1.0$
$\mu/\rho = 0.214$

1 cm³ ice
$\mu = 0.196$
$\rho = 0.917$
$\mu/\rho = 0.214$

0.09 cm³

1 gm water vapor (1,670 cm³)

1 gm ice (1.09 cm³)

Fig. 6-5. — Relationship of mass attenuation coefficients and linear attenuation coefficients for 1.0 gm of water as it changes its physical state to ice or to water vapor. Values are for a 50 kev monochromatic photon beam. Ice and water vapor are less dense than water so μ changes proportionally to reflect that density change.

nice, smooth exponential curve. This, however, is not the case. A proper curve used to show this relationship is seen in Fig. 6-6. Note that the curve is not continuous but is broken at specific energy levels. One such break in the curve occurs at 88 kev. The reason for this response is that photons will photoelectrically interact with, and therefore be absorbed by, electrons bearing binding energies closest to their energy. As the energy of the photon increases beyond that binding energy, the probability of the photoelectric effect taking place is reduced; therefore, percent transmission increases. This fall in attenuation continues until the photon energy reaches the binding energy of the next lowest energy shell, at which point a sharp rise occurs in the mass attenuation coefficient and percent transmission once again is drastically reduced. This point of abrupt change is called the *K-edge* or *L-edge*, depending on the photon energy. The curiosity of this phenomenon is that with two radionuclides of different energy, the amount of lead needed to adequately shield the lower energy radionuclide may be greater. For example, since the K-edge for lead occurs at 88 kev, it would require more lead shielding to satisfactorily attenuate an 81 kev radionuclide (xenon 133) than a 140 kev radionuclide (technetium 99m).

Attenuation in the Compton range. Another factor that affects attenuation is the number of electrons per gram. As a general rule, the lower the atomic number, the higher the number of electrons per gram. Just as with the mass attenuation coefficient, even though the term is in units per weight, the unit has little meaning as far as attenuation in the body goes. The number of electrons per gram of water is the same whether it is in the liquid, solid, or gaseous state. To circumvent this problem, the unit should be multiplied by density units to yield electrons per cubic centimeter as follows:

$$\frac{electrons}{gram} \times \frac{grams}{cm^3} = \frac{electrons}{cm^3}$$

In this form, the unit has meaning. The number of electrons per cubic centimeter is especially important to attenuation at energy levels where the Compton reaction predominates. If the photon is not able to be absorbed by way of the photoelectric effect as a result of its high energy, then reliance must be placed on the probability that the Compton interaction will occur and recur, eventually reducing the photon energy to a point where the photoelectric effect will be possible. That probability is directly related to the number of electrons per cubic centimeter. The suggestion by the use of this term is that a less dense material may have the same shielding capabilities as a more dense material because of its increased number of electrons per gram. Or the reverse could be true; a material having fewer numbers of electrons per gram than another material can have significantly different attenuation capabilities associated with differences in the density of the materials, as is evidenced by Table 6-5. This table shows silver (Ag) as being less dense, but as a result of its number of electrons per gram it is a more effective radiation shield. Needless to say, the cost of silver far outweighs this advantage. The reverse is

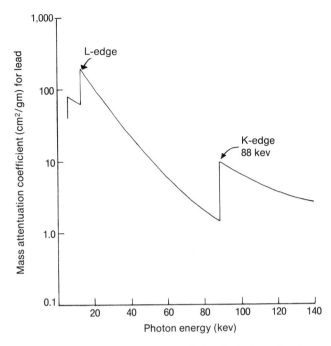

Fig. 6-6. Photoelectric mass attenuation coefficient for lead as related to energy.

Table 6-5. Relationship of density units and electron per gram (e/gm) units to attenuation

Element	Z	e/gm*	Density	e/cm³
Ag	47	2.62×10^{23}	10.5	2.751×10^{24}
Pb	82	2.38×10^{23}	11.35	2.701×10^{24}
U	92	2.33×10^{23}	18.68	4.352×10^{24}

*e/gm $= \dfrac{\text{Avogadro's no. } (6.02 \times 10^{23}) \times Z}{A}$

also true; uranium, which has fewer electrons per gram than lead, is a much more effective shield because of the density differences. Depleted uranium is used at the ports of teletherapy units as "trimmers" designed to reduce ineffective radiation to the therapy patient.

Shielding formula. All the factors influencing the effectiveness of the attenuating material can be expressed mathematically as follows:

$$I = I_0 e^{-\mu x}$$

I = Radiation intensity after shielding
I_0 = Radiation intensity before shielding
e = Base of the natural logarithm, 2.718
μ = Linear attenuation coefficient in cm⁻¹
x = Thickness of shield in cm
Minus sign indicates that the intensity is decreasing

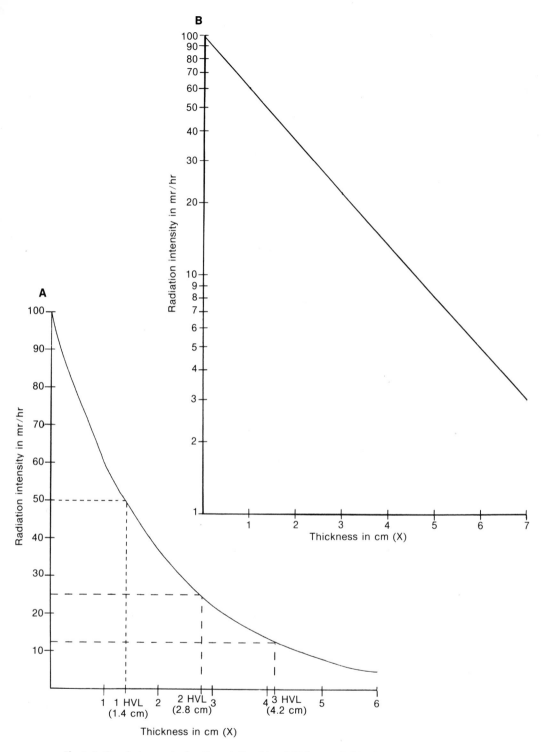

Fig. 6-7. Graph demonstrating the relationship of thickness of shielding to radiation intensity. **A** demonstrates the exponential function of the relationship. **B** reproduces the curve as a straight line plotted on semilogarithmic paper. The half-value layer (HVL) can be ascertained from either part of the graph.

To use the formula, assume that the radiation intensity before shielding is 100 mr/hr and that the density of the shield (absorber) is such that the fractional decrease (μ) is one-half the intensity per centimeter (50% per centimeter, or 0.50 cm^{-1}); the intensity after 1 cm shielding would not be 50 mr/hr as might be expected but greater than that value because of many complicating factors, such as back-scatter and dose buildup, for which all are accounted in the formula. A μ factor of 0.50 cm^{-1} would result in a decrease in the intensity to only 61 mr/hr according to the following:

$$I = I_o e^{-\mu x}$$
$$I = 100 \times e^{-0.50 \times 1}$$
$$I = 100 \times e^{-0.50}$$
$$I = 100 \times .61 = 61 \text{ mr/hr @ 1 cm}$$

Calculations for 2, 3, 4, 5, and 6 cm of the same absorbing media using this formula yield a resultant intensity of 37 mr/hr, 22 mr/hr, 13.5 mr/hr, 8 mr/hr, and 5 mr/hr, respectively. By plotting these intensity values versus thickness on linear graph paper, an exponential curve is received as in Fig. 6-7, *A*. Plotting the same parameters on semilogarithmic graph paper produces a straight line as in Fig. 6-7, *B*.

The formula itself is not of major practical importance in the field of nuclear medicine. It has value in that it makes possible the prediction of the attenuation of a gamma photon.

Half-value layer. It has already been stated that x- or gamma radiation can be reduced to acceptable limits but theoretically cannot be reduced to zero. As is evidenced by Fig. 6-7, it can be attenuated in a predictable manner. This useful information is referred to as the half-value layer (HVL). By definition HVL is the thickness of any particular material necessary to reduce the intensity of a radiation field to one half its original value.

Fig. 6-7 shows that by interposing 1 HVL (1.4 cm) of shielding material between the source and a detector, the radiation field is reduced to one half its original intensity (from 100 mr/hr to 50 mr/hr). Similarly, by interposing 2 HVLs (2.8 cm), the field is reduced by one half again (from 50 mr/hr to 25 mr/hr). Because the exponential curve approaches the abscissa asymptotically, it can be theorized that no amount of shielding could completely stop all the photons. Continuous interpositioning of HVLs results in a continuous halving process that becomes infinite.

Half-value layers for almost all radionuclides in various media are known and can be found in any radiologic handbook. Table 6-6 lists a variety of HVLs for various photon energies in a variety of media. These values provide a quick calculation of the shielding necessary to reduce the radiation intensity to acceptable limits. An example follows.

Problem. A cobalt 60 calibration source producing a radiation field of 24 mr/hr at 1 meter requires protection. If lead is used as the standard shielding material,

Table 6-6. Half-value layers for a variety of media and photon energies*

Attenuator with ρ in gm/cm³	Pb 11.34	Al 2.7	H₂O 1.0	NaI 3.67
HVL (cm) at 20 kev	0.0007	0.0747	0.975	0.011
HVL (cm) at 27.4 kev	0.0015	0.174	1.597	0.029
HVL (cm) at 140 kev	0.0256	1.796	4.530	0.278
HVL (cm) at 364 kev	0.2190	2.646	6.245	1.510
HVL (cm) at 511 kev	0.4021	3.094	7.220	2.120

*Adapted from Gottschalk, A., and Potchen, E. J.: Diagnostic nuclear medicine, Baltimore, 1976, The Williams & Wilkins Co.

Table 6-7. Relationship of radiation intensity to barrier thickness

Attenuation (HVL)	Intensity (mr/hr @ 1 m)	Lead thickness (cm)*
0	24	0
1	12	1.25
2	6	2.5
3	3	3.75
4	1.5	5.0

*Convert to inches: 4.8 cm ÷ 2.54 cm/inch = 1.97 inches. Therefore 2 inches of lead would be adequate to reduce radiation intensity to 2 mr/hr @ 1 m.

how much lead is required to reduce the radiation intensity to acceptable limits? (Pb HVL for ^{60}Co = 1.25 cm.)

Solution. Two inches of lead would be adequate to reduce the intensity to 2 mr/hr measured at 1 meter, the acceptable limit. Table 6-7 demonstrates this relationship.

The respect for half-value layers as a radiation protection device should become tremendously enhanced when it is realized that 1 HVL will reduce intensity to one-half, regardless of the original intensity. Accordingly, 1.25 cm of lead will reduce a cobalt 60 source with an intensity of 1,000 r/hr to 500 r/hr, just as the same 1.25 cm of lead will reduce cobalt 60 from 1 mr/hr to 0.5 mr/hr.

By carefully examining the shielding formula and discussion, a number of general statements may be made regarding it:

1. Four factors influence the efficacy of shielding: density, electrons per gram, thickness, and energy.
2. As density, electrons per gram, and/or thickness of the attenuating medium increases, the after-shielding intensity decreases.
3. As the energy of the photon or particle increases, the after-shielding intensity increases.
4. Any material regardless of the magnitude of these three factors, will absorb

some of the radiation and consequently decrease the after-shielding intensity.

5. The type of radiation is also an important consideration. Alpha radiation intensity can be reduced to zero (completely absorbed) by a sheet of paper. Beta radiation intensity can be reduced to zero (completely absorbed) by $\frac{1}{4}$ inch of plastic or 1 inch of wood. X- and gamma radiation intensity can never be totally reduced, although they can be attenuated in a predictable manner.

6. The shielding material must be of sufficient density and/or thickness to reduce the exposure to acceptable limits. A standard acceptable limit is 2 mr/hr at 1 meter because of the following.

$$2\text{mr/hr} \times 50 \text{ hr/wk} \times 50 \text{ wk/yr} = 5,000 \text{ mr/yr, or } 5 \text{ r/yr*}$$

This value is the MPD for occupational radiation personnel per year. For any length of time, 1 meter is a reasonable working distance from any source of radiation.

Exposure

Exposure formula. A formula that might find utility in the medical management of a therapy patient is one that can predict the exposure rate at some distance from that treated patient. Since exposure rate is proportional to the emission rate of photons and their energy and decreases inversely with the square of the distance, a formula for gamma photons between 70 kev and 4 mev is as follows:

$$\text{Exposure rate (mr/hr)} = \frac{6\,CEf}{d^2}$$

C = Activity of source in mCi
E = Photon energy in mev
f = Fraction of atoms yielding E energy photons
d = Distance from source in feet (centimeters can be used by changing 6 to read 5000)

Example. A patient was treated with 100 mg Eq† cesium 137 brachytherapy sources. What is the exposure rate in mr/hr at a distance of 100 feet? (Mg Eq ^{137}Cs must be multiplied by 2.7 to determine mCi.)

$$\text{mr/hr} = \frac{6 \times 100 \times 2.7 \times 0.662 \times 0.946}{10^2}$$

$$= 10 \text{ mr/hr}$$

If the radionuclide used for therapy had several significant photons, each would have to be calculated in this manner and added as follows.

---

*Actually 5 rems per year, but Title 10CFR20.4 states that, "For the purpose of the regulations . . . a dose of one rem . . . is equivalent to . . . a dose of 1 r due to x- or gamma radiation."
†Eq is equivalent dose to ^{226}Ra therapy.

Example. Patient was treated with 100 mCi of iodine 131. What is the exposure rate from this patient at 10 feet? (Iodine 131 has two significant gamma photons, 364 kev [83.8%] and 637 kev [6.6%].)

$$\text{mr/hr from 0.364 mev photons} = \frac{6 \times 100 \times 0.364 \times 0.836}{10^2}$$

$$= 1.83 \text{ mr/hr}$$

$$\text{mr/hr from 0.637 mev photons} = \frac{6 \times 100 \times 0.637 \times 0.066}{10^2}$$

$$= 0.25 \text{ mr/hr}$$

$$\text{Total exposure rate} = 1.83 + 0.25 = 2.08 \text{ mr/hr}$$

Another formula to express the same relationship within acceptable agreement is as follows:

$$\text{Exposure rate (R/hr)} = \frac{\Gamma A}{d^2}$$

Γ^* = The specific gamma ray constant expressed in R/mCi-hr at 1 cm and found for each radionuclide in appropriate handbooks

A = Activity in mCi

d = Distance in cm

Time

The principle of time is also a very practical method of radiation protection. It is obvious that the longer an individual is exposed to a field of radiation the greater will be the total exposure. Common sense dictates that time should be used as a control of radiation exposure. In diagnostic applications of nuclear medicine, time does not become as important as in therapy.

Three groups of nonoccupational personnel deserve special time considerations: nursing personnel, visitors, and adjacent patients.

In order that time considerations become meaningful, reference must be made to the NRC regulations on the subject (10CFR20.105). These regulations stipulate that "No licensee shall possess, use or transfer licensed material in such a manner as to create in an unrestricted area† . . . radiation levels which, if an individual were continuously present in the area, could result in his receiving a dose in excess of two millirems‡ in any one hour . . . or a dose in excess of 100 millirems in any seven consecutive days."

With respect to these regulations, the three groups of nonoccupational personnel can be treated as two groups: visitors and nursing personnel in one group and the adjacent patient in another.

Visitors and nursing personnel. It is unlikely that any one of these two groups

---

*^{137}Cs = 3.3, ^{60}Co = 13.2, ^{198}Au = 2.3, ^{131}I = 2.2, ^{192}Ir = 4.8, ^{226}Ra = 8.25.

†An "unrestricted area" is any area the access to which is not controlled by the licensee for purposes of protection of individuals from exposure to radiation and radioactive materials and any area used for residential quarters.

‡1 mrem ≅ 1 mr caused by x- or gamma radiation.

would be near the bedside of the patient any longer than 50 hours per 7 consecutive days. (This statement may be erroneous with respect to the immediate family of a seriously ill patient. In these instances, the family visitation privileges must be limited to 50 hours per week per person.) Under these conditions, this group has satisfied both phases of the NRC requirements. Their regulations regarding the exposure in any 7 consecutive days (100 mrems) concur with that of the permissible radiation exposure in any 1 hour (2 mrems) because of the following relationship:

$$100 \text{ mrems} \div 50 \text{ hr} = 2 \text{ mrems/hr}$$

Since both clauses of the NRC regulations calculate to be the same, no clause takes precedence, and any member of this group must be limited to 2 mrem in any 1 hour.

Adjacent patient. The situation of the patient adjacent to a recently treated patient presents another problem with reference to time considerations. The adjacent patient cannot be limited to 50 hours per week as can visitors and nursing personnel. It is conceivable that an adjacent patient could be subjected to this exposure every hour for 7 consecutive days (168 hours). For this group of people, the dose rate must be restricted to 0.6 mrem/hr or less according to the following relationship:

$$100 \text{ millirems} \div 168 \text{ hr} = 0.6 \text{ mrem/hr}$$

Since one clause of the NRC regulations states 2 mrems in any 1 hour and the other clause calculates to a permissible exposure rate of 0.6 mrem/hr, the latter takes precedence. Therefore the exposure rate of all patients adjacent to a recently treated patient must be less than 0.6 mrem/hr.

This regulation automatically rules out placing therapy patients in multibed wards after administration of therapy. The patient requires a private room. This statement is made based on the assumption that all therapies of 30 mCi or less are treated on an outpatient basis.* If, in the opinion of the physician, a patient treated with less than 30 mCi requires hospitalization, the patient may not require a private room. This is entirely dependent on the dose and the subsequent radiation field surrounding the treated patient. These regulations do not apply to the patient receiving x-ray or cobalt teletherapy treatments, since the radiation-emitting material is not placed within the patient. It does apply to radium or cobalt interstitial or intercavitary implants.

A point to be emphasized in the NRC regulations is that which relates to the exposure of 2 mrems/hr. This means 2 mrems in any 1 hour; it does not mean that one could receive 10 mrems in an hour and remove himself from the patient's room for the next 4 hours.

---

*This is a condition placed on all NRC licensees for therapeutic human use of by-product material; that is, patients containing larger amounts of radioactivity shall remain hospitalized until the residual activity is 30 mCi or less.

When the exposure rate exceeds 2 mrems/hr, calculations must be performed to determine the length of time that visitors and nursing personnel can remain there. The following problem will demonstrate the point.

Problem. The survey meter measurement at the bedside of a recently treated patient indicates an intensity of 12 mr/hr. What is the length of time that a visitor or a nurse could remain at the point where the reading was taken?

Solution. According to the following calculation:

$$\frac{12 \text{ mr}}{60 \text{ min}} = \frac{2 \text{ mr}}{x}$$

Solve for *x* when 2 mr is equal to the amount of exposure nonoccupational personnel may receive in any 1 hour:

$$12 \text{ mr } (x) = 2 \text{ mr } (60 \text{ min})$$
$$x = \frac{2 \text{ mr } (60 \text{ min})}{12 \text{ mr}}$$
$$x = 10 \text{ min}$$

If this reading of 12 mr/hr was taken at the bedside of the patient, in a reading 3 or 6 feet from the patient, the radiation dose rate would be decreased in accordance with the inverse square law, and the visitors would be allowed to remain longer. It might also be important to indicate that in some therapeutic applications of radiopharmaceuticals this dose rate will decrease with time because of large eliminations by way of normal biologic processes. If such is the action of the therapeutic agent, readings taken at various times of the day could extend visitation privileges.

BIBLIOGRAPHY

Blahd, W. H.: Nuclear medicine, New York, 1965, McGraw-Hill Book Co.

Bogardus, C. R., Jr.: Clinical applications of physics of radiology and nuclear medicine. St. Louis, 1969, Warren H. Green, Inc.

Chandra, R.: Introductory physics of nuclear medicine, Philadelphia, 1976, Lea & Febiger.

Chase, G. D., and Rabinowitz, J. L.: Principles of radioisotope methodology, ed. 3, Minneapolis, 1967, Burgess Publishing Co.

Goodwin, P. N., and Rao, D. V.: The physics of nuclear medicine, Springfield, Ill., 1977, Charles C Thomas, Publisher.

Gottschalk, A., and Potchen, E. J.: Diagnostic nuclear medicine, Baltimore, 1976, The Williams & Wilkins Co.

Hendee, W. R.: Medical radiation physics, Chicago, 1970, Year Book Medical Publishers, Inc.

Johns, H. E.: The physics of radiology, ed. 2, revised edition, Springfield, Ill., 1964, Charles C Thomas, Publisher.

King, E. R., and Mitchell, T. G.: A manual for nuclear medicine, Springfield, Ill., 1961, Charles C Thomas, Publisher.

Quimby, E. H., and Feitelberg, S.: Radioactive isotopes in medicine and biology, ed. 2, Philadelphia, 1963, Lea & Febiger.

Rollo, F. D.: Nuclear medicine physics, instrumentation, and agents, St. Louis, 1977, The C. V. Mosby Co.

Shilling, C. W.: Atomic energy encyclopedia in the life sciences, Philadelphia, 1964, W. B. Saunders Co.

Shapiro, J.: Radiation protection, Cambridge, Mass., 1972, Harvard University Press.

United States Department of Health, Education and Welfare: Radiological health handbook revised edition, Washington, D. C., September 1960, United States Department of Commerce Clearinghouse for Federal Scientific and Technical Information.

Wagner, H. N.: Principles of nuclear medicine, Philadelphia, 1968, W. B. Saunders Co.

7 Dosimetry

Perhaps the major consideration in all studies in which radionuclides are administered to human beings is the amount of activity administered to a patient and its consequent radiation dose to vital organs. For the diagnostic utilizations of such drugs, this becomes the limiting factor. It is obvious that all these problems of statistics, time involved in any given study, and so on could be resolved immediately merely by increasing the amount of radioactivity administered. Nuclear medicine procedures are not like x-ray procedures in which millions of photons per second are available for a given study. Because of this factor, many radiographic techniques require only fractions of seconds to complete. The magnitude of photons from a nuclear medicine procedure is on the order of hundreds of thousands of photons; therefore minutes or hours are required to obtain enough counts to make a statistical evaluation of a study. In such studies the radioactive materials become lodged, pooled, or incorporated into selective organs and remain there for periods as short as seconds to as long as months or even years. While the radioactive material is in the organ or is being excreted by the body, it is irradiating the exposed tissues even after the study has been completed. X rays, however, originate external to the body and produce effects only during the time that the body or organ or both is exposed to the x-ray unit.

Since this is the case, the radiopharmaceutical user must be able to give thoughtful consideration to the question of radiation dosage caused by the agent during the time that the body and its critical organs are being exposed. It enables the physician to assess benefit versus risk for either a particular radionuclide or a particular application. This is considered important by all three government bodies having at least some form of jurisdiction in the use of radiopharmaceuticals (Nuclear Regulatory Commission, National Institutes of Health, and the Food and Drug Administration). The FDA has authority over all pharmaceutical preparations, whereas the Nuclear Regulatory Commission has authority only over byproducts from a nuclear reactor, and the National Institutes of Health has control of blood derivatives.

For years the knowledge of dosimetry was much too fragmentary to establish exact values of dosage to the body and critical organs as a result of the administration of a known amount of radionuclide. The prevailing compromise was to attempt to predict in the approximate order of magnitude the absorbed radiation dose (in rad units) to the whole body, critical organ (organ in which the radionuclide is primarily collected), and the organs of elimination. Many assumptions were incorporated into such a calculation. In many cases when exact values were unknown, it was customary to use pessimistic assumptions. In this way, the result represented an acceptable figure but on the upper limit of the true value. If this value were adequate, the true value would represent an even smaller radiation dose.

The classic expressions of radiation dosimetry according to Marinelli are as follows:

$$D_\beta = 73.8 \times C \times \overline{E}_\beta \times T_e$$
$$D_\gamma = 0.0346 \times C \times \Gamma \times \bar{g} \times T_e$$

D_β = Dose in rads from beta radiation
D_γ = Dose in rads from gamma radiation
C = Initial concentration of radionuclide in $\mu Ci/gm$
$\overline{E}_\beta$ = Mean energy of β radiations in mev ($\cong \frac{1}{3}E_{max}$)
Γ = Gamma dose constant in r/mCi/hr at 1 cm distance
$\bar{g}$ = Geometric factor to account for variations in
    shape, size, and volume of organ
T_e = Effective half-life in days

The two constants, 73.8 and 0.0346, are conversion factors so that the product appears in rads. $\overline{E}_\beta$ and Γ are parameters that can be found in any handbook of radiation health and in many advanced texts. All other factors are variables. C is a variable because the number of microcuries and the gram weight would both vary among individuals. The adequate calculation of this parameter is compounded when radiopharmaceuticals are used for dynamic function studies, such as rose bengal and sodium iodohippurate (Hippuran) studies. T_e varies from person to person. The $\bar{g}$ values are available for a variety of standard geometric configurations, but no human organ exactly resembles a sphere or a cylinder, so this contributes to the value as something removed from the true value. Other complicating factors include unequal distribution of the radioactive material in the organ, energy of the emission (some gammas are so weak that they are betalike as far as dosimetry is concerned), and irradiation from adjacent organs (pancreas and liver) or companion organs (cross irradiation from one lung to the other or one kidney to the other).

In these equations, Marinelli and co-workers approached the problem of internal radiation dosimetry from the standpoints of penetrating (D_γ) and nonpenetrating (D_β) radiations but did so by grouping all their constants together and all their variables together and solving for each separately. This necessitated many assumptions, usually erroneously high. Total radiation dose was found by adding the penetrating (p) and nonpenetrating (np) radiations together.

The current approach to the problems of internal radiation dosimetry as proposed by the Medical Internal Radiation Dose (MIRD) Committee is still to consider both penetrating and nonpenetrating radiations. The MIRD technique, however, groups all physical data for both penetrating and nonpenetrating radiations together. Furthermore, it groups all biologic data and some of the physical data related to time and radionuclide distribution together. Actually, the average absorbed dose from an administered radionuclide can be determined by the grouping of a variety of factors into three categories:

1. The biologic parameters that describe the uptake, distribution, retention, and release of the radiopharmaceutical in the body
2. The energy released by the radionuclide and whether it is penetrating or nonpenetrating
3. The fraction of the emitted energy that is absorbed by the target

The average absorbed radiation dose resulting from the administration of internally emitting radionuclides is simply the product of these three groups of information.

BIOLOGIC PARAMETERS

To compute the absorbed dose to an individual from an administered radionuclide, one must know where the radionuclide goes, how long it takes to get there, how long it stays there, and the masses of the organs involved. Furthermore, there should always be an interest in the total amount of radiation to the target organs for the entire amount of time that the radionuclide is present. Therefore it would be important to determine the cumulative activity ($\tilde{A}$) in this organ from its entrance until its complete elimination from the system. This cumulative activity can be integrated and expressed as follows:

$$\tilde{A} = 1.443 \times A \times T_e *$$

$\tilde{A}$ = Cumulative activity in μCi hr
A = Maximum activity in μCi
T_e = Effective half-life in hr

ENERGY RELEASED PER DISINTEGRATION

The next consideration is whether the radiations from the internally deposited radionuclide are penetrating or nonpenetrating. Nonpenetrating (np) radiations include alpha particles, beta particles, positrons, conversion electrons, Auger

---

*There are two assumptions in this cumulative activity formula that may or may not be correct. Assumption 1 is that the maximum activity (A) is reached in a negligible amount of time. Assumption 2 is that the elimination of the radionuclide is a single exponential curve, which often is not the case. If Assumption 1 is incorrect, it can usually be corrected by assuming that the uptake of the material to reach maximum activity is approximately exponential in nature. In this case, the A formula would be altered to read:

$$\tilde{A} = 1.443 \times A \times T_e(1 - T_{uptake}/T_e)$$

If Assumption 2 is incorrect and if more than one exponential curve is apparent, the A formula would consist of more than one term. In this way, each term would represent another exponential and would be added as follows:

$$\tilde{A} = 1.443 (A^1T_e^1 + A^2T_e^2)$$

electrons, and x or gamma rays with energies less than 11.3 kev. The penetrating (p) radiations consist of x or gamma rays having energies greater than 11.3 kev and annihilation photons.

To be able to use this information in the MIRD formula, it is necessary to know the number of times that the gamma or x ray occurs, termed *fractional abundance* (n_i), as well as its average or mean energies (E_i) in mev, and add them all together.

The values for n_i and E_i for all the emissions from a variety of radionuclides may be found in MIRD pamphlets 4 and 6.* Furthermore, to simplify the mechanics of calculating absorbed doses, the MIRD Committee has defined an equilibrium absorbed dose constant (Δ) as follows:

$$\Delta_i = 2.13\, n_i\, E_i$$

Δ is in units of $\dfrac{\text{gram} \cdot \text{rad}}{\mu\text{Ci} \cdot \text{hr} \cdot \text{mev}}$

n_i = Fraction of quanta emitted per disintegration
E_i = Energy of the emitted quanta (mev)
2.13† = Conversion factor so that product appears as gram·rad/μCi·hr·mev

A table of this data as related to technetium 99m can be found in Fig. 7-1. Appendix F contains this data for many radionuclides used in nuclear medicine.

ABSORBED FRACTION OF ENERGY (Φ)

The third consideration, the absorbed fraction (Φ), is defined as the ratio of energy absorbed by the target to the energy emitted by the source. Since nonpenetrating radiation loses essentially all its energy within 1 cm of its origin, the absorbed fraction (n) for these emissions is always 1.0 (or 100%). For penetrating radiation, only partial absorption occurs in the tissue containing the radionuclide and in surrounding tissues and organs. The percentages have been determined using a "standard man" phantom.

The phantom has a simple geometric shape that approximates the body shape and dimensions as far as the major forms are concerned (Fig. 7-2). The phantom consists of three principal sections: (1) an elliptical cylinder representing the arms, torso, and hips; (2) a truncated elliptical cone representing both the legs and the feet; and (3) an elliptical cylinder representing the head and neck.

The absorbed fractions were generated by computer techniques relating many photon histories as they pass through an absorbing media. The computer was used to repetitively trace the path of a single photon through an absorbing medium with absorption coefficient data to calculate the energy lost per interaction and the scattering angle. Many such single photon histories were traced to generate a single absorbed fraction value.

---

*Available from the Society of Nuclear Medicine, 475 Park Avenue, South, New York, N.Y. 10017.

†2.13 $\dfrac{\text{gram} \cdot \text{rad}}{\mu\text{Ci} \cdot \text{hr} \cdot \text{mev}}$ = 1.602 × 10^{-6} $\dfrac{\text{erg}}{\text{mev}}$ × 10^{-12} $\dfrac{\text{rad}}{\text{erg/g}}$ × 3.7 × 10^4 $\dfrac{\text{dis/sec}}{\mu\text{Ci}}$ × 3,600 $\dfrac{\text{sec}}{\text{hr}}$

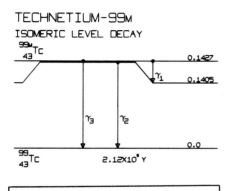

TECHNETIUM-99M

ISOMERIC LEVEL DECAY

$^{99M}_{43}$Tc

0.1427

γ_1 0.1405

γ_3 γ_2

0.0

$^{99}_{43}$Tc   2.12X10^5 Y

••INPUT DATA••

43 TECHNETIUM 99M   HALF LIFE = 6.03 HOURS

DECAY MODE- ISOMERIC LEVEL

TRANSITION	MEAN NUMBER/ DISINTE- GRATION	TRAN- SITION ENERGY (MEV)	OTHER NUCLEAR DATA
GAMMA 1	0.9860	0.0021	E3
GAMMA 2	0.9860	0.1405	M1, AK= 0.104
			K/L= 7.70
GAMMA 3	0.0140	0.1426	M4, AK=23.0
			AL(T) = 9.21

REF.- LEDERER, C.M. ET AL, TABLE OF ISOTOPES,
6TH ED.
LEGRAND, J. ET AL, INT. J. APPL. RAD. AND
ISOTOPES 21, 139 (1970).

••OUTPUT DATA••

43 TECHNETIUM 99M   HALF LIFE = 6.03 HOURS

DECAY MODE- ISOMERIC LEVEL

RADIATION	MEAN NUMBER/ DISINTE- GRATION n_i	MEAN ENERGY/ PAR- TICLE $\bar{E}_i$ (MeV)	EQUI- LIBRIUM DOSE CONSTANT Δ_i (g-rad/ μCi-h)
GAMMA 1	0.0000	0.0021	0.0000
M INT CON ELECT	0.9860	0.0016	0.0035
GAMMA 2	0.8787	0.1405	0.2630
K INT CON ELECT	0.0913	0.1194	0.0232
L INT CON ELECT	0.0118	0.1377	0.0034
M INT CON ELECT	0.0039	0.1400	0.0011
GAMMA 3	0.0003	0.1426	0.0001
K INT CON ELECT	0.0088	0.1215	0.0022
L INT CON ELECT	0.0035	0.1398	0.0010
M INT CON ELECT	0.0011	0.1422	0.0003
K ALPHA-1 X-RAY	0.0441	0.0183	0.0017
K ALPHA-2 X-RAY	0.0221	0.0182	0.0008
K BETA-1 X-RAY	0.0105	0.0206	0.0004
KLL AUGER ELECT	0.0152	0.0154	0.0005
KLX AUGER ELECT	0.0055	0.0178	0.0002
LMM AUGER ELECT	0.1093	0.0019	0.0004
MXY AUGER ELECT	1.2359	0.0004	0.0011

Fig. 7-1. Radionuclide decay schemes and nuclear parameters for use in radiation dose estimates using technetium 99m. (Courtesy Dillman), L. T., and Von der Lage, F. C.: MIRD pamphlet #10, New York, 1975, Society of Nuclear Medicine.)

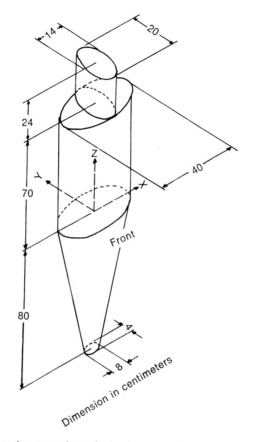

Fig. 7-2. Phantom illustrating approximate body shape and dimensions used to determine absorbed fraction (Φ) by the MIRD Committee.

It is clear, then, that the absorbed fraction is a function of photon energy and the size and shape of the tissue containing the radionuclide. Charts are available in MIRD pamphlets 3 and 8, which contain absorbed fractions for a variety of organs (see Table 7-9).

Calculations

In summary, the absorbed dose to a particular tissue is the product of the three factors just discussed:

$$\text{Absorbed dose} = \text{Cumulative concentration} \left(\frac{\text{Activity}}{\text{Mass*}} \right)$$
$$\times \text{Summation of all energies emitted per disintegration} \times \text{Their absorbed fractions}$$

---

*Mass in grams. Masses for all organs (as agreed on by the MIRD Committee) are found in Table 7-10.

Expressed in mathematical form:

$$D_\infty = \frac{\tilde{A}}{m} \Sigma \Delta_i \Phi_i$$

Substituting for $\tilde{A}$:

$$D_\infty = \frac{A \times 1.44 \times T_e}{m} \Sigma \Delta_i \Phi_i \text{ rads}$$

Problem

A liver scan is to be performed using 2.0 mCi of ^{99m}Tc sulfur colloid. Approximately 85% of the dose is taken up by the liver, 10% by the spleen, and 5% by the bone. Compute the dose to the liver with both the Marinelli and the MIRD formula. Assume immediate uptake of the colloid by the liver, with no biologic elimination, that is, the effective half-life is equal to the physical half-life.

Marinelli—The computation based on the Marinelli formula is as follows:

$$D_\beta = 73.8 \times C \times \bar{E}_\beta \times T_e$$
$$= 73.8 \times \left(\frac{2,000 \times 0.85}{1,833}\right) \times 0.016 \times 0.25*$$
$$= 0.28 \text{ rad}$$
$$D_\gamma = 0.0346 \times C \times \Gamma \times \bar{g} \times T_e$$
$$= 0.0346 \times \left(\frac{2,000 \times 0.85}{1,833}\right) \times 0.56 \times 50 \times 0.25*$$
$$= 0.23 \text{ rad}$$
$$D_\beta + D_\gamma = 0.28 + 0.23 = 0.51 \text{ rad to each gram of the entire liver}$$

MIRD—The computation based on the MIRD formula requires the calculation of the contribution from three sources: the liver itself, the spleen, and the bone. These calculations are as follows.

Contribution from liver (Tables 7-1 and 7-3)

$$D_{\infty \text{ liver} \leftarrow \text{liver}} = \frac{2,000(0.85) \times 1.443 \times 6*}{1,833} \Sigma_i \Delta_i \Phi_i \text{ rads}$$

To determine $\Sigma \Delta_i \Phi_i$ for the dose *to* the liver from ^{99m}Tc sulfur colloid *in* the liver, prepare a table as seen in Table 7-1. The table lists all the penetrating and nonpenetrating contributions from technetium 99m (in gray) multiplied by the absorbed fraction (Φ) for each entry. A Φ value of 1.0 means 100% absorbed, a value that applies to all nonpenetrating radiations. Penetrating radiations vary, their value being taken from tables such as Table 7-9 to receive the $\Delta_i \Phi_i$ of each contribution, all of which are summed at the base of the last column. It is this figure that is used in the MIRD calculation. A compressed version of this table is seen in Table 7-2.

---

*NOTE: In the classic Marinelli formula T_e is in units of days, whereas in the MIRD formula T_e is in hours.

Table 7-1. Effective absorbed energy data for technetium 99m (gray area only) listing all the penetrating and nonpenetrating contributions*

Radiation	η_i	$\overline{E}_i$	$\Delta_i = 2.13\,\eta_i\overline{E}_i$	Φ_i	$\Delta_i\Phi_i$
Gamma-1	0.0000	0.0021	0.0000	–	
M-ice, γ-1†	0.9860	0.0016	0.0035	1.0	0.0035
Gamma-2	0.8787	0.1405	0.2630	0.162‡	0.0426
K-ice, γ-2	0.0913	0.1194	0.0232	1.0	0.0232
L-ice, γ-2	0.0118	0.1377	0.0034	1.0	0.0034
M-ice, γ-2	0.0039	0.1400	0.0011	1.0	0.0011
Gamma-3	0.0003	0.1426	0.0001	0.162‡	–
K-ice, γ-3	0.0088	0.1215	0.0022	1.0	0.0022
L-ice, γ-3	0.0035	0.1398	0.0010	1.0	0.0010
M-ice, γ-3	0.0010	0.1422	0.0003	1.0	0.0003
Kα1 x rays[1]	0.0441	0.0183	0.0017	0.830‡	0.0014
Kα2 x rays[2]	0.0221	0.0182	0.0008	0.830‡	0.0006
Kβ1 x rays[3]	0.0105	0.0206	0.0004	0.784	0.0003
KLL Auger e[4]	0.0152	0.0154	0.0005	1.0	0.0005
KLX Auger e[5]	0.0055	0.0178	0.0002	1.0	0.0002
LMM Auger e[6]	0.1093	0.0019	0.0004	1.0	0.0004
MXY Auger e[7]	1.2359	0.0004	0.0011	1.0	0.0011

$$\Sigma\ 0.0818$$
$$\Sigma_{\eta\rho}\ 0.0369$$
$$\Sigma_{\rho}\ 0.0449$$

*The rest of the data (absorbed fraction, Φ) is compiled for technetium 99m in the liver as a contributor to the radiation dose to the liver.

†Internal conversion electron from M shell as a result of γ-1 interaction.

‡Interpolated values from absorbed fraction tables (Table 7-9).

Key: 1, Kα1 x ray ≡ K-L$_{III}$ transition; 2, Kα2 x ray ≡ K-L$_{II}$ transition; 3, Kβ1 x ray ≡ K-M$_{III}$ transition; 4, KLL Auger e ≡ an Auger electron emitted from the L shell as a result of the transition of another L shell electron to a vacancy in the K shell; 5, KLX Auger e ≡ an Auger electron emitted from the X shell, where X stands for any shell higher than the L shell, as a result of the transition of an L shell electron to a vacancy in the K shell; 6, LMM Auger e ≡ an Auger electron emitted from the M shell as a result of the transition of another M shell electron to a vacancy in the L shell; 7, MXY Auger e ≡ an Auger electron emitted from the Y shell as a result of the transition of an X shell electron to a vacancy in the M shell, where X and Y each stand for any shell higher than the M shell.

Table 7-2. Compressed version of the effective absorbed energy data for technetium 99m in the liver as a contributor to the radiation dose to the liver, listing all the penetrating contributions but combining all the nonpenetrating contributions (compare to Table 7-1)

Radiation	η_i	$\overline{E}_i$	$\Delta_i = 2.13\,\eta_i\overline{E}_i$	Φ_i	$\Delta_i\Phi_i$
Σηρ			0.0369	1.0	0.0369
Gamma-1	0.0000	0.0021	0.0000	–	–
Gamma-2	0.8787	0.1405	0.2630	0.162	0.0426
Gamma-3	0.0003	0.1426	0.0001	0.162	–
Kα1 x rays	0.0441	0.0183	0.0017	0.830	0.0014
Kα2 x rays	0.0221	0.0182	0.0008	0.830	0.0006
Kβ1 x rays	0.0105	0.0206	0.0004	0.784	0.0003

$$\Sigma\Delta_i\Phi_i = 0.0818*$$

*Once determined, this value, the *effective absorbed energy,* will never change; therefore, save for all future liver calculations using 99mTc in which values of absorbed energy by the liver from contributions from the liver are required.

Since all nonpenetrating particles and nonpenetrating photons (those less than 11.3 kev) have an assumed absorbed fraction of 1.0, then Table 7-1 can be greatly reduced by simply adding all the Δ_i values for these nonpenetrating emissions together. In this way, they can be listed as nonpenetrating and the others computed as seen in Table 7-2. (Note that the information in the gray areas is all the same for ^{99m}Tc. This information will always be the same for ^{99m}Tc, regardless of the chemical/physical form or of its use.) Data for other radionuclides used in nuclear medicine can be found in Appendix F.

Using the summation data of Tables 7-1 and 7-2, the dose to the liver as a result of the liver contribution (which accounts for 85% of the dose) is determined by the following formula:

$$D_{\infty \text{liver} \leftarrow \text{liver}} = \frac{2,000 \ (0.85) \times 1.443 \times 6}{1,833} \Sigma\Delta_i\Phi_i$$

$$= \frac{14,719}{1,833} \times 0.0818 = 0.657 \text{ rad}$$

Contribution from spleen (Table 7-3)

The contribution from the spleen (assuming the spleen received 10% of dose) is as follows:

$$D_{\infty \text{liver} \leftarrow \text{spleen}} = \frac{2,000 \ (0.10) \times 1.443 \times 6}{176} \Sigma\Delta_i\Phi_i$$

$$= 9.8386 \times 0.0018 = 0.0177 \text{ rad}$$

Table 7-3. Effective absorbed energy data for technetium 99m in the spleen as a contributor to the radiation dose to the liver

Radiation	η_i	$\overline{E}_i$	$\Delta_i = 2.13 \ \eta\overline{E}_i$	Φ_i	$\Delta_i\Phi_i$
$\eta\rho$ — no contribution				0.00	—
Gamma-1	0.0000	0.0021	0.000	0.00	—
Gamma-2	0.8787	0.1405	0.2630	0.00708*	0.0018
Gamma-3	0.003	0.1426	0.0001	0.00708	—
Kα1 x rays	0.0441	0.0183	0.0017	0.000	—
Kα2 x rays	0.0221	0.0182	0.0008	0.000	—
Kβ1 x rays	0.0105	0.0206	0.0004	0.000	—
					$\Sigma\Delta_i\Phi_i = 0.0018†$

*Interpolated from information on pp. 38-39 of MIRD pamphlet 5.
†*Save for all future determinations.*

Contribution from bone (Table 7-4)

The contribution from bone (assuming bone received 5% of dose) is as follows:

$$D_{\infty \text{liver} \leftarrow \text{bone}} = \frac{2,000 \ (0.05) \times 1.443 \times 6}{10.091} \Sigma\Delta_i\Phi_i$$

$$= 85.7992 \times 0.0013 = 0.1115 \text{ rad}$$

Table 7-4. Effective absorbed energy data for technetium 99m in bone as a contributor to the radiation dose to the liver

Radiation	η_i	$\overline{E}_i$	$\Delta_i = 2.13\,\eta_i\overline{E}_i$	Φ_i	$\Delta_i\Phi_i$
$\eta\rho$ – no contribution				0.00	
Gamma-1	0.0000	0.0021	0.0000	0.00	—
Gamma-2	0.8787	0.1405	0.2630	0.00478*	0.0013
Gamma-3	0.003	0.1426	0.0001	0.00478	—
$K\alpha1$ x rays	0.0441	0.0183	0.0017	0.00060	—
$K\alpha2$ x rays	0.0221	0.0182	0.0008	0.00060	—
$K\beta1$ x rays	0.0105	0.0206	0.0004	0.00083	—
				$\Sigma\Delta_i\Phi_i =$	$\overline{0.0013}$†

*Interpolated from information on pp. 36-37 of MIRD pamphlet 5.
†*Save for all future determinations.*

Total dose to the liver

To determine the total dose to the liver from all implicated organs, the totals of these calculations must be added together as follows:

$$\text{Contribution from liver} = 0.6570 \text{ rad}$$
$$\text{Contribution from spleen} = 0.0177 \text{ rad}$$
$$\underline{\text{Contribution from bone} = 0.1115 \text{ rad}}$$
$$\text{Total radiation dose to the liver} = 0.7862 \text{ rad, or } 0.8 \text{ rad, or } 800 \text{ mrads}$$

Problem

This MIRD method of dosimetry can easily be extended to other organs as well. Suppose the patient who received this dose of ^{99m}Tc – labeled sulfur colloid revealed, at a later date, that she was pregnant at the time of the dosing. The expectant mother now is concerned about the normal maturation of the fetus. The MIRD formula can be used very easily to allay her fears as seen in Table 7-5.

Table 7-5. Effective absorbed energy data for technetium 99m in the liver as a contributor to the radiation dose to the uterus

Radiation	η_i	$\overline{E}_i$	$\Delta_i = 2.13\,\eta_i\overline{E}_i$	Φ_i	$\Delta_i\Phi_i$
$\eta\rho$ – no contribution					
Gamma 1	0.0000	0.0021	0.0000	0.00	—
Gamma 2	0.8787	0.1405	0.2630	0.000123	0.00003
Gamma 3	0.003	0.1426	0.0001	0.0000	—
$K\alpha1$ x rays	0.0441	0.0183	0.0017	—	—
$K\alpha2$ x rays	0.0221	0.0182	0.0008	—	—
$K\beta1$ x rays	0.0105	0.0206	0.0004	—	—
				$\Sigma\Delta_i\Phi_i =$	$\overline{0.00003}$

The dose to the uterus from the liver is as follows:

$$D_{\infty \text{uterus} \leftarrow \text{liver}} = \frac{2{,}000\ (0.85) \times 1.443 \times 6}{1{,}833} \Sigma \Delta_i \Phi_i$$

$$= \frac{14{,}719}{1{,}833} \times 0.00003 = 0.00024 \text{ rad or } 0.24 \text{ mrad}$$

By this computation, the concern of the young mother in this problem can be diminished. A dose of less than 0.25 mrad should be of minimum concern to the normal maturation of the fetus.

"S" tables — absorbed dose per unit cumulated activity (rad/μCi-hr)

As indicated in the footnotes of each of the preceding tabulations, once determined, the effective absorbed energy values should be saved for future determinations. It is obvious that the MIRD committee has arranged a formula so that tables of factors can be generated for all of the organs (or even parts of organs and contents of some organs) with a variety of radionuclides used in nuclear medicine routinely. Once these factors are generated, that value will not change regardless of the patient. The only variable then, in the MIRD formula, is the biologic data necessary for the estimation of the cumulative activity, expressed as $\tilde{A}/M$.

The MIRD committee has even taken it one step farther. They have incorporated the mass of the organ into this single factor, provided the median values for organ weights of a standard 70-kg man can be used and it can be assumed that the activity is uniformly distributed in that organ. That factor is called the "S" factor and is expressed as the absorbed dose per unit cumulated activity in rad/μCi-hr. These tabulations are referred to as the "S" Tables.* The use of these tables has greatly simplified the problems of internal radiation dosimetry by sparing the dosimetrist the agony of generating all of the tables that preceded this section.

The MIRD formula using these tables (for example, Table 7-6) is expressed as follows:

$$\overline{D} = \tilde{A}\ S$$
$\overline{D}$ = Mean dose delivered to target organ,
$\tilde{A}$ = Cumulative activity in μCi-hr
S = Absorbed dose per unit cumulated activity in rad/μCi-hr

The formula is also written as follows:

$$\overline{D}(r_k \leftarrow r_h) = \tilde{A}_h\ S(r_k \leftarrow r_h)$$
r_k = Target organ
r_h = Source organ
$(r_k \leftarrow r_h)$ = Dose to target organ as a result of contributions from source organ

---

*Available as MIRD Pamphlet No. 11 from Society of Nuclear Medicine, 475 Park Ave. S., New York, N.Y. 10017.

Table 7-6. "S," absorbed dose per unit cumulated activity, (rad/μCi-hr), technetium-99m, half-life 6.03 hours*

Target organs	Source organs									
				Intestinal tract						
	Adrenals	Bladder contents	Stomach contents	SI contents	ULI contents	LLI contents	Kidneys	Liver	Lungs	Other tissue (muscle)
Adrenals	3.1E-03†	1.5E-07	2.7E-06	1.0E-06	9.1E-07	3.6E-07	1.1E-05	4.5E-06	2.7E-06	1.4E-06
Bladder wall	1.3E-07	1.6E-04	2.7E-07	2.6E-06	2.2E-06	6.9E-06	2.8E-07	1.6E-07	3.6E-07	1.8E-06
Bone (total)	2.0E-06	9.2E-07	9.0E-07	1.3E-06	1.1E-06	1.6E-06	1.4E-06	1.1E-06	1.5E-06	9.8E-07
GI (stom wall)	2.9E-06	2.7E-07	1.3E-04	3.7E-06	3.8E-06	1.8E-06	3.6E-06	1.9E-06	1.8E-06	1.3E-06
GI (SI)	8.3E-07	3.0E-06	2.7E-06	7.8E-05	1.7E-05	9.4E-06	2.9E-06	1.6E-06	1.9E-07	1.5E-06
GI (ULI wall)	9.3E-07	2.2E-06	3.5E-06	2.4E-05	1.3E-04	4.2E-06	2.9E-06	2.5E-06	2.2E-07	1.6E-06
GI (LLI wall)	2.2E-07	7.4E-06	1.2E-06	7.3E-06	3.2E-06	1.9E-04	7.2E-07	2.3E-07	7.1E-08	1.7E-06
Kidneys	1.1E-05	2.6E-07	3.5E-06	3.2E-06	2.8E-06	8.6E-07	1.9E-04	3.9E-06	8.4E-07	1.3E-06
Liver	4.9E-06	1.7E-07	2.0E-06	1.8E-06	2.6E-06	2.5E-07	3.9E-06	4.6E-05	2.5E-06	1.1E-06
Lungs	2.4E-06	2.4E-08	1.7E-06	2.2E-07	2.6E-07	7.9E-08	8.5E-07	2.5E-06	5.2E-05	1.3E-06
Marrow (red)	3.6E-06	2.2E-06	1.6E-06	4.3E-06	3.7E-06	5.1E-06	3.8E-06	1.6E-06	1.9E-06	2.0E-06
Oth tiss (musc)	1.4E-06	1.8E-06	1.4E-06	1.5E-06	1.5E-06	1.7E-06	1.3E-06	1.1E-06	1.3E-06	2.7E-06
Ovaries	6.1E-07	7.3E-06	5.0E-07	1.1E-05	1.2E-05	1.8E-05	1.1E-06	4.5E-07	9.4E-08	2.0E-06
Pancreas	9.0E-06	2.3E-07	1.8E-05	2.1E-06	2.3E-06	7.4E-07	6.6E-06	4.2E-06	2.6E-06	1.8E-06
Skin	5.1E-07	5.5E-07	4.4E-07	4.1E-07	4.1E-07	4.8E-07	5.3E-07	4.9E-07	5.3E-07	7.2E-07
Spleen	6.3E-06	6.6E-07	1.0E-05	1.5E-06	1.4E-06	8.0E-07	8.6E-06	9.2E-07	2.3E-06	1.4E-06
Testes	3.2E-08	4.7E-06	5.1E-08	3.1E-07	2.7E-07	1.8E-06	8.8E-08	6.2E-08	7.9E-09	1.1E-06
Thyroid	1.3E-07	2.1E-09	8.7E-08	1.5E-08	1.6E-08	5.4E-09	4.8E-08	1.5E-07	9.2E-07	1.3E-06
Uterus (nongrvd)	1.1E-06	1.6E-05	7.7E-07	9.6E-06	5.4E-06	7.1E-06	9.4E-07	3.9E-07	8.2E-08	2.3E-06
Total body	2.2E-06	1.9E-06	1.9E-06	2.4E-06	2.2E-06	2.3E-06	2.2E-06	2.2E-06	2.0E-06	1.9E-06

*Decay data revised – March 1972. Reference – MIRD Pamphlet No. 10. Date of issue – 05-13-75. From Snyder, W. S., Ford, M. R., Warner, G. G., and Watson, S. B.: "S" absorbed dose per unit cumulated activity for selected radionuclides and organs, MIRD Pamphlet No. 11, New York, 1975, Society of Nuclear Medicine.
†The digits following the symbol E indicate the power of ten by which the number is to be multiplied. For example, 3.1E-03 is equivalent to 3.1×10^{-3} or 0.0031.

The foregoing determination of the total dose to the liver involved the summation of contributions from a number of organs; therefore, the total average dose to the target organ is determined by:

$$\overline{D}(r_k) = \sum_h A_h \, S(r_k \leftarrow r_h)$$

DOSE CALCULATIONS USING "S" TABLES (Table 7-6)
Problem 1

Estimate the dose to the *total body*, the *kidneys* and the *testes* due to the presence of 1.0 mCi of ^{99m}Tc in the kidney. Assume that $T_e = T_p$ and there is instantaneous uptake.

Dose to kidney ($\overline{D}_{KID \leftarrow KID}$):

$$(1{,}000 \ \mu Ci)(1.443)(6.0)(1.9 \times 10^{-4}) = 1.64 \text{ rads}$$

Dose to total body ($\overline{D}_{KID \leftarrow TB}$):

$$(1{,}000 \ \mu Ci)(1.443)(6.0)(2.2 \times 10^{-6}) = 0.019 \text{ rad}$$

Dose to testes ($\overline{D}_{KID \leftarrow TES}$):

$$(1{,}000 \ \mu Ci)(1.443)(6.0)(8.8 \times 10^{-8}) = 0.0007 \text{ rad}$$

Problem 2

Compare the dosimetry of iodine 131 and iodine 123 as used for thyroid evaluation studies. Assume the dose to be 100 μCi with a 20% uptake, the uptake period being negligible. Assume biologic excretion as a single exponential with a biologic half-life (T_b) of 90 days. The solution follows:

1. Convert T_b to T_e (90 days = 2,160 hr)

$$^{131}I : T_e = \frac{8.05 \times 90}{8.05 + 90} = 7.4d = 178 \text{ hr}$$

$$^{123}I : T_e = \frac{13 \times 2{,}160}{13 + 2{,}160} = 13 \text{ hr}$$

2. Complete the MIRD formula, given that the only significant dose contribution to the thyroid gland comes from the thyroid tissue itself and the "S" factors for iodine 131 and iodine 123 as taken from MIRD Pamphlet #11 are:

$$^{131}I = 2.2E\text{-}02$$
$$^{123}I = 4.0E\text{-}03$$

$$^{131}I : \overline{D}_{thy \leftarrow thy} = 100(.20) \times 1.443 \times 178 \times 2.2 \times 10^{-2}$$
$$= 113 \text{ rads}/100 \ \mu Ci \ ^{131}I$$

$$^{123}I : \overline{D}_{thy \leftarrow thy} = 100(.20) \times 1.443 \times 13 \times 4.0 \times 10^{-3}$$
$$= 1.50 \text{ rads}/100 \ \mu Ci \ ^{123}I$$

To compare the dosimetry for these two radionuclides that are used to perform identical functions is to justify the use of iodine 123. The tremendous reduction in radiation dose to the thyroid gland far outweighs the increased cost of iodine 123.

Table 7-7. S(embryo ← r$_h$), absorbed dose per unit cumulated activity (rads/μCi-hr), for several radionuclides and various source organs r$_h$ with the embryo as the target organ*

Source organs	Radionuclides					
	^{99m}Tc	^{111}In	^{113m}In	^{123}I	^{131}I	^{133}Xe
Adrenals	4.0E-07†	1.4E-06	8.6E-07	4.9E-07	1.3E-06	7.0E-08
Bladder contents	1.9E-05	5.7E-05	3.2E-05	2.7E-05	4.9E-05	9.8E-06
Bone (total)	7.6E-07	2.3E-06	1.3E-06	9.0E-07	2.0E-06	2.1E-07
GI tract (stom. cont.)	9.7E-07	3.0E-06	1.8E-06	1.1E-06	2.8E-06	2.1E-07
GI tract (SI and cont.)	1.1E-05	3.1E-05	1.8E-05	1.4E-05	2.7E-05	4.8E-06
GI tract (ULI cont.)	6.1E-06	1.8E-05	9.9E-06	7.4E-06	1.5E-05	2.1E-06
GI tract (LLI cont.)	7.6E-06	2.2E-05	1.2E-05	9.2E-06	1.9E-05	2.7E-06
Kidneys	1.2E-06	3.6E-06	2.1E-06	1.4E-06	3.3E-06	2.5E-07
Liver	6.5E-07	2.1E-06	1.3E-06	7.7E-07	2.0E-06	1.3E-07
Lungs	8.4E-08	3.2E-07	2.4E-07	1.1E-07	3.6E-07	1.2E-08
Marrow (red)	2.3E-06	6.6E-06	3.7E-06	2.7E-06	5.8E-06	7.0E-07
Other tissues (muscle)	2.6E-06	8.0E-06	4.6E-06	3.8E-06	6.9E-06	1.3E-06
Ovaries	2.0E-05	5.8E-05	3.3E-05	2.7E-05	5.0E-05	9.9E-06
Pancreas	6.8E-07	2.2E-06	1.3E-06	8.0E-07	2.1E-06	1.3E-07
Salivary glands	4.5E-09	2.4E-08	2.5E-08	7.3E-09	3.9E-08	4.2E-10
Skin	7.0E-07	2.1E-06	1.2E-07	8.3E-07	1.9E-06	1.9E-07
Spleen	5.4E-07	1.8E-06	1.1E-06	6.5E-07	1.7E-06	1.0E-07
Thyroid	4.5E-09	2.4E-08	2.5E-08	7.3E-09	3.9E-08	4.2E-10
Total body	2.8E-06	8.2E-06	8.4E-06	4.1E-06	1.2E-05	5.3E-06

*From Smith, E. M., and Warner, G. G.: Estimates of radiation dose to the embryo from nuclear medicine procedures, J. Nucl. Med. **17**:836-839, 1976.

†The digits following the symbol E indicate the power of 10 by which the initial number is to be multiplied, e.g., 4.0E-07 = 4.0 × 10^{-7}.

Dose estimated for the embryo

Just as the thyroid can be computed for radiation dose/100 μCi to the thyroid, so also can all other organs be computed similarly. One of the more important areas and certainly the area that produces the most anxiety and concern is the dose to the embryo. This is especially true when the dose was administered unknowingly to a woman shortly after the time of conception.

This was the subject of a scientific paper presented at the Sixteenth Annual Meeting of the Southeastern Chapter of the Society of Nuclear Medicine in Atlanta, Ga., in October 1975 and published in the Journal of Nuclear Medicine, vol. 17, pp. 836-839, in 1976 by E. M. Smith and G. G. Warner. Until this time, the dose to the embryo was considered to be equivalent to the dose to the uterus. In this work, "S" factors were generated with the embryo being the target organ from applicable source organs for a variety of radionuclides (Table 7-7).

The dose per administered activity was calculated for several of the radiopharmaceuticals commonly used in nuclear medicine (Table 7-8). Using tables like this and knowing the amount of activity administered, one can easily estimate the dose to the embryo.

Table 7-8. Dose estimates for the embryo*

Radiopharmaceutical	Rads per millicurie administered
^{99m}Tc-sulfur colloid (normal)	0.007
^{99m}Tc-sodium pertechnetate	
resting population	0.037
non-resting population	0.039
^{123}I-sodium iodide (15%)†	0.032
^{131}I-sodium iodide (15%)†	0.10
^{123}I-sodium rose bengal	0.13
^{131}I-sodium rose bengal	0.68

*From Smith, E. M., and Warner, G. G.: Estimates of radiation dose to the embryo from nuclear medicine procedures, J. Nucl. Med. **17**:836-839, 1976.
†Assumed thyroid uptake.

Problem. Using Table 7-7, estimate the dose to the embryo from an injection of 2.0 mCi ^{99m}Tc-labeled sulfur colloid.

$$\text{Embryo dose} = 2 \text{ mCi} \times 0.007 \text{ rad/mCi}$$
$$= 0.014 \text{ rad}$$

• • •

Extension of tables such as Table 7-8 will undoubtedly occur in the near future. At the present time, however, if the radiopharmaceutical does not appear in this table, then the "S" tables (Table 7-7) will have to be used.

LIMITATIONS OF THE MIRD CALCULATION

The MIRD formula has reduced the number of assumptions necessary to perform the dosimetry calculations over that required by the classic expression of dosimetry. The MIRD formula still has some limitations, however. If one looks at the tables in MIRD pamphlet 5, a second set of figures appears next to each absorbed fraction. This number is the coefficient of variation. This is a statistical limitation. A coefficient of variation of 50% or greater represents considerable uncertainty in the estimate of the absorbed fraction. Other limitations are that the kidney model is not divided into cortex and medulla and the bladder and stomach are a fixed size. Furthermore, the MIRD formula presupposes that the source is uniformly distributed within a standard size organ, which, of course, is subject to much patient variation. In the case of the dose estimates for the embryo, radioactivity was assumed not to cross the placenta; therefore, nonpenetrating activity was not included in the calculations. Authors are quick to point out in all discussions of dosimetry that the user should be aware of all the assumptions and limitations used in the generation of the data. However, as techniques develop, and as more information on the actual distribution of these radionuclides becomes available, calculations will become increasingly more accurate. Only in this way can the intelligent approach to radiation dosimetry and reduced radiation dose to the patient be better served.

Table 7-9. Absorbed fractions (Φ) for different photon energies (Eᵢ) from a uniform source in the liver – photon energy, E_i (mev)

Target organ	0.010	0.015	0.020	0.030	0.050	0.100	0.200	0.500
Adrenals			0.183E-03	0.440E-03	0.392E-03	0.270E-03	0.237E-03	0.198E-03
Bladder					0.169E-03	0.275E-03	0.389E-03	0.358E-03
Gastrointestinal tract (stomach)			0.171E-03	0.151E-02	0.360E-02	0.300E-02	0.271E-02	0.280E-02
Gastrointestinal tract (SI)	0.171E-03*	0.495E-03	0.117E-02	0.493E-02	0.108E-01	0.109E-01	0.100E-01	0.971E-02
Gastrointestinal tract (ULI)		0.575E-03	0.927E-03	0.318E-02	0.448E-02	0.401E-02	0.387E-02	0.364E-02
Gastrointestinal tract (LLI)					0.613E-04	0.149E-03	0.211E-03	0.391E-03
Heart		0.112E-03	0.132E-02	0.531E-02	0.762E-02	0.674E-02	0.570E-02	0.573E-02
Kidneys		0.105E-03	0.106E-02	0.437E-02	0.566E-02	0.437E-02	0.390E-02	0.386E-02
Liver	0.967	0.898	0.784	0.543	0.278	0.165	0.158	0.157
Lungs	0.139E-03	0.299E-02	0.859E-02	0.165E-01	0.147E-01	0.101E-01	0.923E-02	0.838E-02
Marrow	0.288E-03	0.182E-02	0.819E-02	0.228E-01	0.325E-01	0.206E-01	0.133E-01	0.107E-01
Pancreas			0.186E-03	0.107E-02	0.130E-02	0.105E-02	0.102E-02	0.822E-03
Skeleton (rib)	0.721E-03	0.447E-02	0.183E-01	0.402E-01	0.366E-01	0.181E-01	0.111E-01	0.867E-02
Skeleton (pelvis)				0.523E-03	0.265E-02	0.308E-02	0.216E-02	0.182E-02
Skeleton (spine)			0.393E-03	0.566E-02	0.217E-01	0.167E-01	0.108E-01	0.857E-02
Skeleton (skull)						0.629E-04	0.140E-03	0.187E-03
Skeleton (total)	0.721E-03	0.458E-02	0.209E-01	0.587E-01	0.803E-01	0.498E-01	0.324E-01	0.260E-01
Skin			0.136E-02	0.468E-02	0.558E-02	0.499E-02	0.507E-02	0.561E-02
Spleen				0.617E-04	0.533E-03	0.606E-03	0.645E-03	0.619E-03
Thyroid								
Uterus					0.564E-04	0.115E-03	0.136E-03	0.130E-03
Trunk	0.996	0.997	0.984	0.905	0.660	0.453	0.413	0.404
Legs					0.159E-03	0.480E-03	0.716E-03	0.141E-02
Head				0.110E-04	0.381E-03	0.493E-03	0.867E-03	0.106E-02
Total body	0.996	0.997	0.984	0.905	0.661	0.454	0.415	0.407

*Read as 0.000171. (E-03 means move decimal point 3 places to the left. E-02 means move decimal point 2 places to the left and so on.)

Table 7-10. Mass of organs used in the MIRD study*

Body organs	Abbreviation	Reference man report	Mass (gm) Phantom
Adrenals	AD	14	15.5
Bladder			
Wall	BLADW	45	45.13
Contents	BLADC	200	200
Gastrointestinal tract			
Stomach			
Wall	STW	150	150
Contents	STC	250	246.9
Small intestine and contents	SI	640 wall	1,044 wall plus contents
		400 contents	
Upper large intestine			
Wall	ULIW	210	209.2
Contents	ULIC	220	200
Lower large intestine			
Wall	LLIW	160	160.1
Contents	LLIC	135	136.8
Kidneys (both)	KI	310	284.2
Liver	LI	1,800	1,809
Lungs (both, including blood)	LU	1,000	999.2
Other tissue	OT	48,000	48,480 (2,800 gm suggested for muscle; 12,500 gm for separable adipose tissue)
Ovaries (both)	OV	11	8.268
Pancreas	PA	100	60.27
Salivary glands	SALG	85	Not represented
Skeleton	SKEL	10,000	10,470
Cortical bone	CORTB	4,000	4,000
Trabecular bone	TRAB	1,000	1,000
Red marrow	RM	1,500	1,500
Yellow marrow	YM	1,500	1,500
Cartilage	CART	1,100	1,100
Other constituents	—	900	1,370
Spleen	SP	180	173.6
Testes	TE	35	37.08
Thyroid	THY	20	19.63
Uterus	UT	80	65.4
Total body	TB	70,000	69,880

*From Snyder, W. S., Ford, M. R., Warner, G. G., and Watson, S. B.: "S" absorbed dose per unit cumulated activity for selected radionuclides and organs, MIRD Pamphlet No. 11, New York, 1975, Society of Nuclear Medicine.

BIBLIOGRAPHY

Blahd, W. H.: Nuclear medicine, New York, 1965, McGraw-Hill Book Co.

Chandra, R.: Introductory physics of nuclear medicine, Philadelphia, 1976, Lea & Febiger.

Dillman, L. T., and von der Lage, F. C.: Radionuclide decay schemes and nuclear parameters for use in radiation-dose estimation, MIRD Pamphlet No. 10, New York, 1975, Society of Nuclear Medicine.

Goodwin, P. N., and Rao, D. V.: The physics of nuclear medicine, Springfield, Ill., 1977, Charles C Thomas, Publisher.

Hendee, W. R.: Medical radiation physics, Chicago, 1970, Year Book Medical Publishers, Inc.

Johns, H. E.: The physics of radiology, ed. 2, revised edition, Springfield, Ill., 1964, Charles C Thomas, Publisher.

Quimby, E. H., and Feitelberg, S.: Radioactive isotopes in medicine and biology, ed. 2, Philadelphia, 1963, Lea & Febiger.

Rollo, F. D.: Nuclear medicine physics, instrumentation, and agents, St. Louis, 1977, The C. V. Mosby Co.

Smith, E. M., and Warner, G. G.: Estimates of radiation dose to the embryo from nuclear medicine procedures, J. Nucl. Med. 17:836-839, 1976.

Snyder, W. S. Ford, M. R., Warner, G. G., and Fisher, H. L.: Estimates of absorbed fractions for monoenergetic photon sources uniformly distributed in various organs of a heterogeneous phantom, MIRD Pamphlet No. 5, J. Nucl. Med. 10:5-52, 1969.

Snyder, W. S., Ford, M. R., Warner, G. G., and Watson, S. B.: "S" absorbed dose per unit cumulated activity for selected radionuclides and organs, MIRD Pamphlet No. 11, New York, 1975, Society of Nuclear Medicine.

Wagner, H. N.: Principles of nuclear medicine, Philadelphia, 1968 W. B. Saunders Co.

8 Biologic effects of radiation

Some of the specific factors involved in radiation protection were discussed in Chapter 6. The reason for various methods of radiation protection is obvious—to decrease the radiation dose to the human body. There is concern about radiation exposure to the human body because of its generally harmful biologic effect. Radiation acts on biologic tissue at the molecular level and therefore on the cell and its constituents. For this reason, exposure to ionizing radiations may result in changes in the highly organized molecular system, destruction of certain cellular elements, and, of greatest concern, altered function or death of the cell. In this chapter, the action of radiation at the cellular level and the somatic and genetic effects of radiation on biologic systems and organs will be discussed.

RATIONALE

Before proceeding into a discussion on the biologic effects of radiation, it should be said that the science of radiobiology is still in its infancy. For this reason, few fundamental principles concerning it are known, and only a few general statements may be made regarding radiobiology. One thing is certain—when biologic material is irradiated, a long chain of events begins to occur, and the biologic material absorbs a certain amount of energy from the radiation. Exactly what occurs and exactly what causes the death of the cell is not completely known. There are several actions of radiation on cells, the most prominent being that *profound changes or damage to the cells can result when a single charged particle passes through the cell nucleus.* This appears to be the case whether the cell is somatic or genetic in nature.

Somatic cells are cells with paired chromosomes; *genetic* (germ) cells, by definition, are cells with unpaired chromosomes. The somatic cells constitute all the cells of an organism with the exception of the reproductive cells. The somatic cells are generally more resistant than genetic cells to the effects of ionizing radiation, although damage to these cells leads to organic damage, loss of function of tissues or organs, and may even result in death of the cell. When damaged, however, they cannot bring about genetic alterations in the organism's offspring. Mutations can occur in somatic cells, but they cannot be transmitted sexually and therefore they disappear when the cell dies. Damage to germ cells, however, can be transmitted to the offspring.

The chain of events leading to cell damage or change begins as an ionizing particle passes through the biologic material. Since charged particles have the capability of ionizing and/or exciting atoms and molecules, the charged particles leave a path of such matter in their wake. In ionizing or exciting an atom, energy is released from the particle as it passes. In this way the particle loses its energy and eventually comes to rest, at which point it is no longer of radiobiologic significance. Energy releases along this track are called LET *(linear energy transfer)*. The LET is known to be a function of the charge and velocity of the ionizing particle. The greater the charge and the lower the velocity, the greater the particle's LET. A comparative example would be that of alpha particles and beta particles. The alpha particle is of low velocity (because of its large mass), and it has a positive charge of $+2$. A beta particle is of high velocity (because of its insignificant mass), and it has a charge of -1. For these reasons, the LET of the alpha particle is much greater than that of the beta particle. There have been many investigations as to the importance of LET in radiobiology. In general, it can be said that as the LET increases (as the number of ionization events increases), the lethal effect of radiation also increases.

As the high-velocity, charged particle enters matter, the LET is relatively small. The velocity is such that fewer ionization events occur. As each ionization event happens, the charged particle becomes reduced in energy and travels more slowly. In traveling more slowly, the possibility for an ionization event to occur is increased; therefore the LET is increased. As the particle is reduced in energy, it loses more and more of its energy per unit path until it finally stops. Just prior to the particle reaching rest mass the LET increases tremendously.

Action of radiation on cells

The way that radiation acts on cells is of two types: *direct action* and *indirect action*. Both actions are involved when a charged particle passes through a cell. Both actions can cause damage to the cell but by different mechanisms.

Direct action. Direct action is when a molecule is ionized and/or excited by the incident radiation itself. It has been already stated that the energy of the ionizing particle is reduced in energy by an average of 34 electron volts. Only a portion of this energy is used to remove an electron from a molecule (10 to 25 ev). The remaining energy excites the molecule. It has been shown that this excitation energy can actually break the molecule into smaller units that are identical because many larger molecules are composed of a chain of smaller molecules bound together chemically. Since the smaller molecules are identical, it appears that the breaks occur at the same bond. Further, since it is highly unlikely that the radiation would strike the same bond each time, it is highly suggestive that the energy is absorbed anywhere in the molecule and transferred down the molecular chain to the weakest bond.

For any significant effect to the cell, the molecule must be of extreme importance to the continued existence of the cell. Such molecules would be the deoxyribonucleic acid (DNA) molecule and the ribonucleic acid (RNA) molecule of the cell. Changes in these and other important molecules can temporarily, or permanently, alter cellular function. If the molecular change can be restored, then cell function is only temporarily lost. If the molecular change cannot be repaired, then the function of that molecule would be lost to the cell. The significance of such an event is related to the importance of the molecule's function and the number of other molecules that remain to perform the same function. The result of the event could vary from insignificant to lethal. If the molecule is not significant (and therefore probably in excess), cellular function may be unaltered. It is possible that these cells may be temporarily reduced or may be changed in function if enough of them are affected. In the latter case, they will be replaced in due course, and total cellular function will be restored. More often, however the radiation energy is absorbed by the molecule and distributed over the entire molecule. In this way, an insufficient amount of energy is able to be concentrated at the weakest bond and the molecule remains intact. For this reason the direct action concept of radiation damage is felt to be the least important of the two actions.

Indirect action. Indirect action is when a molecule reacts with a molecule or the product of a molecule that has undergone direct action. This type of action uses a number of physical and chemical events to describe the death of the cell. Since water is a major constituent of all biologic materials, water enters into the reaction that is believed to eventually cause the death of the cell after irradiation. The death of the cell by water is brought about by the formation of free radicals. The most important process following a series of complicated ionization events seems to be the dissociation of the water molecule into a free hydrogen radical ($H^\bullet$) and a free hydroxyl radical ($OH^\bullet$) according to the following formula:

$$H_2O \xrightarrow{\text{ionization}} H_2O^+ + e^- \rightarrow H^\bullet + OH^\bullet$$

Note that the hydrogen and the hydroxyl groups are not ions but short-lived and highly reactive radicals. The ionization event has broken the covalent bond, and these fragments possess unfilled electron shells. They carry no charge; therefore, they are not ions. They are neutral atoms in search of another atom with which to combine to fill their shells.

What happens to the hydrogen and the hydroxyl radicals after the breaking of the covalent bond is highly dependent on the LET of the particle. Two reactions are possible. The hydrogen and the hydroxyl radical could recombine to form water:

$$H^\bullet + OH^\bullet \rightarrow H_2O$$

This result is always in competition with the possibility of two hydrogen atoms combining to form hydrogen gas and two hydroxyl radicals combining to form hydrogen peroxide according to the following formulas:

$$H^\bullet + H^\bullet \rightarrow H_2$$
$$OH^\bullet + OH^\bullet \rightarrow H_2O_2$$

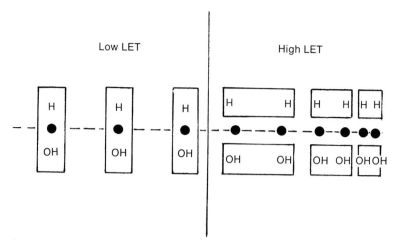

Fig. 8-1. Passage of particulate radiation through biologic matter, illustrating the ionization of the water molecule, the specific ionization, and the predominant recombination reaction that prevails as a result of the spacing of individual radicals.

Primarily, the LET value determines which reaction or set of reactions takes place. If the LET value is low (Fig. 8-1), the spacing of the ionization events will be far apart, and the probability that recombination will occur to form water is increased. If the LET value is high, the ionization events are closer together, and the possibility of the hydrogen radicals combining and the hydroxyl radicals combining is much greater. The resulting hydrogen peroxide is toxic to the cell, and death of the cell can ensue.

While water is an omnipresent molecule in biologic tissue and lends itself well to the discussion of indirect action, it is not the only biologic material that can do this. Any molecule can undergo ionization to yield free radicals. It's just that water is clearly the most abundant molecule in biologic material, and indirect action is considered by most radiation biologists as the most plausible explanation for the majority of radiation effects.

RADIATION EFFECTS AT THE MOLECULAR LEVEL

As indicated in the preceding discussion, the observable effects of radiation occur, either through direct or indirect action, by producing damage to molecules important to the continued existence of the cell. The importance of the molecules depends on the cell's location, number, and function. For instance, the DNA macromolecule (the genes) resides in the nucleus (the most radiosensitive portion of the cell), is few in number (to damage it is to inflict more harm than if it were greater in number), and provides a function that is extremely important (a storehouse for information necessary to the survival of the cell as well as to direct and control cellular activity). Another important molecule is the RNA. The RNA molecules are synthesized by the DNA macromolecule, leave the nucleus, and move into the cytoplasm where they serve as messengers of DNA, directing the synthesis of other proteins that serve in both a structural as well as a functional capacity in the cell. The RNA molecules reside in the cytoplasm, are somewhat greater in number, and provide a function somewhat less important than DNA. While the irreversible damage of one of these molecules would not be as serious as that of DNA, it still could be very damaging to the cell. Contrast this to the hundreds of proteins that are synthesized by the RNA molecule and their individual importance to the continued existence of the cell. Changes in proteins and other important molecules will be discussed.

Proteins. Virtually all activities of the cell involve proteins in some way or other. Some proteins form the structure of the cell. Some are the hormones that regulate metabolic activity. Others are the antibodies used in the body defense mechanism. Still others are the enzymes essential to many chemical reactions in the body.

Proteins can be described as chains of amino acids, each amino acid being composed of an amino group ($-NH_2$) and carboxyl group ($-COOH$) for the acid and a side chain (R) that characterizes the amino acid. These chains can have other molecules separating them, such as carbohydrates (glycoproteins) and nucleic acids (nucleoproteins). Sometimes these amino acid chains will coil on themselves, creating a three-dimensional helix configuration, held in place by cross links composed of various types of bonds (such as disulfide bonds and hydrogen bonds) across the space of the coil.

The amino group usually is the most radiosensitive portion of the amino acid, but because it is locked in so firmly to the carboxyl group, itself quite radioresistant, it becomes the side chain that is the most radiosensitive portion of a protein. Since this is the portion that distinguishes the protein from all other proteins, a change in this portion could reflect a serious change in the entire protein. Other changes would involve the break in the bonds that hold the protein in the coiled configuration. To do this may produce a change in its chemical reactivity because of exposed components of the protein that were not free to react prior to the radiation incident. It might also cause an uncoiling and disorientation of the protein's internal structure as well as destroy some of the spatial relationships important to the side chains. Changes in solubility have been observed following this phenomenon. Precipitation has been also noted as a result of increases in molecular weight when new components chemically reacted with the newly-exposed portions of the molecule following irradiation.

Enzymes. A well-known effect of radiation is the inactivation of enzymes. The exact extent to which such action produces irreversible cell damage is directly related to the dilution of the enzyme. It appears that enzymes are inactivated by the free radicals produced by indirect action of radiation. As the enzyme molecules become more dilute and are spaced farther apart, the likelihood becomes greater that the free radicals will combine with each other and not with the enzymes, producing no change.

Enzymes are an example of proteins that are great in number, are probably excessive in most instances, reside primarily in the cytoplasm, and are used only when needed by the cell to catalyze a reaction. To damage such a protein may not appreciably affect the life of the cell. If called on to perform some function, it might be unable to perform, but the damage would not be irreversible since other enzymes would be able to compensate in time. Damage of the protein does destroy the cell's system of checks and balances, however, for a time. A massive exposure to radiation would ultimately produce an irreversible effect.

Nucleic acids. The importance of two nucleic acids, DNA and RNA, has already been established. They are macromolecules having nitrogen type bases hooked to 5-carbon sugars and linked together by phosphate groups. One of the main differences between the two types of nucleic acids is that the sugar constituent in RNA is D-ribose, whereas the sugar constituent in DNA is 2-deoxy-D-ribose. Changes to these complicated and intricate configurations following irradiation include breaking of hydrogen bonds between chains, change or loss of a base, and breaking of a strand (between sugar and phosphate) resulting in separation of strands or cross-linking of strands to other nucleic acids or other proteins. Not all of these changes produce irreversible damage to the cell. Some of them can be corrected by the molecule itself as a result of its restrictive helix configuration. If separation or cross-linking to other nucleic acids or proteins occurs, irreversible damage has occurred to the macromolecule and possible to the cell itself.

Fats. All biologic materials have some lipid components. These include all sorts of material that are soluble in organic solvents, such as acetone. The major effect of radiation on fats is their conversion to peroxides (organic peroxides). The effect on the living cell is not too unlike the hydrogen peroxides produced during the irradiation of water.

Carbohydrates. Any compounds comprised primarily of carbon, hydrogen, and oxygen fall into the category of carbohydrates. A *monosaccharide* is composed of five or six carbon sugars, either in a ring form or in chain form. Monosaccharides can join to form disaccharides, trisaccharides, and polysaccharides. Very large combinations of these saccharides serve as starches, glycogen, and cellulose. It appears that radiation will cause the breaking of these long chains.

RADIATION EFFECTS AT THE CELLULAR LEVEL

It can be generally stated that *no* living cells are completely resistant to radiation. Cell damage manifests itself in many different ways. The damage may vary from alteration of a single molecule, which can be repaired at once, to death of the cell. Which portion of the cell is most sensitive and is directly responsible for the cellular damage has been a subject of debate for a long time. It is generally assumed that there is a significant difference between the radiosensitivity of the nucleus and of the cytoplasm of the cell. Nuclear structures, particularly the chromosomes at time of division, undergo dramatic changes as a result of radiation. The cytoplasm, however, does not appear to be as radiosensitive under the same radiation conditions.

Growth suppression. One of the most obvious effects on the cell from radiation is growth suppression. Cells decrease in number after radiation because mitosis (the process responsible for cellular division) and therefore growth are interrupted. It is generally agreed that cells with greater mitotic activity are more sensitive to radiation. This mitotic activity depends on the number of cells entering mitosis and the length of time that each cell spends in mitosis. The statement does not imply that the cell must be actually in mitosis at the time of the radiation to be damaged but only that it be mitotically active—one that will enter mitosis at some subsequent time.

This latent form of radiation damage manifests itself at the time of division. The cell loses the ability to divide successfully. This relationship between a mitotically active cell and radiation has a number of paradoxical exceptions. Some tumors, such as malignant melanoma and osteogenic sarcoma, are relatively radio-resistant even though they show considerable mitotic activity. Conversely, seminomas and lymphocytes are radiosensitive although they show no mitotic activity (the lymphocyte is one of the most radiosensitive cells in the human body). Other radiation effects on cells are *restriction of motility, and alterations in gland secretions.*

Effect on chromosomes. Another readily demonstrable effect of radiation is the effect on chromosomes. After irradiation, chromosomes become adherent. Varying amounts of radiation cause chromosome adhesions, nuclear clumping, and chromosome breakage. Chromosome breakage results in new arrangements of a higher general mortality in these groups of heavily irradiated people. They remain open, or they may unite with another chromosome. The genes of the chromosomes may be locked, duplicated, inverted, or moved to a new position on the same chromosome. Mutations may occur at the site of a chromosome break. Mutation-like changes may result from rearrangement of gene sequences. It is known that breakage can have a lethal effect on the cell. The hypothesis at this point in the science of radiobiology is that damage to chromosomes is the basis of lethal effects of radiation on dividing cells.

Giant cells. One of the outstanding effects of irradiation of cells is the production of the giant cell. This type of cell is produced in the radiation therapy of tumors. Cells may be damaged to the point where they are not capable of cell division, but the irradiated cell may not die immediately. It still may be able to carry on its metabolic activity. For this reason the cell becomes larger and larger. Since the cell can never divide, however, it ultimately dies.

Environmental factors. Environmental factors also play a role in the effect of radiation on living cells. The mechanism of action is not completely known, but oxygen content, temperature, and pressure can increase or decrease radiosensitivity. A general statement can be made regarding the three environmental factors. Radiosensitivity of a cell is directly proportional to the amount of *oxygen, temperature,* and *pressure.* As any of the environmental factors increases, so also does radiosensitivity; as it decreases, radiosensitivity decreases.

RADIATION EFFECTS ON BIOLOGIC SYSTEMS

When discussing radiation effects to biologic systems, it is necessary to divide all cells into three basic groups in order to understand radiosensitivity. The three categories are precursor cells, differentiating cells, and mature cells. Each organ system falls into a radiation response category because of the predominance of cells in each of these categories.

Precursor cells are regarded as stem cells or immature forms of the final form that the cell is going to take but very much undifferentiated. These are mitotically active cells used to reproduce cells that require replacing. These cells are very sensitive to radiation.

Differentiating cells arise from stem cells when they begin to specialize by losing their general character and assuming special characteristics. In this way, they can better serve in their specialized function. This usually involves considerable cell division. These cells are also very sensitive to radiation.

Mature cells are the cells that perform the necessary function of each cell. Very little mitotic activity occurs here, so these cells are relatively radioresistant. Function of organs continues following irradiation and is reduced only by the inability of the organ to produce stem or differentiating cells. The greater the life span of the mature cell, the longer the organ will continue to function and the less radiosensitive the organ will be.

The effects of radiation vary considerably from one organ system to another. The following discussion of some of the major systems will provide a basis for anticipating problems in a radiation accident.

Hematopoietic system

Organs that produce blood cells, such as the bone marrow, spleen, and lymph nodes, are extremely radiosensitive, as are the blood cells themselves. The mature circulating cells are relatively radioresistant in contrast to the blood cell precursors. The latter are highly radiosensitive, and this radiosensitivity is demonstrable within a few hours after irradiation by the effect on the subsequent circulating blood cells. The white blood cells (leukocytes) are the most radiosensitive and disappear from circulation first. The first type of white blood cell to disappear is the lymphocyte, followed by the granulocytes. The red blood cells (erythrocytes) disappear next, followed by the platelets.

The drop in lymphocytes, since they are the most radiosensitive components of the blood, becomes an irradiation indicator. If the lymphocyte count decreases to a level of 100 to 200/mm³ within 12 to 24 hours, the radiation dose is probably lethal. (The normal average lymphocyte count is 2,100/mm³.) A decrease to 500/mm³ in the first 24 to 48 hours is indicative of a questionable prognosis. If the count remains above 1,000/mm³, the prognosis is good; if the count increases after the first week, recovery is almost assured. Death may occur with no measurable drop in the number of circulating red blood cells, since a drop in cellular components is caused by nongeneration by the hematopoietic system. Lymphocytes disappear rapidly because they have a life-span of about 2 days, whereas erythrocytes have a life-span of about 120 days, so radiation effects are not as observable.

Hemorrhage is directly related to the circulating blood platelet level and the effects of radiation on capillaries. Since radiation causes a decrease in platelet count, hemorrhage is a symptom of radiation exposure. Bleeding rarely becomes severe until the platelet count is less than 20,000/mm³ (the normal average is 240,000/mm³). A decreased platelet count is clinically observed as a reduced coagulation time. Hemorrhaging can lead to circulatory embarrassment and ultimate cardiac failure.

Blood plasma is highly radioresistant, and there have been no predictable changes in its constituents to date. Furthermore, there have been no functional changes in circulation observed, such as changes in cardiac output or blood pressure, until after several thousand roentgens of radiation have been administered to the whole body. Circulatory embarrassment has been known to occur with lesser amounts of radiation because of tissue destruction of the vascular bed, fragility of the vascular walls, and occlusion of the vessels. The latter has been the cause of gangrene in the extremities of irradiated persons. One of the mechanisms here is that following irradiation the endothelial cells lining the lumen of the capillaries and small arteries will swell and block the lumen. Another mechanism is that sometimes the radiation damages some of the endothelial lining cells. These cells will eventually slough off, fall into the lumen, and be removed by such organs as the liver and spleen. However, before sloughing, the presence of these damaged cells will stimulate the undamaged endothelial cells to reproduce. Sometimes more cells are produced than were destroyed resulting in a pile-up of lining cells, occluding the capillaries, a phenomenon referred to as *overcompensatory hyperplasia*. Other mechanisms include capillary collapse produced by nearby inflammatory processes and clot or fibrotic formations at the site of destroyed cells. Whatever the case, the end result is the same — blocked blood supply to the area that the arteriole or capillary served. Cells in this area soon die for lack of oxygen and nutrients. Often, the only cure is amputation.

Reproductive system

The gonads (the ovaries in the female and the testes in the male) are highly radiosensitive. Mutations and aberrations occur in the chromosome system in either the ova or the sperm after irradiation. Sterility is also known to be a radiation effect. The latter can be either permanent or temporary. Both degrees of sterility occur at lesser doses in the female of a species than in the male. Temporary sterility occurs in female mammals after exposure to doses less than 200 r; permanent sterility occurs after exposure to doses exceeding 300 r. In the case of the male mammal, temporary sterility occurs when the testes are exposed to radiations exceeding 300 r; permanent sterility occurs after exposure to doses greater than 1,000 r. In the female mammal the ova and precursor follicular cells are the highly radiosensitive elements. Spermatogonia are the most radiosensitive element in the male mammal; the spermatocytes, spermatids, and spermatozoa are highly resistant. In the male mammal there is a noticeable loss of sperm motility and an increased incidence of sperm abnormalities after irradiation. One outstanding feature in male mammals, however, is the capacity for complete testicular regeneration after radiation exposure and the formation of functional spermatozoa.

Occupational radiation personnel and the radiation therapy patient are constantly worried about radiation causing sterility or impotency. Sometimes the two terms become confused and are used synonymously. They actually are two distinct entities. Sterility is defined as the involuntary, total inability to reproduce; potency is defined as the ability of the male to perform the sexual act. Radiation will affect sterility both on a temporary basis in low levels of radiation and on a permanent basis in higher levels of radiation exposure. Human potency, however, does not seem to be affected by radiation exposure except in lethal doses. Potency may be affected by fatigue accompanying radiation illness and by the psychologic factors that are always involved on exposure to any degree of radiation. However, the radiation itself does not produce impotency. Radiation to the testes depresses or prevents spermatogenesis, but it does not affect hormonal secretion; therefore, potency is not affected.

Lymphatic system

The spleen, lymph nodes, and thymus all exhibit high degrees of radiosensitivity, since all of them are related to the lymphatic system. The spleen shows inhibition of mitosis in less than an hour after medium doses of radiation. This is followed shortly by severe damage to the lymphocytes. Another radiation effect on the spleen is loss of splenic weight. In fact, this weight loss becomes a sensitive indicator of the dose of radiation to which the organ has been exposed. A most profound observation in the function of a spleen exposed to radiation is the cessation of the production of both red blood cells and white blood cells. During this period the precursor cells completely atrophy. If the radiation is such that hemorrhage occurs throughout the entire body, bleeding into the spleen becomes marked.

Lymph nodes and other lymphoid tissue are also highly radiosensitive at very low levels of radiation. After radiation, lymph nodes initially decrease in size. Then, depending on the amount of radiation, they either reconstitute themselves and regain their function or they become swollen, edematous, and hemorrhagic.

The thymus gland also shows a highly radiosensitive response caused by a large lymphocyte content. Special note is made of the thymus because in the 1920s many children were given x-ray treatments for enlarged thymus glands to reduce the gland's size and activity. There is evidence now that such treatment has increased the incidence of leukemia and thyroid cancer.

Gastrointestinal tract

The mucosal epithelium of the gastrointestinal tract is quite radiosensitive but not as highly sensitive as that of the hematopoietic system and the gonads. The first change to be seen after irradiation is the cessation of mitosis, followed by edema, degeneration, and necrosis of the mucosal epithelial cell. These early changes are responsible for the gastrointestinal syndrome of radiation sickness. This syndrome exhibits itself through anorexia, nausea, vomiting, and diarrhea. There are also functional changes that include the depression of pepsin and acid secretion by the stomach, increased mucus production by the small intestine and the colon, and impaired intestinal absorption. Another common symptom is dryness of the mouth caused by a decrease in salivation. As the radiation dose increases, the intestine becomes inflamed and bizarre forms of mucosal cells are produced. The diarrhea produced by the gastrointestinal syndrome appears thin, mucoid, or bloody. The latter is usually controlled by drugs such as paregoric. Vomiting occurs after very low radiation doses and can be of diagnostic importance. Early onset of vomiting is usually an indication of heavy doses of radiation, and it carries a poor prognosis. This symptom is also of diagnostic importance in ruling out psychosomatic causes and malingering. The vomiting can be controlled by antiemetic drugs if it is not of psychosomatic origin.

Skin

The skin is a relatively radiosensitive tissue of about the same magnitude as that of the gastrointestinal tract. Radiation effects on the skin are usually exhibited by a redness (erythema) and changes in its appendages (hair and nails). Loss of hair (epilation) is noticeable at fairly low exposure doses. With higher doses, depigmentation, ulcerations, and dermatitis occur. Treatment for skin contamination consists of prompt decontamination of the skin and hair with the use of detergents and copious amounts of water. Treatment of actual burn lesions is similar to the treatment of thermal burns. The burn is cleansed, itching and pain are reduced, and antibiotics are applied.

Eye

Protection of the eye has long been the concern of radiation workers. The most radiosensitive area of the eye is the lens. It is a well-known fact that opacities of the lens of the eye (cataracts) result from exposure to ionizing radiation. This fact is of primary concern to radiologists and x-ray technologists and is especially applicable to those working with fluoroscopic equipment. The protection of the eye is one of the primary considerations in the design of such equipment. Cataract formations have been noted in radiation workers who were involved in the development of the cyclotron and in Japanese survivors of the atomic bombing of Hiroshima and Nagasaki. The lens is such a simple structure from a histologic standpoint that cataract formations are the only lesions of radiobiologic significance. Inflammation of the cornea, increased photosensitivity, pain, and redness of the eye have been caused by radiation.

Central nervous system

The central nervous system is the most radioresistant organ system in mammals. Furthermore, the brain is considered more radiosensitive than the spinal cord; however, this radiosensitivity exhibits itself only after exposure to thousands of roentgens. Radiation effects on the central nervous system are usually caused by localized radiation exposure, such as that used in therapy, not by exposure to the total body. Under conditions of localized exposure, radiation may permanently injure the blood vessels of the brain or spinal cord, resulting in a lack of blood supply (ischemia) to the brain. Several thousand roentgens of radiation have also been known to destroy certain elements in the central nervous system, causing a dysfunction of vital nerve centers, after which death ensues. In general, however, the central nervous system is a highly radioresistant organ system.

All other organs

All other organs, including the heart, kidney, liver, and pancreas, are extremely radioresistant. The only changes found in these organs are caused by high radiation doses. Such changes include hemorrhage, infarcts, necrosis, and edema.

RADIOSENSITIVITY

According to the preceding discussion of biologic systems, all organs can be placed in one of three rather ill-defined groups: radiosensitive, radioresponsive, and radioresistant. All blood-forming organs, including the bone marrow and lymph organs, and reproductive tissues comprise the radiosensitive category. The radioresponsive group includes the epithelium of the gastrointestinal tract and the skin. The radioresistant group includes all other organs.

At the present time this division into three categories of response to radiation is a qualitative rather than a quantitative categorization. It is not well understood why such a range of response exists. An even more difficult phenomenon to understand is the tremendous degree of species variation regarding the amount of radiation causing death. Familiar medical terminology involving dose to mortality is LD_{50}. This term refers to the lethal dose whereby 50% of a species die. A similar term, $MLD/30$ (sometimes written as $MLD_{50}/30$), is used to describe mortality caused by radiation. This term refers to the median lethal dose whereby 50% of those exposed die in 30 days. This tremendous species variation is exemplified by two extremes: the guinea pig and the bat. Guinea pigs have an MLD/30 of 250 rems, whereas the MLD/30 value for bats is 16,000 rems. The paramecium, one of the most radioresistant forms of life, has an MLD/30 value of 300,000 rems. In man the MLD/30 value is 400 ± 100 rems. All other organisms have MLD/30 values that vary between that of the guinea pig and the paramecium.

Mammals seem to be more radiosensitive than birds, fish, and reptiles. The fact that they are *warm-blooded* organisms may contribute to this increased sensitivity. *Age* is an extremely important factor in that the adult organism or the adult cell is much more resistant than the embryo or the newly formed cell. This is the rationale for radiation therapy of cancer. A cancer is an uncontrolled growth and is therefore made up of predominantly newly formed cells. Increases in *temperature, pressure,* and *oxygen* content also increase radiosensitivity. *Unicellular* organisms are generally more resistant to radiation than multicellular organisms. Those tissues that *proliferate cells* needed for maintenance and function of the organ seem to be the most susceptible to radiation. Such tissues include the blood-forming components, the gastrointestinal tract mucosa, the precursors of the germ cells, the skin, and the lens of the eye. Mature cells of cartilage, bone, muscle, and the central nervous system are relatively insensitive to radiation.

Law of Bergonié and Tribondeau

According to the law of Bergonié and Tribondeau, radiosensitivity of tissue depends on a number of factors. According to these early radiobiologists (1906), radiation response in tissue was a function of (1) a high number of undifferentiated cells in the tissue, (2) a high number of actively mitotic cells, and (3) the length of time that the cells remain in active proliferation. It is not clear why lack of differentiation of the cell enhances radiosensitivity. It has been shown, however, that undifferentiated cells or cells in the process of differentiating are easily killed by radiation. The length of time that cells remain in active proliferation refers to the number of divisions between the most immature stage and the final mature stage. These stages vary between different types of cells. The longer the cell remains in active proliferation, the greater is its sensitivity to radiation.

While the law of Bergonié and Tribondeau remains fairly accurate in predicting tissue radiosensitivity, there are many exceptions to this law. These exceptions are usually related to (1) the oxygen content of the cell and/or (2) the ability of the normal tissue to recover following irradiation, to repopulate, and to assume tissue function. Increased oxygen content in the cell allows for the increased production of hydrogen peroxide by virtue of the oxygen combining with the hydrogen and hydroxyl radicals even in low LET areas.

Of even greater significance to loss of tissue function, perhaps, is the relationship of recovery between tumor and nontumor cells. If the tissue is irradiated and the normal tissue can recover and regenerate faster than the tumor cells, the effect on tissue function can be minimal. If the reverse is true, even though the tumor tissue is supposedly more radiosensitive than normal tissue, according to the law of Bergonié and Tribondeau, then the tumor tissue can recover and regenerate cells faster than normal tissue and the tumor growth is retarded, not stopped. For these reasons, tissue repair is extremely important to tissue function.

Cytoplasm

Radiosensitivity has also been linked to cytoplasmic factors. The ratio of nuclear volume to the volume of cytoplasm has been linked to radiosensitivity by many observers. The more cytoplasmic volume a cell has in contrast to nuclear volume, the more radioresistant is the cell. Further, cells with a large amount of cytoplasm are generally more radioresistant than those with smaller amounts of cytoplasm. It has also been noted that cells containing large numbers of mitochondria in the cytoplasm are more radioresistant than those with fewer numbers of mitochondria.

Organ function

Loss of organ function is considerably harder to predict because organs are comprised of a number of tissues, all having differing rates of radiosensitivity and differing ranks of importance to the normal functioning of the organ. As has already been seen, some organs are extremely sensitive to radiation, while others are resistant. Sometimes organ impairment is associated with radiation to the organ itself; sometimes it is induced by radiation to supportive tissues, such as blood and lymph. All of these factors play a role in organ function, making loss of organ function highly unpredictable.

Embryo

In modern day medicine, most of our attention dealing with radiation and radiobiologic effects focuses on the developing embryo. The reasons are numerous. Many of the occupational workers in a medical field are females of child-bearing age. Many studies utilizing radiation are performed on pregnant women in an effort to ensure a complication-free birth. More multiple studies using radiation are being performed on the general public as a whole, some of whom knowingly or unknowingly are pregnant. The age and marital state of the female patient is no longer a clue to potential pregnancy. Abortions are now available legally. And most important, many medicolegal cases center around the suspected radiation dose to the fetus. All of these conditions have made the general public and the medical community very much aware of radiation as a potential hazard to the proper development of the embryo.

In following the law of Bergonié and Tribondeau, it is no surprise that the embryo is highly sensitive to radiation. It has all the elements of high radiosensitivity. The cells are undifferentiated, particularly in the initial stages of development. The cells are undergoing mitosis at an extremely high rate. Further, these embryonic cells are the "parents" of millions of other cells just like them in the adult and any damage to any of these cells is multiplied by that order of magnitude. Much of the information regarding radiation effects to human embryos is extrapolated from animal research. The number of abnormalities produced in humans as a result of radiation exposure is far too small to accurately represent the true picture. The rational for extrapolation from animals is that every known malformation in the human fetus has been demonstrated by the irradiation of animals at various stages of development.

The stages of fetal development in the first three months (first trimester) are very important. One stage is that of preimplantation. Another stage is the period of major organ development. Still another stage is the period of neuroblast and germ cell development. Time of irradiation and the amount of irradiation with respect to these stages determines the effect on the developing fetus.

The preimplantation period (0 to 11 days after conception) is the time when the ovum has already been fertilized in the tubes that lead from the ovaries to the uterus. During the next 11 days, the fertilized egg will move down the ovarian tubule to the uterus where it will ultimately adhere (implant). All during this time the fertilized egg is starting to divide. Any major radiation damage during this period usually results in *prenatal death*. This can be as a result of death to the fertilized ovum caused by the radiation or failure of the embryo to implant in the uterus (also as a result of radiation to the embryo). One phenomenon that the embryo possesses to a remarkable degree and that becomes less active with time is that of regeneration and repair. If radiation were to kill a cell, the embryo has the capability of phagocytizing the dead cell and allowing one of the remaining undifferentiated (and undamaged) cells to assume the function of the dead one. In this way, the function is not lost to the developing embryo; however, the embryo will usually exhibit this change by being smaller. Obviously, this ability to have other cells assume these functions, decreases as more and more cells become differentiated. For these reasons, irradiation to the fetus during this stage, results in death, rather than abnormalities.

The stage of major organogenesis (11 to 38 days after conception) carries with it a high incidence of many types of abnormalities. During this phase, the cells are fairly well differentiated but formation and growth of the organs predominate with much mitotic activity. The key to determination of the extent of the abnormality lies in when, in the mitotic process, the cell damage occurred. If it occurred early in the formation of the organs, the organ may be so greatly deformed that it cannot function at all. If the organ is important to the survival of the organism (the embryo), then the damage would be inconsistent with life and the embryo would die. If the radiation incident occurred later in the maturation cycle, then a deformity may result with no organism death. During this stage, then, abnormalities predominate but the incidence of *neonatal death* is quite high.

Beyond 40 days after conception, the embryo is considered to be fairly radio-resistant. During this time, neuroblasts and germ cells are maturing. Irradiation of the fetus at this time may result in damage to the nervous system and reproductive organs.

In March of 1975, the NRC (Nuclear Regulatory Commission) addressed the question of fetal radiation in the occupational worker by way of their NRC Guide 8.13, *Instruction Concerning Prenatal Radiation Exposure*. This guide was to be used for instruction of all female workers regarding prenatal exposure risks to the developing embryo and fetus prior to employment. The intent of this publication was to stress the keeping of radiation exposures to pregnant women as low as reasonably achievable (ALARA*) even though the National Council on Radiation Protection and Measurements (NCRP) had recommended that the occupational exposure of the mother should not exceed 0.5 rem per 9-month gestation period (same exposure limit of nonoccupational workers per year). Evidence suggests a causal relationship between prenatal exposure and increased risk of childhood cancer (especially leukemia). Based on this knowledge, the female worker should be aware of her alternatives:

1. Decide not to accept assignments in these areas
2. Use more distance, more shielding, and less time to decrease the amount of occupational radiation received
3. On getting pregnant, ask for reassignment to areas of less radiation
4. Delay having children
5. Continue working and accept the small risk

The latter implies that nothing is going to be changed now that the female is pregnant. This is rarely the case. Thousands of female workers have been made aware of these concepts and have chosen to continue working in a radiation field. However, during pregnancy it is only natural to be more cautious of radiation areas and more precise with radiation protection techniques. This is the spirit of ALARA. It is no different than attempting to curtail smoking, drinking, and extremely strenuous activities during pregnancy. All of these agents and activities have been shown to have a causal relationship to fetal problems and should be discouraged as much as possible.

ACUTE SOMATIC EFFECTS OF RADIATION

When man is exposed to a large, single, short-term (from several minutes to a few hours) whole-body dose of ionizing radiation, the resulting injury is expressed as a complex of clinical symptoms and laboratory findings. These are collectively termed the *acute radiation syndrome*. This syndrome represents a clinical expression of the damage to many important organs simultaneously by depletion of ra-

---

*The subject of another NRC Guide (8.18) that had been published "for comment" at publishing time of this edition.

diosensitive cells resulting from their inability to reproduce themselves. From studies of survivors of nuclear bombing attacks, radiation therapy patients, and occupational radiation accident victims, the sequence of events following large whole-body radiation exposure can be divided into four clinical stages:

1. Initial stage — 0 to 48 hours after exposure
2. Latent stage — 48 hours to 2 or 3 weeks after exposure
3. Severe illness stage — 2 to 3 weeks to 6 to 8 weeks after exposure
4. Recovery stage — 6 to 8 weeks to several months after exposure

The clinical findings in the initial stage include loss of appetite (anorexia), nausea, sweating, and fatigue. In the latent period, which begins about 2 days after exposure, these clinical findings may become normal and remain that way for 2 to 3 weeks. The severe illness stage may include fever, infection, sensitive scalp, loss of hair, hemorrhage, diarrhea, lethargy, disturbances in consciousness and perception, and cardiovascular collapse. These symptoms depend entirely on the dose to which the human being was exposed.

Although responses of a patient to a given dose are difficult to itemize, Table 8-1 is presented to give some idea of what symptoms to expect in approximate dose ranges. According to this table, the first system to stop functioning is the highly radiosensitive hematopoietic system. If the radiation injury is more severe, gastrointestinal symptoms become predominate. Finally, as the radiation dose becomes extremely severe, damage to the relatively radioresistant central nervous system causes almost immediate death, although the exact cause of death is subject to controversy at the present time. The predominance of gastrointestinal symptomatology with doses of 600 rads and central nervous system complications after exposure to 3,000 rads does not indicate that severe hematologic damage has not taken place at these levels of exposure. These patients simply do not survive long enough to display the full manifestation of their hematologic injury. The information in Table 8-1 is based primarily on cases of external radiation exposure. Similar manifestations of this acute radiation syndrome may accompany the administration of internal radiation emitters, such as gold 198 and phosphorus 32, when given in very high doses. In general, however, the true acute radiation syndrome is not seen after exposure to internal emitters. The effects of internal emitters are usually chronic and occur after long-term, low-level exposure.

Hematopoietic syndrome

The hematopoietic syndrome occurs as a result of a single radiation insult in the 500 rad range given with a time period of a few minutes to a few hours and given uniformly over the whole body. The primary target in the hematopoietic syndrome is the bone marrow.

Immediately following the radiation, the bone marrow becomes rapidly reduced in cellular material, which is replaced with extravascular red blood cells and fatty substances. Depending on the severity of the radiation damage, fatty

Table 8-1. Summary of the acute radiation syndrome

Group	Dose (rads)	Symptoms	Treatment	System involved	Time of death
I	100	Anorexia; nausea; vomiting	Antiemetics	(Leukemia?) Increased aging?	Approaches normal life-span
II	200	Same as group I, plus slight anemia; infection; hemorrhage; conjunctivitis; sweating; purpura; scalp pain; hair loss, weight loss	Antiemetics; aseptic isolation (masked and gowned attendants); antibiotics and transfusions, if warranted	Same as above	Approaches normal life-span
III	500	Same as groups I and II: plus disorientation; shock; coma	IV feeding (calories and electrolyte balance); transfusion of whole blood and platelets	Hematopoietic system	10 to 30 days
IV	500 to 1000	Increased shock; increased hemorrhage; severe infection; fever	IV feeding (blood diet); bone marrow transplant, steroids and vasopressors; hemodialysis, if needed; antibiotics	Gastrointestinal tract	3 to 14 days
V	>5000	Immediate burning sensation over entire body; immediate vomiting and diarrhea; cyanosis; acute respiratory distress; papilledema; oliguria; WBC 41,000 by 16 hours; lymphocytes disappear by 7 hours	IV fluids; steroids; pressor agents	Central nervous system (?)	Hours to 2 days after exposure

substances can ultimately fill the entire bone marrow spaces. Regeneration of bone marrow will take place eventually, the success and speed with which it occurs being dependent on the amount of radiation. Although mitotic frequency might be restored, the cells that are so produced might be abnormal. This results in a reduction in number and a change in the kind of circulating blood cell. If the cell is abnormal (shrunken nuclei, clumped chromatin, aberrant chromosomes), it will be quickly removed from circulation. This anemia continues to worsen because of breakdown in capillary wall integrity with resultant hemorrhage (petechiae).

Lymph nodes are also affected by severe depletion of cells and disruption of architecture. This results in a decrease in white blood cells and the loss of the body's natural defense mechanism against infection. Another problem is the deficiency in the number of platelets that the radiation causes, resulting in increased clotting times and leading to the possibility of uncontrolled bleeding.

In the treatment of a patient exhibiting the hematopoietic syndrome, infection can be controlled by broad-spectrum antibiotics and the increased clotting time can be reversed by an injection of platelets. Death resulting from the hematopoietic syndrome takes longer than that caused by other radiation-caused syndromes. It is ultimately caused by the failure of the bone marrow to recover sufficiently to maintain its function. The red blood cell has an expected life span of 120 days. Those that were not destroyed or altered by the radiation accident will eventually die and be removed from circulation. Others are lost through hemorrhage. With only a few normal erythrocytes being produced by the bone marrow and a larger number of immature forms being produced, life for the organism will soon stop. If death occurs from this syndrome, it will occur within 10 to 30 days after irradiation.

Gastrointestinal syndrome

The gastrointestinal syndrome is seen as the predominant cause of organism death in ranges of 500 to 2,000 rads total body irradiation. The critical organ is the gastrointestinal tract — more specifically, the lining cells of the GI tract, both small and large intestine. These cells eventually become stripped from their villi. The villi themselves lose cells and become smaller, so that, at death, the intestinal villi are flat and completely void of cells. Regeneration is possible, and its success is a function of the radiation dose. Just as with the bone marrow, damaged cells will attempt to regenerate, resulting in abnormal forms.

The denuded villi play a role in two major areas of concern; fluid and electrolytes and infections. In the organism succumbing to the gastrointestinal syndrome, severe diarrhea, loss of intestinal absorption capabilities, and leakage of fluids through the denuded intestinal walls into the lumen of the intestine result in a critical fluid and electrolyte imbalance. One factor contributing to this problem is a reduction in food and water intake resulting from the loss of appetite exhibited by victims of this syndrome. Another factor is that the diarrhea has been shown to be largely the result of irritation of bile salts to the colon produced by a lack of resorption of these materials by the distal end of the ileum. The diarrhea can become so severe as to be hemorrhagic.

Infections certainly also play a significant role in the final stages of this syndrome. In the terminal stages, the entire body defense mechanism is practically destroyed. The white blood cells are depleted and the nutritional and electrolytic balance of the organism is destroyed. Under these conditions, the bacteria that are not normal residents of the GI tract can enter the body through the denuded villi and become life-threatening.

Death, if it occurs by this syndrome, will occur 3 to 14 days after irradiation, with a mean survival rate of 6 days in humans.

Cerebrovascular syndrome

The cerebrovascular syndrome is seen as the predominant cause of organism death in ranges in excess of 5,000 rads whole body radiation. It is possible to have radiation doses so high that the cerebrovascular syndrome and, therefore, cerebrovascular death occur as the radiation is being given.

The organism exhibits problems with irritability first, which is sometimes followed by apathy. Serious stages are manifested by problems in equilibrium and coordination and by convulsions, seizures, coma, and finally death. Many of these problems are a result of the breakdown of the blood-brain barrier, resulting in liquid infiltration and cellular infiltration into the meninges and choroid plexus, with edema occurring throughout the brain. Vasculitis plays a major role inasmuch as it is probably a contributor to the breakdown in the blood-brain barrier. All of these infiltrations appear to contribute to cell death by causing damage to the nerve cells (neurons) by way of increased intracranial pressure.

CHRONIC SOMATIC EFFECTS

Chronic somatic effects caused by exposure to radiation are more difficult to demonstrate with certainty. It was not until about 10 years after the discovery of the x ray and of natural radioactivity that it was realized that somatic effects from overexposure to ionizing radiation might not be evident until years or decades after the event. The discovery that radiation could have a chronic effect was based primarily on the evidence of changes in the skin. Burns and dermatitis, known to be a result of radiation exposure, progressed eventually to cancer of the skin. Knowing the positive agent for the burns, it was hypothesized that not all of the effects of radiation were acute in nature but that they could occur at some later time. This has since been supported by evidence from laboratory animal experiments. Other chronic effects of radiation are shortening of the life-span, early aging, increased incidence of leukemia, and increased incidence of benign and malignant tumors.

Shortening of life-span. Animal experimentation has demonstrated very clearly that shortening of the life-span follows single or repeated doses of radiation exposure. There is not, however, conclusive evidence that this is a general manifestation of radiation exposure in man. It is known that there is an increased incidence of leukemias and malignancies after radiation, and these are obviously going to reduce the life-span of individuals having these diseases. The problem is further complicated because it is difficult to extrapolate results of animal experimentation to man. It is also difficult to obtain such information in human populations. At the present time it can be generally stated that there is very little evidence of human life shortening from radiation exposure. Furthermore, there are as yet no data from man that provide a satisfactory basis for quantitative estimation of overall life-shortening effects. The atomic bombing survivors (60,000 still living in 1950, including 7,000 who demonstrated the major symptoms of the acute radiation syndrome) have been and are being carefully studied. Thus far, there is no evidence of a higher general mortality in these groups of heavily irradiated people. There has been some controversial evidence presented that radiologists die 5.2 years earlier than physicians not occupationally exposed to radiation. With improvements in radiation safety practices and radiation safety devices in recent years, this deficit in life-span has been shown to decrease.

Early aging. Early aging, the enhancement of the physiologic aging process, has been associated with radiation exposure. It has been shown that fibrosis of the skin, heart muscle, lymphoid organs, and endocrine glands follows irradiation. Chronic lung inflammation has been observed. Atrophy and defective development in the skin, lymphoid organs, bone marrow, and gonads have also been seen. There have been alterations in the pigment deposition in the skin and hair. These are all processes associated with aging. This whole concept of premature aging, however, is subject to controversy.

Leukemia. Increased incidence of leukemia has been reported in a number of groups of individuals exposed to radiation—radiologists, survivors of atomic bombing, children who were treated with x rays for thymus gland abnormalities, persons who received intravenous Thorotrast, and persons who were treated by x rays for rheumatoid arthritis of the spine. The body load of internal emitting radionuclides is kept to a minimum because of the possibility of their leukemogenic (leukemia-producing) effects in man.

Cancer. Development of cancer from radiation exposure has definitely been shown to be one of the chronic effects after total body irradiation. There seems to be little evidence contrary to this conclusion. Carcinomas have been noted in several groups of occupational radiation workers, as well as that large group of people injected with Thorotrast. Cancer, since it was first observed as a skin lesion on pioneers of the x ray, has appeared as lung carcinoma in miners of radioactive ores and as carcinoma of the mouth in some radium dial painters.

Current evidence supports a relationship between thyroid cancer and early childhood irradiation of the neck area. Clinical conditions in which such treatments were used included x-radiation of the thymus gland for "thymus enlargement," x-radiation for middle ear infections and acne, and the use of radium plaques for birthmark removals in the neck area. This situation has become so prevalent, records are so incomplete, and people living in the United States are so mobile that all persons living during the pre1940 era who suspect that such treatment was performed on them are not ill-advised to have a complete thyroid evaluation.

The radium dial painters were girls who painted luminous watch dials in New Jersey, Connecticut, and Illinois from 1914 to 1925. It was their habit to put a fine point on their brushes by shaping them with their lips. In so doing, they ingested the radium, and osteogenic sarcoma developed. Many of these radium dial painters (over 500 of the exposed have been studied) died with severe anemia and destructive lesions of the mouth and jaw. Of particular significance is the fact that no leukemia has been demonstrated in these cases of radium ingestion. It has been estimated that about 2,000 such luminous dial painters are still living, most of them in good health. It is known that about 50 have died as a result of this internal exposure to radiation. These cases have now become classic examples of the destructive effects of radioelements in humans.

Another source of information on the internal dose problem is the large group of persons who were injected with Thorotrast. This suspension of ThO_2 was injected for the purposes of diagnostic radiology from 1928 to 1945. In these patients, hepatic tumors seem to be the predominant neoplasm. There is a long induction period for cancer, ranging from 10 to 20 years.

GENETIC EFFECTS

Every human individual develops from a single cell formed by the fusion of two germ cells from the two parents. Each cell contains a number of microscopic, threadlike structures called *chromosomes,* which in turn contain genes. Genes constitute the material that determines the hereditary characteristics of the individual. The germ cell receives half its genes from each parent, and these determine the family likenesses.

Occasionally, something happens to the gene, and the likeness is altered. This alteration is called a *mutation,* and the characteristic that it governs may be changed in the offspring. These mutations may be of thermal or chemical origin, or they may be induced by ionizing radiation.

Some mutations are beneficial. The evolution of man is an example. Man has evolved to his present state through small changes from the average. Other mutations are harmful. Approximately 2% of all defects in the present population are of genetic origin: defects such as congenital malformations, idiocy, and so on. Some of the defects are undoubtedly caused by ionizing radiation, but the exact percentage is uncertain. There are two types of mutations—dominant and recessive.

Dominant mutations change the characteristic in the next generation, if either parent develops the mutation. Recessive mutations change the characteristic only if both parents develop the mutation and pass it on to their offspring. Dominant mutations are much rarer than recessives, and the chance of passing the altered characteristic to the offspring is even more rare. The transmission of the more common recessive mutations becomes progressively less in subsequent generations. If both parents have the recessive trait, the probability is that 50% of the children would receive it, 25% of the grandchildren, and 12.5% of the great-grandchildren. It is well known that everyone carries his share of recessive mutations from his ancestors. This is one of the arguments against "blood" marriages — the possibility that both parents would have the same recessive gene from their ancestors would increase the probability that their offspring would exhibit the recessive trait.

No accurate data exist on the genetic effects of ionizing radiation in man. Much work has been done on insects and animals in this regard, but extrapolation to man must be done with caution. The survivors of the atomic bombings in Hiroshima and Nagasaki are being carefully studied, but very little information is available from these studies. Some general statements may be made, however, regarding the genetic effects of ionizing radiation.

1. Any amount of radiation can produce some mutation; there is no lower threshold.
2. The rate of mutation is proportional to the radiation exposure.
3. There is rarely recovery by the gene after its mutation.
4. Damage to genetic material is cumulative. Long continued exposure to low-intensity radiation produces as much genetic damage as a single exposure to an equal dose of higher intensity. This is unlike somatic damage.
5. Radiation increases the frequency of gene mutation but produces no new kinds of mutations.

Doubling dose. One way to look at the effects of genetic mutation is by way of the doubling dose. At the present time, there are approximately 2 million spontaneous defective persons in a generation. A defective would include anyone with congenital malformation, idiocy, heart defect, and so on. If a doubling dose (between 15 and 30 rads in an acute exposure) was applied to the entire population, the number of defectives in that generation would increase to 4 million. Because of the nature of these mutations, that number would be reduced to 3 million in the next generation, 2.5 million in the next, and so on until the rate would return to 2 million defectives (Fig. 8-2). It is believed that the only way to maintain a level of 4 million defectives would be to continually irradiate the populace with a doubling dose. After many applications, the population would reach an equilibrium value twice the spontaneous value. But this would require many applications of the doubling dose.

· · ·

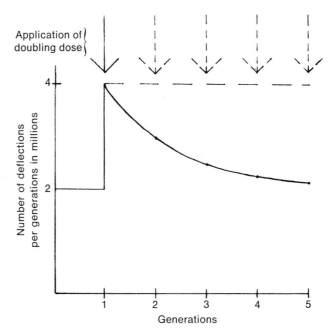

Fig. 8-2. Graph showing effects on mutations after one doubling dose (solid line) and after more than one doubling dose (dotted line).

Conclusions at the present time are that the genetic effects of radiation do not constitute a serious consideration in the production of damaging mutations. The studies of the Japanese bomb survivors reveal in one generation only a very few types of mutations. Furthermore, everyone carries a large number of damaging mutations received from ancestors. A few additional ones as a result of exposure to radiation will not alter the hereditary pattern significantly.

BIBLIOGRAPHY

Blahd, W. H.: Nuclear medicine, New York, 1965, McGraw-Hill Book Co.

Casarett, A. P.: Radiation biology, Englewood Cliffs, N.J., 1968, Prentice-Hall, Inc.

Chandra, R.: Introductory physics of nuclear medicine, Philadelphia, 1976, Lea & Febiger.

Dalrymple, G. V., Gaulden, M. E., Kollmorgen, G. M., and Vogel, H. H., Jr.: Medical radiation biology, Philadelphia, 1973, W. B. Saunders Co.

Hall, E. J.: Radiobiology for the radiologist, New York, 1973, Harper & Row, Publishers.

Johns, H. E.: The physics of radiology, ed. 2, revised edition, Springfield, Ill., 1964, Charles C Thomas, Publisher.

Pizzarello, D. J., and Witcofski, R. L.: Medical radiation biology, Philadelphia, 1972, Lea & Febiger.

Pizzarello, D. J., and Witcofski, R. L.: Basic radiation biology, Philadelphia, 1975, Lea & Febiger.

Prasad, K. N.: Human radiation biology, New York, 1974, Harper & Row, Publishers.

Shilling, C. W.: Atomic energy encyclopedia in the life sciences, Philadelphia, 1964, W. B. Saunders Co.

Shapiro, J.: Radiation protection, Cambridge, Mass., 1972, Harvard University Press.

Wagner, H. R.: Medical radiation physics, Chicago, 1970, Year Book Publishers, Inc.

9 Principles of radiation detection

Since ionizing radiations cannot be perceived by any of the human senses, it is advantageous to have some sensory device that can detect their presence. Furthermore, it is desirable to be able to quantitate the amount of ionizing radiation present, which is useful not only for radiation protection but also for diagnostic and therapeutic applications. A large number of such devices are available, and all have specific applications. These devices have been grouped into three main categories: gas detectors, scintillation detectors, and miscellaneous detectors.

GAS DETECTORS

The counting function of a gas detector depends on the collection of ion pairs produced in the gas volume by the passage of radiation to the detector. These ion pairs are collected by the walls of the gas chamber, which are electrically conductive. An external circuit consists of a DC voltage source in series with a sensitive current meter.

As ion pairs are produced by radiation passing through the enclosed volume of gas, the positive ions begin to migrate to the negative wall and the negative ions (electrons) begin to migrate to the positive wall of the detector, provided an external voltage is applied. The positive ion, which has a mass many thousand times greater than that of the electron, is accelerated toward the negative electrode at a slow rate compared to the rate at which the electron will travel to the positive electrode (anode) (Fig. 9-1).

The operation of gas detectors may best be explained through pulse heights. The number of ions collected at their respective poles is a function of voltage and is directly proportional to pulse height. A characteristic curve for gas detectors may be received by plotting pulse height versus voltage (Fig. 9-2). Fig. 9-2 outlines six regions defined by changes in pulse height response to changes in voltage. These areas are called the *recombination, ionization, proportional, nonproportional, Geiger-Mueller,* and *continuous discharge regions,* respectively. The two curves, denoted by alpha and beta symbols, are typical pulse height responses to these two particles. In Fig. 9-2 the alpha curve, because the alpha particle is more ionizing, corresponds to a level having 100 times the number of ion pairs initially produced by a beta particle. Each of the regions will be discussed individually. The kind of machine used is determined by the intensity of the radiation field and whether a specific particle is responsible for the intensity.

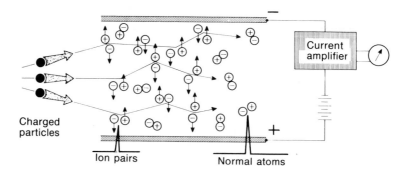

Incoming particles ionize atoms

Electodes attract ions

Arrival of ions constitutes current

Current is measure of particles

Fig. 9-1. Diagram of a gas detector and its method of radiation detection by attracting the products of ionization events to oppositely charged electrodes. (Courtesy U. S. Nuclear Regulatory Commission.)

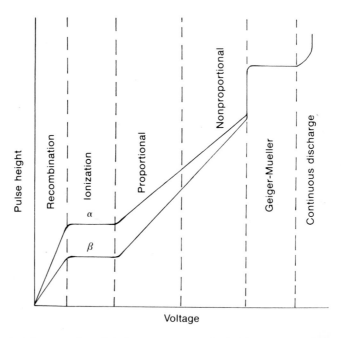

Fig. 9-2. Characteristic curve of gas detector responses to pulse height versus voltage. The curve demonstrates the response expected from two different particles passing through each of the three fundamental types of gas detectors: ionization, proportional, and Geiger-Mueller.

Recombination region. If no voltage is applied between the two electrodes, no direction is given to ion pairs produced by the passing radiation. With no voltage, no ions are collected by the respective poles and no pulse is produced. This is indicated by the curve beginning at the lower left-hand corner of Fig. 9-2. The initial application of a voltage permits the collection of some ion pairs; other ion pairs recombine. The latter will not affect the current and will not be observable on the meter. As the voltage is increased, the number of ion pairs collected increases rapidly because, by increasing the voltage, the probability of an ion reaching an electrode before it combines with a positive ion also increases. This increase in pulse height continues until eventually the region of ionization is reached.

Ionization region. In the ionization region the increase in pulse height as a function of voltage no longer exists. The curve flattens out. This area is called a *plateau,* or *saturation voltage.* No increase in pulse height is seen because the voltage is sufficient to collect all ions produced by the passing radiation. There is no longer a probability of recombination. Once this region is reached, further increases in voltage serve only to collect the ionized particles more rapidly.

The device used to measure radiation in this region is called an *ionization chamber.* When it is operated at the proper voltage (saturation voltage), the current (flow of electrons) going through the meter is a direct measure of the total number of ion pairs produced per unit time in the enclosed volume of gas. It is therefore a measure of the ionization produced by radiation.

The ionization chamber is used primarily in areas of high radiation intensity, such as measuring the output of an x-ray tube. Since one ion pair is produced and collected per ionization event, the pulses from single ionization events are much too small for even the most delicate electric meter to register. The proportional pulse heights of the alpha and beta curves allow differentiation between the types of emissions.

The ionization chamber may be a portable dose rate meter, such as the "Cutie Pie," which measures the intensity of radiation per unit time (r/hr), or it may be a dose meter such as the condenser-r meter (a calibration instrument) or a pocket dosimeter (a personnel monitoring device). Most dose calibrators also employ the ionization principle.

Dose rate meter. The portable dose rate meter is an enclosed volume of gas with a sensitive current meter and a voltage usually supplied by dry cells. The dry cells are such that a few hundred volts are supplied to the system so that the saturation voltage is reached. Although generally used in high-intensity radiation fields, dose rate ionization meters that measure very low intensities are available. These are ordinarily very expensive and heavy. The usual ionization type survey meter is seen in Fig. 9-3, *A.*

Dose meters. Other ionization chambers are available that measure just the quantity (dose) of radiation rather than intensity (dose delivered over a certain unit of time).

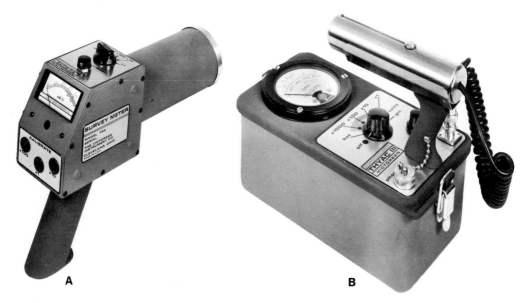

Fig. 9-3. A, Ionization type dose rate survey meter. **B,** Geiger-Mueller type dose rate survey meter. (Courtesy Victoreen Instrument Co., Cleveland, Ohio.)

An ionization chamber can be charged to a certain voltage and the voltage source disconnected. When this chamber is exposed to ionizing radiation, the ions are collected at their respective poles, and the collection decreases the voltage (discharges) proportionally. The discharge is measured on a voltage meter that is calibrated to read in units of radiation intensity.

The dose meter must be initially charged to predetermined voltage. This is accomplished by a charger. Some chambers require a separate reader, in which case the charger and reader are in a self-contained charger-reader unit. Other chambers (dosimeters, primarily) are self-reading. In this case the chamber incorporates a quartz fiber voltage meter, which, when held up to the light, casts a shadow on a scale calibrated in units of dose (Fig. 9-4).

Proportional region. As the voltage is increased beyond the saturation voltage, another rise in the number of ion pairs collected is seen. This area is called the region of proportionality. It has already been stated that in the ionization region all ion pairs formed are collected. With additional voltage, however, there is an increase in the number of ion pairs collected (Fig. 9-2). This increase in number of ion pairs collected cannot result from increased primary ion collections, since all have been accounted for in the region of ionization. The increase is caused by the phenomenon called *gas amplification*. At higher voltages, the increased speed or energy acquired by the ions during collection eventually gives them the capability of ionizing other gas atoms in their path to their collecting electrode (Fig. 9-5). The path of the electron as it makes its way to the positive electrode becomes tor-

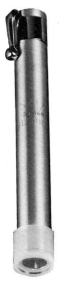

Fig 9-4. Ionization type self-reading dose meter, commonly called a dosimeter. (Courtesy Victoreen Instrument Co., Cleveland, Ohio.)

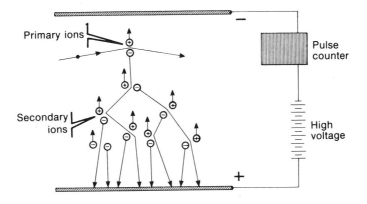

Electrons receive enough energy to ionize

Avalanche of secondaries

Current multiplied by 1,000 to 1,000,000

Fig. 9-5. Diagram of a gas detector illustrating the phenomenon of gas amplification that follows the primary ionization event. This occurs when the voltage between the electrodes is sufficiently high, which is the case in the area of proportional counting. (Courtesy U. S. Nuclear Regulatory Commission.)

tuous, since it rebounds from one neutral molecule to another. If the electric field is sufficient, as it is in this proportional region, these electrons can obtain enough energy to ionize a neutral molecule on collision and thus create an additional ion pair, which in turn will be collected also. Because of this phenomenon, an amplification occurs whereby *more than one* ion is collected per ionizing event, in contrast to that which occurs in the ionization region. As the voltage increases in this region, the gas amplification phenomenon becomes even greater. The secondary ions also acquire enough energy to ionize other neutral atoms on their path to the positive electrode, thereby creating other secondary ion pairs. This phenomenon is called an *avalanche.*

The device used in this region is called a *proportional counter.* Many have a continuous flow of gas through the detector. This counter has a distinct advantage over the ionization chamber in that the current pulse height produced by the passage of a single charged particle is large enough to be detected. Furthermore, the pulse heights have maintained a proportionality, so that low-intensity radiation can be detected as to alpha or beta emissions by the sorting of the pulses. A problem arises because, even though the current pulses are detectable, they are so small that only the most delicate and elaborate electronic devices are used. These are generally not used in a routine nuclear medicine laboratory. They are used for detecting low-level contamination of alpha particles, as in the case of a possible leak of a radium needle used in therapy.

Nonproportional region. Further increases in the voltage result in the two curves of Fig. 9-2 coming closer together. This region is called the region of nonproportionality. In this region true proportionality between primary ionization and the number of ions collected is no longer maintained. Instead, the pulse height becomes more and more a function of the applied voltage and less and less a function of the amount of initial ionization, as the curves in Fig. 9-2 come together and lose proportionality entirely. This region is not important from the standpoint of radiation detection.

Geiger-Mueller region. Further increases in voltage result in a sharp rise in the curve in Fig. 9-2. This is called the Geiger-Mueller region. In this region the pulse height shows no difference as to primary ionization events, so there is no distinction between ionizing particles. Gas amplification is so intense in this region that a limiting value has been reached. High acceleration in this region produces a catastrophic avalanche of ions delivering a mass of electrical pulses to the collecting electrode. The avalanche of ions results from the production of low-energy photons due to Bremsstrahlung. The voltage in the region is so high and the energy acquired by the negative member of the ion pair (electron) is so great that they create Bremsstrahlung photons on their path to the positive electrode (anode). The photons have the ability of striking the negative electrode (cathode) and knocking off electrons from its surface. They traverse the entire gas volume on their way to the anode, creating more Bremsstrahlung and secondary ion pairs. In this way, ionization is spread throughout the entire gas volume.

The size of the pulse is no longer in proportion to the initiating event. This is called the *Geiger effect*. The voltage at which Geiger-type counting becomes established is called the *threshold*. It is followed by a *plateau*, over which the counting rate increases slowly. The device for measurement of radiation in this region is called the Geiger counter, or G-M counter. The Geiger counter is applicable to areas of low-intensity radiation, such as determining the extent of a radioactive spill in a routine nuclear medicine laboratory, because a tremendous number of electrons are collected per single ionization event. This is in sharp contrast to the ionization chamber where only one electron is collected per single ionization event.

The Geiger counter (Fig. 9-3, *B*) has some disadvantages. Since one ionization event spreads ionization through the entire gas volume, a second ionization event may go undetected. The time during which the counter cannot respond to another ionizing event is called its *dead time*, which makes the Geiger counter grossly inefficient. Another disadvantage is that proportionality is lost. The life of a counter is the number of counts that can be accumulated before deterioration of the gas takes place. The counting life of a G-M tube is ordinarily in the range of 1 billion to 10 billion counts. This means that in the usual applications of such a counter, the shelf life would be several years. As the tube ages, the plateau of the Geiger counter becomes shorter until eventually stable operations can no longer be maintained.

Continuous discharge region. If the voltage is raised significantly beyond the G-M region, a rapid rise in numbers of ions collected is seen. This is the region of continuous discharge. Up to this point the discussion has been devoted primarily to the collection of electrons at the anode. Meanwhile, however, the positive ions, because of their mass, move slowly toward the cathode, where they are eventually neutralized.

As the positive ion approaches the negative electrode, it acquires an electron and is deionized. Since it requires energy to ionize the gas, energy must be released on deionization. This energy is released in the form of ultraviolet light, which has sufficient energy to cause another electron to be ejected from the cathode. These additional free electrons enter the gas volume and proceed toward the anode just as did the initial electrons from the primary ionization event. Furthermore, these electrons initiate avalanches on their path to the positive electrode just as did the primary ionization event. The collection of electrons from these events results in an increased number of ion collections, accounting for the sharp rise in the continuous discharge region. If this is allowed to continue, the electrode surfaces of the counter are damaged, and the counter may even be destroyed. The continuous discharge can be stopped to a certain degree by a process called *quenching*. This process limits the discharge process. It can be done by momentarily reducing the voltage on the tube or by incorporating a suitable constituent into the counting gas.

SCINTILLATION DETECTORS

Certain materials have the property of emitting a flash of light or scintillation when struck by ionizing radiation. A scintillation detector is a sensitive element used to detect ionizing radiation by observing the scintillation induced in the material. When a light-sensitive device is affixed to this special material, the flash of light can be changed into small electrical impulses. The electrical impulses are then amplified so that they may be sorted and counted to determine the amount and nature of radiation striking the scintillating materials. Scintillators are used to determine the amount and/or distribution of radionuclides in one or more organs of a patient for diagnostic purposes.

The procedure of recording a scintillation involves several systems: the detector, the photomultiplier, a high-voltage power supply, the preamplifier, the amplifier, gain controls, a pulse height analyzer, and the display mode. All these will be treated individually, showing the sequential stages of the detection and recording process of a disintegration.

Detector. Two major types of scintillation detectors are currently being used: crystal and liquid. Since the liquid scintillation detector is not as common in routine nuclear medicine laboratories, it will be discussed only briefly.

Liquid detector. Scintillating solutions can be prepared so that when radioactive materials are added to the solution, the radiations are detected through light production. The light is detected and measured through a system of one or more photomultiplier tubes and ancillary electronic equipment to analyze and count the radiations. The liquid solution contains the material being counted, a solvent, and a scintillator. There are a variety of liquid scintillator materials, most of which are organic compounds. The solvents are primarily aromatic hydrocarbons, which efficiently transfer energy from the point of emission to the scintillator molecule. The use of liquid scintillation materials has its greatest advantage in its ability to detect β^- emissions or weak energy gamma rays, since the radioactive material is mixed with the scintillating material so that there is little loss of emissions by absorption before they reach the detector. Such absorption could be by the cover of the detector or by self-absorption.

Crystal detector. The most widely used scintillation detector is the solid type—a sodium iodide (NaI) crystal activated with thallium, commonly written NaI(Tl). Pure sodium iodide crystals do not scintillate at room temperature. However, if impurities such as thallium are added, centers of luminescence are produced that can be excited at room temperature by ionizing radiation.

Sodium iodide is hygroscopic (retains water) and must be kept in a moisture-free atmosphere. Consequently, the crystal is hermetically sealed. It is enclosed by an aluminum container on all sides except that side attached to the photomultiplier tube (Fig. 9-6). A glass or plastic window protects it on this end. The inside surfaces of the container have reflective capabilities. More recently, the crystal and photomultiplier have been produced as an integral assembly, eliminating the necessity for the glass or plastic shield, and the entire assembly is hermetically sealed. Should the crystal or the assembly become damaged so that there is a break in the seal and moisture enters, the crystal shows a yellow discoloration (probably caused by free iodine).

The process of detection is initiated when an incident gamma ray enters the crystal. Under ideal conditions the energy is eventually totally absorbed. This is usually accomplished through a series of Compton collisions with subsequent total absorption of the energy by a photoelectric collision. (Pair production is also possible if the incident gamma ray is greater than 1.02 mev of energy.) Each time such a Compton collision occurs, some of the energy of the incident gamma ray is

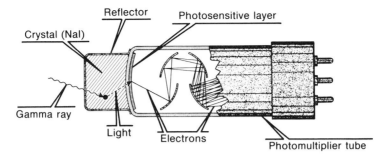

Total light to tube nearly proportional to gamma ray energy

If 1 electron ejects 5 from a dynode, 11 dynodes result in 5^{11}

or

about 50 million electrons output

Fig. 9-6. Crystal photomultiplier assembly illustrating the detection of a gamma ray by the crystal and its subsequent amplification through the photomultiplier tube. (Courtesy U. S. Nuclear Regulatory Commission.)

transferred to an electron that will produce luminescent light in proportion to its energy. The light is in the form of small flashes following the interactions of the ejected electrons. If the energy of the incident gamma ray is high, many Compton collisions will occur before the energy is totally absorbed. The increased number of Compton collisions will produce more secondary electrons that will, in turn, produce more flashes of light. If the energy of the gamma ray is low, fewer collisions will occur before total absorption; therefore, there will be fewer flashes of light. These small flashes of light, although emitted in a sequential manner, appear to the human eye or on the photomultiplier tube as a single flash or shower of light. The intensity of the light is directly proportional to the number of flashes of light. Since the number of flashes increases with energy of the gamma ray, it can be said that the intensity of the light is proportional to the energy of the incident gamma ray. This flash of light is eventually directed to the photomultiplier tube, either by reflection from the interior surface of the aluminum housing or by the direction in which it was emitted.

Photomultiplier. The photomultiplier is a light-sensitive device that is optically connected to the sodium iodide crystal. Its purpose is to convert the light energy from the crystal to electrical energy and amplify the resultant pulse of electricity. The photomultiplier tube consists of a photocathode and a series of 10 dynodes. The photocathode receives the flash of light from the crystal. The photocathode consists of a material that responds to waves of light energy, much like any atom responds to waves of gamma energy in the Compton effect; the incident light wave hits the atoms of the photocathode and causes electrons to be ejected. This is called *photoemission*. The principle of this operation is not unlike that which occurs in "electric eye" applications. The number of electrons released from the photocathode is directly proportional to the intensity of the light from the crystal.

As the electrons are emitted from the photocathode, they are drawn to the first of the 10 dynodes in the photomultiplier tube (Fig. 9-6). They are drawn to the dynode because of an applied voltage between the photocathode and that dynode. This voltage accelerates the electron, impinging it on the dynode with such force that more than one electron is released from the dynode. This is called *secondary emission*. These electrons are then drawn to the second dynode by a similar increase in applied voltage, whereupon secondary emission occurs again. This process continues throughout the entire photomultiplier tube. By the time the electrons have left the tenth dynode, the number of electrons released may be on the order of millions. The photomultiplier tube therefore possesses the ability to convert one flash of light to a burst of millions of electrons—hence the name photomultiplier. The usual terminology to describe this burst of electrons is a voltage pulse, and the number of electrons collected at the last dynode is proportional to the voltage pulse height.

A system of proportionality exists throughout the entire crystal photomultiplier assembly. This can be summarized by the following:

1. The pulse height is proportional to the number of electrons received at the last dynode, which is in turn dependent on the number of electrons released by the photocathode.
2. The number of electrons released by the photocathode is directly proportional to the intensity of the light received from the crystal.
3. The intensity of the light received from the crystal is directly proportional to the energy of the incident gamma ray.
4. *The pulse height is directly proportional to the energy of the incident gamma ray.*

High-voltage power supply. In any standard counting device (scaler or rate meter) almost invariably there is a separate voltage supply unit to provide high voltage to the photomultiplier tube. The total high voltage applied to the tube is divided among the various dynodes. For instance, if the voltage is 500 v, a 50 v potential difference exists between successive dynodes (voltage and potential difference are synonymous). If 1,000 v were applied to the photomultiplier tube, a potential difference of 100 v would exist between successive dynodes. The purpose of the high-voltage power supply is to provide enough "attraction" of the electrode that secondary emission will occur each time an electron hits a dynode. It is important that this high-voltage power supply be very stable. Instability of this voltage power supply is called *drift*. It may be caused by temperature change, change in line voltage, and so on. The reason for being concerned with drift, or rather the lack of it, is its effect on secondary emission. The number of secondary electrons produced by each electron that strikes a dynode is directly dependent on the voltage that exists between the two dynodes. Should the voltage at time of calibration be such that 5 electrons are released by secondary emission for each electron striking the dynode, then a drift in the voltage might cause only 4 electrons to be given off by secondary emission. This would alter the clinical results considerably. (This will become clearer during the discussion of pulse height analysis.)

The drift may occur upward as well. If it is sufficient, the voltage becomes so great that electrons are pulled off the dynodes without other electrons striking the dynode. This is referred to as *thermal emission,* or "noise." This phenomenon is easily demonstrated by increasing the voltage without a source of radioactivity. Eventually a high count rate is received, caused by thermal emission.

Preamplifier. The preamplifier is generally found at the rear of the detector assembly. The word "preamplifier" is a misnomer because it implies that the size of the voltage pulse is amplified in some manner. The actual result, however, is that it is usually a little less in amplitude because of the phenomenon of transmission of electrical power known as *impedance*. This is a fairly complicated principle, the definition of which is not of particular importance to nuclear medicine personnel. Impedances between the photomultiplier tube and amplifier must be matched so that there is no loss of power. For this reason, a reduction in pulse height is sometimes necessary. The preamplifier also provides a driving force, characteristics of which are such that the pulse will not be lost in the several feet of cable connecting the detector to the main scaler chassis. The pulse is then fed into the amplifier.

Amplifier. The pulses that are fed into the amplifier have a wide variation in pulse height because there is a wide variation in energies of gamma rays striking the scintillation crystal. All of these pulses must be increased in amplitude by a constant factor so that the final pulse is still proportional to the energy lost by the gamma ray in the crystal. This is called *linear amplification*. Nonlinear amplification would defeat the purpose of pulse height analyzers (p. 180) because all pulses, regardless of their size, would be amplified to the same height. The amplifier consists of four tubes or transistors in two successive sections. The voltage gains for the two sections are approximately 70 to 120, so that the overall amplification is something more than 8,000. The amplifier receives pulses on the order of millivolts. If 1 mv were sent through this amplifier, it would be increased to 8 v. The amplifier is capable of amplifying to 100 v or more with negligible distortion.

Gain control. Between the two sections of the amplifier there is a stepped gain control. This allows the operator to increase or decrease the amplification as desired. In scalers there are usually five such positions represented in a variety of ways, depending on the manufacturer of the detector. Gain control values are usually represented by the numbers 32, 16, 8, 4, and 2 or 4, 2, 1, 0.5, and 0.25. Regardless of their value, they do the same thing. The five steps on the gain control represent full gain, one half, one fourth, one eighth, and one sixteenth of the maximum gain; at each step the amplification is one-half that of the next higher step. This type of gain is called an *inverse gain*. Other numerical sequences are also possible, not always representing the halving process. Equipment manuals should be consulted.

The exact opposite is true in the utilization of gain settings on most scanners. These settings are represented by the numbers 1, 2, 5, and 10, which, rather than decreasing the amplification by factors of one half, actually increase the amplification by the factor indicated by the number. Therefore a pulse of a certain height on a gain of 1 would be increased to twice the height on the gain of 2, five times the height on the gain of 5, and ten times the height on the gain of 10. This is called a *true gain*.

A simplified explanation of gain settings is shown in Fig. 9-7. The dark line (third from the top) represents the actual settings on the gain control. This is expressed as a range of 0 to 100 v, equivalent to 0 to 1,000 kev on that gain setting. The usual procedure is to calibrate on midgain (a value of 8 or 1, depending on the settings available). By calibrating on this gain, the operator has essentially set each small division on the discriminator dials (which have 1,000 small divisions) to be equal to that number in kev. The gain setting essentially expands or contracts that scale, depending on the gain settings used. If the operator has amplified the pulse to 50 v (500 kev), by changing the gain setting to 16 (or 2) that same pulse would no longer be found at the 500 units setting, but would be found at approximately the 250 setting. If the settings are changed to 32 (or 4), that same pulse will now be found at a 125 value. The converse is also true. If, going back to the gain settings of 8 (or 1), the operator is analyzing a 10 v pulse (100 kev), the pulse would be found at 100 kev. If the gain settings are changed to 4 (or 0.5), the pulse will now be seen at a setting of 200 kev, or if the gain setting is changed to 2 (or 0.25), that same pulse will be seen at 400 kev units. By the increasing of the numerical value of the gain setting, the pulse height has actually been decreased, and therefore the operator must go down scale to receive it; conversely, by the decreasing of the gain settings, the pulse height has actually been increased, and the operator must go up scale to receive the pulse.

In using the true gain settings as found on some scanners, the figures to the right in Fig. 9-7 apply. As the gain setting is increased, the pulse amplitude is also increased; therefore, the operator must go up in analyzer units to receive the pulse. A 100 kev pulse on range 1 would be found at 100 kev units; however, on range 2 the same pulse would be found at 200 kev units, on range 5 at 500 kev units, and on range 10 at 1,000 kev units.

Most linear amplifiers will only analyze pulses from 0 to 100 v high. This ability to analyze is most accurate from 10 to 15 v high to 100 v high. If low-energy pulses are to be amplified correctly and subsequently analyzed, they must be amplified further by the gain settings. For example, if an operator were using iodine 125, which has 35 kev (3.5 v), inaccuracies would result if it were to be analyzed on gain settings of 8 (or 1) or on scanner settings of 1, since the pulse is not high

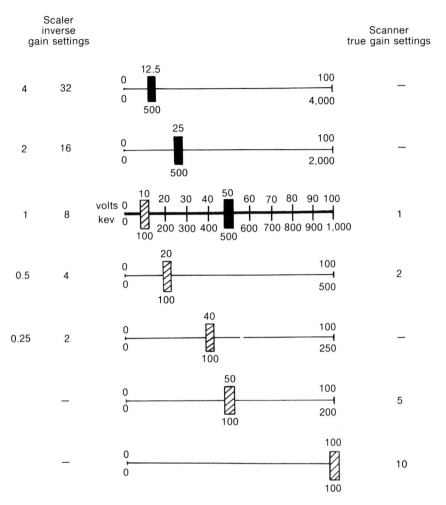

Fig 9-7. Diagram demonstrating the principle of gain control, using various settings. The values to the left of the diagram represent the principle of inverse gain as seen on most scalers. The values to the right of the diagram represent the principle of true gain as seen on most scanners and other electronic equipment.

enough to be analyzed correctly. The alternative is to change the gain settings to 4 (or 0.5), at which point the pulse would be seen at 140 kev units (14.0 v). The same is true for the scanner. For the 77 kev (7.7 v) of mercury 197 gammas a gain setting of 1 would be inadequate; however, a gain setting of 10 would be more accurate. By the judicious use of gain settings, low-energy electromagnetic radiations would not be all squeezed down into a range of a few volts where they are not discernible. The same is true of energy radiations greater than 1,000 kev. For example, cobalt 60 decays with a gamma emission having an energy of 1.17 and 1.33 mev. This is representative of 117 v and 133 v and is greater than the range of the analyzer. In this case the pulse height will have to be decreased so that it will fall within the analyzer's capabilities. This could be accomplished on a scaler by changing the gain settings to 16 (or 2) or 32 (or 4). In this way the pulse height would be halved or quartered, respectively, for correct analysis.

It becomes clear that each spectrum to be investigated must be treated individually, and the operator must choose the most advantageous gain setting for the radionuclide to be utilized to its fullest advantage. After the appropriate gain settings and voltage settings have been chosen, the pulse is now capable of being correctly analyzed.

Pulse height analyzer. The pulse height analyzer is an electronic device that enables the operator to select pulses of a certain height and reject all pulses of a

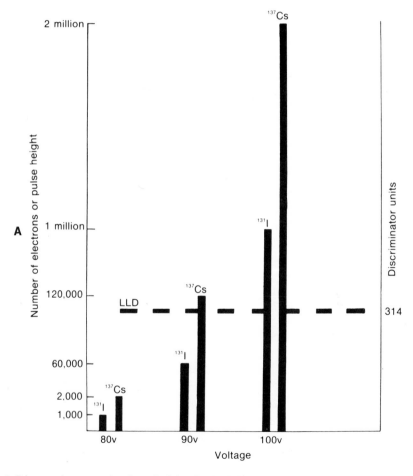

Fig. 9-8. Diagram demonstrating the principle of pulse height analysis. **A,** Lower level discrimination only. Only pulses rising above the LLD setting will be accepted and counted. **B,** Spectrometer. Only pulses that rise above the LLD and fall below the ULD will be accepted and counted.

different height. There are two types of pulse height analyzers: lower level discriminators and spectrometers. The former do not recognize any pulse height below a predetermined level; the spectrometers do not recognize any pulse heights below one level and above another level, recognizing only those which fall between the two settings. A device that isolates only one set of pulses is called a *single-channel analyzer*. Most analyzers on instrumentation used in a routine nuclear medicine department are single-channel analyzers. (A multichannel analyzer is a circuit combining two or more single-channel analyzers to provide simultaneous and sequential counting of radioactivity in more than one energy range or more than one pulse height.)

Since pulse heights are directly proportional to the number of electrons collected at the last dynode, a pulse height analyzer might best be described by comparing that number of electrons to the energy of incident gamma as a function of voltage (Fig. 9-8). Suppose a sample of activity is being used that contains two

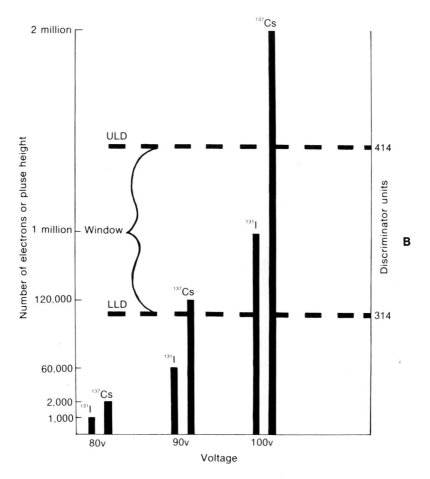

Fig. 9-8, cont'd. For legend see opposite page.

isotopes of varying energies, for example, iodine 131 (364 kev) and cesium 137 (662 kev). Assume total absorption in the crystal and that the intensity of the light was such that 1 photoelectron was emitted from the photocathode for ^{131}I and that 2 photoelectrons were emitted for ^{137}Cs. If a potential difference existed between each dynode of 80 v (800 v to the entire system), the attraction force of the dynode to the electron might provide sufficient energy to release 2 secondary electrons for each primary electron striking each dynode. Since there are ten dynodes, the number of electrons accumulated at the end of the photomultiplier tube would be 2^{10}, or approximately 1,000 electrons. Similarly, if each of the 2 cesium 137 photoelectrons releases 2 electrons by secondary emission, the end result would be 2×2^{10} electrons, or 2,000 electrons accumulated at the end of the photomultiplier tube. The pulse heights are represented in Fig. 9-8 above the units 80 v.

Should the voltage to the dynodes be increased so that a potential difference of 90 v exists between each dynode, the attraction force would be greater and the number of electrons released by secondary emission might increase to 3 electrons for each electron striking the dynode. The iodine 131 single electron from the photocathode would be multiplied to a factor of 3^{10}, or 60,000 electrons, and the cesium 137 would be 120,000, as seen in Fig. 9-8, above 90 v. Should the voltage be increased to 100 v per dynode, the number of electrons produced by secondary emission might increase to 4, therefore 4^{10} or approximately 1,000,000 electrons for the iodine 131 absorption and 2,000,000 electrons for the cesium 137 absorption, as in Fig. 9-8 above 100v.

Lower level discrimination. By the arbitrarily setting of a threshold that a pulse must rise to or exceed in height to be counted, a lower level discriminator (LLD) has been established. In Fig. 9-8, *A*, at 80 v, neither iodine 131 nor cesium 137 would have been counted because neither pulse height attains the lower level discriminator setting. At 90 v, however, the cesium 137 pulse rises higher than the lower level discriminator setting, and therefore it would be counted; the iodine 131 pulse would not. At 100 v, both the iodine 131 and the cesium 137 would be counted because both rise above this lower level discriminator setting.

It is important to note that the use of a lower level discriminator allows the separation of a higher energy radionuclide from a lower energy radionuclide, but the reverse is not true. At 90 v, only the pulses from ^{137}Cs are seen and counted and therefore discriminated from ^{131}I pulses. There is no voltage setting, however, which will separate ^{131}I from ^{137}Cs. Any setting that includes the lower energy radionuclide must necessarily include the higher energy radionuclide too. This is termed *integral counting.*

Spectrometer. The spectrometer is an electronic device that enables the operator to reject any pulse whose height falls below one analyzer setting or above another. Should an upper level discriminator be introduced, as in Fig. 9-8, *B*, placed at a level higher than the lower setting, such a device has been electronically arranged. The lower level discriminator continues to reject any pulses that do not rise to that level, and the upper level discriminator (ULD) will reject any pulses rising higher than its level. This is called *differential counting*. By using this two-level arrangement, both high-energy radionuclides and low-energy radionuclides can be separated from each other by varying the voltage. If 90 v are applied to each dynode, only the higher energy cesium 137 will be detected and recorded. If 100 v are applied, iodine 131 would be the only radionuclide to be counted. The area between the upper level and the lower level discriminators is called a *window*. Accordingly, pulse height analysis can be a function of voltage. This is not the general use of a pulse height analyzer; however, in some instruments this is the case. The windows are automatically preselected, and the voltage is varied to accomodate the window.

The usual method of describing an upper level discriminator is to say that it discriminates against all pulses above a certain pulse height. This approach to an explanation is simply describing an effect. A spectrometer is actually two lower level discriminators acting in combination with an anticoincidence circuit. Figs. 9-9 and 9-10 will help explain their operation.

Fig. 9-9 illustrates schematically the pathway that a pulse travels after the absorption of a photon by a sodium iodide crystal. It passes the preamplifier at the end of the photomultiplier tube and goes through the cable to the amplifier, where

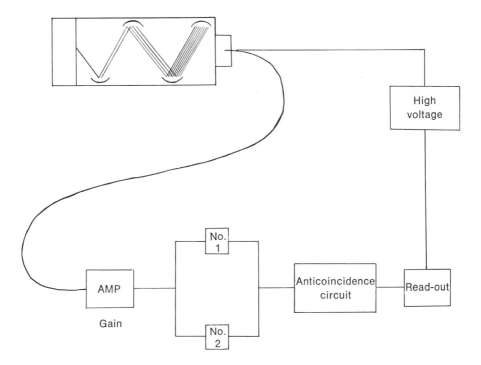

Fig. 9-9. Schematic of a scintillation detection system.

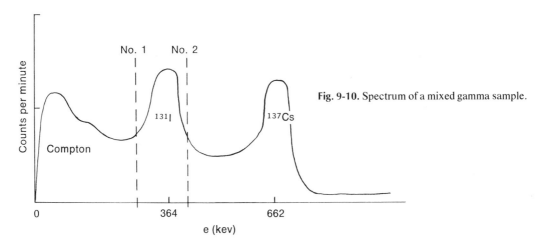

Fig. 9-10. Spectrum of a mixed gamma sample.

it is further amplified. The pulse is then divided and sent to LLD No. 1 and LLD No. 2. If the pulse(s) is not rejected by either one of the LLDs, it will pass to the anticoincidence circuit for acceptance or rejection. If it is accepted by the anticoincidence circuit, it will go on to the read-out system, where one event (count) will be recorded.

Fig. 9-10 displays a gamma spectrum of two radionuclides. The placement of the LLDs indicates a desire to count only iodine 131 photons. Such will be the case because of the following: If a Compton event is "seen" by the detector, both LLDs will reject the pulse because the pulse is lower than either LLD setting. If a cesium 137 gamma ray is detected, both LLDs will accept the pulse because the pulse is higher than either LLD setting; however, since both pulses will arrive into the anticoincidence circuit in coincidence, they are rejected at that stage. If an iodine 131 gamma ray is absorbed by the crystal, the pulse is accepted by LLD No. 1 but rejected by LLD No. 2. By this electronic technique, only pulses from iodine 131 pass the anticoincidence circuit. Therefore only pulses from iodine 131 will activate the read-out mechanism, where one event will be recorded.

The normal use of a pulse height analyzer is to predetermine the voltage setting and change the window to see the different pulses. This is accomplished by presetting the LLD and ULD, placing a source near the crystal, and adjusting the voltage until the highest count is reached. The dials governing the settings of the lower level and the upper level discriminators are usually ten-turn, 1,000 unit potentiometers. These are two main control dials listed as the lower level setting, or base (E dial), and the window, or upper level setting (ΔE dial). The lower level dial is usually calibrated to read from 0 to 100 v (0 to 1,000 kev).* The upper level dial, if designated as window, is usually calibrated on scalers to read from 0 to 30 v (0 to 300 kev)* or, if ULD, to read from 0 to 100 v (0 to 1,000 kev).* (Window

*This is true only with proper gain settings.

is found on scalers; ULD is found on most scanners.) There are two different types of upper level discriminators, since on scalers the upper level discriminator is dependent on the LLD and exists as a window riding on top of the lower level discriminator setting. For instance, it is known that cesium 137 (actually, barium 137m) has a gamma energy of 662 kev. If the machine were to be properly calibrated using this source, a suggested lower level discriminator setting would be 652 units on the 1,000 unit potentiometer and the window would be set at 20 units, meaning that the window would be from 652 to 672 units. In the case of most scanners the upper level discriminator is completely independent of the lower level discriminator, in which case the LLD would read 652 units and the ULD would read 672 units to calibrate the same source. This calibration procedure would be used on the scanners that have variable window control. Some scanners have preset windows set in arbitrary units, and pulse height analysis is a function of varying voltage for each radionuclide.

It can be seen from Fig. 9-8 that by increasing the high voltage, the pulse height of any event that occurs in the sodium iodide crystal can also be increased. Rather than setting the window at arbitrary settings and varying the voltage, the usual procedure is to calibrate the voltage setting so that the 1,000 units on the ten-turn potentiometer become equivalent to kev units. Cesium 137 is the usual standardizing source because of its monoenergetic gamma at 662 kev. The procedure of calibration is to set the arbitrary units on the analyzer to 652 units and 672 units. If a ^{137}Cs source is placed near the crystal and the voltage is increased, eventually the pulse will be built up to such a point that it will be received by the preset window. The voltage at which the maximum count is received would be equivalent to seeing all energies between 652 and 672 kev. If the voltage is increased any further, the pulse heights will be driven above the upper level discriminator setting and rejected. That point at which the highest count is received is the proper operating voltage, for it has essentially calibrated the arbitrary units on the analyzer control dials to read in terms of kev and no longer in arbitrary units. It is important to point out that this is true only at the gain setting used at the time of calibration. Should the gain be changed, these units have a new meaning in energy units dependent on that gain control.

After the usual calibration procedure, each unit on the potentiometer is equal to 1 kev. Since the voltage has produced pulse heights proportional to the energy of the incident gamma ray, it is now possible to slide the window up-scale or down-scale to accept pulses from other radionuclides of different energies. By calibration, 662 potentiometer units have become 662 kev units; therefore, 364 potentiometer units are now 364 kev, and pulses from ^{131}I will be recorded. Similarly, ^{198}Au will be recorded at 411 potentiometer units, ^{99m}Tc will be recorded at 140 units, and so on. This suggests a linearity between pulse height and voltage. This is generally true for all energies above 100 kev (10 v). Below that level, adjustments must be made either in gain, voltage, or window settings. This is often a cause of decreased count rate in the use of ^{125}I (35 kev). The voltage determined for counting ^{137}Cs and all energies above 100 kev often does not apply to ^{125}I. Either the voltage must be redetermined for this radionuclide using the ^{137}Cs voltage as a base (the voltage, although representative of many lost counts, should only be slightly deviated from the value found for ^{137}Cs), or the window must be changed. Which of these procedures should be used is the subject of much controversy. Whatever the procedure, it should include gain, since its use would be most advantageous in this situation.

Most commercially available pulse height analyzers provide the flexibility of using just the lower level discriminator or the spectrometer. These may be simply an "in-out" switch. The "out" position signifies just the lower level discriminator; the "in" position signifies a window. It may also be listed as "integral" and "differential," respectively. When the switch is in the "integral" or "out" position, it essentially cuts out the operation of the upper level discriminator.

Gamma spectrum. A gamma spectrum is a linear graph of the number of counts received per unit(s) of kev. Another way of expressing a gamma spectrum is the number of times a pulse of a certain height occurs per unit of time. In Fig. 9-8, *B,* the lower level discriminator may be designated as having units of 314 kev and the upper level discriminator as having units of 414 kev. At a voltage setting of 100 volts per dynode the iodine 131 pulse height is exactly in the center of the window. Although this is theoretically correct, not all pulses of iodine 131 are represented by exactly 364 kev energy. Since the highest percentage of iodine 131 decays by the emission of a gamma ray of 364 kev, this should be the case. The fact is that most of these pulses are near the 364 kev energy peak but do not always reach it exactly. Actually, they extend from approximately 314 to 414 kev.

The reasons for this are several. If the gamma ray was not totally absorbed in the crystal, which is possible, the intensity of the light emitted in the crystal and the pulse height would indicate this. These pulses would probably not occur anywhere near the main peak of iodine 131. They are referred to as *scatter*. Those that would occur near the main peak but that would represent a slight increase or a slight decrease in energy are primarily those that have been totally absorbed but that for some reason have not been faithfully reproduced by the instrumentation. A gamma ray that was totally absorbed near the outside edge of the crystal, for example, would have to pass its light all the way through the crystal for it to be seen by the photocathode. Consequently, some of the intensity of the light would be lost through transmission. This would appear to be slightly lower in energy than one that was totally absorbed in an area of the crystal immediately adjacent to the photocathode.

Another reason for pulse variation would be the dynodes. It is impossible to expect each dynode to faithfully multiply the number of electrons each time an electron strikes it. In some cases, if the voltage was such that 4 secondary electrons were supposed to be released and only 3 were, the pulse height would actually be lower, giving the illusion that the energy of the incident gamma ray was less. In other cases the number of secondary electrons released from the dynode may be 5 instead of 4, at which point the pulse height would be increased, giving the illusion that the energy of the incident gamma ray was greater than 364 kev. If one more or one fewer electron were released at the first dynode, it would have considerably more effect than if this discrepancy existed on the last dynode; the deficiency or abundance of electrons would be changed by a power of 10 if it occurred on the first dynode, a power of nine on the second, and so on. For this reason, the end result is a variety of slightly different pulse heights; all represent valid counts from iodine 131 and should be used in the analysis of the radionuclide.

A sample of the variety of pulse heights is seen in Fig. 9-11. If the number of times a pulse height occurs were counted and plotted versus the representative energy of that pulse height, a graph would be produced similar to that shown in Fig. 9-12. This is exactly the case of the gamma spectrum. Rather than showing the gamma spectrum as just the main energy peak, it shows the numbers of pulses of energy from 0 to 1,000 kev, as seen in Fig. 9-13.

PLOTTING A GAMMA SPECTRUM. An analogy may be made between plotting a

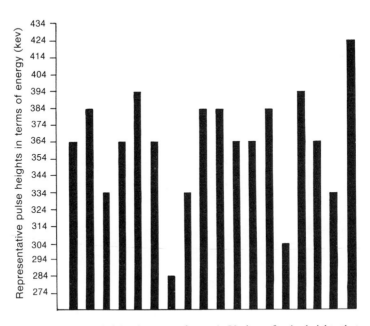

Fig. 9-11. Representative pulse heights in terms of energy. Variety of pulse heights that might be received from the interaction and complete absorption of 18 ^{131}I gamma photons with a crystal detector. Their absorption and subsequent amplification represent energies other than 364 kev even though every one of these pulses is from a 364 kev ^{131}I gamma photon.

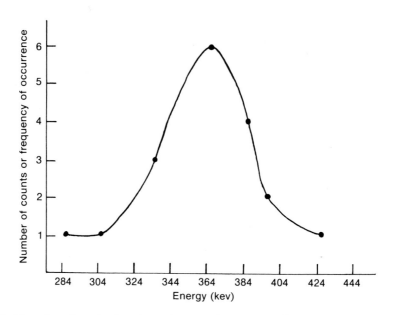

Fig. 9-12. Plot of number of pulses (counts) versus the representative energy of each pulse from Fig. 9-11.

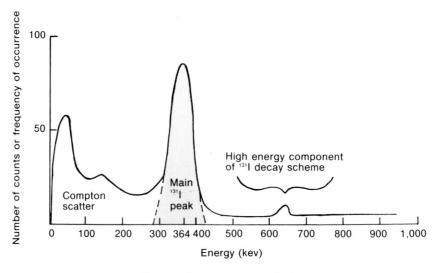

Fig. 9-13. Gamma spectrum of [131]I.

gamma spectrum and plotting the heights of a random sampling of 50 men. Of the 50 men, the heights may be as follows:

Height	Number of people
6'4''	1
6'2''	2
6'1''	6
6'	9
5'11''	13
5'10''	9
5'9''	7
5'8''	2
5'6''	1

By plotting number versus height, a curve would be received (as in Fig. 9-14) similar to the iodine 131 main energy peak.

The gamma spectrum can be plotted much like counting the number of men in the example just given. The men would have been asked to line up according to increasing height and then counted according to height. The same principle is applied in plotting a gamma spectrum. With the proper voltage, a very narrow window is set. Only those gammas within the narrow window would have been counted for a predetermined period of time. The process is repeated changing only the window until the entire spectrum is displayed. With Figs. 9-11 and 9-12, a window

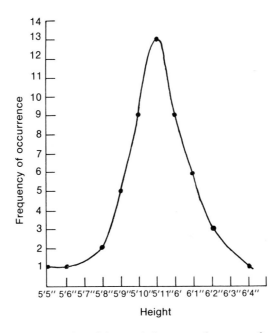

Fig. 9-14. Plot of heights of a sampling of the population versus frequency of occurrence. A graph of this nature is analogous to a gamma spectrum in which pulse heights (representative of different energy levels) are plotted against frequency of occurrence.

could have been set with an LLD at 324 and the window set at 20, therefore, counting a window of 324 to 344. In a preset period of time three counts would have registered, and the number would be plotted in the center of the window (334). If the same window is retained but the LLD is increased to 354, the window would be reading all pulses having the height representative of 354 kev to 374 kev, at which point six counts would have registered and that number would be plotted in the middle of the spectrum (364). This would be continued until the entire spectrum is displayed. In actual practice a smaller window is usually preferred, and the LLD is usually increased in smaller increments than has been shown in this example. A typical peak may be run with a 10 kev window and increases in increments of two units.

Narrow windows used for calibration purposes are *not* the windows used for routine nuclear medicine procedures. Routine studies require a larger window. The reason for using a larger window is the stability of the lower level discriminator and the window width. This is very important for the accurate performance of the system. Narrow window counting requires the ultimate in stability. By increasing the window width to include most of the peak, two purposes are served — to increase the counting rate and therefore obtain better statistics and to reduce the effect of possible analyzer instability. According to the graph in Fig. 9-12, appropriate analyzer settings would be an LLD of 314 and a window of 100 (or a ULD of 414). This determination of working window width should be performed on all scintillation detectors for each radionuclide and checked periodically. Although this is a relatively long procedure with a standard single-channel analyzer, a gamma spectrum can be accomplished very rapidly by using a single-channel analyzer in series with a count-rate meter or by using a multichannel analyzer.

Multichannel analyzers (MCA). A multichannel analyzer is a circuit that combines two or more single channel analyzers to provide simultaneous or sequential counting of radioactivity in more than one energy range. The number of channels can be as many as there are numbers of picture elements (pixels) in the computer in one direction, for example, 64, 128, 256, 512, and so on. The MCAs have a multitude of uses in clinical applications of nuclear medicine. Gamma spectra can be performed very quickly on the MCA because each channel is analyzed individually but is recorded at the same time. Most commercially available camera systems are capable of doing this now. It is used very effectively and efficiently to set and to check proper window settings. MCAs are used very effectively in radionuclides with more than one energy peak (such as ^{67}Ga and ^{111}In) to bracket each peak and enhance image quality. Prior to this use of MCAs, the image was received by accepting all peaks in one large window, which meant accepting large amounts of background and scatter counts to degrade the image, or, in the case of multipeak radionuclides, accepting counts from only one peak and therefore accepting fewer counts, which also meant degrading the image or accumulating counts for a much longer period of time. With the advent of triple peak capabilities, an optimum window could be set for each peak, reducing background and increasing count rate. Radionuclide identification or, even more significant, determination of radionuclide contamination by way of gamma spectrum is another excellent use of this multichannel capability.

Display modes. There are two types of display modes, the scaler and the count rate meter.

Scaler. A scaler is an electronic circuit that accepts signal pulses from a radiation detector and counts them. Scalers provide a unit for rapid counting of electrical pulses that result from light flashes from ionizing radiations interacting in the crystal. This method of counting is far superior to the dark-adapted eye. The scaler is usually electronically devised so that the operator has a choice between accepting a certain number of counts (preset count) or a predetermined period of time over which counts can be accumulated (preset time). With preset time, the scaling device will count the number of events that occur during a set interim of time and will then shut off automatically; the number of counts becomes the variable. With preset count, the predetermined number of counts are accumulated, after which the scaler is automatically shut off; time becomes the variable.

USE OF SCALER AS A COMPUTER. A scaler may be used as a computer provided it has both preset time and preset count accommodations. This can be accomplished by setting the scaler for a preset number of counts (10,000) and noting the time required to accumulate the preset number of counts. This is usually done with the standard sample. This time value is then used in the preset time section (preset count must be manually eliminated), and all unknowns are counted for that preset period of time. The answer can be read directly as percent by moving the decimal point over the required number of spaces. (In the case of 10,000 the decimal point must be moved two places to the left.)

Count rate meter. Another type of display mode is the count rate meter. This is a radiation detector connected to an indicator that continuously shows the average rate of counts coming from the detector per preselected time periods. Count rate meters have wide usage in survey meters and laboratory monitors, since their usual purpose is to promptly indicate increases in activity. The count rate meter also has extensive use for clinical work in dynamic studies in which the accumulation and transportion of radiopharmaceuticals is followed by external detectors, such as renograms and cardiac outputs.

There are two types of rate meters currently in use: the analog rate meter and the digital rate meter. The fundamental difference between the two types is in the kind of memory used to store information from the incoming pulses. The analog rate meter stores a *charge* that is proportional to the number of pulses received per unit time. A digital rate meter stores the *count* in digital form much like the scaler. Since rate meters are so dependent on time constants, a discussion of time constants is warranted.

TIME CONSTANT. The time constant is an electronic averaging property of the circuit for determining the time interval over which the summation of the incoming pulses is taken. Since the nature of radioactive decay is one of random events, fluctuations will be seen in the count rate meter. The degree of fluctuation is dependent on the time constant or the count rate or both. It is similar to taking subsequent counts on a scaler and plotting them. If a radioactive source counted 10,000 cpm, variations between readings would not be appreciable; the counts will not vary by much more than 2% from the true count rate. Plotting the results of subsequent 1-minute counts would yield almost a straight line. The count rate meter with the time constant set for 1 minute performs this accumulation and averaging automatically. When the meter is connected to a stripchart recorder, the results are graphed as in Fig. 9-15, *A*. Note that there is a delay in reaching the true count rate. Actually, the rise in count rate is an exponential function of time. For this reason, the rate meter reads only 50% of the true count rate value at the time indicated by the time constant; that is, the time constant is 1 minute, but at 1 minute only a count rate of 5,000 cpm is indicated. The true count rate (10,000 cpm) is not realized until after approximately 4 minutes (four times the time indicated by the time constant). With such a long time constant in this count rate situation, statistical variations are not a factor.

By using the same source of radioactive material but reducing the time constant to 0.01 minute (100 counts per 0.01 minute), a stripchart record similar to that in Fig. 9-15, *B*, will be obtained. The statistical fluctuation now becomes a

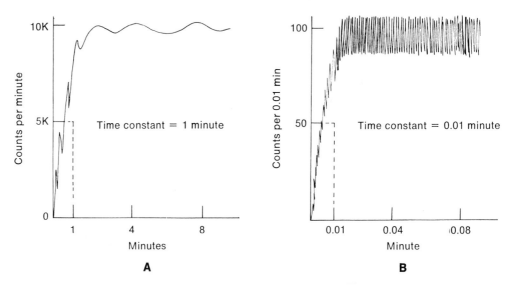

Fig. 9-15. A, Effect of a time constant on the response of a count rate meter. A long constant of 1 minute at the indicated count rate allows only slight deflection of the needle, but it requires four times the time constant setting to achieve 100% value. **B,** Effect of a much shorter time constant but the same count rate. The vascillation of the needle is greater, but four times the time constant is still necessary to achieve the 100% value.

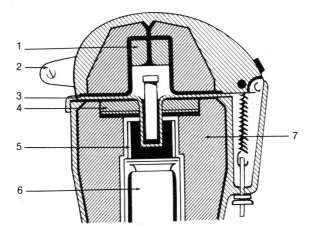

Fig. 9-16. Cross sectional view of scintillation well detector. *1,* Removable lid plug; *2,* handle; *3,* splash guard; *4,* lead beaker plate; *5,* large well crystal; *6,* photomultiplier tube (6292); *7,* lead shield. (Courtesy Picker Nuclear, White Plains, N. Y.)

crystal immediately surrounding the counting sample is a variable. For these reasons, the ability to count higher energy radionuclides varies considerably and the efficiency with which lower energy radionuclides are counted varies, but to a lesser degree. Other sizes of crystals are available that accommodate larger volumes or have a greater thickness of sodium iodide for greater counting efficiencies. The detection of pulses from this type of scintillation detector is the same as with any scintillation detector.

Organ imaging devices. In 1950 Cassen and his associates found that by using the newly developed scintillation counter, mounting it on an automatically moved carriage, and attaching a dot-producing mechanism that would respond to the electrical impulses from a scintillation counter, the spatial distribution of radioactive iodine in the thyroid gland could be printed mechanically. As a result, Cassen opened up a whole new area of isotope utilization in medicine. Until this discovery, the only means of scanning the organs of the body containing any radioactive material was manual scanning. A manual scan was performed by placing the probe as close to the skin as possible, moving in small increments over the gland or area to be scanned, and recording a count as each new area was surveyed. A "hot" or "cold" area would be indicated by an area with count rates that were increased or decreased, respectively, as compared to the count rates seen over the normal functioning areas of the organ. An anatomic map of the organ could be made by plotting the areas having the same count and by connecting these points by lines. These lines, called *isocount lines,* represented the shape of the organ and the distribution of the radioactivity. This procedure was long and painstaking.

Automatic scanners, called *rectilinear scanners,* were designed to perform this scanning procedure automatically, making a map of the location of radioactive materials in the patient's body. The scanner moves across the organ in one or more planes until the organ or the area in question has been completely surveyed by the scintillation counter. As it moves back and forth across the organ containing radioactivity, the scanning mechanism produces electrical impulses proportional to the amount of activity present in the area that, at that instant, is covered by the scintillation probe. It creates a picture by a number of read-out systems. Parameters are set for lateral movement, and through the use of microswitches the detector head is automatically indexed upward or downward and begins again on its path across the body. In this way the entire organ can be visualized. The speed with which the detector moves laterally and the distance that it moves laterally or indexes up or down can be manually controlled.

Read-out systems. The map of the organ containing radioactivity can be presented as a visual display by several methods. One of these methods (and one of the first used) is a paper known as *teledeltos*. This paper is capable of electrical conductivity and is coated with a white, chalklike substance. As the electrical impulse is received by the stylus of the dot-producing mechanism, this chalklike compound is burned away by the electric current. This exposes a black material beneath, producing a black dot on white paper. The paper is held stationary, and the dot-producing mechanism moves synchronously with the detector head over the teledeltos paper.

Another device for the same purpose uses a solenoid-operated "tapper," which strikes the record paper through a carbon ribbon (much like a typewriter ribbon) to produce dots. The number of dots is proportional to the amount of radioactivity present in the area under the detector. As the radioactivity increases, the number of dots also increases.

Another type of visual display is the display on x-ray film. As in the dot mechanism, a small cathode tube moves synchronously with the scintillation detector over x-ray film. As scintillations are received, a collimated cathode light source produces a spot on the film, flashed on for a preset length of time. On completion of the scan, the x-ray film is developed in the usual manner. The developed x-ray film demonstrates the organ and its concentrations of radioactivity as dots or squares of darkening on the film. These film images are generally thought to be superior to teledeltos or tapper images because the image is produced by the overlapping of dots as well as density control of the dots. Consequently, variations in concentrations of activity can be seen as dots ranging from white (not seen on film) through shades of gray to black. The black areas represent high concentrations of radioactivity, and the varied gray areas represent lesser concentrations of radioactivity. A variety of light sources have been used, including an incandescent lamp and a cathode tube. The latter has been used as the light source of choice because of its quick response.

Another display system found on some imaging devices is that of a color dot print-out. This displays a range of color from blue, indicating a cold area, through intermediate colors to red, indicating a hot area. It was designed because, theoretically, the ability to discern colors is much easier than variations in shades of gray. The color print-out is accomplished by a ribbon similar to a typewriter ribbon with several adjacent bands of different colors that move transversely under a fixed tapper. The position of the ribbon and therefore the color of the dot are dependent on the counting rate. If the count rate is low, the blue color band slides under the tapper. If the count rate is around 50% of the maximum, then the green band falls under the tapper, and if the count rate is the maximum count rate, then the red band falls under the tapper.

Types of organ imaging devices. There are several devices designed to show radionuclide distribution in the body and in the organs. One such device is the rectilinear scanner. Some of these scanners consist of one probe that moves back and forth across the organ; others have two probes that move back and forth synchronously, with the body or the organ positioned between the two probes. Other forms of organ imaging devices are stationary devices that visualize the entire organ at one time. These devices are of two types: (1) those that contain a single crystal (camera) and (2) those that contain multiple crystals (autofluoroscope), each of which is capable of visualizing the entire organ. Although these types differ considerably in construction, they all have many basic features in common. All imaging devices, whether rectilinear or stationary, have a collimator. In addition to this, they all have a detector unit, which for scintillation imaging devices consists of a crystal(s) and photomultiplier tube(s). They also have a linear amplifier, pulse height analyzer, and a scaler or rate meter or a combination of both.

Rectilinear imaging devices. There are a variety of factors that influence the results of the read-out system of a rectilinear imaging device, whether it is the dot record or the photographic record. It is important to realize that each patient presents a new set of variables for which the operator of the imaging device must supply a new set of factors to receive the optimum results. The imaging of organs is not an exact science by any means. Formulas are available to assist nuclear medicine personnel in producing an adequate image, but an element of art exists in the production of a better than adequate image. The establishment of such empirical values requires experience. The next section is included to provide the student of nuclear medicine with an understanding of the function of these various parameters so that these empirical values might be learned with a minimum of experience.

PARAMETERS APPLICABLE TO BOTH PHOTO AND DOT RECORDINGS. There are four settings applicable to both the photo recording and the dot recording of a rectilinear image. These are the pulse height analyzer, speed, line spacing, and time constant. The pulse height analyzer has already been discussed, and appropriate settings are necessary for the radionuclide being detected. The *speed control* is an adjustable potentiometer that controls the speed at which the detector traverses the organ. The speed is dependent on the count rate determined from the area of highest activity, the line spacing, and desired information density (ID).* Speed can be calculated by the following formula:

$$\text{Scan speed} = \frac{\text{Maximum counts per minute}}{\text{Line space} \times \text{ID}}$$

The *line spacing* adjustment is a variable control that determines the distance the detector indexes before it attempts another sweep across the organ being visualized. The choice of line spacing is usually determined by the choice of light collimator on the cathode ray tube of the photo recording section. The usual procedure is to display as much information in as small an area as possible. This requires that the top of the spot on the film in one row be touching the bottom of the spot in the row above it. If they do not approximate each other in this manner, a line is produced with no information, referred to as the venetian blind effect, and in most cases this interferes with interpretation. The standard small light collimator requires 0.2-cm spacing, whereas the large light collimator requires from 0.35- to 0.4-line spacing. Some investigators have preferred square light collimators so that interpretation is not distributed by the wavelike effect between the tops and bottoms of subsequent dots.

The *time constant* has already been discussed at some length with regard to rate meters, but its utilization in rectilinear scanning deserves special attention. It has been stated that the buildup of a rate meter is an exponential function so that there is a delay before the true count rate is indicated. There is also an exponential decrease in output of the count rate so that, should the detector move into an area containing no radionuclide, the reading on the rate meter is not immediately zero. This presents a unique problem in rectilinear scanning because the increase or decrease in count rate must be quickly indicated or a possible lesion will be obscured. This is especially true in a scan that is performed on a long time constant setting. The value of rectilinear scanning lies in the fact that as the detector moves across the organ, it almost immediately presents the information consistent with the amount of activity in that area of the organ. However, this is not true if the time constant is too long, since the information will be presented from an area that was previously under the probe. Consequently, as the detector reaches the edge of an organ, the count rate does not decrease immediately. Information continues to be presented beyond the organ edge because of the exponential release of the higher count rate. As the detector indexes and begins to make another sweep across the organ, it does not present information until after it has gone some distance across the organ because of the exponential buildup. It continues across the organ displaying information from a previous scanning area. It continues to display beyond the other edge of the organ until the count rate decreases. This procedure continues throughout the entire scan. This defect of scanning produces an irregular outline of the organ and makes it appear larger than it actually is. This defect is commonly referred to as *scalloping*. If there were a small lesion in the

---

*ID = Number of observed events per square centimeter (see Chapter 11).

organ itself, the scalloping would tend to mask the lesion. Scalloping can also occur if the scan speed is too fast and therefore inconsistent with the time constant.

PARAMETERS APPLICABLE ONLY TO THE DOT RECORDING. There are two settings related to the dot recording: the dot factor and the background erase. The *dot factor* is a numbered dial that indicates the number of events seen by the detector to produce a dot. If the dot factor were 4, four events would have to be seen in order that one dot be produced; if the dot factor were 16, sixteen events would have to be seen to produce one dot. The choice of a dot factor is contingent on the count rate at the area of highest radionuclide concentration, and it must be consistent with the response of the dot-producing mechanism and its subsequent record. The dot factor for teledeltos paper is always greater (more events per dot) than for the tapper systems. If a dot factor of 1 were used in the teledeltos system of recording, the record would be nothing but a straight line in areas of high activity with no difference in count rate suggested. Furthermore, the dot pattern consists of lines of small dots. These are difficult to interpret because of the spaces between consecutive scan sweeps. Also, variations in dot density are difficult to recognize. The tapper systems are easier to interpret because these systems display a narrow vertical line that allows the lines to touch each other from one scan sweep to the other and the eye of the interpreter can distinguish differences more easily. Although graphs are available for this purpose, the dot factor can be mathematically determined by the following formula:

$$DF = \frac{\text{Maximum counts per minute}}{\text{Scan speed} \times 10}$$

Every scan includes areas in which counts are received from areas other than the organ of interest (natural background or radioactivity in other portions of the body). Since these counts are not of primary interest and since they only disrupt the interpretive process, a technique of *background erase* is used to prevent any data recording of count rate below a preselected level. Lack of judicious use of this parameter can result in loss of valuable information. An example is a liver scan. The edges of the liver are very thin, and the concentration of radioactivity approaches body background. If the background erase selector is set too high, the liver can actually be made to look smaller than it is because the liver edge is treated as background and is erased. Continual increases in background erase can cause the liver to appear to become continuously smaller.

Misuse of the background erase can also result in loss of information from different parts of an organ. The scanning of an autonomous thyroid nodule is an example. The area of highest concentration is not difficult to visualize in these clinical states, but visualization of the rest of the organ can present problems. The rest of the thyroid gland may have received some of the radionuclide, but the nodule acquired the major portion of the dose, resulting in the rest of the organ having activity levels only slightly greater than the surrounding extrathyroidal tissue. Too much background erase will present the autonomous nodule as the only functioning tissue in the gland.

PARAMETERS APPLICABLE ONLY TO PHOTO RECORDING. The photo record has in general become the record of choice. The photo record displays the information as dots varying in density from white through an infinite number of shades of gray to black. The variations in density reflect the variations in concentration of the radionuclide in the organ being studied. The interpreter is usually better able to distinguish variations in shades of gray on the photo record than on the dot record, which is black or white.

The photo record frequently employs a cathode ray tube (CRT). The CRT flashes a beam of light directly onto an x-ray film, which, when developed displays a dark area at the point of exposure. The size of the dark area is controlled by a light collimating device. The amount of film darkening can also be controlled. It can be accomplished by several methods: (1) by varying the brightness of the light flash, (2) by varying the "on" time of the cathode ray tube, or (3) by a combination of both. Furthermore, the degree of darkening is dependent on scan speed and count rate.

Parameters used to regulate the record on the x-ray film include the density, the range differential, the light source voltage (as opposed to the photomultiplier voltage), and the rate meter range. Some of these parameters are automatically adjusted on some instruments, some are manually adjusted on other instruments, and some instruments can be adjusted either manually or automatically. In any of these cases the principles are not altered, and a basic understanding of their function will help the nuclear medicine student understand their use.

The *density control* indicates the duration of time the cathode ray tube is on per detected pulse. It therefore determines the length of time that the x-ray film is exposed. The longer the film is exposed, the darker the area on the film becomes. Furthermore, a density setting that would produce a black dot if the cathode ray tube were stationary would produce a less intense dot (gray) if the cathode ray tube were moving. The light rays would be superimposed on each other in the former instance but not perfectly superimposed in the latter. The same reasoning prevails if a scan is performed at a predetermined scan speed and density setting and is repeated at a faster speed. In order that the *film density* be duplicated, the density setting must be increased proportionally; to double the scan speed, the density must also be doubled. (Note: *density control* and *film density* are two separate entities. Density control relates only to the duration of the light flash. Film density relates to the degree of darkening of the film, which is governed by several factors, including the density control, the count rate, the scan speed, and the size of the light collimating device.)

Density is an automatically controlled device in some instruments. Graphs are available to determine the adjustment of this parameter in manually controlled instruments, or the value can be calculated as follows:

$$\text{Density} = \frac{\text{Scan speed} \ \times \ \text{Light collimator conversion factor}}{\text{Maximum counts per minute}}$$

Conversion factor for small light collimator $= 4{,}000$
Conversion factor for large light collimator $= 2{,}500$

X-ray film, regardless of the type, possesses a known useful film density range. This is the range from white to black, beyond which the dot does not become darker. It is generally considered desirable to manipulate the various parameters so that the maximum count rate area is represented by maximum film density (black) and the background is represented by minimum film density (white). In this way, intermediate count rate areas will be represented by intermediate shades of gray. This is called the *range differential*. To accomplish this, the percentage of full scale deflection from maximum to minimum count rate must be ascertained. If the maximum count rate showed as 80% of the entire scale and minimum count rate showed as 20% of the entire scale (background representing 0% to 20%), the differential between the two extremes would be 60%. This value becomes the range differential. Note that the range differential becomes a background erase mechanism for the photo record. If more background is desired, the range differential value may be increased. By erroneously calculating the range differential, information can be lost, just as in the background erase for the dot record. Range differential is calculated by the following:

$$RD = \% \text{ maximum deflection} - \% \text{ minimum deflection}$$

The use of this parameter is a form of *contrast enhancement*. Just as the name implies, contrast (from white to black) is enhanced as the range differential is reduced. It requires less of a change in the count rate to proceed from the white to the black range, with fewer gradations of gray. On some equipment this is referred to as *suppression*.

The *light source voltage* is a parameter that adjusts the brightness of each light flash to the output of the count rate meter. The voltage is adjusted so that the area of maximum count rate provides maximum film density as well. This parameter must be determined after the range differential has been calculated.

Using the range differential example of 60 with no light source voltage applied, this value could represent a range of 0 to 60, 10 to 70, 20 to 80, 30 to 90, or 40 to 100. The purpose of the light source voltage is to ensure that the range differential of 60 represents the deflection of the count rate needle from 20% to 80% of the full scale.

Another parameter in setting up a scan is the use of the *count rate meter range* adjustment, which must be selected prior to calculation of the range differential. This parameter has a variety of selections, which change the values of the scaled units. The same position on the scale could represent 1,000, 10,000 or 100,000 counts per minute, depending on the range switch value. Furthermore, some units have an ancillary switch separate from the range selector control that expands the scale by a factor of 2. Therefore a maximum count rate of 10,000 cpm could be represented on the meter as 10,000 on the standard scale (meaning 10,000 cpm) or 5,000 on the expanded scale (meaning 5,000 × 2 = 10,000 cpm). The former would represent 100% full-scale deflection on the appropriate scale, and the latter would represent 50% full-scale deflection on the same scale, expanded. This would mean that the range differential could be no greater than 100% on the standard scale, whereas the range differential could be no greater than 50% on the expanded scale.

CONTRAST ENHANCEMENT. It has been shown that contrast enhancement can be produced by varying the range differential. The phenomenon of contrast enhancement is generally considered to be of less and less significance as instrumentation and radiopharmaceuticals are improved. Contrast enhancement has been used in the past to accentuate areas with changes in count rate that because of the lack of statistics actually represented very little change in count rate at all. It is currently believed that all information should be recorded, with few exceptions, and the contrast enhancing techniques performed postfactum. (There is a certain degree of innate contrast enhancement in x-ray film, oscilloscopes, and so on, provided the information presented falls within a good statistical range.) Postfactum contrast enhancement is accomplished in a variety of ways. It can be performed by the use of ancillary equipment as expensive as computers and closed-circuit television or as inexpensive as a piece of ordinary nonglare glass, the type used in picture frames.

The reason contrast enhancement has fallen into disrepute can be exemplified in pulmonary imaging. A pulmonary scan demonstrating *decreased* perfusion is suggestive of pulmonary embolism, whereas *no* perfusion suggests tumor. Since contrast enhancement demands a decision before the image is realized, an erroneous setting by the technologist may result in an erroneous interpretation by the physician.

Single crystal rectilinear imaging devices. A single crystal rectilinear scanner consists of a centrally located chassis containing most of the electronic components and the photo recording unit. All the controls for the parameters just discussed are also found in this central section. The detector assembly is mounted on one arm of the unit, and the dot recording mechanism is mounted on the other arm above a platform on which the required paper is placed.

The detector arm continually moves back and forth parallel with the front of the scanner and indexes stepwise in a direction perpendicular to the front of the scanner until the entire organ has been visualized. The person under study lies on a patient cart under the detector head.

Dual probe rectilinear imaging devices. There are several commercial products currently available using differing combinations of crystals, photomultiplier tubes, and associated electronics in a dual probe arrangement. The instruments differ in that each probe contains 1 crystal-1 photomultiplier tube, or 10 crystals-10 photomultiplier tubes, or a single crystal-7 photomultiplier tubes. All three types have advantages over the single probe, single crystal device.

Dual probe scanner. The dual probe scanner, as the name implies, is a scanner that has two standard scintillation detectors (one crystal-one photomultiplier tube) instead of one. The scintillation detectors are opposite one another so as to view opposite sides of the same subject. The usual method of operation is to have the patient lie on a table. One detector traverses over the table, and the other traverses under it. The patient therefore lies between the two detectors. This system offers the obvious advantage of obtaining two scans during the time required to obtain one. There is very little difference in the operation of the dual probe scanner from the single probe. Each detector has its own system of detection, amplification, pulse height analysis, and read-out devices. The only difference is that both probes are linked mechanically so that they share the same mechanical moving facilities and therefore move in synchrony.

Several features of using a dual scanner deserve special mention. Commercially available dual probe scanners have a feature of minifaction by changing the gear ratio of the motors. Consequently, an image can be reduced through a series of stepped reductions (2:1, 3:1) to as small as one-fifth the original size. In using this feature, a 14- by 17-inch x-ray film, ordinarily just large enough to include a lung scan, is able to display an entire body scan. Another feature of dual probe scanners is that they allow the summation of all the events from both detectors to yield one image. This is especially applicable to scans involving low concentrations of radionuclides. Another feature is that a dual probe scanner allows the subtraction technique. The subtraction technique is used to delineate organs that accumulate only one of two injected radionuclides from superimposed organs that accumulate both radionuclides. An example is the pancreas. Selenium 75–labeled selenomethionine localizes in both the liver and the pancreas, whereas technetium 99m sulfur colloid localizes in the liver. The concentration of selenium 75 in the pancreas can be visualized by subtracting any areas that contain both selenium 75 and technetium 99m. In this manner a liver-pancreas scan can be performed in which the liver will be subtracted and the pancreas will be visualized. Another advantage to the dual probe scanner is the possibility of using the opposing heads to detect positron emissions. In this utilization a coincidence mode must be used so that only those pulses detected simultaneously (the two gamma rays resulting from annihilation reactions) will be recorded.

Multicrystal whole-body scanner. This rectilinear imaging device consists of two opposing detector heads, with each head consisting of 10 sodium iodide crystals and 10 associated photomultiplier tubes (Fig. 9-17, *A*). Each crystal measures 4.9 inches in length, 2.2 inches in width, and 1.0 inch in thickness, allowing for a crystal area of 107.8 sq in (Fig. 9-17, *B*). Each crystal has its own photomultiplier tube and focused collimator. The action of the heads are to move in synchrony along the entire body while the 10 crystals, working as a unit, move back and forth across the body. This movement allows for a scan width of 24 inches, with a 119-hole collimator focal distance of 4.7 inches. Collimators are designed for low-energy nuclides, up to 350 kev. The images generated by the upper and lower detector heads are displayed on a CRT simultaneously, where area brightness is a function of the number of photons detected in that area. Each increment of travel of the detector causes a trace of the distribution across the patient's body to be re-

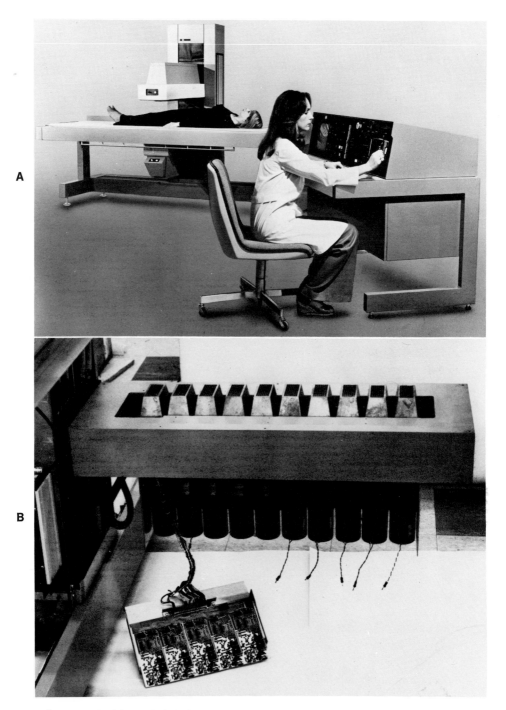

Fig 9-17. A, Multicrystal whole-body scanner. **B,** Cut-away view of the lower probe of a multicrystal whole-body scanner showing crystals and photomultiplier tube assembly. **C,** Each increment of travel of the detector assemblies causes a trace of the distribution of activity across the patient's body to be displayed on the television monitor and recorded on magnetic disc, Polaroid, and/or transparency film. Patient identification, date, isotope used, and other pertinent information are recorded with the simultaneously obtained anterior and posterior images. (Courtesy Union Carbide, Norwood, Mass.)

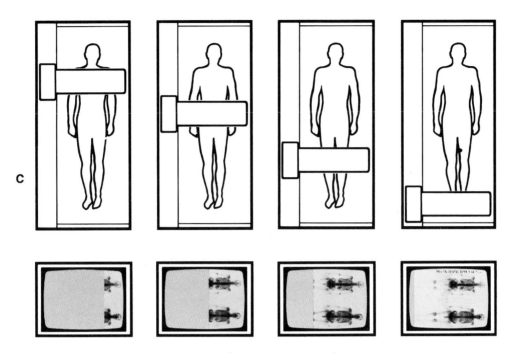

Fig 9-17, cont'd. For legend see opposite page.

corded on that portion of the oscilloscope face corresponding to the position of the detector (Fig. 9-17, *C*). Data can also be recorded on magnetic disk as a permanent record or for playback and display purposes. The obvious advantage of this unit is speed and, with a 1-inch thick crystal and high-energy collimation, better efficiency and resolution with higher energy radionuclides such as gallium 67.

Multiplane tomographic scanner. This rectilinear imaging device (Fig. 9-18, *A*) consists of two opposing detector heads with each head composed of a single 8½-inch diameter by 1-inch thick sodium iodide crystal viewed by a bank of seven 3-inch photomultiplier tubes arranged in a hexagonal array. Each of the two detectors is actually a small scintillation camera. A variety of converging collimators for different energy radionuclides are available, all having a focal distance of 3½ inches.

The head of the scanner moves the length of the patient as the detector itself moves from side to side. As it moves, it creates six longitudinal tomographic whole body images from each probe. Each tomographic image is a view of the patient or organ at a different focal plane (none of which fall at the geometric focal plane of the collimators), totaling 12 tomoplane images per study.

The principle of action of the complicated piece of electronics has been simplified by its inventor, Mr. Hal O. Anger. When the detector scans across the patient, radioactive objects at different depths produce images that move across the detector at different velocities. Speed depends on the proximity of the object to the geometric focal plane of the collimator and the direction depends on whether the radioactive object is above or below the geometric focal plane of the collimator (Fig. 9-18, *B*).

Signals from seven photomultiplier tubes proceed through conventional gamma ray circuitry producing position signals for each detected gamma ray. These signals are then directed to a CRT, which displays them as "flashes" on continuous display—called *field display*. There are six field displays for each detector,

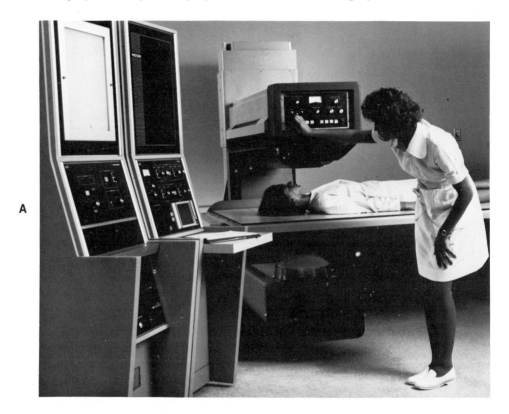

A

Fig. 9-18. A, Multiplane tomographic imager. (Courtesy Searle Diagnostics, Inc.) **B,** Schematic showing the method by which the detection head views four-point sources at four different focal planes. In the top part of the figure, with the detector in this position, all point sources at all planes are in view of the detector. The bottom portion of the figure is intended to show how any standard detector with converging collimation would view these point sources. The point sources farther away from the geometric focal plane will appear to be more out of focus and will appear to move across the face of the detector at a greater speed. The direction that these point sources move across the detector (arrows) is a function of their position relative to the geometric focal plane. Had a point source been placed at the exact geometric focal plane, the dot would appear in focus with no direction. Computer reconstruction techniques are capable of using these factors of speed and direction of travel to identify position and depth, and in the case of a clinical study, reconstruct six different images of the body (or organ) at six different tomoplanes. With two detector heads, the commercially available model is capable of presenting information in 12 tomoplanes, six from each head.

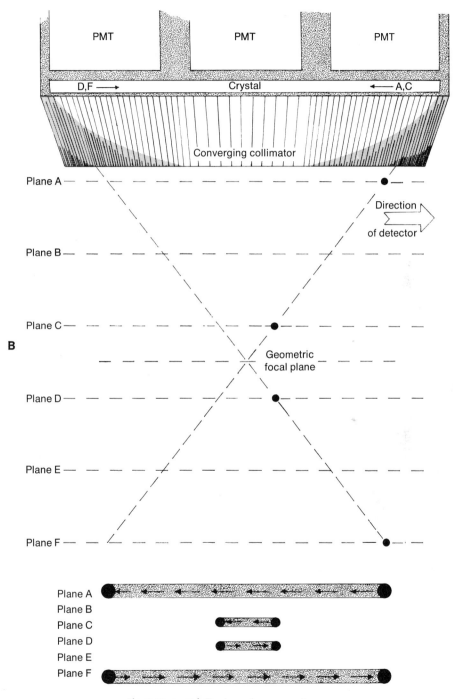

Fig. 9-18, cont'd. For legend see opposite page.

one for each focal plane. All six field displays are scanned in synchrony with the detector head and therefore are a rectilinear scan. To produce the final readout, a time exposure of the CRT is taken on film.

The principle is analogous to taking a time exposure of moving cars. If the camera is aimed at a car and follows the car, the image of the car will be sharp but the images of all other cars, moving at different speeds and in different directions, will be blurred. The multiplane tomographic scanner is similar. The six different field displays in the scanner are analogous to six different cameras following cars moving at six different velocities.

Single crystal imaging devices. The single crystal imaging device, commonly called the *scintillation camera,* or *Anger camera,* is a device that views all parts of the radiation field continuously, rather than scanning the subject point by point. Today, commercially available scintillation cameras employ a single sodium iodide crystal measuring from 11 inches to 16 inches in diameter and from $1/4$ to $1/2$ inch in thickness as the detector unit. This crystal is viewed by a bank of 19, 37, 61, or 91 photomultiplier tubes arranged in a hexagonal array. In some systems the photomultiplier tubes are separated from the crystal by a transparent optical "lightpipe." This lightpipe is critical to the resolution of the entire system. The thinner the lightpipe and the closer the material to the index of refraction of the crystal, the better the resolution. In both instances the light collection from the scintillation crystal is enhanced, contributing statistically to the ease with which the position and pulse-height information can be processed.

In the single crystal imaging device, gamma rays pass through the holes of the collimator and are totally absorbed in the scintillation crystal. The light that is produced is emitted in all directions and is received by many of the photomultiplier tubes (Fig. 9-19). The closest photomultiplier tube to any given scintillation event receives the most light. Since it receives the most light, that photomultiplier tube also produces the largest pulse, in comparison to the surrounding photomultiplier tubes, which also produce a pulse but of decreasing height. The output signal from each of the phototubes goes directly to a capacitor network where impulses from all the phototubes are modified, processed, and converted to four output signals that carry all the necessary position information, as well as the pulse-height information. The position information is obtained from four of the output signals, called the X^+, X^-, Y^+, and Y^- signals. A fifth signal, the Z signal, is the pulse-height signal. It is proportional only to the brightness of the sum of the scintillations from all the involved photomultiplier tubes having no regard whatsoever to where the scintillation occurred in the scintillation crystal. This Z signal is obtained by adding the pulses from all the photomultiplier tubes involved in the detection of the event to determine, after all the processing of the position signals has taken place, whether the spectrometer is going to accept or reject the event.

The position signal that is derived from the four output signals can best be described by envisioning the crystal as a pie cut into four equal parts (Fig. 9-20).

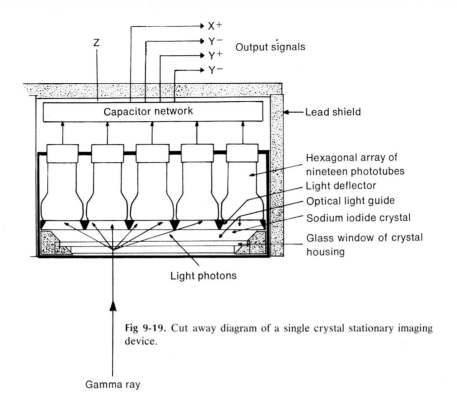

Fig 9-19. Cut away diagram of a single crystal stationary imaging device.

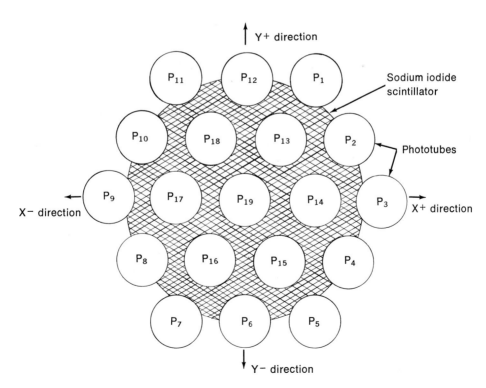

Fig. 9-20. Bird's-eye view of the arrangement of the photomultiplier tubes and the scintillation crystal divided into four equal parts.

Using the center of the pie as zero, the four cuts now represent four different axes, the X+, X−, Y+, and Y−. The magnitude of the signal taken from each phototube to form the X+ signal is proportional to the position in the X+ direction. The X−, Y+, and Y− position signals are obtained by adding signals from the phototubes in their respective directions. Signals are then sent to ancillary data presentation equipment, which is discussed later in this chapter.

Multiple crystal stationary imaging device. The multiple crystal stationary imaging device, commonly called the *Autofluoroscope,* is an instrument with multiple crystals on the detector assembly. The detector head is made up of a matrix, measuring 6 by 9 inches and consisting of 294 separate scintillation crystals that form a grid of 14 by 21 crystals (Fig. 9-21). Each crystal is 7/16-inch wide and 1½-inch thick. These crystals are mounted in a mosaic pattern and are separated from one another by lead. These lead separators help stop gamma and light rays from crossing into adjacent crystals. This "cross talk" is further reduced by the use of a multihole collimator having 294 tapered holes. Each hole corresponds to each crystal element in the mosaic. The purpose of the thick mosaic scintillator is to obtain high detection efficiency for medium- and high-energy gamma rays, which is not possible with the scintillation camera.

Each of the 294 crystals in the 9- by 6-inch mosaic is optically connected by a pair of Lucite lightpipes to two of the bank of 35 photomultiplier tubes. (See Fig. 9-22.) One lightpipe goes to the *x* axis, and the other lightpipe goes to the *y* axis. In this way, simultaneous pulses from the two photomultiplier tubes identify the crystal element in which the scintillation occurred. A light is then produced on the

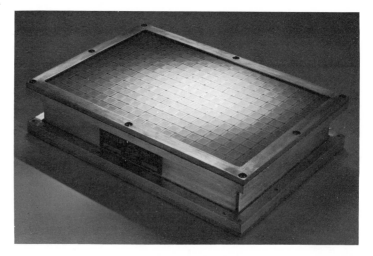

Fig. 9-21. Detector head of the multiple crystal stationary imaging device. (Courtesy Harshaw Chemical Co., Cleveland, Ohio.)

recording oscilloscope face corresponding to the original location of a gamma ray or scintillation of light resulting from the gamma ray. With this arrangement, only 294 discrete storage locations for gamma quanta are available. Position of these gamma quanta therefore takes place in a digital fashion. The information is registered on a two-dimensional core memory (p. 234) conforming to the detector matrix. The contents of the core memory can then be transferred to magnetic tape (p. 231). An anticoincidence circuit eliminates gamma rays scattered between one crystal and another in the mosaic. This technique eliminates scintillations caused by both the original gamma ray and the scattered gamma ray. As in the Anger camera, the signals from the two photomultiplier tubes are summed and fed to a pulse-height analyzer for acceptance or rejection.

Since this instrument has only 294 storage locations, the original instrument was such that each image was composed of 294 units of information. This camera now is used in conjunction with a programmed bed that moves 16 times within each individual crystal, yielding 4,704 independent data points that are used for

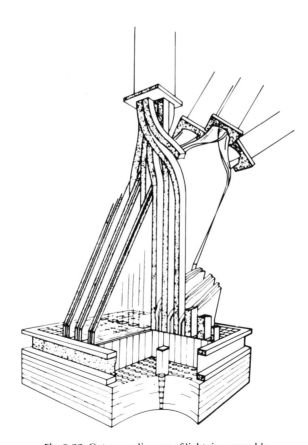

Fig. 9-22. Cut-away diagram of lightpipe assembly.

image construction (Fig. 9-23). Each move is equal to 2.78 mm per move. This bed motion allows each detector crystal to scan a square area with 1.11-cm sides. Bed motion is visibly undetectable.

This arrangement combines the data acquisition principles of both the camera and the scanner. The information for each move is collected on core memory but transferred to magnetic tape. This transfer clears the core memory to accept information from a subsequent move by the programmed bed. The 16 single pictures of the scan are combined into one complete picture by means of a computer.

The nature of this detection system lends itself to obtaining digital data by a unique "flagging" technique. The areas of interest that are to be selected are addressed by means of a photocell light pen, called a *wand*. The photocell generates control signals synchronized to the memory timing system. This synchronized signal generates a "flag" that keeps track of the selected memory locations and displays the stored information as a digital presentation on command.

Camera data presentation equipment. Both types of scintillation cameras yield X and Y position signals that must be utilized by some ancillary data presen-

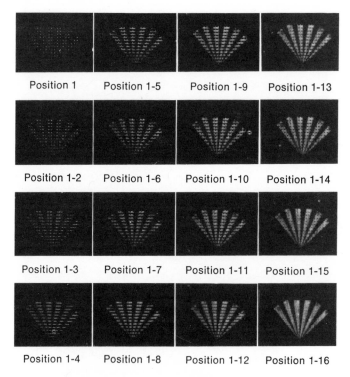

Position 1	Position 1-5	Position 1-9	Position 1-13
Position 1-2	Position 1-6	Position 1-10	Position 1-14
Position 1-3	Position 1-7	Position 1-11	Position 1-15
Position 1-4	Position 1-8	Position 1-12	Position 1-16

Fig. 9-23. Static image accumulation. These actual Polaroid photos show the results of the imager's programmed bed, which indexes 16 times within each individual crystal 2.78 mm per move—and you have in effect a matrix of 4,704 individual detectors. Each detector accumulates events to form an image with valid information content.

tation equipment. Four such ancillary pieces of equipment are (1) a cathode ray tube oscilloscope, (2) a multiformat programmer, (3) a variable persistence scope, and (4) a whole-body imaging table.

CATHODE RAY TUBE OSCILLOSCOPE. X and Y position signals generated by the scintillation camera can be sent to the cathode ray oscilloscope to direct the beam of the oscilloscope to the position of the original scintillation in the crystal. Just like the scintillation camera, the oscilloscope can also be thought of as a pie cut into four pieces, with the cuts serving as *x* and *y* coordinates. The normal position of the electron beam of the oscilloscope is in the center of the phosphor (Fig. 9-24, *dotted line*). When in this "resting" position, the electron gun is not activated (called *blank*); therefore, no electrons strike the phosphor of the oscilloscope face. The activation of the electron gun requires an accepted Z pulse from the pulse-height analyzer, now called the *unblank* pulse. This unblank pulse will turn the electron beam on for a short period of time (a function of the unblank pulse width), only after the X and Y position signals have been allowed to stabilize. This assures that the electron beam will strike at the point on the phosphor representative of the point on the detector crystal. Should that event be in the exact center of the crystal, then the electron beam is not moved and the unblank pulse turns on the electron beam. However, if the event occurred anywhere other than in dead center, the electron beam will require a change in direction. This is the purpose of the horizontal (X) and vertical (Y) deflector plates.

Since electrons will change their directions slightly in an electric or magnetic field, the magnitude of the position signals will change the course of the electron beam. This is accomplished by making the poles within the oscilloscope either more positive with respect to one another or more negative with respect to one another in all four directions. This affords an infinite number of positions on the

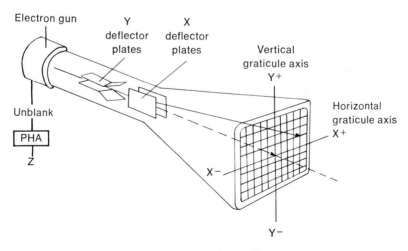

Fig. 9-24. Schematic of an oscilloscope.

oscilloscope face for the electron beam to be directed. The total resolution of the scintillation camera system depends on the collimation (extrinsic resolution) and the crystal and its associated electronics (intrinsic resolution) to properly adjust the polarity of these signals to the oscilloscope. By so doing, it correctly directs the electron beam to a position on the oscilloscope that corresponds with the position of the original scintillation in the crystal. The electrons striking the phosphor on the oscilloscope will excite the atom comprising the phosphor, which produces

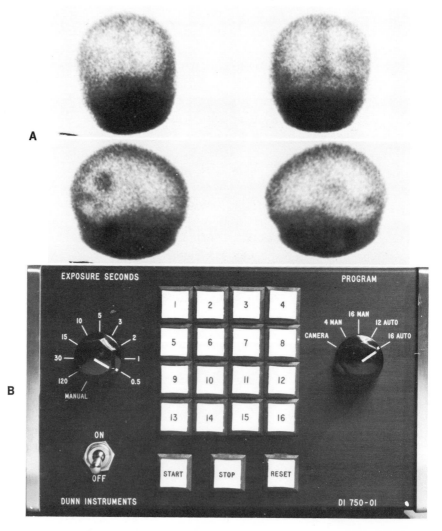

Fig. 9-25. A, Multiple views of brain image displayed on one piece of standard size x-ray film using multiformat programmer, **B.**

a flash of light. This flash of light can then be recorded on film. Each dot on the oscilloscope is a result of that electron beam being directed to a new location on the oscilloscope screen. Each change in location is produced by another event that occurred in the detector. The recording of these events over a period of time results in an image on film that displays the distribution of the radionuclide within an organ.

MULTIFORMAT PROGRAMMER. An adaptation of this process of placing one whole image on one piece of film is to place more than one image on a single film. A unit that allows this is termed a *multiformat programmer*. The concept of this system is to apply a constant gain to each signal that enters the oscilloscope. This changes the magnitude of the position signal so that in effect the center of the electron beam has been changed. Furthermore, its movement will be restricted to one section of the oscilloscope face and therefore one section of the film. This gain change also minifies the image. During a second exposure the position of the image can be changed automatically or by manually pressing a position button (Fig. 9-25). This automatically sets another gain, allowing the second exposure to be restricted to another portion of the oscilloscope face. In this way many smaller views can be placed on one piece of film (Fig. 9-26). This has been found to be particularly useful with dynamic flow images, where less information is lost by the electronic change in position than the automatic mechanical advancement of photographic film.

VARIABLE PERSISTENCE SCOPE. Oscilloscopes, as generally used in medicine, have phosphors that stay excited for a known amount of time; therefore, light is emitted by this phosphor for a predetermined length of time. There was no way in which this "persistence" time could be varied. Since different phosphors persist for different amounts of time, an oscilloscope was selected for a particular use by the persistence time of the phosphor. Phosphors having a short persistence are commonly selected for general use because most signals are repetitive and occur at a rate fast enough that flicker is not bothersome. However, long persistence is often sought to display slowly moving biomedical phenomena and applications in which the traces must persist after the moving spot. Although many long persistence phosphors are available, most do not properly accommodate the signal and are easily burned. Other applications could take advantage of the ability to vary the persistence so as to have a phosphor that would persist for a long period of time when needed and then alternately persist for a very short period of time. Since persistence is an inherent property of the phosphor, this is not possible except by artificial means.

The ability to vary the persistence is achieved by what is now called a *variable persistence scope* (Fig. 9-27). This type of scope consists of three surfaces and two electron guns. The three surfaces are: (1) a collector mesh that acts as a device to orient electrons so that they travel perpendicular to the phosphor and parallel to the CRTs longitudinal axis, (2) an electron storage mesh that is an elec-

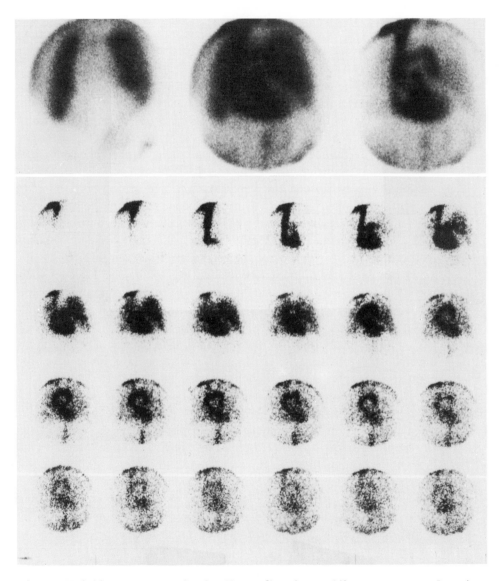

Fig. 9-26. Varied format as presented on 8 × 10 x-ray film using a multiformat programmer. Large image in the upper left is a transmission image of the lungs. Large image in the middle is a transmission image combined with a static flow image through the heart. Large image in the upper right is just the static flow image. The 24 smaller images represent a cardiac flow, reading from left to right. (Courtesy Holy Family Hospital, Des Plaines, Ill.)

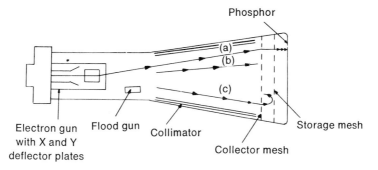

Fig. 9-27. Schematic of a variable persistence scope: *a* represents the high-energy "writing" beam of electrons being oriented by the collector mesh and knocking off several secondary electrons from the storage mesh; *b* represents electrons being absorbed by the collector mesh; *c* represents electrons passing through the collector mesh but being repelled by the negative charge on the storage mesh, to finally be absorbed by the collector mesh.

trostatic surface on which an image is written or generated, and (3) the phosphor itself. The two electron guns are the writing gun, which writes with a focused high-energy beam, and a flood gun, which continually sends a cloud of electrons toward the three plates.

The writing gun produces a focused stream of high-energy electrons that passes through the collector mesh (some are collected) and "writes" a channel of positive charges on the electron storage mesh. This is accomplished by the high-energy electron beam knocking off electrons from the storage screen by secondary emission similar to that which happens on the dynodes of the photomultiplier tube. The absence of these electrons makes the area where the electron beam struck positive with respect to the other areas of the screen. The electrons produced by secondary emission are accelerated toward the phosphor, where they strike and excite their atoms with the subsequent release of energy in the form of visible light. The degree of brightness of the recorded event on the phosphor is a function of the voltage *(growth rate)* applied to the cathode of the CRT. As this voltage is increased, the energy of the "writing" electrons is increased. As these higher energy electrons strike the electron storage mesh, a greater number of secondary electrons are emitted from its surface. These are then accelerated to the phosphor, creating an increasingly larger and increasingly brighter spot on the oscilloscope phosphor.

Persistence is a function of the flood gun. This electron gun continually sends a cloud of electrons toward the phosphor. Since the electron storage mesh is usually negatively charged in its entirety, the cloud of electrons is prevented from getting to the phosphor and being collected by the collector mesh. It is only when the writing gun generates its relative positive charge on the electron storage mesh that these electrons from the electron cloud are attracted to it and through it. These electrons then are accelerated to the phosphor to persist the image by continuing to excite the phosphor. The usual length of time that light is visible on a cathode ray tube oscilloscope screen (that is, from the time that the light is first seen through the inherent decay time of the phosphor) is 0.2 second. The variable persistence scope allows one to extend that time up to 60 seconds. *Variable persistence* is achieved by varying the rate of erasure of the electron storage mesh. This erasure is controlled by varying the rate of discharge of the electron storage mesh, thereby making the area that possessed a relative positive charge more negative. The rate at which this discharge occurs is the variable. As the positive area becomes less positive, fewer electrons from the flood gun are allowed through to the phosphor, and the dot gets lighter and lighter. Eventually the positive area is completely discharged, and the dot of light disappears. In reality, then, increased persistence is a result of decreasing the erasure rate. "Blooming," or phosphor flare-up, occurs in a variable persistence scope when the erasure time is faster than the inherent decay time of the phosphor. When these conditions exist, the phosphor responds by a flare-up caused by the overwhelming number of events striking the phosphor.

WHOLE-BODY IMAGER. Another adaptation to electronically manipulating position information is the *whole-body imaging table* (Fig. 9-28). With this system

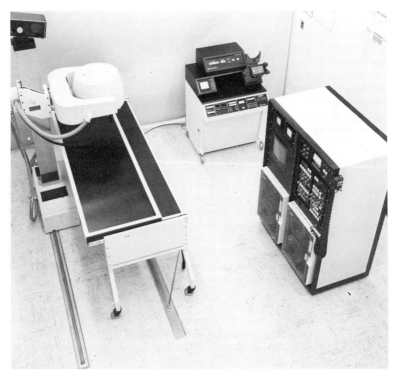

Fig. 9-28. Scintillation camera with whole-body imaging table. (Courtesy Ohio Nuclear, Inc., Solon, Ohio.)

the patient, the detector, or both, on a specially designed scanning platform, are moved lengthwise past the scintillation detector. The detector "sees" one longitudinal section of patient anatomy as defined by the limiting edges of the detector field of view. Integrated data from the longitudinal section is presented to the cathode ray tube as a "minified" display to accommodate the total body image. An indexing mechanism within the table allows for subsequent longitudinal sections, dependent on patient width. Either one, two, or three passes are electronically selected. The electronics keeps the image from overlapping, which would result in a blurring of the image. Consequently, these lines represent a displacement rather than a loss of information. "Single pass" whole-body cameras are also available. These cameras view the whole body in one pass by the detector as opposed to a composite image made by three passes over the whole body. Altered electronics and special fan-shaped collimators make this technique possible.

To ensure high sensitivity and constant uniformity over the entire scan area, it is necessary that each portion of the body appear in the detector's field of view for the same amount of time. This depends on three essential factors that are automatically controlled. First, the crystal must be electronically masked to restrict the area of sensitivity to a rectangular format, which eliminates the integration of counts from the otherwise overlapping edges of a circular aperture detection system. Second, the patient must be "overscanned" at the head and feet to assure uniform exposure of these areas to the detector. Third, the speed of the platform or crystal and movement must be kept constant and smooth, regardless of the patient's weight and the position of the scanning platform.

As the drive mechanism moves the scanning platform or the detector head in a continuous motion, a digital shaft encoder electronically transmits to the oscilloscope the platform positive relative to the detector. The information is then recorded on film relative to the position of the detector at the time that the event occurred. The composite picture as a result of the camera data presentation equipment is seen in Fig. 9-29.

Converters: ADC or DAC. It is important to remember that the signal coming from the scintillation detector is as a result of a single discrete photon interacting with the crystal. This is true whether it be a well, an uptake probe, an Anger scintillation camera, or a rectilinear scanner. However, by the time the light that is produced in the sodium iodide crystal is collected by the photocathode and amplified by the dynodes of the photomultiplier tube, the resultant electric signal is not a discrete electric "spike" but is more of an electric "peak," its highest point representing some value in voltage (Fig. 9-30, *A* and *B*). This is an *analog* signal and can be defined as any signal in which voltage changes with time.

In the case of the scanner, the analog pulses from the detector are generated through an averaging process since they are usually relayed through a count-rate meter governed by a time constant. As already indicated, this arrangement allows counts to be accumulated over some predetermined period of time (time constant)

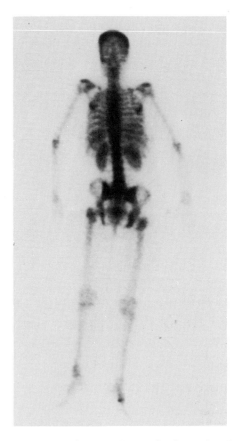

Fig. 9-29. Whole-body image as presented on 5 × 7 x-ray film by a whole-body imaging table associated with a scintillation camera.

and averaged with previous but similar periods of time. Pulses from an Anger camera can also be displayed on an oscilloscope as signals whose voltage value changes as a function of time.

Any of these analog signals can be converted to digital signals through the use of an *analog-to-digital converter (ADC)*. While there are many ADC techniques, the most usual technique in nuclear medicine because of the importance of pulse-height analysis is through a pulse height–to–time conversion. Digital pulses are given the same voltage value regardless of the pulse height. Variations in pulse height are expressed as variations in the length of time that the pulse is allowed to exist (Fig. 9-30, *C*). In this form, the information is easily stored and retrieved in computer systems. By reversing the process, it is easy to see that information in digital form can also be changed to an analog signal. The systems that perform this function are called *digital-to-analog converters (DAC or D/A)*.

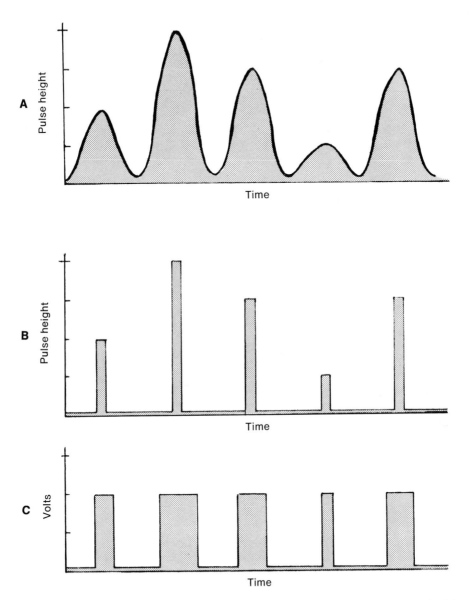

Fig. 9-30. A and **B**, Representative pulses from the detector in analog form. **C**, Same pulses in digital form as seen following a conversion by way of ADC. Note that the variations in pulse height are reflected as a difference in time. Most ADCs currently used in nuclear medicine use this pulse height – to – time conversion technique.

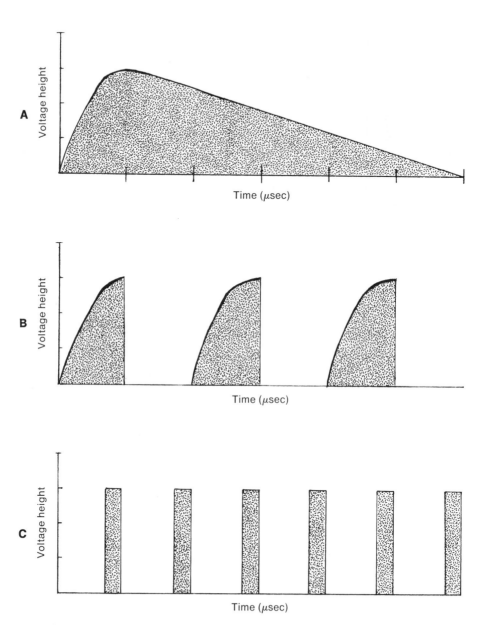

Fig. 9-31. Effects of pulse-shaping through a charge-to-voltage converter. **A,** The integrated voltage waveform. **B,** Same voltage waveform terminated at its maximum voltage height, allowing for more events to be processed during the "decay time" of the waveform in **A. C,** Same waveform shaped differently, allowing for even more events to be processed during the "decay time" of the waveform in **A.**

Pulse shapers. Other signal manipulations are also being carried out by the electronics of nuclear imaging equipment. These manipulations are referred to as *pulse shaping*. The purpose of this function is to increase the signal-to-noise ratio, which would enhance the validity of recording a detected event. In so doing, count rate capability is usually increased.

One of the most effective areas in which pulse shapers can be used in nuclear medicine equipment is following the use of a charge-to-voltage converter in which the current generated by the detector is changed to a voltage pulse. The electronic components are better able to use the information in this form. During the detection of a single photon event, the largest number of electrons from the photomultiplier tube arrives at the anode of the tube at approximately the same time, and the rest of the electrons generated by that same detection event arrive at a decreasing rate with time. The conversion of this current information to voltage results in a characteristic curve (Fig. 9-31, *A*). This curve is referred to as an *integrated voltage waveform*. The most important part of the waveform is its maximum height. Therefore, if it were electronically possible to terminate the waveform at its maximum height, more time would be available to process a subsequent event (Fig. 9-31, *B*). Further refinements could result in a square waveform (Fig. 9-31, *C*).

There are many techniques used to perform these corrections and pulse manipulations, the description of which is felt to be beyond the scope of this book. Needless to say, this concept of pulse shaping is much more complicated than as presented here. There are an infinite number of waveforms possible, and these have to be matched to a particular component for proper efficiency and function. The time for integration of the voltage waveform must be adequate to ensure statistical accuracy. If the waveform being shaped is that of the X or Y position signal, the integration time must be adequate for proper positioning of the CRT electron beam or the resolution of the clinical image would be poor. These decisions are the job of the electronics engineer designing the instrument. Suffice it to say that this concept of pulse shaping has allowed the count rate capabilities of these imaging devices to increase by at least one order of magnitude since the development of the original commercially available instrument.

MISCELLANEOUS DETECTORS

In addition to the gas detectors and the scintillation detectors, there are other detectors that do not use either of these operating principles. Radiologic film detection and thermoluminescent dosimetry are two other possibilities.

Film badges. The film badge is probably the most commonly used radiation detection device today. It provides a reasonably accurate means of determining doses from beta, gamma, and x-radiation. Most film badges consist of a plastic holder containing radiation-sensitive film, usually of dental film size or 35-mm photographic film. The film badge also contains a variety of filters used to absorb certain radiations of varying energies. The variety of filters placed at different points on the film badge allows identification of a specified type of radiation. The use of these absorbers gives an indication of the penetration and energy of the radiation producing the exposure. There is also an area on the film badge that has no filter and is not covered by even the plastic holder. Beta as well as very weak energy gamma radiation can be detected in this area.

Films are developed and then evaluated by measuring the density of the blackening on the film. These measurements are compared to standard films that have been exposed to known radiation doses. Generally, film badges are capable of measuring doses from 50 mr to 500 r.

The film badges are worn on the pocket or the belt of nuclear medicine personnel. The same film may be worn for a week to, usually, a month. The length of time depends on the sensitivity of the film and the amount of radiation to which the radiation worker is exposed. Since nuclear medicine personnel are usually exposed to very low levels of radiation, the longer the film is worn, the greater will be the accuracy of the measurement. The film badge is not sensitive to radiation exposures much below 50 mr. It is suggested that nuclear medicine personnel wear their film badge for periods of 1 month at a time so that the radiation level will fall into the sensitive area. With the advent of radionuclide generator systems the Nuclear Regulatory Commission has suggested that the radiation worker use finger or wrist badges as well.

Film badges have an advantage over other types of monitoring devices in that they provide a reasonably accurate record at a low cost. Furthermore since the film badges are not developed, evaluated, or recorded in the nuclear medicine laboratory, the film badges provide a permanent unbiased record of exposure. The disadvantage of a film badge is that since the mailing, evaluation, and return of the report requires approximately 3 weeks, an immediate record of exposure is not available. Other disadvantages include the fact that film badges may become darkened if improperly handled, such as when left on a radiator or on clothes that are sent to the laundry.

Thermoluminescent dosimetry. Thermoluminescent dosimetry is a method of radiation detection that is rapidly gaining acceptance as a personnel monitoring device. Materials used for thermoluminescence are primarily calcium fluoride and lithium fluoride. These materials, when exposed to ionizing radiation, absorb the energies released in the material. This energy is liberated only on subsequent heating of the material. As the temperature reaches a characteristic value, the energy is released in the form of light, and this light is analyzed for exposure intensities — hence the name thermoluminescence.

Thermoluminescent dosimetry offers a variety of uses in the radiation medicine field. In addition to personnel monitoring applications, it is used in the measurement of doses in tissues surrounding a therapeutic tissue implant source. The thermoluminescent method appears to be much more sensitive than the film badge.

BIBLIOGRAPHY

Blahd, W. H.: Nuclear medicine, New York, 1965, McGraw-Hill Book Co.

Bogardus, C. R., Jr.: Clinical applications of physics of radiology and nuclear medicine, St. Louis, 1969, Warren H. Green, Inc.

Chandra, R.: Introductory physics of nuclear medicine, Phildelphia, 1976, Lea & Febiger.

Chase, G. D., and Rabinowitz, J. L.: Principles of radioiosotopes methodology, ed. 3, Minneapolis, 1967, Burgess Publishing Co.

Goodwin, P. N., and Rao, D. V.: The physics of nuclear medicine, Springfield, Ill., 1977, Charles C Thomas, Publisher.

Gottschalk, A., and Potchen, E. J.: Diagnostic nuclear medicine, Baltimore, 1976, The Williams & Wilkins Co.

Hendee, W. R.: Medical radiation physics, Chicago, 1970, Year Book Medical Publishers, Inc.

Hine, G. J.: Instrumentation in nuclear medicine, vol. 1, New York, 1967, Academic Press, Inc.

Hine, G. J., and Sorenson, J. A.: Instrumentation in nuclear medicine, Vol. 2, New York, 1974, Academic Press, Inc.

Johns, H. E.: The physics of radiology, ed. 2, revised edition, Springfield, Ill., 1964, Charles C Thomas, Publisher.

King, E. R., and Mitchell, T. G.: A manual for nuclear medicine, Springfield, Ill., 1961, Charles C Thomas, Publisher.

Quimby, E. H., and Feitelberg, S.: Radioactive isotopes in medicine and biology, ed. 2, Philadelphia, 1963, Lea & Febiger.

Rhodes, B. A.: Quality control in nuclear medicine, St. Louis, 1977, The C. V. Mosby Co.

Rollo, F. D.: Nuclear medicine physics, instrumentation, and agents, St. Louis, 1977, The C. V. Mosby Co.

Shilling, C. W.: Atomic energy encyclopedia in the life sciences, Philadelphia, 1964, W. B. Saunders Co.

Shapiro, J.: Radiation protection, Cambridge, Mass., 1972, Harvard University Press.

Strauss, H. W., Pitt, B., and James, A. E., Jr.: Cardiovascular nuclear medicine, St. Louis, 1974, The C. V. Mosby Co.

Wagner, H. N.: Principles of nuclear medicine, Philadelphia, 1968, W. B. Saunders Co.

Wagner, H. R.: Medical radiation physics, Chicago, 1970, Year Book Medical Publishing Co.

10 Computer fundamentals

William Pavlicek, B.S.

The tremendous developments that have occurred during the past 20 years in the field of electronics have led to the increased use of special-purpose, or so-called dedicated, digital computers. A computer with the ability to handle a very large number of electronic signals quickly and accurately finds a logical application when *interfaced* (connected) with a scintillation camera during the visualization of organs. This logic becomes apparent if one considers nuclear medicine procedures, electronically speaking, as (1) accumulation, (2) processing, and (3) presentation of data. In fact, simply restating these steps in computer terminology will describe the operational sections of a modern digital computer. (See Fig. 10-1.)

Every modern digital computer contains the same five basic sections. These are as follows:

1. *Input* section
2. *Memory* section
3. *Control* section
4. *Arithmetic* section
5. *Output* section

The middle three of these sections, the *memory, control,* and *arithmetic* sections, are usually termed the *central processing* unit, or simply the *central processor.*

The general flow of data starts with the input section. This section accepts the raw data (analog electronic signals from the detector) and converts it into a form (digital) that can be readily used by the central processing unit. The data is then stored in the memory section until such time as the control unit directs its processing. The control unit, always acting under a specific set of instructions called a *computer program,* directs the appropriate raw data from the memory section to the arithmetic section. Here the data may be added, subtracted, or otherwise acted on in the manner prescribed by the computer program. The control unit then directs the return of the processed data to the memory section, where, depending on the program, it may temporarily remain or be transferred to bulk storage. Eventually, however, this information will continue to the output section, where it will be translated from the machine language of the computer to the language of its human operator.

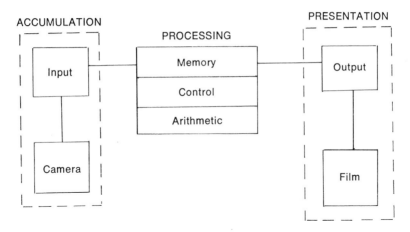

Fig. 10-1. Block diagram of a digital computer interfaced with a scintillation camera.

Although all the various instructions used by the control section to direct the flow of data are termed *computer software*, the electromechanical devices and electronic gadgetry that make up the physical construction of the computer are aptly termed *computer hardware*.

BASIC COMPUTER CONCEPTS

In a computer, information is always conveyed by means of electrical pulses. As an example, the 10 digits of the decimal system can be represented by electronic pulses of equivalent voltage levels. Computation may then be performed in the manner familiar in decimal mathematics. For example, if the digit 5 is represented by a pulse of 5 v and the digit 6 represented by a pulse of 6 v, then the sum of these two digits may be obtained by simply adding their voltages and measuring the result as 11. This is descriptive of an *analog* method of addition; computers that employ this technique are analog computers.

One difficulty with such a method is that the computer must be able to transfer its data from one section to another. This makes for complicated electronics in the analog computer and permits the possible introduction of errors induced by noise or other variations in voltage levels.

Although the analog computation as just discussed utilized a continuously variable physical quantity, a *digital computer* is designed to use pulses having only *two* discrete voltage levels. To represent any of the various possibilities of different numbers, a *code* is developed and used by the computer in substitution. In mathematics, such a number system with only two values (0 and 1) is termed a *binary* system.

For example, two commonly used voltage states in the digital computer are 0 v (no pulse) and +5 v (pulse). The 0 v pulse may represent the binary 0, and the +5 v pulse may represent the binary digit 1. The term *BI*nary digi*T* indicates a single character of the binary system and is always referred to by the computer term *bit*. Any number of the familiar decimal system may now be converted easily into the binary system for use by the computer. (See Fig. 10-2.) The decimal value in column one is represented by an equivalent binary number as shown in column two. The binary numbers were generated by counting in the binary system shown in column three. A bank of lights is electrically connected in such a manner that an incoming pulse will cause a change of status. That is, if the light is off, then it will be lit, and if it already is lit, then it will go out, with the pulse continuing to the left.

Number	Equivalent binary number	Binary counter							
		128	64	32	16	8	4	2	1
0	0	N	O	L	I	G	H	T	S
1	1								*
2	10							*	
3	11							*	*
4	100						*		
5	101						*		*
6	110						*	*	
7	111						*	*	*
8	1000					*			
9	1001					*			*
10	1010					*		*	
11	1011					*		*	*
12	1100					*	*		
149	10010101	*			*		*		*
etc.	etc.				etc.				

Fig. 10-2. Binary counting.

Each possible combination of lights and no lights (pulse and no pulse) is then generated and corresponds to a number in the decimal system.

It is apparent that large numbers in the decimal system would be even larger numbers in the binary system. However, the computer easily compensates for this apparent unwieldiness because of its ability to handle the binary numbers with incredible speed.

To follow the digital computer's method of addition, the reader should return to the mathematical problem given previously – the addition of 5 and 6. To perform this operation in the binary mathematical system, one first substitutes the decimal numbers with the binary numbers and completes the addition by following the appropriate rules.

Binary mathematical rules of addition

1. $0 + 0 = 0$, with no carry
2. $0 + 1 = 1$, with no carry
3. $1 + 0 = 1$, with no carry
4. $1 + 1 = 0$, with a carry of 1

Substituting,

Decimal	*Binary*
5	101
6	110
11	1011

The equivalent of the decimal 11 is the four-bit answer, *1011*.

All other problems in mathematics are simply treated by the digital computer in the same manner by following the other rules of the binary number system.

The binary answer obtained from the problem just given (1011) can be treated by the computer as one piece of information. This is a definition of the computer term *word*, which is the basic unit of information in the computer. Computer *word length*, then, is simply the number of bits contained in the word and is dependent on the physical construction of the hardware.

In addition to the *data* word just explained, two other words are used by the computer: the *instruction* word and the *address* word. The instruction word, as its name implies, contains bits of information indicative of the particular procedure to be carried out. The address word, on the other hand, contains bits of information indicating the location of the data word(s) that are to be processed.

In the example of a computer interfaced to a scintillation camera the data word can be composed of bits indicating the number of counts obtained at a specific location by the crystal. The address word will contain information indicating the location of these counts, whereas the instruction word can contain the directive to add to this data word any future counts occurring in the same area of the crystal.

Generally speaking, the data words of information are stored in the memory section of the computer, whereas the instruction and address words are associated with the arithmetic and control sections.

Different computers vary in their method and ability to handle words of information that are fed to them. These differences are purposely built into the computer to provide a more efficient or better suited approach to a particular application. Regardless of these differences, some underlying principles of hardware are common from computer to computer.

COMPUTER HARDWARE

Computer hardware may be defined as all the electronic or electromechanical devices, components, and gadgetry that comprise the physical makeup of the computer. The first device that is encountered by the electronic signals generated by a scintillation camera is the analog-to-digital converter (ADC). This circuitry converts the analog voltages of the camera to the digital needs of the computer. Since a scintillation camera will produce two signals for a gamma event (x and y coordinates), some nuclear medicine computers are supplied with two ADCs, one for each signal. Digital-to-analog converts (DACs), on the other hand, perform the opposite function by converting the digital signals back to analog form as needed for image presentation and display.

Although each of the five basic sections of a digital computer has its own associated hardware, often the input and output sections utilize the same instrumentation and for this reason are usually discussed together.

Input/output

Magnetic media is a general term used to classify any of the forms of information storage or transfer that incorporate the magnetic properties of iron or ferrous material. This includes the use of magnetic tape, drums, discs, and core (magnetic core is discussed on pp. 231-234).

Paramount, however, to a discussion of the uses of these types of devices is an understanding of some basic properties of magnetism. One may demonstrate these properties by collecting two ordinary sewing needles and a bar magnet. The two needles when placed together will initially show no attraction for each other. Stroking one of the needles with the bar magnet in a continuous fashion will induce this needle to become magnetized , and it will then be able to attract the other needle. The needle that is magnetized will exhibit the common property of having one end, perhaps the point of the needle, become the "north" pole, whereas the "eye" of the needle will become the "south" pole. Striking the needle or dropping it will result in a loss of its induced magnetic properties. If desired, the needle may be remagnetized in the opposite direction. That is, the point of the needle will then become the "south" pole and vice versa.

This simple experiment describes the properties inherent in magnetic media that are incorporated by the input/output section for use with a digital computer. Specifically, these properties are as follows:

1. The ability to have two distinct states (magnetized and nonmagnetized, or north and south poles), the "code" of the binary numbers 0 and 1

2. The ability to magnetize or demagnetize (or change the direction of the magnetic field) with *enormous* speed
3. The ability of one piece of ferrous material to determine (sense) the magnetic state or field direction of another, which permits the transferring of information from one section to another

Magnetic tape. Magnetic tape is the most widely used of the magnetic family. Its use is similar to the familiar tape recording systems of home entertainment units. Both systems have tape transports, recording heads, and playback heads. Magnetic tape used for digital computers differs from that of home entertainment units because the information placed on the tape is in a digital form rather than the analog forms used for music or voice. This is performed by recording on a present or absent basis with regard to its magnetic state.

The tape itself is made of plastic and coated on one side with a ferrous oxide. It is often 1 inch wide, with common lengths of 2,400 or 3,600 feet. Spaced across the tape width and running the entire length are tracks. These tracks simply serve as designated areas for locating the magnetized spots and typically are six or eight in number. A six-track tape has six possible locations for writing information, whereas an eight-track tape has eight such areas. The tracks are arranged in random order simply to increase the overall wear of the tape. (See Fig. 10-3.)

The pattern of the magnetized spots (represented by dashes) across the width of the tape and along its length is a coded representation of the data stored on it. As may be seen, many possible different combinations of "spots" (bit) and "no-spots" (another bit) are available. On a section of tape that has been used to record a nuclear medicine study one may find the pattern of magnetized spots to be the binary equivalent of the number of counts (gamma events) that occurred in a certain portion of the detector.

In computer terminology the recording of information on magnetic media is called *writing*, whereas the playing back of any of the magnetic media to retrieve information is called *reading*. Both these functions are carried out by a system

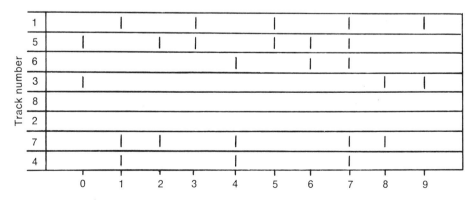

Fig. 10-3. Magnetic tape.

that is appropriately called the *read/write head*. Read/write heads perform their function by making use of the magnetic properties as discussed. The write head will record its information by inducing specific locations of tape to become magnetized, whereas the read head will perform the reverse of this operation by sensing which of the spots are magnetized.

The writing of information and its subsequent reading can be performed with great speed. Tape transporting systems operate at 90 inches per second, with a common packing density of 800 bits per inch. Multiplying these two values together will determine a tape *transfer rate* of approximately 72,000 bits per second. Once information is recorded on magnetic media, the magnetic state is fixed, and it may be kept as a permanent record of a study. Thus one may speak of magnetic tape (and drums and discs) as having an indefinite *archival quality*.

Magnetic drums. Magnetic drums are constructed of aluminum and coated with a ferrous oxide on their outer surface. The surface of the drum, like the magnetic tape, is divided into a number of tracks or channels, each track or channel serving as a location for the induction of a magnetized spot. Unlike magnetic tape, however, drum systems usually have multiple read/write heads, one for each track. The drum will rotate past the heads at a common speed of 3,600 rpm. (See Fig. 10-4.)

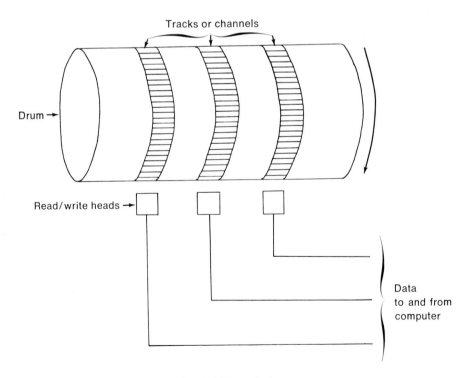

Fig. 10-4. Magnetic drum.

The information is coded in much the same manner as information on magnetic tape. Any single piece of information on one track, however, is never more than one revolution away. Thus the use of magnetic drums will decrease the *access time* for obtaining information over that of magnetic tape. What the drum offers in terms of speed, however, is lost with regard to storage capacity and thus cost.

Magnetic discs. Magnetic disc devices are general-purpose, random-access storage units. They normally are used as input/output devices in medium-to large-size computers for applications requiring large-volume data transfer with immediate accessibility. As shown in Fig. 10-5, the magnetic disc is similar to the 45 rpm "jukebox" record playing system. The individual discs are made of plastic and coated on both sides with ferrous oxide. The typical rotational speed for magnetic discs is about 1,000 rpm.

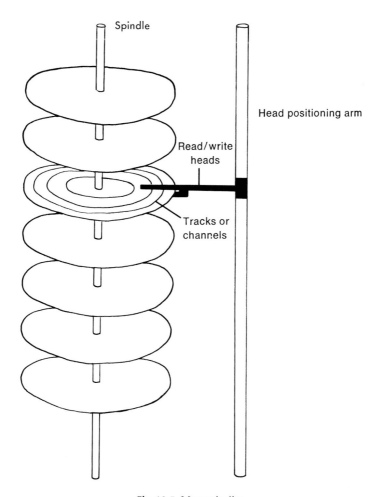

Fig. 10-5. Magnetic disc.

This system can consist of a single disc or a series of discs, arranged vertically on a spindle. Some disc models have permanently attached discs, whereas others use a detachable set of discs called a *disc pack*. The disc pack is popular because it permits the data to be moved to other locations for processing by other computers.

Each disc face is divided into a number of concentric tracks or channels for the storage of information. The discs are separated from one another with sufficient room to permit the movement of the read/write heads. This method of information storage allows for extremely quick transfer of data.

Many other forms of input/output devices are in great use. Included among these are the familiar punched card and paper tape, both of which use a series of punched holes to code information for digital use. The operation of these and the other input/output devices is not within the scope of this discussion. Regardless of the type of input, however, once the information has been coded in the proper form it is transferred to the memory section to begin the desired manipulation.

Computer memory

The hardware of the computer memory basically consists of small ferrite rings arranged on a matrix. These metal rings, or "cores," are very small—10,000 of them would fit in a thimble. Each one of the ferrite cores has four very thin wires passing through it, with each of the wires at a 45-degree angle from the others. (See Fig. 10-6.)

Unlike the magnetic media that store information on the basis of the presence of absence of a magnetized area, a magnetic core indicates the information it contains by changing the *direction* of its magnetization. Being formed in the shape of a ring, core memory has but two directions in which to alter directions—clockwise and counterclockwise, each corresponding to one of the two values of the binary number system.

The two wires running in the north-south and the east-west direction through any of the metal rings are called *address wires*. These are the wires labeled X and Y in Fig. 10-6. The two wires serve the function, for a computer interfaced to a scintillation camera, of reproducing in this memory core matrix the exact location of the gamma ray absorption that occurred within the crystal. For example, if the scintillation camera passes along the coordinates (X and Y values) of the location of a gamma event, then a current will be applied to both of the address wires in memory that corresponds to the origin of that event in the crystal. The current passing through either of these wires will attempt to change the direction of all the ferrite cores along its path. However, each ferrite core is so constructed that only a current of a certain value will cause it to change direction. The currents applied to the X and the Y wires are purposely reduced to half that value. This results in only the one memory core (the one at the site of the X and Y intersection) receiving the combined current of the wires, thus enabling it to change direction.

The remaining two of the four wires run diagonally along the matrix. These are

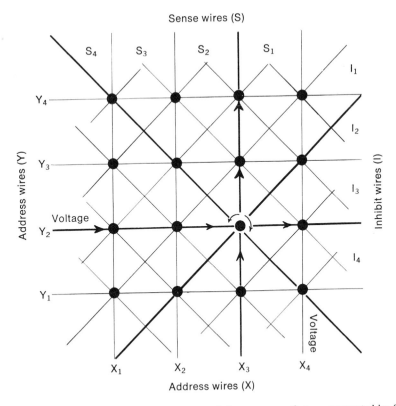

Fig. 10-6. A single matrix is composed of many metal rings or cores that are connected by four thin wires. The two address wires (X_3 and Y_2) have a voltage applied to them that results in a change of magnetic direction (a 0 to a 1 or vice versa) of the core located at their intersection. The sense (S_4) and inhibit (I_2) wires pass through this core and effect the reading of information from memory.

termed the *sense* and *inhibit wires*. A current will pass through the inhibit wire only when a particular address is not to change states, whereas the sense wire is so positioned that it will produce an output pulse whenever a change of magnetic direction occurs. Generally speaking, then, the address wires write information in the memory, whereas the sense and inhibit wires read the information from the memory.

Note that Fig. 10-6 shows a matrix that is 4 bits × 4 bits, with a total of 16 different locations or addresses. In reality, a more common matrix size is 64 bits × 64 bits, or a total of 4,096 separate addresses. Memory core is always built of many such matrices, stacked one on top of another. Very often 8 such matrices stacked on one another will comprise the memory section, each of the 4,096 addresses now referencing 8 cores or bits. In this example, each group of 8 bits can be referred to as a *memory address,* a *memory cell,* a *memory location,* or a *computer word.*

Fig. 10-7 shows a simplified illustration of building up counts in memory as radionuclide activity is absorbed in a scintillation crystal. The accumulation of

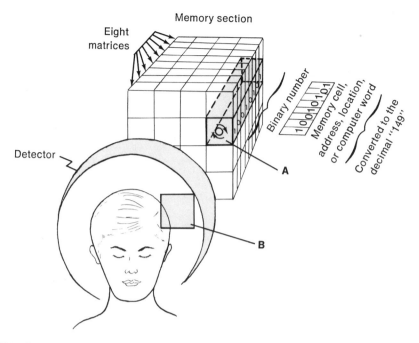

Fig. 10-7. Computer memory. *A*, A 0 or 1 can be written in core; *B*, 149 gamma events occur within this area. For a memory section of 4,096 addresses, this area would measure 4.4 mm × 4.4 mm on a 10-inch crystal.

counts is achieved by alternating the direction of magnetization on the core to indicate the appropriate binary values (1 and 0) of decimal equivalents *(A)*. Thus the 149 gamma events that occur at area *B* are represented in memory as the 8-bit computer data word 10010101. The entire organ image is simply the extension of this sample principle to the other addresses in computer memory. The greatest number of total counts that can be written in a single memory cell is simply the largest number that can be presented with eight characters of the binary system (that is, 2^8, or 256). For a memory of 4,096 separate cells or addresses, each would reference an area of approximately 4.4- by 4.4-mm on a scintillation camera having a 10-inch field of view.

In expressing the storage capacity of a computer memory, one always gives both the number of addresses (rounded to the nearest thousand) and the word length (number of bits per word). For example, the memory unit just described is referred to as a 4K (4,000, but actually 4,096) 8-bit word computer.

Once the data is accumulated in memory, its processing is carried out under the direction of the control unit.

Control section

The most important component of the control section is an electronic oscillator, commonly referred to as the *clock*. The clock generates a stream of pulses, on a regularly timed basis, that open and close all the other circuits in the computer. In this manner the control section is able to regulate the external and internal operations of all the sections. Since it initiates and synchronizes everything in the computer, the clock is sometimes likened to a heartbeat.

Clock rate is the frequency with which these regularly timed pulses are generated and may be on the order of nanoseconds for a modern computer. As an example of how incredibly short a nanosecond is, the distance that light will travel (at 3×10^{10} cm/sec) during this time (10^{-9} seconds) is 3×10^1, or 30 cm.

Another portion of the control section is the control panel or console for direct human to machine communication. This will contain a number of "start" and "stop" buttons, as well as the individual controls for the various input/output devices and displays. For a scintillation camera interfaced with a dedicated computer, some common control would be available for (1) cathode ray tube (CRT) display, (2) image orientation (X, Y, and Z planes), (3) area of interest (AOI), (4) uniform field correction, (5) addition and subtraction, (6) smoothing, and (7) graph generation.

In addition, there will be the usual controls to display or indicate the number of the study, patient identification, time of the study, and counts obtained.

Although the control section directs the implementation of instructions, the actual performance of nuclear medicine data manipulation is carried out in the arithmetic section of the computer.

Arithmetic section

The various electronic circuits of the arithmetic section are scattered throughout the computer. There are *registers* used as temporary storage locations, *comparers* used in mathematical operations, *counters* to tally items of information such as instructions, and *flip-flops* used to perform logic statements. Interconnecting all these elements is a network of other electronic and logic circuits that directs the signals along their appropriate paths.

COMPUTER SOFTWARE

As previously mentioned, the control section always acts under the direction of a computer program. Computers that are termed *general purpose,* or *programmable,* permit the introduction of different sets of instructions for the performance of different tasks. On the other hand, a computer may be preprogrammed to perform only specific tasks. This type of computer is called a *dedicated,* or *hard-wired,* computer and will lack the hardware necessary to accept additional sets of instructions without an alteration of electronics.

COMPUTER PROGRAMMING

Regardless of the type, any digital computer will solve problems only in a step-by-step manner. Therefore the program that is written into the computer memory (a computer program may have its own memory) for usage must necessarily be

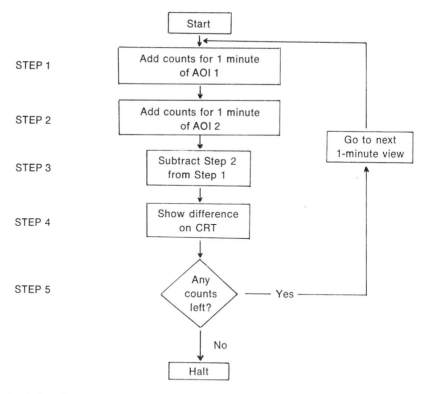

Fig. 10-8. A flow chart is a block diagram of the steps involved in solving a problem and is an invaluable aid to a programmer. This example illustrates the sequence of events in developing a background-corrected, organ uptake curve. Note that if the answer to Step 5 is yes, a loop would direct the computer to return to Step 1.

broken down into the smallest possible series of sequential and logical steps. It is the job of a *computer programmer* to analyze a problem to determine a best suited approach. As an aid to this task, a programmer first draws up a block diagram of the problem, laying out the proper sequence of events and indicating with arrows the direction of data flow. A diagram so produced by programmers for their use is termed a *flow chart* (Fig. 10-8).

Fig. 10-8 is a simplified flow chart that shows the basic steps involved in generating a graph or histogram of background-corrected organ uptake, as may occur in a dynamic study. Assume that 1-minute images were obtained for 15 minutes and that two electronic areas of interest (AOI) have been established. The first AOI is located over the organ of interest, whereas the second one is positioned over background activity. The graph is to be presented on the cathode ray tube of the computer system for photographing. Following is the sequence of events as diagrammatically shown on the flow chart in Fig. 10-8:

Step 1 — The control section of the computer finds the addresses of those gamma events located in memory that are delineated by the first electronic area of interest. The number (binary) of gamma events at those addresses accumulated during the first minute are totaled by the arithmetic section of the computer. This value is temporarily stored in a register.

Step 2 — The control section of the computer finds the addresses of those gamma events located in memory that are delineated by the second electronic area of interest. The number (binary) of gamma events at those addresses that were accumulated during the first minute are totaled by the arithmetic section of the computer. This value is temporarily stored in a register.

Step 3 — The control unit directs the arithmetic section to subtract the number of background counts from the number of organ counts.

Step 4 — The control unit directs this number to be presented to the digital-to-analog converter for display on the cathode ray tube.

Step 5 — The control section directs the arithmetic section to sense the number of counts in both registers and compare that value to the total number of counts in memory at the addresses of the areas of interest. If the number of counts in the register is equal to the number of counts in this section of memory, then the program is finished. If, however, the number of counts in the register is less than the number of counts in the portion of memory, the control unit is directed by the computer program to go to the second minute of the study and continue as in Step 1. Eventually the comparison of the two values will be equal, and the computer will stop.

It should be noted that when Step 5 is reached and more counts are yet to be processed, a rerouting on the flow chart occurs. This technique is known as a *loop* and is employed to great use by programmers. It not only saves programming time but also can save a large amount of valuable memory space as well.

Once a programmer has determined the best suited approach to a problem, the program is coded in a language compatible with the computer. These languages are known as *compiler languages* and represent a compromise between human and machine languages. Examples of compiler languages are FORTRAN, which is especially suited for scientific applications, and COBOL, a business-oriented language.

NUCLEAR MEDICINE APPLICATIONS

Although many applications of the digital processing of images are currently being developed, several uses are common. These uses may be classified under the general headings of system applications, dynamic study applications, and static study applications.

System applications

Field uniformity correction is the process of digitally correcting organ images for nonuniformities inherent with a scintillation camera. A key point, however, is that differing nonuniformities may exist with usage of different collimators or with different energy radionuclides. In its best usage, therefore, a computer-corrected field would be developed for each combination of collimator and radionuclide. Indeed, since the developed values are collimator dependent, care must be taken to align the collimators in the same manner during day-to-day usage. Techniques for field uniformity correction will be discussed separately in this chapter.

Internal controls is a general term that covers all the various system identification abilities. These include (1) patient identification, (2) the date, (3) the type of study, (4) the collimator used, (5) the time of the study, (6) the counts obtained, and (7) the radiopharmaceutical employed.

Three-dimensional views may be obtained, since the computer develops a digital representation of radionuclide distribution in memory. It is a simple matter to rotate the Z orientation on a CRT to receive an indication of the activity "depth."

Dynamic study applications

Smoothing can be effected during flow studies by a digital process. This can be achieved by instructing the computer to arithmetically alter each of a sequence of images. For example, to the counts of one memory cell of one image may be added half the difference (increase or decrease) of the counts for that same memory cell of the next image. An "in-between image" is thus developed, which when displayed in rapid sequence will give the appearance of a "movie."

Graphs or *histograms* are a commonly used analytical tool for describing the inferred physiologic progresses. The electronic areas of interest are located over the appropriate organ (for example, kidney), and the graph is developed by the computer as described in the discussion of the flow chart.

Temporal comparisons of radionuclide activity can be made by subtracting early views from those taken at a later time. If the early distribution of a tracer is largely vascular and the agent slowly leaks into a pathologic region, the differences in counts between these studies may outline the pathologic site in sharp relief.

Static study applications

Smoothing may be performed by arithmetically manipulating a stored image in memory. This can be performed in different ways, but the technique commonly employed is to have the counts of a memory cell and its neighboring cells added together, a mean average determined, and this value substituted for the original counts accumulated in the cell. As this is performed on every cell, the final image will have a "smoothed" appearance.

In its most used form, *addition* and *subtraction* is simply the process of increasing or decreasing the number of counts in each cell by a constant value to permit the observer to best *perceive* the desired information in the location of possible pathology. This form of image enhancement (perhaps a more descriptive term would be "perceptibility enhancement") can be used to subtract background or to add counts to a low count image.

Another form of subtraction occurs with the use of two radionuclides. The two radionuclides are judiciously chosen for their complementary presence in a scintillation image. Two images are obtained, one from each of the radionuclides, and then the desired image is shown in relief by the subtraction of the other.

In certain circumstances useful *comparative studies* can be made (for example, left and right hemispheres, lungs). This can be done by simply placing regular or irregular areas of interest over the comparative locations and determining their respective counts.

A more sophisticated method is to employ a statistical tool to determine the probability of the difference between these counts having occurred by chance alone. The standard formula for this operation is as follows:

$$N(\gamma) = \frac{N_1 - N_2}{\sqrt{N_1 + N_2}}$$

N_1 = Count obtained from one AOI
N_2 = Count obtained from the other AOI
$N(\gamma)$ = Significance of the difference between the counts

This technique can provide a range of values (similar to the method employed for thyroid uptakes) to support a physician's suspicions that unequal amounts of activity are present.

Nonuniformity correction techniques

Uniformity, or rather the lack of it, has been a constant problem since the advent of the scintillation camera (Anger type). The cause of this nonuniformity is largely twofold: (1) the variations in sensitivity across the face of the crystal and (2) nonlinearities in the position signals, resulting in spatial distortions caused by generation of an area of apparently decreased radioactivity surrounded by an apparent ring of increased radioactivity. The latter defect causes bar phantoms to "barrel" and data from linearity phantoms to be malpositioned, to say nothing of the effects on clinical results. This can be true in a uniform flood system and often is the case in a nonuniform flood situation. The reverse is even more often the case, that is, a nonuniform flood study with no appreciable spatial distortions.

The enigma of the design engineer regarding this problem is that uniformity has always been a compromise with resolution; as resolution is increased, uniformity decreases and vice versa. It becomes the job of the engineer to decide at what point both facets will be compromised to give an acceptable clinical result. With the advent of nonuniformity correction techniques, this dilemma has been solved with a design for resolution and a correction for nonuniformity.

There appear to be at least four different techniques of correcting for nonuniformity. These techniques can apply correction to areas as great as 20% deviation from the average and are as follows:

1. Matrix division, using the computer to either subtract counts from the "hot" areas of a stored image or add counts to the "cold" areas of a stored image
2. Count skimming (also known as count skipping)
3. Z pulse modulation
4. Sliding energy window (also known as micro-Z processing)

Matrix division. This nonuniformity correction technique divides the camera face into squares. Each square corresponds to a location in the computer memory (Fig 10-7). This location should be no smaller than a 64 × 64 matrix or a total of 4,096 picture elements (called "pixels" or words). Each detected event (called a bit) from a flood will be recorded in its corresponding pixel location in the computer memory. The collection continues until there is a statistically significant number of counts in each memory location or until such time as a preselected number has been recorded. Then the recording of events stops. The computer, then, is capable of searching each location and determining the total number of counts stored in each location. If all locations have the same number of stored events, then nonuniformity correction is not necessary. This is rarely the case. In the usual situation, computers will identify the magnitude of the deficiency in each location and correct for it by equalizing all points to no greater than ± 5%, either by the addition of counts or the deletion of counts. Suppose that the computer program was such that in a 64 × 64 matrix, the program would turn off whenever a single pixel received 500 counts (64 × 64 × 500 = 2 million total counts in the flood). Further, suppose that the computer, in its systematic search of each pixel, notes that some pixels have accumulated only 450 counts; the computer will calculate the deficiency to be a 10% reduction from the maximum counts. The computer will record that and will, in future studies (either floods or clinical images), correct those locations by either randomly adding 10% more counts to each of them (and therefore decreasing the time of the study) or randomly rejecting 10% of the counts in each of them (and therefore, increasing the time of the study). This procedure will be carried out for all memory locations, with appropriate correction techniques generated for each.

Count skimming. This nonuniformity correction technique is an attempt to avoid the long dead time necessary in the matrix division-rejection technique. This system uses an *analog derandomizer circuit* in conjunction with a *sample and hold circuit* and a minicomputer. The X and Y position signals and the unblank pulses go directly to an analog derandomizer (Fig. 10-9) rather than to the CRT. This derandomizer is capable of storing up to eight random events from the camera and releasing them at a rate of 200,000 counts per second. In this way, the events are derandomized and put into a form that the ADC and the computer can handle easier and faster. The other advantage is that since pulses (counts) from the camera are random, sometimes a second pulse will arrive during the dead time of the system (called *pulse pile-up*) and not be counted. The derandomizer will be able to count these pulses; therefore, the count rate capabilities of the system are

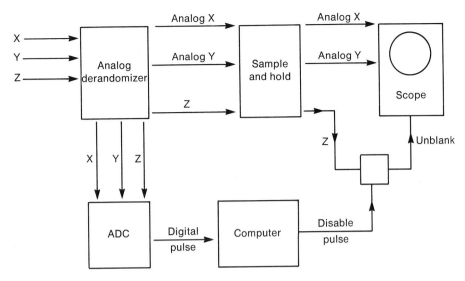

Fig. 10-9. Modified version of a schematic of a count-skimming circuit.

increased. The signals are then sent out of the derandomizer and divided—one set going to the ADC, the other to a sample and hold circuit. The latter is composed of two capacitor memories that serve to delay the analog signal from reaching the CRT. During the delay period, the second set of signals is being sent to the ADC, digitized, and made accessible for the computer to either store as a flood or allow for correction from the stored flood by rejection of counts in "hot" areas. If the event is to be rejected, the correction circuit will release a signal to disable the unblank pulse that is being released at the same time (along with the X and Y position signals) by the sample and hold circuit; therefore, no event is recorded on the CRT. If the computer accepts the event, no disable pulse is generated and the event is allowed to record on the CRT.

Z pulse modulation. Another technique for nonuniformity correction is that of Z pulse modulation. The Z pulse, or unblank pulse, is typically of a uniform width (Fig. 10-10, *A*). This allows the response of the electron gun in the CRT to be the same for each event and, therefore, to be displayed with the same intensity on film. The approach to Z pulse modulation is to vary the pulse width of the Z signal (Fig. 10-10, *B*), thereby varying the response of the electron gun in the CRT. The resultant film then will appear uniform because Z signals from hot areas will be shorter and displayed with less intensity than those from cold areas, while Z signals from cold areas will be longer and therefore displayed with increased intensity on film. This system also uses an analog delay system to allow the memory to develop a correction factor for the event and modulate the Z pulse. This technique does not involve either addition or rejection of counts; therefore, the time for individual clinical studies has not changed whether on or off correction. It is important to note that since the correction occurs at the CRT on the analog signal, this ap-

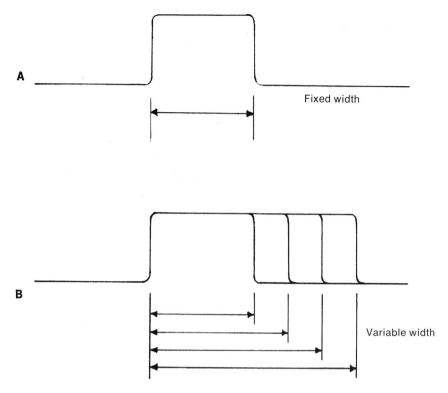

Fixed width

Variable width

Fig. 10-10. A, Typical Z pulse width. **B,** Pulses of various widths as a result of Z-pulse modulation.

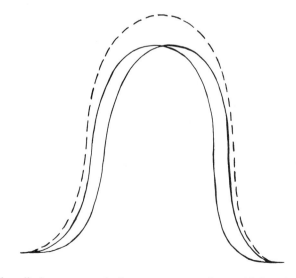

Fig. 10-11. Solid lines display energy peaks from two separate photomultiplier tubes, while dotted line displays a composite energy peak. In order to encompass both energy peaks from these two separate PMTs, a larger window would be necessary, resulting in reduced resolution of a clinical image.

proach would not allow for correction of a computer-generated image. Another program, such as matrix division, would be required for the computer itself.

Sliding energy window. Another approach to correction circuits is that of a sliding energy window. This approach is based on the belief that the major contributors to nonuniformities in the flood study are the crystal, the photomultiplier tubes, the "light pipes," and the interfaces among them. The variations in light distribution relating to these factors result in a slight shift of the photopeak on each of the photomultiplier tubes. The spectrum seen in "peaking in" the instrument is a composite of all of these individual peaks (Fig. 10-11). Since each peak varies slightly, the composite peak is a broader peak. To accept a clinical window based on this composite image, then, is to accept more scatter and degrade the image. A better solution would be that a window be set for each energy peak of each photomultiplier tube. Ideally, since a computer is used, a window could be set for the energy peak received by each pixel. Therefore, a 64×64 matrix computer would be likened to 4,096 individual pulse height analyzers, each setting its own optimum window. This is the case with the sliding energy window technique. In this way, uniformity is improved and energy resolution is optimized because each window is treated separately, rather than in common. Any causes for nonuniformity not related to energy are corrected by any of the other correction techniques already mentioned.

Multigated acquisition techniques

Organ motion in nuclear medicine studies has long been a distressing problem for the interpreter of nuclear medicine procedures. Liver and lung motions have been irresolvable problems since the advent of the rectilinear scan. Scintillation cameras have helped, but not solved, the problem. Early attempts to limit liver motion during a scanning procedure ranged from strapping the patient across the diaphragm and to the cart so tightly that diaphragmatic breathing (the cause of liver motion) was discouraged to "freezing" the phrenic nerve, which innervates the diaphragm. Attempts were made to image lungs with the camera only during the short pauses of inhalation or exhalation. Composite images were formed by manually turning on the camera each time the patient inhaled and held and manually turning off the camera during exhalation. A statistically valid image was achieved by repeating the process many times. This on-off procedure is referred to as *gating*. All of these attempts met with little success because there was no easy way to signal the imager to automatically turn on at any specific time and turn off at some other preordained time.

Another organ that would require some sort of gating mechanism in order to be visualized is the heart. The acquisition of a composite camera image of the heart at end systole (end of the contracting and pumping phase) or end diastole (end of the relaxing and filling phase) or both was considered unattainable by most. The reason is obvious. It was humanly impossible to gate the heart manually. Counts were always recordable at the various stages of action, using something as simple as an external probe and a strip chart recording device, but not images.

The first significant change was the advent of the Brattle Physiological Synchronizer. This device accepted the leads from an electrocardiogram (ECG) machine and used the ECG signals, such as the R or T wave, to automatically signal the camera to turn on at the beginning of a wave and off at its end. In this way, a composite image could be made of the heart in the same stage of contraction or relaxation. Clinically significant images were formed by accumulating counts during that short portion of the cardiac cycle over several hundred heartbeats. Similar leads were used to signal inspiration or expiration cycles for automatic gating of lung images.

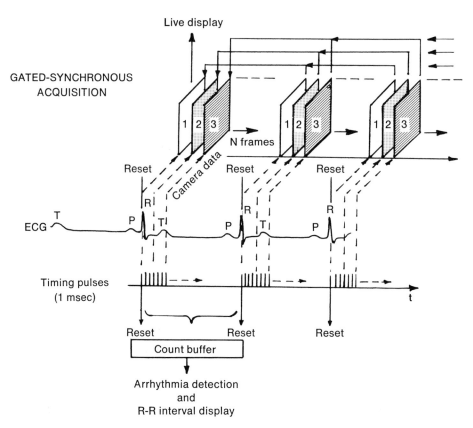

Fig. 10-12. Diagrammatic representation of gated frame mode data acquisition for cardiac studies. Data from the gamma camera are in N frames between each R wave with the R wave causing the reset to frame 1. N may be up to 48 in 32 × 32 acquisition or up to 12 in 64 × 64 acquisition. The data collected during each heartbeat are added to those from the previous beats so that valid statistical images result. A continuously updated display of the first frame together with R-R interval, number of cycles collected, and number of cycles rejected is displayed on the computer display screen. (From Cradduck, T. D., and MacIntyre, W. J.: Camera-computer systems for rapid dynamic imaging studies, Semin. Nucl. Med. 7(4):323-336, October 1977. By permission.)

The computer extended the capabilities of the Brattle gater even further. With the computer, in combination with the ECG and the internal clock (see "Control section" in this chapter), the cardiac cycle can be framed into many segments (for example, 48), each segment representing a different position of the heart during one complete cycle (Fig. 10-12). A composite image of each position is possible when interfaced with a multiformat programmer. This is accomplished by preselecting the number of frames desired, which sets up the 1-msec clock to allow for a certain number of pulses to occur before moving the image to another computer frame or another position on the CRT or TV. The imaging is triggered by the first R wave after the system is started. Each subsequent frame is opened for collection under the control of the internal clock until another R wave causes data collection to reset and begin again with the first frame. This is termed multigated acquisition (MUGA). The procedure continues for 300 to 500 heartbeats, with each frame of each heart cycle adding to its previous counterpart to provide a series of clinically significant images of the heart in each position of the cardiac cycle. Rejection circuits are available to disallow the recording of information from arrhythmic heartbeats.

From this recorded information several determinations can be made. Since the computer image is based on numbers, it is easy to recall numbers for the determination of ejection fraction and stroke volume. The computer can generate left ventricular volume curves of counts versus time. Single pass calculations as well as multigated calculations can be used. Wall motion studies can be performed by recalling all frames of data sequentially at a rate of speed that is variable, termed *ciné mode*. With all this data on computer, many more studies will be available in the future. Especially significant is the fact that with the advent of mobile cameras and minicomputers, the entire cardiovascular recording capabilities can be arranged on a mobile unit to bring modern, state-of-the-art nuclear medicine to the bedside of the critically ill patient.

BIBLIOGRAPHY

Gottschalk, A., and Potchen, E. J.: Diagnostic nuclear medicine, Baltimore, 1976, The Williams & Wilkins Co.

Hine, G. J.: Instrumentation in nuclear medicine, vol. 1, New York, 1967, Academic Press, Inc.

Hine, G. J., and Sorenson, J. A.: Instrumentation in nuclear medicine, vol. 2, New York, 1974, Academic Press, Inc.

Lapidus, S. N.: A new method of correcting for detection non-uniformity in gamma cancers, Stanford, Conn., Raytheon Medical Electronics.

Rhodes, B. A.: Quality control in nuclear medicine: radiopharmaceuticals, instrumentation and in-vitro assays, St. Louis, 1977, The C. V. Mosby Co.

Rollo, F. D.: Nuclear medicine physics, instrumentation, and agents, St. Louis, 1977, The C. V. Mosby Co.

Strauss, H. W., Pitt, B., and James, A. E., Jr.: Cardiovascular nuclear medicine, St. Louis, 1974, The C. V. Mosby Co.

Technical Data Sheet NTD-002 and NTD-004: Solon, Ohio, Ohio Nuclear, Inc.

Todd-Pokropek, A. E., Erbsmann, F., Soussaline, F.: The Non-uniformity of imaging devices and its impact in quantitative studies, IAEA-SM-210/154.

Wagner, H. R.: Medical radiation physics, Chicago, 1970, Year Book Medical Publishers, Inc.

11 Considerations of counting and imaging

The detection and subsequent count rate obtained from a radioactive source is governed by many factors. These factors include the operating voltage, resolving time, geometric relationship between the source and the counter, scatter, absorption, background radiation, efficiency of the counter, collimation, and the use of statistics. All these factors depend on the detector itself, the counter, the source of radiation, and the material surrounding the source.

OPERATING VOLTAGE

The count rate obtained from a given source with a Geiger or scintillation detector is highly dependent on the voltage applied to the detector. This has already been discussed at great length, and in this chapter it will be assumed that the proper operating voltage has been determined.

RESOLVING TIME VERSUS DEAD TIME

Every counting system, whether ionization or crystal, requires a certain recovery period after the detection of a pulse before the system is capable of counting a second pulse. In the discussion of G-M tubes it was stated that after an ionization event the electrons travel quickly to the anode, but the positive ions travel at a much slower rate to the cathode. During the travel time of the positive ions, any other ionization events will not be seen by the detector. This description of a G-M counter will help to distinguish the fine differences between dead time, resolving time, and recovery time. The time period during which ions are traveling to their respective poles and therefore no pulse of any kind can be generated is called the *dead time*. The time period during which sufficient numbers of gas atoms have recombined and, therefore, partially restored the gas, at least sufficiently to record an event, is called *resolving time*. The time period required for all atoms to recombine and, therefore, for the detector to return to its full potential (actually, potential difference) is the *recovery time*.

Scintillation detectors have resolving times from 10^{-5} to 10^{-6} seconds, and the scaler has a resolving time of 10^{-5} seconds. In the case of a scintillation crystal, it is often the scaler that is the limiting component in the system, rather than the detector.

As a result of the phenomenon of dead time, the observed counting rate is always less than the true counting rate. There is a certain probability that one or more pulses will follow a detected event within the interval of the resolving time and will not be counted. As the counting rate increases or the resolving time increases, this probability will become greater. If the counting rate and resolving time are known, the number of events that are lost can be predicted, and the observed counting rate can be corrected.

In these days of high–count rate imaging techniques, the way that these systems handle this problem of resolving time becomes very important. Some early G-M counters and scintillation cameras were such that if the count rate was high, the events would be recorded for awhile, then the system would shut down and no events would be recorded. Needless to say, this was disastrous for a cardiac flow study. The reason for this phenomenon was that the events were being seen by the detector but the associated electronic component was not having sufficient time to recover from each recording. If the system cannot recover from one event, it cannot record another. These systems are said to be *paralyzable.*

These paralyzable systems are such that each event resets the recovery process before it has had sufficient time to recover to the point that another event can be recorded. With no events being recorded, the system shuts down. Advanced electronics in cameras and self-quenching G-M survey meters have improved this situation. They allow the recording of only those events that occur after the system has had sufficient time to recover. These systems are called *nonparalyzable.* In these systems, if the count rate exceeds the saturation point of the system, there will be a reduction in count rate/unit activity but not a shutdown of the system.

GEOMETRY

The geometric relationship between source and counter has a profound influence on the count rate obtained for a given activity. The count rate is particularly sensitive to the size and shape of the source and detector and to the distance between the source and detector.

The inverse square law (discussed in detail in Chapter 6) has a profound influence on count rate. Using a point source, the counting rate is decreased by one fourth if the distance is doubled and is increased by a factor of 4 if the distance is halved. In the case of a source of activity that is not a point source, this relationship does not hold exactly, but the relationship between count rate and distance is still profound.

This principle is important in routine nuclear medicine procedures such as the thyroid uptake study and the renogram. An uptake study, for instance, that does not use the same distance between detector and thyroid as between the detector and the standard will represent a gross change in count rate, and therefore, the results will be erroneous.

Perhaps the greatest disregard for proper geometry considerations is not in the correct use of a probe but in counting samples in a well detector. Distance and inverse square are not so readily recognized in this type of detection procedure. A common problem is comparing the counts from a 4-ml standard to a 2-ml unknown, where it was possible to collect only 2 ml of serum. To obtain a correct count, the *geometry must be identical,* unless a correction factor is known. This means that the technologist cannot compare the two samples by counting the 2-ml sample and multiplying by 2. The 2-ml sample must be diluted with an activity-free solution to 4 ml, then the count multiplied by 2, since more of the emissions from the 2-ml sample are being exposed to the detector than from the 4-ml sample (Fig. 11-1). The gray area in Fig. 11-1 represents percentage of counts that are not exposed to the detector from the 4-ml sample but are exposed from the 2-ml sample. Since more of the emissions are allowed to go undetected by the 4-ml sample, the count could not be accurately compared to a 2-ml count.

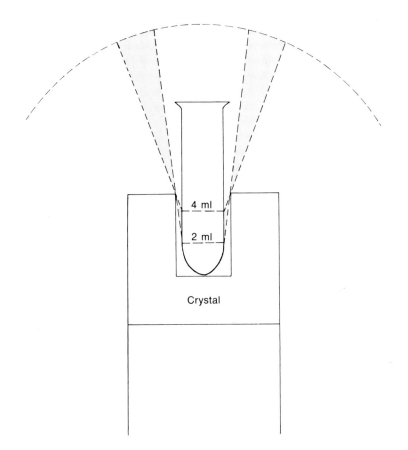

Fig. 11-1. Diagram illustrating the importance of geometry considerations in well counting. A 2 ml sample will have greater than one-half the count rate of a 4 ml sample of the same material because a greater number of photons will go undetected (gray area) from the 4 ml specimen.

This principle is dramatically proved by taking a count of a 1-ml sample, then making several 1-ml additions of water and counting after each addition. As the water is added (the water is activity-free), the count rate decreases until the level of the liquid reaches the top of the crystal. After that point the changes are not as great.

Errors in well counting can occur in comparing two sources in unlike containers. A 4-ml sample counted in a narrow test tube and compared to a 4-ml sample counted in a wide test tube will represent a considerable error for the same reason as different volumes.

The size and shape of the detector also influence the count rate. For example, some counters, called 4π counters, completely surround the source and are geometrically able to count all radiations emitted. Two π counters detect only 50% of the radiation emitted, since they surround only half of the source. Probe type detectors count only a small fraction of the emitted radiations, and well type detectors, by partially surrounding the source, can detect 50% or more.

SCATTER

Scatter is the term applied to radiation that is diverted from its original path by some type of collision. Radiation is emitted in all directions from its source. Those radiations emitted directly toward the detector may be counted. Those radiations emitted in any direction other than directly into the detector may be deflected in such a way that they will eventually strike the detector and also be counted. Since a collision of some kind was necessary, these emissions are reduced in energy. Barring pulse height analysis, this type of scatter would *increase* the count rate. The degree of scatter is influenced by the atomic number and the thickness of the backing material. Scatter will increase as either of these factors increases. Beta particles can be deflected by heavy nuclei through angles greater than 90 degrees and therefore can increase the count rate. Gamma ray back-scatter is caused either by Compton collision, resulting in a photon of lower energy traveling in a different direction from the primary gamma, or by pair production, wherein two 0.51-mev photons are ultimately produced. This scatter phenomenon is extremely important in understanding the principles of collimators. Scatter can reduce the count rate if it occurs in the material between the source and detector when gamma rays or charged particles are deflected out of the beam.

ENERGY RESOLUTION

Theoretically, since all gamma rays emitted from a monoenergetic gamma-emitting radionuclide such as ^{137}Cs have exactly the same energy, all pulses resulting from their detection would have the same amplitude. Furthermore, having the same amplitude, they should all appear at exactly the same point on a gamma spectrum. As has been seen in the section entitled "Gamma spectrum" in Chapter 9, this is not true. The display of gamma photons on a gamma spectrum resembles more a bell-shaped curve, representing gamma photons of many energies, than a "spike," representing gamma photons of a single energy. Although a "spike" is what should be displayed, this could happen only if the entire system of scintillation detection were perfect. Such is not the case. *Apparent* increases and decreases in pulse amplitude occur as a result of incomplete gamma absorptions in the crystal, losses of light intensity during crystal transmission, nonproportional release of electrons at the photocathode, infidelity of electron multiplication at the dynodes, and imperfections in the linearity of pulses in the amplifier. Defects in any of these components causes a widening in this bell-shaped curve, an undesirable effect that, if serious enough, is incompatible with continued use. Resolution is the term describing the limitations of such a spread of the primary photopeak. It is calculated as the ratio of the width of a photopeak (measured at a point equal to one-half the amplitude of the peak) to its energy. This value varies depending on the energy of the radionuclide.

ABSORPTION

Absorption of radiation differs from scatter in that the total energy of the radiation is dissipated in the absorbing material. Three sites of absorption exist in any counting situation: the source itself, the media between the source and detector, and the detector. All influence the resultant count rate.

Absorption occurring in the source, called *self-absorption,* reduces the count rate. This can be very significant in particle counting. In some cases self-absorption limits the number of counts that can be detected from a source material. As more radioactive material is added, the added material absorbs as many radiations as it emits. Gamma ray detection does not usually involve problems with self-absorption. However, if the gamma ray energy is less than 0.1 mev or if the source is large, such as a human body or an organ, then self-absorption must be considered.

Absorption of radiation occurring in the media between the source and detector also reduces the count rate. An example would be the air and the window of the detector in beta or alpha particle detection. For gamma ray detection it is usually unnecessary to take into account those gamma rays absorbed by the air or the detector window. However, a material of high density may absorb many of the gamma rays.

The final site of absorption occurs in the detecting medium. The detection of radiation depends on the absorption or transfer of energy from the radiations to the detector. Particulate radiations will, in general, be absorbed by the detector if they have sufficient energy to penetrate into the detecting medium. Therefore precautions must be taken not to allow the particles to be absorbed before they reach the sensitive volume of the detector. This is the rationale behind liquid scintillation counting. With gamma rays the problem is different. It is possible for a gamma ray to travel through a detector without interacting to complete absorption and therefore, using correct pulse height analysis, go undetected. The chance of this happening decreases as the mass or density of the detector increases. Therefore gaseous detectors such as Geiger tubes stop only a few gamma rays, whereas scintillation detectors stop many more.

BACKGROUND

All counters will record some activity without a source present. This activity is known as room background activity. It is caused both by radiation from natural radioisotopes and cosmic rays entering the detector and by instrument noise. The *gross count* of a source also includes background counts. Thus to obtain the *net count* from the source alone, the background count rate must be determined and subtracted from the gross count rate.

Many times the room background activity does not represent a significant change in the count, in which case it is a waste of time to consider it at all. In most of the recently developed instruments, background count rate never exceeds 100 counts per minute. Generally, any background count less than the square root of the total count can be disregarded because it will not introduce a significant amount of error into the procedure. For example, if the count rate were 10,000 cpm, a background count rate less than 100 dpm would be considered insignificant ($\sqrt{10,000} = 100$).

The primary purpose of a background determination is assurance that the instrument is operating properly. A room background count is performed *daily* by determining the proper operating voltage and allowing the unit to count for a predetermined unit of time without a source of activity near or in the detector. Background counts should be taken in the approximate clinical situation. For instance, the background count for the thyroid uptake probe should be taken with the probe pointing in the same direction as it would if it were being used for a patient count; the room background count of a well detector should be taken with the lid closed if this is the way it is being used with patient samples or with the lid of the well open if the clinical use of the unit dictates this procedure.

EFFICIENCY OF COUNTING

The factors just discussed are all a part of counting efficiency. The efficiency of any system is loosely defined as that which is obtained from the system divided by that which is put into the system. It can also be expressed as a formula:

$$\text{Efficiency} = \frac{\text{Counts/unit time}}{\text{Disintegrations/unit time} \times \text{Mean number/disintegration}}$$

To determine the efficiency of a well counter, it is possible to purchase a calibrated solution (iodine 131, for example) in which the disintegrations per second are known. For example, $1.0\mu\text{Ci}$ of a calibrated solution of iodine 131 can be used to determine the efficiency of counting. A microcurie has already been defined as 2.22×10^6 dpm, but this sample has been counted using the 364 kev gamma, which is *83.8%* abundant, and determined to be only 222,000 (2.22 × 10⁵) cpm. The efficiency can be determined as follows:

$$\text{Efficiency} = \frac{2.22 \times 10^5}{2.22 \times 10^6 \times 0.838} = 0.119 = 11.9\%$$

This result would indicate that the unit is capable of counting only 11.9% of all disintegrations and therefore is only 11.9% efficient. It is important to realize that the measurement of any radionuclide in a given sample need not be determined as its absolute value of disintegrations per unit time. In a routine nuclear medicine department the only concern is usually for relative values—the relative comparison of the activity in one sample with the relative value of the activity in another sample. The physician need not have the absolute value to make a valid diagnosis. The point can be demonstrated by the following examples.

A blood sample having an *absolute* value of 200 cpm was obtained from an injected dose having an absolute value of 20,000 cpm, representing 1% in the sample. The same samples counted on an entirely different instrument may represent *relative* values of 100 cpm from an injected dose having a relative value of 10,000 cpm—also 1% in the sample.

In both examples, whether absolute or relative values are used, the percentage of administered dose recovered in the blood sample is the same. The factors that influence the count received are presented in this discussion in an effort to make the technologist aware of these influencing factors so that in using relative values, these factors are kept constant. In this way the relative comparisons reflect a true comparison.

Coincidence counting

Once efficiency has been established for a certain set of circumstances, this percentile will remain fairly constant as long as these parameters do not change or until some major repair is indicated on the detector–read-out assembly. There is one exception to this statement, however. It is possible to exceed the capabilities of the detection system by increasing the radioactivity in the source being counted. Count rates may continue to increase with each subsequent increase in radioactivity but not in proportion to the increase in activity. This phenomenon may better be explained by simply stating that two highly radioactive but equal sources placed simultaneously near a scintillation crystal will result in a count rate less than both samples placed in identical geometrics but counted separately and then summed. The reason is that as the radioactivity increases, the probability of simultaneous gamma interactions in the crystal increases. When this occurs, a coincident pulse is registered as only one event by the recorder or, if the magnitude of the coincidence pulse height exceeds the upper-level discriminator setting, there is no registry of the interaction at all. As a result, the efficiency of the scintillation detector will decrease as the activity increases. In fact, at the point where coincidence loss begins, a second energy peak of twice the energy of the incident photons will begin to develop and will continue to build as activity increases. As suggested, 2 primary energy photons interacting with the scintillation crystal at the same time are being seen as 1 photon of twice the energy (for example ^{99m}Tc at 140 kev will also have a second peak at 280 kev). In fact, if the increases in activity continue, the actual count rate will also decrease. In some of the older paralyzable type imaging systems this would result in complete electronic shutdown of the instrument. In most of the new nonparalyzable types of imaging systems this point is reached with significant loss in resolution. It is important, therefore, to know these capabilities of the equipment and not to exceed them.

COLLIMATION

Electromagnetic radiation of longer wavelengths, such as light, can be focused by bending rays through lenses or by reflection from polished surfaces. Electromagnetic radiations of shorter wavelengths, however, will not respond to such mechanical manipulations. The only way a gamma ray can be removed from its path is by absorption or scatter of the ray. Therefore a device must be used that can eliminate from detection all gamma rays except those of interest. This device is called a *collimator*. The collimator is generally constructed of lead and extends in front of the scintillation detector. The lead is arranged in a configuration that allows it to perform the desired function. In the usual nuclear medicine laboratory two types of collimators are used, the flat-field collimator and the multihole collimator. There are four types of multihole collimators: parallel hole, focused (converging), diverging, and tomographic. Each of these types of collimators has different characteristics since each is used for a different purpose. In addition, there are straight-hole collimators and pinhole collimators.

Perhaps the most informative method of demonstrating the characteristics of these collimators is by the use of isocount lines (Fig. 11-2).

Flat-field collimators

In the event that a whole organ such as a thyroid or kidney is to be seen by the detector, the collimators must be designed to eliminate not only a portion of the background radiation but also radiation coming from other parts of the patient's body. The collimator chosen for this use must be able to detect radiations coming from any part of the organ of interest. A flat-field collimator would be used, since a flat response is received at a certain distance from the face of the collimator (Fig. 11-2). In Fig. 11-2 the isocount (same count) or isoresponse is demonstrated as having a flat portion, which increases in diameter as the distance from the face of the collimator is increased. A point source lying anywhere along such a line would result in the same number of counts. A line drawn directly across the face of the collimator with the point source centrally placed would represent 100%, the maximum count detectable. The same source located anywhere on the 80% isocount line would give a count equal to 80% of the maximum count.

When this collimator is used to visualize a whole organ, the distance that the

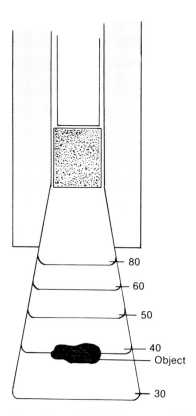

Fig. 11-2. Flat-field collimator whose characteristic is demonstrated by the construction of isocount lines, indicating uniform "vision" through organ under investigation.

collimator is placed away from the organ must be great enough to enable the detector to see the whole organ and to have a relatively uniform sensitivity to the entire organ. The flat-field collimator serves the uniform sensitivity criterion very well because of its flat response. The distance required to see the entire organ depends on the collimator and the diameter of the detector. For example, a 1½-inch diameter detector requires a 36-degree collimator to include a large thyroid at a distance of 20 cm. At a distance of 35 cm the same detector requires a 20-degree collimator.

Straight-bore collimator. In other nuclear medicine applications it is more desirable not to view the entire organ as a whole but to study particular segments of an organ independently from the rest of it. This requires a detector that views only a small area at a time, a special collimator.

The collimator used to view small areas of an organ is one that can also distinguish between small areas of differing count rates. Such a collimator is rated by *resolution*. Resolution is the minimum distance between two radioactive objects that can still be distinguished as two distinct sources by the collimator. The degree

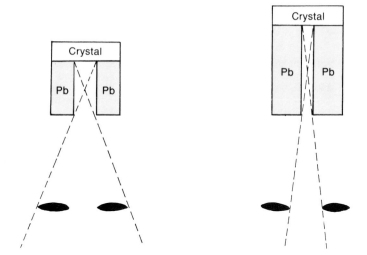

Fig. 11-3. Straight-bore (single-hole, single-channel) collimator illustrating the effects of size of hole and depth of hole on resolution. Dotted lines define the solid angle of inclusion. These same limits are analogous to penumbral limit lines in radiation therapy. (See Fig. 11-5, *B*.)

of resolution varies with the physical design and material of the collimator, as well as with the energy of the gamma rays being counted. A collimator is chosen according to the requirements of a specific application. In general, one with good resolution should be used for studies of small organs and one with poorer resolution can be used for larger organs.

One of the first collimators used for viewing small areas of an organ was the straight-bore collimator (Fig. 11-3). The straight-bore collimator is nothing more than a large piece of lead with a small hole bored through it. The piece of lead is attached to the face of the scintillation detector. The resolution of the collimator is influenced by the diameter and the length of the hole; the smaller the bore and the longer the collimator, the greater its resolution. Fig. 11-3 displays in a simple manner the effect of collimator length and bore size to resolution. All radiations emitted in the direction of the crystal and within the dotted lines will be detected in their pure energy state. Both detectors are aimed at two ⅝-inch areas of activity situated ⅝ inch apart and at a depth of 3 inches from the face of the collimator. The first detector, which has a shorter collimator with a larger bore size, is unable to differentiate between the two lesions because the *solid angle of inclusion* encompasses both lesions. This detector would have very poor resolution. The second detector has a collimator that is increased in length and decreased in bore size. The same two areas of activity, situated identically with respect to each other and to the collimator, are resolved as the detector unit passes over them. Emissions from the two areas of activity are not detected in their pure energy state if the detector is situated as depicted. As the detector moves to the right or to the left, pure emissions are seen only from the right or left areas of activity, respectively. Resolution is then greatly enhanced, and the system could be expressed as having a resolution of ⅝ inch. Another very important fact regarding resolution is that as resolution increases, statistics suffer. The collimator sees fewer and fewer events as resolution increases.

These principles of resolution are basic to understanding the influencing factors of any collimator, be it single-bore, focused, or parallel hole. These principles are easy to understand in the straight-bore collimator, but they often seem more complex when extended to the multibore or multichannel type collimator. However, there is no difference. The principles are the same, only the number of holes has changed.

Multihole collimators

Characteristics. The *number of holes* in a collimator is determined by the crystal size of the detector and the required septal thickness. In general, it can be stated that the number of holes for any given size crystal increases as the resolution increases. A decrease in number of holes suggests either nonutilization of the entire crystal, larger holes, or thicker septa.

There are both low-energy collimators and high-energy collimators available today. As gamma rays increase in energy, the ability of the collimator to absorb or deflect them becomes less. High-energy gamma rays require greater septal thickness than do low-energy gamma rays. This reduces sensitivity because the greater the thickness of lead, the smaller the area of crystal utilization. Consequently, two types of collimators are available based solely on their septal thicknesses: (1) a low-energy collimator, which is designed for all radionuclides having gamma energies less than 150 kev, and (2) a high-energy collimator for all radionuclides having energies greater than 150 kev. High-energy collimators can be used for imaging an organ containing a low-energy radionuclide, but the reverse is not true. Sensitivity, of course, is much less with the high-energy collimator and a low-energy radionuclide than with a low-energy collimator and a low-energy radionuclide.

Multibore focused collimators. Although the straight-bore collimator, as originally designed, had good resolution between two distinct lesions, tremendous amounts of radioactivity had to be administered to the patient for the count to be statistically adequate. For this reason, there had to be an increase in the number of events detected while limiting the detection area so that the resolution did not suffer tremendously. Such a compromise led to the production of a multibore focused collimator.

This collimator consists of a series of holes in a piece of lead that are angled in such a way that their holes are aimed at approximately the same spot. This spot is called the *focal point*, or *focal depth*, and represents the 100% isocount area. Unlike the other collimators discussed, the 100% area is not at the face of the collimator but at a point distant to the face. Another feature of the focused collimator is that the diameter of the holes is tapered; the larger end is closest to the crystal to increase the detection efficiency. The isocount lines proceed in a somewhat elliptical fashion around the focal point as indicated in Fig. 11-4.

The same two factors of collimator length and bore size affect the resolution of the focused collimator. In addition, special consideration must be extended to the energy of the emission. The resolving ability of the collimator decreases as the energy of the gamma ray increases. As the resolution decreases, a gamma ray is allowed to begin its path up one channel toward the detector, to pass through the lead septa without its energy being altered appreciably, and to enter into another channel where it strikes the crystal and is counted. This crossing into another channel is called *cross talk*. Since that gamma ray did not come from the area to-

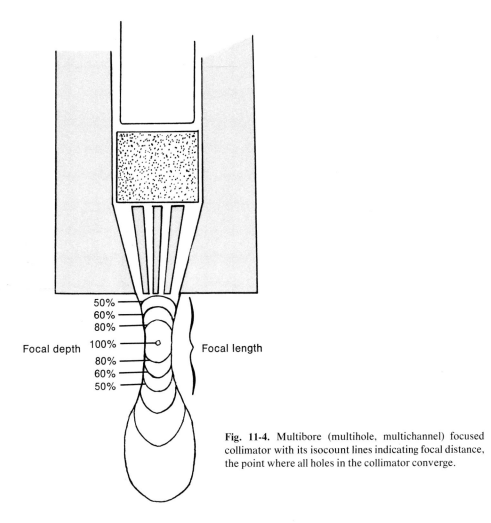

Fig. 11-4. Multibore (multihole, multichannel) focused collimator with its isocount lines indicating focal distance, the point where all holes in the collimator converge.

ward which that hole was aimed, the collimator did not do its job in defining the area from which the gamma ray came. This represents erroneous information and in effect reduces the resolving power of the system. Therefore the more energetic the gamma, the more absorbing material (usually lead) required between the holes to stop all the gamma rays.

Cross talk is not permitted if a collimator is to be effective. The principle behind collimators and their use is to either absorb or scatter gamma rays in such a fashion that they either go undetected or are scattered to such a degree that the detection event will not be accepted (a function of pulse height analysis). Scatter is represented by gamma rays emitted from some other area of the organ not immediately under the view of the collimator; therefore, these rays do not have a clear path to the scintillation detector. In coming in from an angle, they must pass through lead before reaching one of the holes. The resultant secondary gamma is one of decreased energy and changed direction (Compton effect). The direction may be such that the gamma ray is directed up the hole of the collimator. In such instances the correct utilization of pulse height analysis will reject the detection event because the gamma ray is no longer of sufficient energy to produce an acceptable pulse height. It is for this reason that the operator of any imaging device must understand and correctly use pulse height analysis. If the pulse height analyzer is arranged in such a manner that the detection unit would accept and count this secondary gamma coming from an area not in the view of the collimator, it is possible to mask a cold lesion.

It can be argued that pulse height analysis is not as important in well detection systems because the percentage of gammas from Compton collisions (scatter) remains as a constant percentage of the pure gammas emitted. This argument cannot be extended to any other utilization of radionuclides. Correct pulse height analysis in areas such as thyroid uptakes, renal studies, and imaging techniques is extremely important to the value of the study.

Focal depth is a variable with focused collimators. The focal depth is the distance from the face of the collimator to the point where all the holes converge. Standard focal depths are 3 inches and 5 inches. The focal depth cannot exceed the diameter of the scintillation crystal. Therefore 3-inch–diameter crystals have only 3-inch–focal depth collimators, whereas 5-inch–diameter crystals have collimators available in both 3-inch and 5-inch focal depths.

Two other terms used to define the utility of the focused collimator are *focal width* and *focal length*. As shown in Fig. 11-4, the isoresponse pattern of a focused collimator resembles an hourglass, the smallest portion being at the focal depth. A cross section of that isoresponse pattern at the focal depth and parallel to the face of the collimator indicates that sensitivity falls off very rapidly with distance. The distance from the 50% isoresponse curve on one side of the focal point (the 100% point) to the 50% isoresponse curve on the other side of the focal point is generally referred to as the *focal width*. This varies with the resolution of the collimator and is the parameter by which resolution is usually determined. The smaller the distance, the better the resolution.

A cross section of that same isoresponse pattern at the focal depth but this time in a plane perpendicular to the face of the collimator indicates a much slower decrease in sensitivity with distance from the focal point. The distance from the 50% isoresponse line going toward the collimator and the 50% isoresponse line going away from the collimator is generally referred to as the *focal length*. This also varies with the resolution of the collimator. The better the resolution, the smaller the focal length. Furthermore, the focal length defines the primary region of interest during a scan. It is the path, or "swath," that the crystal "sees" through any organ.

The terms *coarse focus* and *fine focus* are used to qualitatively describe the degree of resolution that can be expected from the use of a collimator. These terms describe the isoresponse of a collimator. A fine-focused collimator is one in which the isocount curves are shortened both in width and in length and are used primarily for definition of very small lesions in small organs. The coarse- (or broad-) focused collimator is one in which the isocount curve is larger both in length and in width and therefore does not have as high a resolving power. These are generally used in large organ imaging techniques in which the definition of small lesions is not so rigid. The fine-focused collimator usually has a larger number of small holes. A coarse-focused collimator usually has a smaller number of large holes. The names of the collimators describe their function.

Another way of looking at focused collimators is by applying terms that are already being used extensively by radiation therapists, *umbra* and *penumbra*. A line drawn from the edge of the crystal to the opposite edge of the hole of the collimator defines the penumbral limits (Fig. 11-5, *B*). A line drawn from the edge of the crystal to the edge of the hole on the same side defines the umbral limits. The area between the umbral limits represents the region through which the isoresponsive curve is the same. A point source drawn parallel to the face of the collimator would have a uniform response in this area. The rest of the area defined by the penumbral lines represents a gradual decrease in isoresponse as the point source moves from center until it reaches 0% at the penumbral limit. Umbral and penumbral effects have been likened to a flashlight directed at a wall from a relatively short distance. The center bright area where the majority of the light is concentrated is analogous to the umbra, whereas the less bright area surrounding it is analogous to the penumbra.

One can easily imagine how a tapered hole with the larger opening at the face of the collimator could decrease the penumbra and increase the umbra to the advantage of increased sensitivity of the system. The focused collimator uses a different concept. This collimator uses tapered holes, but the taper is in the opposite direction. In this situation (Fig. 11-5, *A*) the larger opening is at the crystal, and the smaller opening is at the face of the collimator. The penumbral lines still define

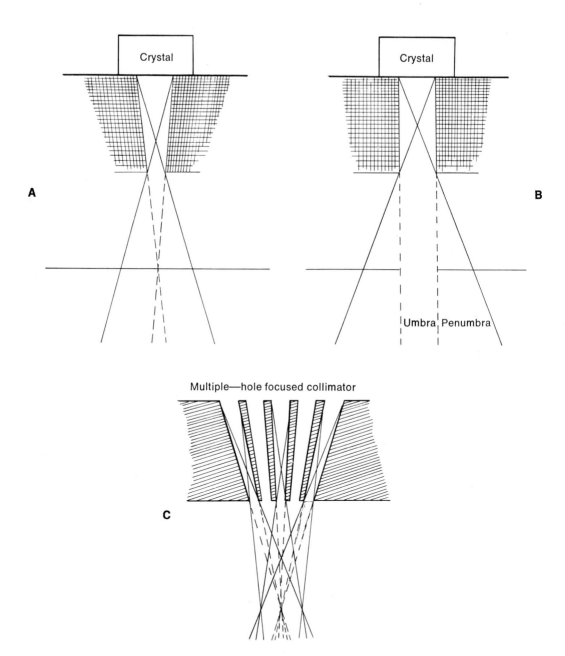

Fig. 11-5. Vision characteristics of various collimators. **A,** Tapered hole demonstrating cross-over of penumbral lines. **B,** Parallel hole demonstrating parallel umbral lines. **C,** Multihole collimator demonstrating convergence of umbral lines at a point in space and convergence of penumbral lines at the same distance in space.

the area seen by the crystal, but the umbral lines cross at a point in space. As a single-hole collimator, this has the effect of increasing the penumbral effects of the collimator and decreasing the umbral effects. This sounds disadvantageous. However, by the addition of more similarly tapered holes (Fig. 11-5, *C*) and the arrangement of them in a tapered configuration, all holes (that is, umbral lines) become focused at the same point in space. This type of collimator serves as a method to increase the resolution of the system by increasing the detection of a greater number of events from a small area and to decrease the penumbral effects of this type of tapered hole. Furthermore, as the tapered holes become more and more angled with respect to one another, the collimator becomes more and more sensitive to the focal depth. It is obvious that the center hole is totally focal-depth insensitive. As more and more holes are added around this center hole, the correct selection of the proper focal depth becomes more critical.

As is evidenced by Figs. 11-5, *C*, and 11-6, penumbral lines have commonalities as well. Penumbral lines define the field of view of the collimator. Fig. 11-6 indicates that as the area encompassed by the penumbral lines decreases by a factor of 2 and therefore the resolution increases by a factor of 2, the count rate (sensitivity) decreases by a factor of 4. Sensitivity is related to the *total area* viewed by the collimator, whereas resolution is related to the *diameter of the area*

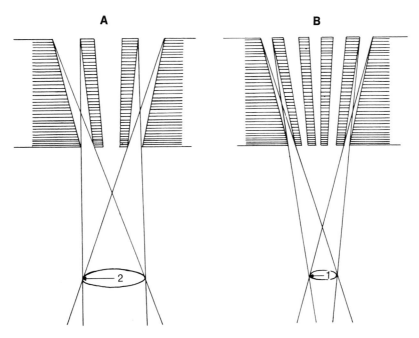

Fig. 11-6. Two collimators showing penumbral lines. Collimator in **B** will provide approximately twice the resolution of collimator in **A**, but collimator in **A** will provide four times the count rate.

viewed by the collimator. Resolution, then, is achieved only at a tremendous sacrifice of count rate.

Knowing the interrelationships of the many holes of a focused collimator makes it easier to understand why the count rates received by a point source are highest at the focal depth and decrease if the point source is moved in *any* direction away from that point in space. Imagine a point source of light held at the focal point of a collimator. All holes are viewing the light source, therefore each hole would contribute light photons to a piece of paper held to the back of the collimator. As the point source of light is held in a central position but moved toward the collimator, the light source is moved "out of view" of the collimator holes around the perimeter. This reduces the overall light intensity (number of light photons) to the same piece of paper. Further changes in position of the light source toward the collimator will result in a further decrease in the number of holes viewing the light source and therefore further decrease the overall number of light photons striking the piece of paper. Conversely, movement of a point source of light away from the focal point will reduce the number of light photons striking the paper, but the reduction in this direction is caused by inverse square relationships. Gamma rays from a point source react no differently with such a collimator.

Once this relationship is understood, the concept of *line spread functions* as a method of collimator comparison and evaluation is not a difficult one (Fig. 11-7). A radioactive point source moved across the collimator at the face will yield a broad count rate curve (Fig. 11-7 at 6 cm) as it moves from one side of the collimator to the other.* As the source is moved away from the collimator and the study repeated, the rapid rise and subsequent decrease in count rate occurs closer together because the "vision" of the holes at that distance is getting closer to the central axis. This in effect increases the spatial resolution because the response to a change in count rate is quicker and therefore a lesion would be more clearly defined in this plane. As the point source moves across the focal plane (Fig. 11-7 at 12 cm), the quickest response occurs, indicating the best resolution. A measurement of line spread function at this point will provide a measurement of collimator resolution, termed *full width, half maximum* (FWHM). The maximum count rate at this focal plane is 100%. The FWHM is determined by moving the sources to each side and noting the point where the count rate falls off to 50%. The distance between these two points is the FWHM, a measurement of collimator resolution. A more precise measurement, however, is that of modulation transfer function (MTF), a subject treated in Chapter 12. Movement of the source farther away causes the line spread function to deteriorate again, indicating poor spatial resolution for lesions beyond the focal plane.

Multichannel parallel-hole collimators. A multichannel parallel-hole collimator, as is used in a stationary imaging device ("camera"), consists of a lead plate

---

*The usual method of performing this determination is to have the collimator move across a stationary radioactive line source.

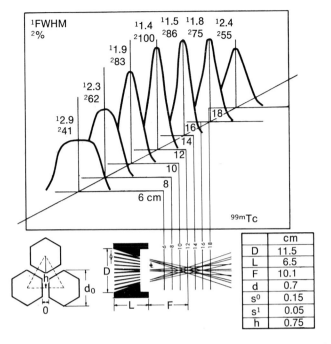

Fig. 11-7. Line spread function of a collimator for a rectilinear scanner, showing where the point source crossed penumbral lines (bottom).

with thousands of channels that are parallel to one another. Each channel accepts only vertically oriented gamma rays from one specific area. Unlike the focused collimators, the holes do not converge on one area at a fixed distance but are aimed through the organ and through the body at an infinite distance. A gamma ray image of the subject is then projected onto the scintillaton crystal detector.

In normal use of this collimator, the subject is positioned as close as possible to the face of the collimator. The reason for this practice is that the resolution of the collimator, termed *extrinsic resolution,* is best for organs or parts of organs closest to the collimator. Sensitivity is not a factor. Resolution decreases with increasing distance from the collimator for the reasons depicted in Fig. 11-8. It is curious that with parallel-hole collimators there is only little loss in count rate as the organ is moved farther away from the face of the collimator. This curiosity can be explained by the fact that although it is true that radioactivity *decreases* by the inverse square of the distance, the area "seen" by each individual hole *increases* by approximately the square of the distance. These two opposing phenomena tend to cancel each other out, resulting in only a slight loss in sensitivity with increased distance.

The factors affecting resolution in parallel-hole collimators are exactly the

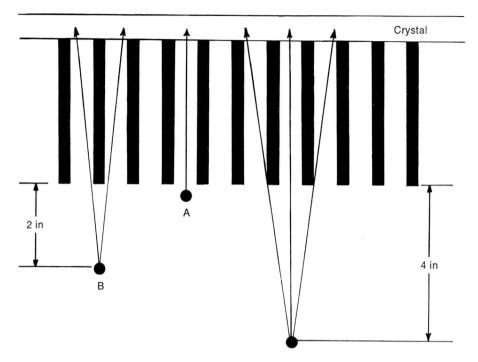

Fig. 11-8. Parallel-hole collimator illustrating loss of resolution with depth.

same as those affecting resolution in focused collimators, that is, the length of the hole and the size of the hole. The advantage of such a collimator is that the predetermination of the correct focal depth is not necessary and the possibility of error from an improperly calculated focal depth is eliminated. The technologist only has to be sure to have the patient as close to the face of the collimator as possible (Fig. 11-9).

Multichannel diverging collimators. Scintillation camera systems that have 9- or 10-inch effective viewing areas present a problem for many patients when performing pulmonary studies or studies in which it is desirable for both liver and spleen to be viewed on the same image. The problem is that many patients are larger than the 9- to 10-inch effective crystal area. The problem can be resolved by going to a larger crystal camera or by the use of a diverging collimator (Fig. 11-10). This collimator is the opposite of focused collimators as used in rectilinear scanners, in that the center hole is perpendicular to the crystal and the holes all begin to diverge at an increasingly greater angle. In this way a greater field of view is capable. Unlike parallel-hole collimators, the image gets smaller as its distance increases from the face of the collimator. Furthermore, the resolution decreases at a more rapid rate as the organ moves away from the detector. It is apparent by the construction of the diverging collimator that the center of the collimator

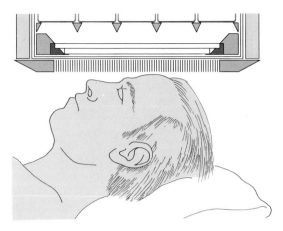

Fig. 11-9. Multichannel parallel-hole collimator as used with brain images. (From Anger, H. O.: Instruments: specific devices. In Wagner, H. M., Jr., editor: Nuclear medicine, New York, 1975, HP Publishing Co. Originally published in Hospital Practice.)

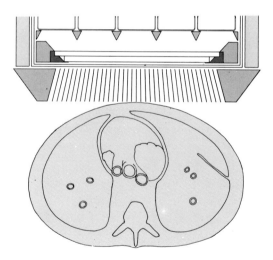

Fig. 11-10. Multichannel diverging collimator as used with lung images. (From Anger, H. O.: Instruments: specific devices. In Wagner, H. M., Jr., editor: Nuclear medicine, New York, 1975, HP Publishing Co. Originally published in Hospital Practice.)

has the best resolution with depth because it approximates the parallel-hole collimator. Furthermore, the resolution of the crystal itself (termed *intrinsic resolution*) is better in the center; therefore, the total resolution of the camera is better in the center. (This fact is useful with camera systems larger than 11 to 13 inches, where for better resolution the image can be visualized by using only the center section of the system.) Both intrinsic and extrinsic resolution (and therefore total resolution) deteriorate as information gets farther and farther away from the center of the crystal.

Multichannel converging collimators. Some manufacturers of diverging collimators have arranged it so that the collimator can be reversed to create a converging collimator. When the collimator is inverted, it takes on the resemblance of a focused collimator. On a scintillation camera, however, it is used to magnify small objects, just as the pinhole collimator is (Fig. 11-11). The converging collimator takes advantage of the two detracting features of the diverging collimator, poor intrinsic and extrinsic resolution away from the center of the crystal. The inversion of the diverging collimator allows the technologist to restrict information to

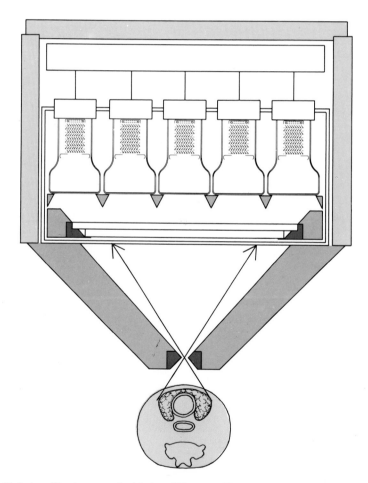

Fig. 11-11. Pinhole collimator as used with thryoid images. (From Anger, H. O.: Instruments: specific devices. In Wagner, H. M., Jr., editor: Nuclear medicine, New York, 1975, HP Publishing Co. Originally published in Hospital Practice.)

the center of the crystal, thereby enhancing intrinsic resolution, and to utilize the tapered hole to its best advantage, increasing extrinsic resolution. This collimator has been used to advantage for imaging of the thyroid, imaging of posterior fossa tumors, and pediatric studies.

Pinhole collimator

The pinhole collimator operates on the old-fashioned box camera principle (Fig. 11-11). It consists of a single small aperture at the end of a lead shield. The collimator is so designed that x rays entering at any angle through the pinhole will be seen by the scintillation detector. This is unlike the single-bore collimator, in which the gamma ray must enter at an angle perpendicular to the face of the crystal to be detected. This principle does not involve the refraction and convergence of rays, therefore focusing is not a problem. Regardless of its distance from the camera, a source appears on the image with as much sharpness as the aperture size and the distances involved permit. It is also apparent that when the distance of the subject to the pinhole is equal to that of the pinhole to the detector, a 1 : 1 relationship of size exists. When the subject is moved farther from the pinhole, a reduction of size occurs, and when the subject is moved closer, magnification occurs. In a comparison of a pinhole collimator to a converging collimator, the pinhole collimator provides the best resolution for small subjects who are positioned a short distance from the aperture; however, the pinhole collimator does this at the expense of sensitivity. The converging collimator has greater sensitivity. Pinhole collimators have been used to take pictures of very large organs but much less effectively. This is accomplished by positioning the subject at great distances from the aperture. This principle has been used for entire lung fields, liver imaging, and so on. Pinhole collimators have greater resolution than parallel-hole collimators, but sensitivity is decreased. Another disadvantage of the pinhole collimator is that it falls off in efficiency at the edges of the image.

STATISTICS

When a source of radioactivity is designated as having a certain number of microcuries or millicuries, it is in effect designated as having a certain number of disintegrations per unit time taking place, since units of activity are defined as the number of disintegrations per unit time (Table 4-1). When such a source is designated as having a certain number of disintegrations per unit time, it is only an average, not a constantly reproducible number. The disintegration of a radioactive atom is a *random* event; therefore, the number of disintegrations is a random variable. It is impossible to predict exactly which atom is going to decay next and exactly how many will disintegrate per unit time; it is possible only to determine an average.

For this reason, a very basic knowledge of statistics is indispensable to both the technologist and the physician for correct utilization of radionuclides and the interpretation of the results of counting or imaging procedures. The physician must use statistical knowledge in evaluating the precision and accuracy* of the counting data. Decisions must be made as to the number of counts to be accumulated (preset count) or the time necessary to accumulate a certain number of counts (preset time), the minimum dose that should be administered, and the travel speed of a rectilinear imaging device. The likelihood that a difference between counts of two different samples or two different areas on an organ image represents a significant difference rather than the random variability between two identical samples or areas must also be determined.

This discussion of statistics will treat the statistics of sample counting and the statistics of imaging as two separate entities because they are not easily related to one another. In both cases, however, the number of events recorded (counts) must be *adequate* to be certain that major differences in the results are not a function of poor statistics.

Statistics of sample counting

Since the number of disintegrations per unit time is a variable, it is to be expected that the counts from the same sample for the same period of time will not be identical. In fact, they can vary considerably, depending on the number of counts accumulated. *As the number of counts increases, the variation between subsequent counts on the same sample also increases but the percent error between subsequent counts decreases.*

An explanation of this statement requires a discussion of the Poisson distribution principle, a principle that is applicable to the observation of random events. The Poisson distribution principle states that the standard deviation is proportional to the square root of the number of observed events. This can be expressed as a formula as follows:

$$\sigma = \sqrt{N}$$
σ = Standard deviation or standard error
N = Number of observed events (counts)

If the number of counts is 100, one standard deviation is $\sqrt{100}$, or 10 counts. (Note that the 100 counts is a quantity, not intensity. It makes no difference as to the length of time required to accumulate that 100 counts.) This is usually expressed as plus or minus one standard deviation, or ± 10 counts from the true count of 100. Furthermore, it is an accepted principle from the Poisson distribution that 68% of all counts will fall within this range of 90 to 110 counts (Fig. 11-12). In other words, if a count were taken 100 times on a sample that emitted 100 counts, 68 of the counts would fall somewhere within a range of 90 to 110 counts,

---

*Precision and accuracy are two entirely different entities. A practiced rifleman can shoot a target four times in a row in almost the exact same spot but outside the bull's eye—precise but not accurate. Another rifleman may possess enough experience to have all four shots hit the bull's-eye—precise and accurate.

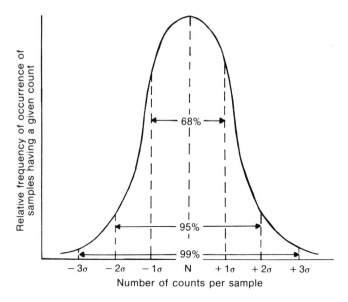

Fig. 11-12. Poisson distribution curve. Curve is plotted as number of counts per sample versus number of times that sample count occurs. In a series of 100 like samples (or the same sample counted 100 times), a 10,000 count sample would result in the largest number of counts having a value of 10,000 per predetermined time period. However, not all counts in this time period would be 10,000 because of the phenomenon of random decay. Some will be larger, some smaller. The above figure predicts that 68 of the 100 counts will fall within $\pm 1\sigma$ (9,900 to 10,000), 95 between $\pm 2\sigma$, and 99 between $\pm 3\sigma$.

and 32 of those counts would fall outside that range. Another way of expressing this relationship is that if a sample were counted only long enough to accumulate 100 counts, the observer could be confident that 68% of the time (approximately two thirds of the time) that count would be within ± 10 counts.

Furthermore, if $1\sigma = \pm 10$ counts, then $2\sigma = \pm 20$ counts and $3\sigma = \pm 30$ counts. The Poisson distribution principle also states that 95% of all counts will fall within $\pm 2\sigma$ and 99% of all counts will fall within $\pm 3\sigma$. In this case, 95 of the 100 counts would fall within a range of 80 to 120 counts, and only one of the counts would fall outside the range of 70 to 130 counts. Accordingly, the observer could be 95% confident that any count on a 100-count sample would be within ± 20 counts of the true value and 99% confident that it would be within ± 30 counts. These relationships are depicted in Fig. 11-12, in which $\pm 1\sigma$ is the 68% level, $\pm 2\sigma$ is the 95% confidence level, and $\pm 3\sigma$ is the 99% confidence level.

The value of the material just presented lies in the percent error that a certain number of counts is likely to introduce into the study. For instance, the 100 counts used in the example just given shows that the observer is only 68% sure that the count that is received is within ± 10 counts of the true value. This is not many counts per se, but it represents a $\pm 10\%$ error. This is totally unacceptable as far as the results are concerned. To go to the higher confidence levels of 95% or 99% introduces an error of ± 20% and ±30%, respectively, which is even worse.

To correct this problem and since the whole area of statistics is based on the number of counts, the situation could be helped by counting 1,000 events instead of 100. In this situation, $\sigma = \sqrt{1,000}$, or 32. Therefore 68% of all counts would be within a range of 968 to 1,032, which represents an error of ±3.2%. Notice that by increasing the number of counts the range has increased (from 20 to 64 for ±1σ), but the percent error has decreased. Furthermore, a count of 10,000 would present a standard deviation of ±100 but would represent a percent error of only ± 1%. These relationships are summarized in Table 11-1 and the following:

> 50% of all counts fall within ±0.675σ
> 68.3% of all counts fall within ±1.0σ
> 90.0% of all counts fall within ±1.65σ
> 95.4% of all counts fall within ±2.00σ
> 99.7% of all counts fall within ±3.00σ
> Probable error = ±0.675σ (50%)
> Standard error = ±1.000σ (68.3%)
> Reliable error = ±1.650σ (90%)

In routine nuclear medicine work the decision must be made by the observer as to how many counts must be accumulated to have reasonable confidence that the count is within an acceptable degree of error. A common solution to the problem is to accumulate enough counts that the observer is 95% confident that the count received is within ±2% error. Table 11-1 shows that a count of 10,000 represents a 68% chance of being within ± 1% error. Since 2σ represents the 95% confidence level, the continuation of the table would read as follows:

Number of counts	2 σ (95%)	Range	Percent error
10,000	±200	9,800 to 10,200	±2%

Accordingly, if the operator accumulated 10,000 counts, he or she would be 95% certain that any such count would be within ±2% of the true value. This is reasonably good statistics for routine nuclear medicine procedures and is the rationale behind the rule of thumb that *regardless of the time required, 10,000 counts should always be accumulated.*

The relationships between the number of counts and percent error, as related to the desired confidence level, can be expressed mathematically as follows:

Table 11-1. Summary of relationship of counts to percent error

Number of counts	1 σ (68%)	Range	Percent error
100	± 10	90 to 110	±10.0%
1,000	± 32	968 to 1,032	± 3.2%
10,000	±100	9,900 to 10,100	± 1.0%
100,000	±317	99,683 to 100,317	± 0.3%

$$\text{For 68\% confidence level: N} = \frac{10,000}{V^2}$$

$$\text{For 95\% confidence level: N} = \frac{40,000}{V^2}$$

$$\text{For 99\% confidence level: N} = \frac{90,000}{V^2}$$

$$N = \text{Number of counts}$$
$$V = \%\,\text{error}$$

The 68% confidence level is generally used for preliminary studies when an approximate statistical evaluation is warranted. The 95% confidence level is used for routine work, and the 99% confidence level is used for research work.

A research project might require the best statistics possible without sacrificing too much time in counting. This would generally mean a statistical accuracy of $\pm 1\%$ error 99% of the time (99% confidence level). The question of how many counts must be accumulated would be solved as follows:

$$N = \frac{90,000}{V^2} = \frac{90,000}{(1)^2} = \frac{90,000}{1} = 90,000 \text{ counts}$$

This formula could also be used to substantiate the 10,000 counts rule of thumb, which states that by accumulating 10,000 counts, the result has a 95% chance of being within $\pm 2\%$ of the true value. Using the 95% confidence level formula and substituting 2% for the percent error, the number of counts to be accumulated is as follows:

$$N = \frac{40,000}{V^2} = \frac{40,000}{(2)^2} = \frac{40,000}{4} = 10,000 \text{ counts}$$

In some studies, such as the Schilling test, it may take as long as 25 to 30 minutes to accumulate 10,000 counts.

Background counts must also be considered when making the final decision of how much time to allow for the count or how many counts must be accumulated for a statistically valid result. There are methods to mathematically calculate the background count value, but they are not practical to use. As mentioned previously, if the total count is at least the square of the background count, background need not be considered statistically (background must be considered when using net counts per minute). In most clinical situations the background is never that high. If it is, the background count is subtracted from the gross counts and counting is continued until 10,000 *net* counts are received.

Statistics of imaging

Statistics also play a major role in imaging techniques with the use of either the rectilinear scanners or stationary cameras. The importance of statistics in both imaging techniques is similar to its importance in sample counting, since an adequate number of events must be recorded to be certain that the lack of a statistical count does not influence the results (diagnosis). The exact number of counts varies in both instances from the rule-of-thumb value of 10,000 used in sample counting.

Rectilinear imaging techniques. Three parameters on a rectilinear scanner influence the statistical evaluation of an imaging technique. They are (1) maximum count rate, (2) the speed at which the detection device moves over the organ, and (3) the space that the detection unit indexes after making one complete pass (line spacing). The count rate has the same relationship to the final evaluation of an image as the number of observed events has to a counting study; that is, the higher the count rate, the better the statistics. However, if the speed is such that the detector unit is not over the area long enough to detect a predetermined number of counts or if the line spacing is such that a lack of continuity exists, then an ideal maximum count rate becomes less than adequate. The position that the operator of the rectilinear imaging device must take is to accumulate and display a predetermined number of counts as quickly as possible for the comfort of the patient. If the maximum count rate is high, a faster speed can be used; if the maximum count rate is low, the speed must be reduced to allow the detection unit to remain over any given area for a longer period of time. Line spacing is largely a matter of esthetics.

The predetermined number of counts has become known as *information density* (ID). The minimum quality scan from the standpoint of statistical evaluation is one in which the ID value is 800 ID, 800 indicating that there are 800 events (counts) detected per square centimeter.* Scans having an ID of less than 800 are poor in quality. Fig. 11-13 illustrates the effects of count rate, speed, and line spacing in statistical evaluation of a scan. In the example in Fig. 11-13, the detector unit would have to make five passes of 0.2-cm distance each. A speed of 60 cm/min would indicate that one pass would require 1 second. The count rate at the area of highest concentration (hot spot) is 6,000 cpm (or 100 counts/sec). Since one pass requires 1 second, it would detect 100 events per pass. In five passes, 500 events would be detected, and this technique would net an ID value of 500.

Since an ID of 500 is considered inadequate statistically, one of the three parameters must be altered: the line spacing must be decreased, the speed must be decreased, or the counts must be increased. The easiest solution would be to decrease the speed so that 160 events would be detected per pass over the one square centimeter area. This can be found by using graphs available

---

*For some equipment this value must be translated into counts per square inch or counts per lineal inch as follows:

$$\text{Counts/in}^2 = \text{Counts/cm}^2 \times 6.5$$
$$\text{Counts/lineal inch} = \text{Counts/in}^2 \times \text{Line spacing in inches}$$

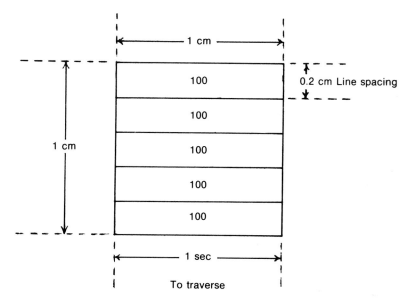

Fig. 11-13. Enlargement of one square centimeter of a scan with an information density of 500 to illustrate the effects of line spacing, speed, and the count rate on the quality of the scan. Line spacing = 0.2 cm; speed = 60 cm/min. (1 cm/sec); count rate = 6,000.

from instrument companies or solving for speed with the following formula:

$$ID = \frac{\text{Maximum cpm}}{\text{Speed (cm/min)} \times \text{Line spacing (cm)}}$$

$$800 = \frac{6,000}{(x)\,0.2} \text{ where } x = \text{Speed in cm/min}$$

$$0.2x = \frac{6,000}{800}$$

$$0.2x = 7.5$$
$$x = 37.5 \text{ cm/min}$$

Accordingly, the speed of the detector will have to be decreased from 60 cm/min to 37.5 cm/min to achieve an ID value of 800.

From this formula, it is apparent that damage to statistical values would occur if the line spacing were increased to 0.4 cm, as some techniques suggest, and the count and speed settings remained the same. Increasing the line spacing would decrease the ID by half. The only compensatory move is to also decrease the speed by half. Therefore by choosing a larger line spacing, the time required to complete the imaging study is not decreased, as many might think. It becomes a matter of the type of scan the physician is trained to interpret.

Stationary imaging techniques. The statistics involved in stationary imaging techniques have been entirely different from those used for rectilinear scanners or sample counting until recently. The purpose of stationary imaging is to detect and record a certain number of events for an entire organ, rather than a segment of an organ, although one can easily be related to the other.

In older instrumentation a predetermined number of counts (thousands or hundreds of thousands of counts) is agreed on prior to a study. Each type of organ study varies as to the number of counts necessary to be accumulated to effect a study of diagnostic value. In addition to the preceding, many new scintillation cameras now offer the capability of using ID to ensure the acquisition of a statistically significant image. This new capability consists of a 1 cm² area of interest that can be moved to any portion of the image. A number is then selected to represent the desired ID, and only those counts originating in that 1 cm² area are registered. The acquisition of image information automatically terminates when the proper ID is reached.

Three different parameters are of concern in establishing such a value: saturation effects, background cutoff, and dot size. The saturation effects come into play when two flashes of light occur at the same place. If the detection device has reached a state of saturation, the second event, which becomes superimposed on the first, is not displayed as a change in the intensity of the dot. Since under usual conditions the intensity would become brighter if two flashes occurred at the same place (suggesting a greater concentration in that area), information is lost if the saturation point has been reached.

Background erase (cutoff or suppression) also affects the image quality. This parameter is generally used to intentionally prevent recording from areas of an organ in which the concentrations of activity are no more than background level. This device is generally used to reduce the interpretive complications of background radiation. However, if the setting of the background erase is too high, more counts than desired are lost.

The size of the dot on the image is also important and is directly dependent on the number of counts to be accumulated. As the accumulation increases, the size of the dot decreases and vice versa. Small density differences in the dots become more difficult to detect if the dots are small with large spaces between them. Conversely, large dots result in the loss of resolution.

These three factors must be taken into consideration when arriving at a statistical value. It has been stressed throughout this discussion of statistics that statistical accuracy increases with increased number of observed events. This is true only to a point with a stationary imaging device. Eventually, principles such as saturation and coincidence loss reduce the image quality and efficiency of detection, and, as a result, the study suffers.

Fig. 11-14 is a study with a thyroid phantom showing how too few or too many counts affect the image. Too few counts result in a very poor image, if any at all. As the counts are increased, the quality of the image also increases. Eventually saturation occurs, and image quality is lost. This could be corrected by reducing the intensity.

A 1,000 counts   **B** 2,000 counts   **C** 5,000 counts

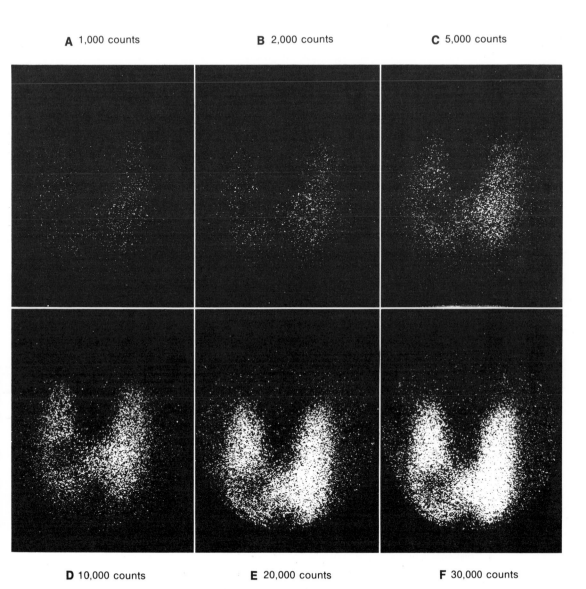

D 10,000 counts   **E** 20,000 counts   **F** 30,000 counts

Fig. 11-14. Effect of statistics using a stationary imaging device. As the number of accumulated counts increases, the image becomes more informative, and diagnosis is easier. A point can be reached, as evidenced by views **E** and **F**, where too many counts are accumulated, the detection device becomes saturated, and information is lost.

PHOSPHORS, FILMS, AND PHOTOGRAPHIC DEVICES
David T. Williams, B.Ed.

The end result of the nuclear imaging study is what is recorded as a permanent record, a photographic display of the imaging systems activities. In most cases this "final form" is a photographic film that, after being exposed to flashes of light from the face of a cathode ray tube (CRT) and properly developed, represents the distribution of radioactive material throughout the area of interest. The three parameters affecting photographic quality are the CRT phosphor, the photographic device, and the film.

The phosphor

CRTs have been thoroughly described earlier in Chapter 9. The phosphor is an inorganic crystal that can absorb electromagnetic energy as provided by the electron beam of the CRT. As this electromagnetic energy is absorbed by the phosphor crystals it is converted to energy of the visible and near visible light spectrum and is emitted by the phosphor. This luminescence is called fluorescence or phosphorescence, depending on the time required to convert energy and become luminescent. Luminescence in less than 10^{-8} second is fluorescence. Luminescence in greater than 10^{-8} second is phosphorescence.

Inorganic crystal phosphors luminesce more efficiently if they contain a metallic impurity called an activator. The two most common phosphors used in nuclear imaging devices are the ^{11}P and the ^{31}P phosphors.

The ^{11}P phosphor is a silver-activated zinc sulfide phosphor with its peak intensity at 425 nm, in the blue light spectrum. Although the ^{31}P phosphor is also a zinc sulfide crystal, it is copper activated. The ^{31}P phosphor peaks at approximately 525 nm and is in the green light spectrum. Therefore, we can see that it is the metallic activator that gives a phosphor its characteristic light emission.

Phosphors continue to luminesce after the energy source ceases. This phenomenon is referred to as persistence. A phosphor's decay constant is the time it takes for the luminescence to decrease to 10% of its initial intensity. Decay constants vary greatly among different phosphors.

The following characteristics of a specific phosphor will effect its ability to be used in an imaging system: persistance, color of light emitted, and whether or not the phosphor is fluorescent or phosphorescent.

Equipment and film designers have gone to great lengths to achieve optimum compatibility between phosphor, film, and photographic devices.

Photographic devices

Multiformat devices have been described previously and need only brief explanation here. Most of these units have a CRT, a lens system, a photimeter, and a film cassette. The CRT is unusual only in that many multiformat CRTs have very fine crystalline phosphors that meet high specification as to dot size and shape.

The photimeter is a device that controls the uniformity of dot brightness for a given technique.

A "photoscope" is a device that attaches to the face of the CRT and, with a system of mirrors, allows the "dots" to be photographed on regular sheet size film (that is, 11×14, 5×8, and so on). Because they rely on reflected light, the intensity settings on the CRT are usually higher.

Camera backs for 105-mm cut film, 70-mm roll film, and Polaroid film are devices that hold bulk packages of film in place for exposure and allow for the manual or mechanical advance of film from frame to frame. Such devices also have a lens (or multiple lens) system that allows the operator to control such things as focus and aperture opening (*f*-stop). The "triple lens" system provides for three exposures on one frame at different densities by allowing three different *f*-stops to be set. (The *f*-stop or aperture setting is simply the width of the lens opening; the wider the opening, the more light can get through and vice versa.)

One other photographic device in common use is the 35-mm, motor-driven, single lens reflex camera. This system is very useful in performing dynamic studies. It has the same general characteristics of the other camera backs described with the additional advantages of more refined lens systems and the ability to operate at a fast frame rate (that is, 1 frame/second).

In dealing with photographic devices the operator should be aware of potential problems and take steps to avoid them by frequent cleaning and maintenance.

Film

Since the end result of any imaging system must be a permanent visual record of the image created on the CRT, the film used is an important component of any imaging system. All negative films vary as to photographic contrast, fog, photographic speed, and (spectral) sensitivity. These photographic characteristics are easily depicted by plotting photographic densities versus the logarithm of the exposures used to produce them. Such plots are known as characteristic curves (sometimes called H & D curves or D-log-E curves).

Characteristic curves show the specific photographic characteristics of a specific film that has been exposed to a specific source of electromagnetic radiation and processed according to a specific protocol. Changing any of the conditions listed will change the characteristic curve of that film.

Fig. 11-15 shows the characteristic curve of negative film commonly used in multiformat devices. Note that the plot is S shaped and is composed of several different components.

The density contributed by the film base and the density of the unexposed but processed emulsion (net fog) are called "gross fog." This is shown on the characteristic curve as the portion of the plot in the lower left quarter paralleling the horizontal axis.

The next portion of the plot is called the "toe". It represents the threshold

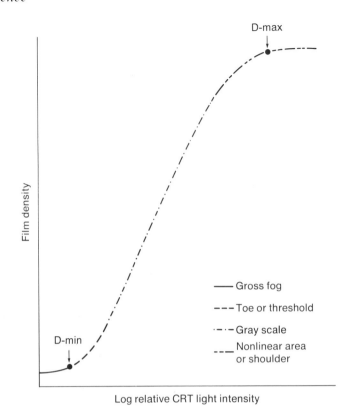

Fig. 11-15. Characteristic H & D curve showing its various components. This response was first described by Hurter and Driffield in 1890.

exposure, that is, how much exposure it takes to create a density above gross fog. This portion of the plot is curved.

The next section of the curve is the most important. This section shows a linear relationship between density and the logarithm of exposure. It is this portion of the plot that represents the "gray scale" of a film. The density increases a linear proportion to the intensity of exposures (brightness).

The last part of the plot is again nonlinear and parallels the base of the graph. In this portion of the plot, density does not change with increases in exposure and details become blurred.

Two more points to be considered are the D-min (minimum) and D-max (maximum) densities. These points are the lowest and highest densities that a film will record.

Negative films used in nuclear medicine have a low-density base and silver halide crystal emulsions. The base is of low density to decrease the amount of gross fog a given film has. Silver halide emulsions are inherently sensitive to

DOUBLE EMULSION FILM

Photons

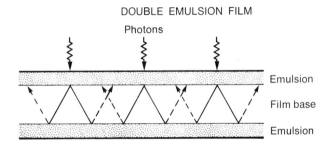

Emulsion

Film base

Emulsion

SINGLE EMULSION FILM

Photons

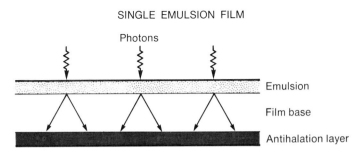

Emulsion

Film base

Antihalation layer

Fig. 11-16. Schematic illustrating the differences between single and double emulsion films. Dotted arrow symbolizes the light being reflected back to the emulsion, thereby degrading the film image.

blue light. By adding sensitizer dyes, these same films can be made sensitive to green light.

Spectral sensitivity is the photographic response of a film to radiation as a function of wave length and again is plotted in curve form. Films used in nuclear medicine must have a spectral sensitivity that includes the spectral output of the phosphor. This output, again expressed in curve form, should be matched to the spectral sensitivity curve of the film for optimum efficiency and photographic clarity. Nuclear medicine films must also be compatible with automatic processing devices. These two parameters hold true, regardless of the negative film format (that is, roll film or sheet film).

Most investigators now agree that, when obtaining a film from a CRT, it is best to use a film with the emulsion on one side (single emulsion film) and an antihalation layer on the other side of the base. The antihalation layer is a light-absorbing substance that prevents light radiations from being reflected back to the emulsion from the base, thus creating sharper "dots" when developed. The difference between single and double emulsion films and the importance of antihalation layers are shown in Fig. 11-16.

Polaroid film

Although Polaroid film does not have the spectral sensitivity of negative films, it serves a practical use in nuclear medicine because of the convenience of instant developing. However, the equipment is subject to misuse and therefore must be properly cared for. The spreading rollers in the Polaroid back must be cleaned with an appropriate solvent after each roll is empty. Polaroid prints must be given adequate time to develop but not be allowed to overdevelop. Finally, when removing the print from the emulsion, one should take care to do so in a smooth and even fashion.

BIBLIOGRAPHY

Blahd, W. H.: Nuclear medicine, New York, 1965, McGraw-Hill Book Co.

Chandra, R.: Introductory physics of nuclear medicine, Philadelphia, 1976, Lea & Febiger.

Chase, G. D., and Rabinowitz, J. L.: Principles of radioisotope methodology, ed. 3, Minneapolis, 1967, Burgess Publishing Co.

Conway, T. T., and Weiss, S.: Polaroid film artifacts, J. Nucl. Med. Tech. 4(4):183-188, 1976.

Fundamentals of instrumentation and imaging in nuclear medicine, copyright Eastman Kodak.

Gottschalk, A., and Potchen, E. J.: Diagnostic nuclear medicine, Baltimore, 1976, The Williams & Wilkins Co.

Hendee, W. R.: Medical radiation physics, Chicago, 1970, Year Book Medical Publishers, Inc.

Hine, G. J.: Instrumentation in nuclear medicine, vol. 1, New York, 1967, Academic Press, Inc.

Hine, G. J., and Sorenson, J. A.: Instrumentation in nuclear medicine, vol. 2, New York, 1974, Academic Press, Inc.

Johns, H. E.: The physics of radiology, ed. 2, revised edition, Springfield, Ill., 1964, Charles C Thomas, Publisher.

King, E. R., and Mitchell, T. G.: A manual for nuclear medicine, Springfield, Ill., 1961, Charles C Thomas, Publisher.

Merrigan, J. A., Sanderson, G. K., and Miale, A.: Selection of film for imaging in nuclear medicine, Med. Radiogr. Photogr. 53(2):22, 1977.

Quimby, E. H., and Feitelberg, S.: Radioactive isotopes in medicine and biology, ed. 2, Philadelphia, 1963, Lea & Febiger.

Rhodes, B. A.: Quality control in nuclear medicine: radiopharmaceuticals, instrumentation, and in-vitro assays, St. Louis, 1977, The C. V. Mosby Co.

Rollo, F. D.: Nuclear medicine physics, instrumentation, and agents, St. Louis, 1977, The C. V. Mosby Co.

Shilling, C. W.: Atomic energy encyclopedia in the life sciences, Philadelphia, 1964, W. B. Saunders Co.

Shapiro, J.: Radiation protection, Cambridge, Mass., 1972, Harvard University Press.

Strauss, H. W., Pitt, B., and James, A. E., Jr.: Cardiovascular nuclear medicine, St. Louis, 1974, The C. V. Mosby Co.

Wagner, H. N.: Principles of nuclear medicine, Philadelphia, 1968, W. B. Saunders Co.

Wagner, H. R.: Medical radiation physics, Chicago, 1970, Year Book Medical Publishers, Inc.

12 Modulation transfer function*

Martin L. Nusynowitz, M.D.
Robert J. Lull, M.D.

BASIC CONCEPTS

Many methods have been employed to describe the resolving capabilities of nuclear imaging systems. Of all these methods, determining the system modulation transfer function (MTF) is generally considered the best index of resolution because it allows reproducible quantitative comparisons between different imaging systems. The basic concept of how MTF measures resolution is straightforward and requires no special background in mathematics or electronics.

MTF and sinusoidal sources

MTF defines resolution by measuring a system's ability to reproduce a three-dimensional source, the intensity of which varies spatially in a sinusoidal pattern as shown in Fig. 12-1. The term *sinusoidal* refers to the "washboard" type surface of the source, which varies like a trigonometric sine wave function.

A system with perfect resolution produces an image that exactly duplicates the sinusoidal pattern of the source. Systems with poorer resolution cause flattening of the image's sinusoidal amplitude, making the distinction between the sinusoidal pattern and the background level more difficult.

This flattening may be quantitatively described by measuring the source and image modulation.

Defining modulation

The concept of modulation is central to an understanding of the MTF. Modulation is merely the ratio of the sinusoidal amplitude to the average background value, as shown in Fig. 12-1. These values are calculated as follows:

$$\text{Sinusoidal amplitude} = \frac{\text{Max value} - \text{Min value}}{2}$$

$$\text{Average background} = \frac{\text{Max value} + \text{Min value}}{2}$$

---

*The material presented in this chapter is extracted from a monograph entitled "A Clinician's Guide to Modulation Transfer Function" by Martin L. Nusynowitz.

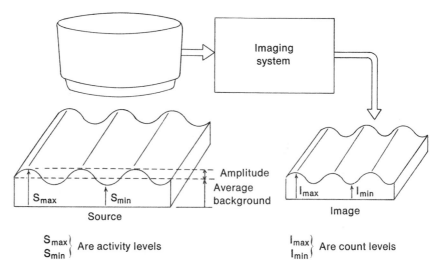

Fig. 12-1. Imaging a sinusoidal source. A three-dimensional sinusoidal source and a representation of its image are depicted.

The source modulation (M_S) and the image modulation (M_I) are calculated by the following:

$$M_S = \frac{\text{Source amplitude}}{\text{Source background}} = \frac{S_{max} - S_{min}}{S_{max} + S_{min}}$$

$$M_I = \frac{\text{Image amplitude}}{\text{Image background}} = \frac{I_{max} - I_{min}}{I_{max} + I_{min}}$$

When poor resolution causes flattening of the sinusoidal image, there is a proportionate decrease in the value of M_I. This change in M_I provides the basis for measuring resolution by the MTF, which is defined as the ratio of image modulation to source modulation:

$$\text{MTF} = \frac{M_I}{M_S}$$

Transferring modulation

MTF, as just calculated, provides a numerical index of the resolution capability of the imaging system. How these numerical values for MTF relate to image quality is demonstrated in Fig. 12-2, which shows a sinusoidal source and the images produced by three systems with differing resolving abilities.

Any loss of modulation during the imaging process is reflected by corresponding image degradation. As system resolution worsens, more and more image flattening occurs. This progressive image degradation is detected and quantitated by the decrease in MTF value.

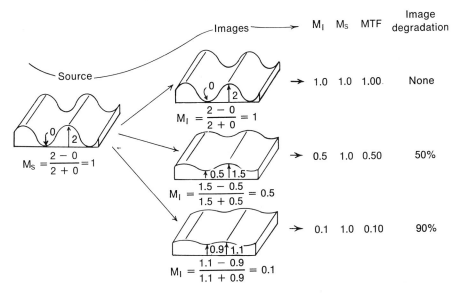

Fig. 12-2. Sinusoidal source and images obtained from three systems with differing resolving abilities. As flattening of the sinusoidal component occurs, M_I and MTF decrease. Note that the average background for each image is the same.

Thus MTF may be considered as measuring an imaging system's ability to transfer modulation from the source to its image. The MTF value is the fractional percent of source modulation that has been successfully transferred. Thus in Fig. 12-2 one system transfers all source modulation to the image so that MTF = 1.00 and there is no image degradation. The other two systems have less successful transfer of modulation, and the resulting image degradation is reflected by the MTF values.

FACTORS AFFECTING MTF

The MTF of an entire system is affected by a variety of factors both extrinsic and intrinsic to the imaging system.

Extrinsic factors include source frequency, distance between source and detector, the nature of any intervening scattering medium, and photon energy of the source radionuclide.

The imaging system itself is made up of various components that cause characteristic modulation losses. Each of these intrinsic components affects overall system MTF, especially when that component causes significant modulation losses. Every component can be thought of as having its own characteristic MTF value, which represents the fraction of modulation successfully transferred through that component. The total system MTF becomes the product of the MTF values of all its components. To illustrate, consider a system composed of components A, B, and C, with the following MTF values: $MTF_A = 0.90$, $MTF_B = 0.90$, and

$MTF_C = 0.20$. The total system MTF will be $(MTF_A) \cdot (MTF_B) \cdot (MTF_C) = (0.9) \cdot (0.90) \cdot (0.20) = 0.162$. Improving the MTF of a poor component, such as component C in the example just given, will markedly improve overall system resolution. This is of significant practical importance when choosing between collimators, since this is the only component that the user can readily change to alter system resolution. Comparing changes in system MTF with different collimators provides a rational basis for collimator selection.

How these important extrinsic and intrinsic factors influence MTF is demonstrated in the following pages.

Source frequency (lesion size)

Sinusoidal sources are not only characterized by peak amplitude but also by frequency (ν) in cycles per centimeter or its reciprocal, wavelength (λ), in centimeters per cycle. Fig. 12-3 shows two sources with the same modulation ($M_S = 0.5$) differing only in frequency.

If both sources are imaged by the same system, M_I and thus MTF will be lower for source B. This occurs because it is more difficult to distinguish activity peaks that are narrow and closely packed. For this reason, each MTF value is specific for a particular source frequency and is expressed as MTF (ν). Consequently, the MTF of an imaging system is usually determined at several source frequencies, and a curve describing MTF as a function of ν is drawn. Fig. 12-4 is a typical MTF curve showing such a relationship. Large lesions correspond to low frequencies (large wavelengths), whereas small lesions correspond to high frequencies (small wavelengths). Since MTF decreases as ν increases, smaller lesions are more poorly imaged than large lesions are.

Distance (Z)

The distance (Z) from the source to the imaging system detector is a major variable affecting MTF. For scintillation cameras with parallel-hole collimators, MTF decreases as Z increases. This fact is demonstrated by the MTF curves shown in Fig. 12-5. The three curves were obtained at Z = 0, 10, and 20 cm from the collimator face and show for any value of ν a decrease in MTF as Z increases.

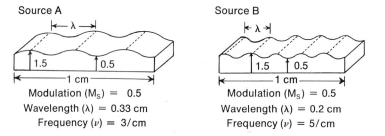

Fig. 12-3. Sinusoidal sources shown differ only in wavelength (λ) and frequency (ν). Note that $\nu = 1/\lambda$.

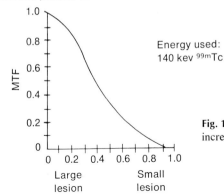

360 kev parallel-hole collimator

Energy used:
140 kev ^{99m}Tc

Fig. 12-4. Effect of source frequency on MTF. As source frequency increases (smaller lesions), resolution decreases.

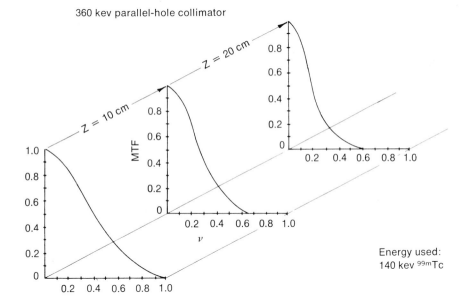

360 kev parallel-hole collimator

Energy used:
140 kev ^{99m}Tc

Fig. 12-5. Effect of source distance on MTF. The curves were obtained with the source at 0, 10, and 20 cm from the collimator face. With a parallel-hole collimator, resolution decreases as distance increases.

Thus for this type of system there will be more image degradation the deeper the lesion. The situation with focusing collimators for rectilinear scanners is different; here MTF will be maximum at the focal plane of the collimator and will decrease as one moves away from the focal plane.

Photon energy

For a given imaging system an increase in photon energy of the radionuclide source generally causes image degradation. This is largely because of increasing

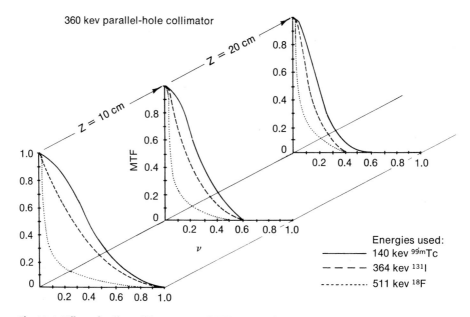

Fig. 12-6. Effect of radionuclide energy on MTF. Resolution decreases as photon energy increases.

septal penetration effects in the collimator. Fig. 12-6 shows how increased photon energy causes a decrease in MTF. The MTF curves are depicted at distance Z for three energy ranges: 140 kev, 364 kev, and 511 kev. Note that at each distance and for each value of ν, MTF decreases as energy increases.

Collimator effects

MTF curves provide an excellent method for comparing collimator resolution. This point is illustrated by Fig. 12-7, which compares the MTF curves of three commonly used low-energy collimators. It can be seen that resolving differences are more apparent away from the detector face and that the high-resolution collimator produces the highest MTF of the three, whereas the high-sensitivity collimator produces the lowest value.

MEASURING MTF

Although MTF is defined in terms of sinusoidal radioactive sources, its actual measurement with such sources is impractical because they are physically very difficult to construct. This problem may be circumvented in several ways. One popular method only requires the data from a line spread function (LSF) obtained with the imaging system. Using a mathematical principle called the *Fourier Theorem*, this LSF data can be used to derive the MTF curve for the imaging system. For a more comprehensive discussion of the theoretic and practical

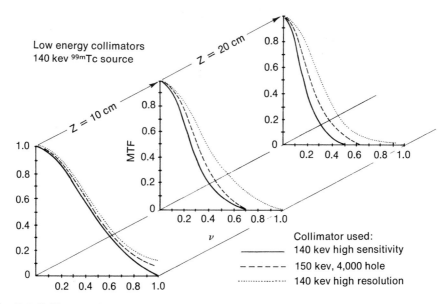

Fig. 12-7. Collimator effects on system MTF. Three collimators, designed for use with 140-kev energy sources, were used to obtain these images. The high-resolution collimator yields the highest MTF curve (at a cost in sensitivity), whereas the MTF curve obtained with the high-sensitivity collimator is lowest.

details of deriving MTF values, the reader is referred to the monograph cited at the beginning of this chapter.

BAR PHANTOM IMAGES AND MTF

Bar phantom images are frequently used to demonstrate system resolution. Resolving ability is measured in terms of the smallest bar width that can be distinguished on the image.

Although simple to obtain, bar phantom results are necessarily subjective, system dependent, and difficult to quantitate. On the other hand, MTF is an objective, system-independent, and precise measure of resolving ability. Thus MTF has significant advantages over the bar phantom method as an index of resolution. Yet direct comparison between MTF and bar phantom images provides valuable insight into both methods of determining system resolution and allows for correlation of the MTF with an actual image.

The basis for comparing MTF and bar phantom images is the fact that a relationship can be established between bar width and source frequency.

Fig. 12-8 illustrates that one bar width can be equated to half a cycle length. A bar phantom consisting of ½-, ⅜-, ¼-, and ³⁄₁₆-inch bars was laid over a flood source and imaged at $Z = 10$ cm using a pinhole collimator. The MTF for fre-

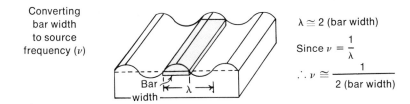

Converting
bar width
to source
frequency (ν)

$\lambda \cong 2$ (bar width)

Since $\nu = \dfrac{1}{\lambda}$

$\therefore \nu \cong \dfrac{1}{2 \text{ (bar width)}}$

Thus each bar width of the bar phantom corresponds
to a particular frequency (ν) on the MTF curve:

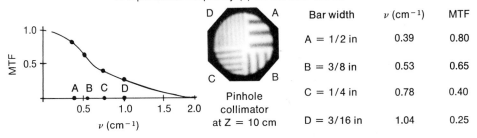

Bar width	ν (cm^{-1})	MTF
A = 1/2 in	0.39	0.80
B = 3/8 in	0.53	0.65
C = 1/4 in	0.78	0.40
D = 3/16 in	1.04	0.25

Pinhole
collimator
at Z = 10 cm

Fig. 12-8. Converting bar width to source frequency. The image was made using a bar phantom of 4 bar widths overlaid on a ^{99m}Tc flood source at Z = 10 cm. The source frequency corresponding to each bar width is tabulated. Direct comparison may be made between the bar phantom image and the MTF.

quencies corresponding to each bar width were tabulated from the MTF curve derived from a line source containing the same radionuclide at the same distance. Thus, as seen in Fig. 12-8, the bar phantom images can be directly related to a corresponding MTF value. Note that the smallest bars are readily discerned, although the image quality (as determined by MTF) at this frequency is 75% degraded. This demonstrates the relative insensitivity of the bar phantom method for detecting even significant image degradation.

SUMMARY

Since the modulation transfer function meets the criteria for a precise and representative parameter of system resolution, it is the generally accepted index of system resolution. The MTF measures the ability of an imaging system to reproduce a three-dimensional source, the intensity of which varies spatially in a sinusoidal manner.

Source and image modulation (contrast) are defined as the signal-to-noise ratio of the sinusoidally varying source and image, respectively. MTF is defined as the ratio of image modulation to source modulation and represents the ability of the imaging system to transfer modulation from the source to the image. Various factors affecting MTF have been illustrated and discussed; among these are source spatial frequency, distance, photon energy, and collimator effects. Finally, a method of comparing MTF values to bar phantom images has been described so that the reader can gain an appreciation of the physical correlation of the abstract concept of MTF.

BIBLIOGRAPHY

Chandra, R.: Introductory physics of nuclear medicine, Philadelphia, 1976, Lea & Febiger.

Hendee, W. R.: Medical radiation physics, Chicago, 1970, Year Book Medical Publishers, Inc.

Hine, G. J., and Sorenson, J. A.: Instrumentation in nuclear medicine, vol. 2, New York, 1974, Academic Press, Inc.

Johns, H. E.: The physics of radiology, ed. 2, revised edition, Springfield, Ill., 1964, Charles C Thomas, Publisher.

Nusynowitz, M. L.: A clinician's guide to the modulation transfer function: monograph.

Rollo, F. D.: Nuclear medicine physics, instrumentation, and agents, St. Louis, 1977, The C. V. Mosby Co.

13 Radiation health safety

The principles of radiation protection were discussed in Chapter 6. The actual implementation of these principles depends on the caliber of radiation health safety programs employed in the individual departments of nuclear medicine. Procedures such as monitoring, record keeping, and waste disposal all place a burden on the nuclear medicine personnel involved. These procedures are time consuming and tedious, but they are very important to the safety of both occupational and nonoccupational personnel. Any technique that will reduce the radiation exposure to occupational personnel is to be considered highly desirable, provided the time and cost factors necessary to achieve the desired results are reasonable. In fact, at the time of this writing, a draft (NUREG-0267) has been proposed by the Office of Standard Development, United States Nuclear Regulatory Commission (NRC), entitled "Principles and Practices for Keeping Occupational Radiation Exposures at Medical Institutions as Low As Reasonably Achievable" (ALARA), which addresses this problem. Since the ALARA philosophy should be a guiding force in establishing radiation safety practices, much material and many forms in this chapter are quoted or modified from this document, even though, as a draft and therefore subject to comment and change, parts of it may be amended in the months to come. It is not felt to be presumptuous to state that future NRC license approvals will be based on this document.

MONITORING

One of the most important health safety procedures is monitoring both the personnel and the work area. The purposes of monitoring are several: (1) to detect radioactive contamination, (2) to evaluate shielding arrangements, and (3) to measure personnel exposure.

Personnel monitoring

Personnel monitoring is usually performed through the use of film badges for whole body exposures and either TLD finger badges or film wrist badges for extremity exposures. The latter is of particular importance to those persons involved in the elution of generators, in the injection of doses in the millicuries or larger range, and in the manipulation of brachytherapy sources such as radium or cesium 137 cervical implants. Pocket dosimeters are found to be useful in situations in which large exposures are expected on a very infrequent schedule. This

292

condition rarely occurs in a routine nuclear medicine practice. Whatever the method used, *personnel monitoring records must be continuously maintained and, in accordance with CRF 20. 401(c) (1), preserved until the NRC authorizes disposition.*

The ALARA philosophy suggests that finger badges, not wrist badges, should be worn by all nuclear medicine personnel who prepare and administer radiopharmaceuticals and by all personnel who receive exposures greater than 10% of the maximum permissible dose. In nuclear medicine operations in which lead aprons are worn as protection against ^{99m}Tc, the whole body badge should be worn outside the apron in order to monitor parts of the body that have the same exposure limits as the whole body. It also suggests that dosimeters be used as monitoring devices in any areas subject to high exposures (such as ^{60}Co teletherapy) and that the dosimeter be read daily. Remote stations should be made available for storage of film badges (when not in use), control badges, and other equipment.

Instruction to workers. In order that personnel understand radiation health safety, Title 10 of the Code of Federal Regulations, part 19 (10CFR19.12) indicates that these individuals be instructed in the following:

1. Where radioactive materials are stored, transferred, or used and the radiation levels in those areas
2. Health protection problems associated with radioactive materials or radiation and the minimizing of those problems through the judicious use of protective devices and precautionary procedures
3. The provisions and conditions of the Code of Federal Regulations and the NRC or state license for personnel protection
4. The responsibility to report any infractions of these rules
5. The proper response to any malfunction or unusual occurrence that may involve contamination or overexposure of personnel
6. The right of any occupational personnel to request a summary of his or her exposure. In fact, it is a requirement by the OSHA regulations (Occupational Safety and Health Act 29CFR1910.96n, 10CFR19.13, and 10CFR20.01) that personnel be advised *annually* of these exposures.

These instructions should be reviewed with all occupational personnel at the time of job orientation and then no less than annually thereafter.

The ALARA philosophy suggests that in-service training be given to all personnel before they are assigned to a restricted area and annually (as a minimum) thereafter. These training sessions should include the presentation of the ALARA philosophy and specific instructions to meet the requirements. Further these sessions should include a review of Title 10 of the Code of Federal Regulations, part 20, a discussion of NRC Regulatory Guides 8.10, "Operating Philosophy For Maintaining Occupational Radiation Exposures As Low as Reasonably Achievable," and 8.13, "Instruction Concerning Prenatal Radiation Exposure," a discussion of the NRC license and its conditions, and a review of institutional procedures used to satisfy all of these documents.

Exposure records. Title 10 of the Code of Federal Regulations (parts 20.101, through 20.105) outlines the procedures for the maintenance of exposure records. This has been discussed in detail in Chapter 6. Title 10CFR19.13 addresses the notification and reporting practices to occupational personnel. Exposure records that are considered reportable to personnel and regulatory agencies are those dealing with the whole-body or finger/wrist measurements or the results of any measurements, analyses, or calculations of radioactive material deposited or retained in the body of the individual. Each report should be in writing and, in addition to the data and results, should contain the name of the licensee, the name of the individual, and his or her social security number and birth date. These reports must be furnished to the following:

1. Any currently employed occupational worker who requests it—on an annual basis
2. Any formerly employed occupational worker who requests it—within 30 days
3. The NRC and the individual in the case of an overexposure—within 30 days

Overexposures. A summary of the NRC regulations regarding notification proceedings of a radiation incident (Titles 10CFR20.402 and 10CFR20.403) is seen in Table 13-1, which is divided into two major sections: an incident large enough to require immediate notification and lesser incidents that require notification within 24 hours. In either case, the regulations further stipulate that the licensee will also submit a written report within 30 days. That report must include the following:

1. Description of the incident
2. Extent of exposure of persons to radiation, whether contained or widespread
3. Estimates of individual exposures to each person involved. Each person must be properly identified with name, social security number, and birth date.
4. Cause of the exposure
5. Corrective steps taken to assure against a recurrence

This report must be sent to:

1. Director of Inspection & Enforcement, United States Nuclear Regulatory Commission, Washington, D.C. 20555.
2. Director of appropriate NRC regional office.
3. The individual exposed and, therefore, named in the report.

Area monitoring

Another important aspect of radiation health safety in nuclear medicine department is the performance of environmental surveys in each working area.

Table 13-1. Summary of Nuclear Regulatory Commission regulations regarding notification of incidents

Conditions of notification	Person(s) notified	Time element	Mode of notification	Remarks
Theft of radioactive materials	Director of nearest NRC Regional Office	Immediately	Telephone *and* telegraph	If substantial hazard may result to persons in unrestricted areas
Loss of radioactive materials	Director of nearest NRC Regional Office	Immediately	Telephone *and* telegraph	If substantial hazard may result to persons in unrestricted areas
Large overexposure	Director of appropriate NRC Regional Office	Immediately	Telephone *and* telegraph	Whole body—≥ 25 rems; skin of whole body—≥ 150 rems; hands, forearms, feet, ankles—≥ 375 rems
Release of highly concentrated radioactive materials	Director of appropriate NRC Regional Office	Immediately	Telephone *and* telegraph	Concentrations $>5,000$ times limits in Appendix B, Table II of 10CFR20, averaged over 24-hour period
Large operational shutdown	Director of appropriate NRC Regional Office	Immediately	Telephone *and* telegraph	Loss of one working week or more of operation of any facilities affected
Large property damage	Director of appropriate NRC Regional Office	Immediately	Telephone *and* telegraph	Loss in excess of $200,000
Small overexposure	Director of appropriate NRC Regional Office	Within 24 hours	Telephone *and* telegraph	Whole body—≥ 5 rems; skin of whole body—≥ 30 rems; hands, forearms, feet, ankles—≥ 75 rems
Release of moderately concentrated radioactive materials	Director of appropriate NRC Regional Office	Within 24 hours	Telephone *and* telegraph	Concentrations >500 times limits in Appendix B, Table II of 10CFR20, averaged over 24-hour period
Small operational shutdown	Director of appropriate NRC Regional Office	Within 24 hours	Telephone *and* telegraph	Loss of one working day or more of operation of any facilities affected
Small property damage	Director of appropriate NRC Regional Office	Within 24 hours	Telephone *and* telegraph	Loss in excess of $2,000

These working areas should include the injection preparation area, the "hot" sink, the storage area, the radioactive waste disposal area, and all surfaces where radioactive material is being used or stored. The instrument generally used in this type of an area survey is a Geiger-Mueller survey meter.

The regulations for surveys are covered in Title 10 of the Code of Federal Regulations, Part 20.201.

A "survey" means an evaluation of the radiation hazard incident to the production, use, release, disposal, or presence of radioactive materials or other sources of radiation under a specific set of conditions. When appropriate, such evaluation includes a physical survey of the location of materials and equipment and measurements of levels of radiation or concentrations of radioactive materials present. Each licensee shall make or cause to be made such surveys as may be necessary for him to comply with the regulations in this part.

Weekly surveys are recommended for all laboratories and other areas in which radioactive materials are handled routinely. Any surface or article reading in excess of twice the background radiation is considered contaminated and should be treated as such. Readings in excess of this value may be received when the reading is taken in proximity to areas containing large quantities of radioactive materials.* The surveyor cannot assume this to be the case, however, since such an area would mask an area of contamination. The latter can easily be ruled out by a "wipe" test in which the area is wiped with a piece of paper toweling and the toweling is subjected to the survey meter in an area where there are not large amounts of radioactivity. Therefore, these wipes should be a part of the weekly routine. *These records must be maintained for 2 years.*

Daily surveys are recommended in the "hot" laboratory area where generators are eluted and where radiopharmaceutical kits are prepared. It is also important to ensure that, following any kit preparation, dose preparation, or dose injection, hands are free of contamination. A wall-mounted laboratory monitor equipped with a G-M probe and an alarm would be adequate for these daily survey needs. Records of these daily surveys are not necessary. The ALARA philosophy suggests, however, that a simple logbook of daily readings in specified areas be kept by the user so that the user may be continuously made aware of changing radiation levels. It further suggests that a continuously operating laboratory monitor be mounted immediately outside the door to the "hot" lab to check for hand contamination. The probe should have sufficient cable to check shoe contamination. It can also serve as a wipe test indicator. Any wipe tests yielding greater than 10,000 dpm/100 cm^2 of surface area is considered contaminated and therefore subject to a decontamination procedure immediately.

---

*In these cases the value should not exceed 2 mr/hr.

DECONTAMINATION
Personnel decontamination

Nuclear medicine personnel contaminated by radioactive material must be quickly decontaminated because of the obvious dangers to the individual from radiation. There are two reasons for immediate decontamination: (1) to prevent the possible transfer of radioactivity to internal organs either by absorption through the skin or ingestion and (2) to prevent spread of the contamination to other persons or to the environment.

Some general considerations to be used in determining the extent and immediacy of the decontamination process are as follows. If there is a break in the skin, decontamination must be prompt because radiation can be absorbed immediately into the body. If there is bleeding associated with the break in the skin, the bleeding should be encouraged while rinsing the skin with water. All contaminated clothing should be removed at once. (This is the reason for wearing long lab coats in the nuclear medicine department.) Decontamination is of secondary importance if the contaminated material is strongly acid or strongly basic; concern for chemical burns to the skin takes precedence in this case. Steps should be taken immediately to neutralize the skin with an appropriate neutralizing agent; then skin decontamination should be undertaken.

Decontamination of the skin is effectively carried out by large amounts of soap and water. The soap should not be of an abrasive nature or highly alkaline. It is best to use warm water, rather than hot, because the latter encourages increased blood flow to the area and therefore increased absorption of the contaminating material. Any materials and clothing that are contaminated or involved in the decontamination process should be checked with appropriate survey meters and treated according to the radiation level. If the radiation level is greater than the accepted level, the materials should be labeled and transferred to the radioactive waste storage area until the radiation decays to acceptable levels.

Equipment and working area decontamination

Decontamination of equipment or the working area is initiated with the use of absorbent material to remove as much of the liquid contaminant that has spilled as possible. The contaminated area is then scrubbed with soap and water until acceptable radiation levels are reached. A simple but effective procedure is to tape a piece of paper over the area to remind people that it is contaminated and to discourage people walking on the area, which would transfer the radioactivity to other parts of the laboratory.

A serious contamination problem occurs if the patients vomits or urinates in the bed after a therapeutic application of radionuclides. The patient must be immediately bathed; bed linen, rubber sheets, and so on must be collected carefully to reduce further contamination to the area and to personnel; contaminated materials are transferred to the waste storage area for decay to safe levels.

RADIATION AREAS

Since the use of radioactive materials represents a possible radiation hazard, laboratories, work areas, and storage areas must be labeled appropriately to aid individuals in minimizing their exposure to radiation. There are three signs approved by the United States Nuclear Regulatory Commission as warnings. The type of sign indicates the dose rate of the area. All three signs use the conventional three-bladed design. The design is purple or magenta on a yellow background. The three signs are as follows:

1. *Caution — Radioactive Materials* is a warning sign used anywhere the amount of radioactive materials exceeds ten times the quantity found in Appendix C of Title 10CFR20. It is best used wherever *any* amount of radioactivity is found.

2. *Caution — Radiation Area* is a warning sign to be placed in the room or area in which the concentration of radioactive materials is such that the radiation intensity would be from 5.0 to 100 mr in any 1 hour or 100 mr in 5 consecutive days.

3. *Caution — High Radiation Area* is a warning sign used in areas in which the radiation intensity would be in excess of 100 mr in any 1 hr.

Each container in which licensed material is transported, stored, or used and that contains a greater quantity of radioactive material than that specified in Appendix C of Title 10CFR20 shall bear a clearly visible label giving the radiation caution symbol, the appropriate words, the name of the radionuclide, the activity, and the date. A label is not required if the concentration of the material in the container does not exceed that specified in Appendix B, Table 1, Column 2 of Title 10CFR20. Further labels are not necessary for laboratory containers such as beakers, flasks, and test tubes used transiently in laboratory procedures when the user is present.

Several exceptions to these posting requirements are recognized by the NRC. One such exception concerns radioactive materials packaged for shipment. These materials are packaged and labeled in accordance with the regulations of the Department of Transportation (DOT). The DOT stipulates that shipment of radioactive materials should provide enough protection so that the radiation intensity is no greater than 200 mr/hr at the surface of the package or 10 mr/hr at a distance of 3 feet from the surface of the package. The DOT regulations further state that the radiation intensity should be expressed in units in which 1 unit is equal to the radiation intensity in millirems per hour at a distance of 3 feet from the surface of the package. The shipment should be labeled as to the principal radionuclide and the activity of the contents. Other exceptions are as follows.

1. In the event of the storage of a sealed source, the room or area in which it is housed is not required to be posted provided the radiation level 12 inches from the surface of its container does not exceed 5 mr/hr.

2. Rooms of patients containing radioactivity need not be posted and control

of entrance to these rooms is not required *provided* that there are personnel in attendance who will observe acceptable radiation health safety practices.

3. Rooms or areas containing radioactivity for periods of less than 8 hours need no signs provided the materials are constantly attended and good radiation health safety practices are observed.

4. Rooms containing radioactive materials ready for shipping need no signs.

HANDLING OF RADIOACTIVE SHIPMENTS

Procedures for the receipt, distribution, and, ultimately, the handling of shipments of radioactive materials require the concern and education of other hospital and clinic personnel not directly related to the nuclear medicine department. The reason is obvious. Radioactive shipments are received by nonoccupational personnel in the receiving department, emergency room, or the switchboard, who have no knowledge of its radiation hazard.

Receipt of shipments

The receipt of packages containing radioactive materials is, in many instances, by personnel who have very little knowledge of radiation and radiation protection practices. If the package is received during off-duty hours, the personnel receiving these materials would have even less knowledge of radiation health safety. As indicated previously, the DOT regulations stipulate that the outside of the package be protected to only 200 mr/hr. Title 10CFR20.105(b) (1) allows a maximum radiation level in an unrestricted area such that nonoccupational personnel do not receive greater than 2 mr in any hour. To allow a condition in which someone could sit on this shipment of radioactive material for longer than 36 seconds would be a violation of the Code of Federal Regulations and, therefore, the NRC license. This could conceivably be the situation in a busy Emergency Room. Therefore, directives must be issued, and nonoccupational personnel must be educated to expedite these shipments as quickly as possible, at any time of day or night, to secure them in a controlled area. The best way is to instruct the security guard or his or her designate to escort the courier with the package to the nuclear medicine department where it will be placed in the hot lab behind lead bricks and the doors to the lab locked. An alternate method would be to have security personnel deliver the package to the controlled area. Whatever the method, before the package leaves the receiving area, it should be visually examined for evidence of damage and/or leakage. If the package is wet, the Radiation Safety Officer should be contacted and the courier asked to remain until it can be determined that neither he or she nor the delivery vehicle is contaminated. Furthermore, the package should be placed immediately in a leak-proof plastic bag by gloved hands for removal from the area to an area approved for decontamination or decay.

The ALARA philosophy suggests that a storage area be available and identified as such in the receiving area for acceptance of radioactive materials. This area should be located in such a way that the time needed to transport the package to a controlled area is minimal and that the need to carry the package through crowded areas of the hospital is avoided. A transport cart should be made available to transport these radioactive packages, further reducing radiation exposure during the transport period.

Opening of shipments

Once the radioactive shipment has been delivered to the controlled area and secured behind protective shielding, it is important that someone open the package, ensure the integrity of its contents, verify the completeness of the order, and secure the contents in its appropriate protective area as soon as possible. This is especially true if some of the material requires refrigeration or, even more important, freezing. The following is a procedure for opening such packages.

1. Visually inspect the package for any sign of damage (for example, wetness, crushed appearance). If damage is noted, stop the procedure and notify the Radiation Safety Officer.
2. Measure the exposure rate at 3 feet from the package surface and record. If it is 10 mr/hr, stop the procedure and notify the Radiation Safety Officer.
3. Measure the surface exposure rate and record. If it is 200 mr/hr, stop the procedure and notify the Radiation Safety Officer.
4. Put on gloves.
5. Open the outer package (following manufacturer's directions, if supplied) and remove packing slip. Open inner package to verify contents (compare requisition, packing slips, and label on bottle) and check the integrity of the final source container (inspect for breakage of seals or vials, loss of liquid, discoloration of packing material). Check also that shipment does not exceed possession limits as stipulated on the NRC license.
*6. Wipe external surface of final source container with moistened cotton swab or filter paper held with forceps; assay and record.
7. Monitor the packing material and packages for contamination before discarding.
   a. If contaminated, treat as radioactive waste.
   b. If not contaminated, obliterate radiation labels before discarding in regular trash.

The only shipments that would be received by a routine nuclear medicine de-

---

*These procedures are specific for any shipment specified in Title 10CFR20.205. Further, these procedures must be performed as soon as practicable after receipt but no later than 3 hours after the package has been received, if received during normal working hours, or 18 hours after receipt, if received after normal working hours. *These records must be maintained for 2 years following disposal or transfer* according to Title 10CFR30.51(c)(1).

partment and that would require the procedures marked with asterisks are as follows:

1. Greater than 100 mCi ^{131}I
2. Greater than 100 mCi "instant" ^{99m}Tc (generators are specifically exempt)
3. Greater than 10 mCi ^{125}I, ^{14}C, ^{3}H, or ^{35}S
4. Greater than 1 mCi ^{75}Se or ^{169}Yb

STORAGE OF RADIOACTIVE MATERIALS

When radioactive materials are not being used, they should be stored in an area such that radiation levels are reduced to a minimum for the occupational personnel. Another consideration for storage is that these radionuclides be stored in such a manner as to discourage the inadvertent exposure of individuals to their emissions. Provision of adequately shielded storage locations is a necessity to good radiation health safety. These areas should be designated by the appropriate caution signs, and access to the areas should be limited to those individuals who work with the materials. This may mean that a lock be provided to prevent deliberate or inadvertent entry into the area if the area is not constantly supervised. A lock is not necessary if entrance into the area is controlled.

Perhaps the easiest approach to the shielding of stored sources of radioactivity is the use of lead bricks. If the lead bricks are placed on a counter top abutting one another two or three bricks high (a standard brick is 2 inches by 4 inches by 6 inches), adequate protection is provided for the whole body. A top or bottom shield is not necessary under these circumstances because the radiation personnel are always working in the "shadow" of the lead bricks. The only time that protection would not be maintained is when the radiation worker would have to search for one of these stored radionuclides for use. This would not present a radiation hazard in the usual nuclear medicine laboratory. Radiation limits are kept to an intensity of 2 mr/hr outside the lead storage area, which is not at all difficult in the usual nuclear medicine department with the use of standard size lead bricks. The design of the storage area should be such that adequate space is available for storing the radionuclides and, even more important, that identification and ready accessibility are provided for each source.

ISOTOPE DISPOSITION RECORDS

Another important series of records is an inventory of all radioactive material, which lists activity received, activity used, and activity disposed of.

Single-dose disposition forms

There are a number of ways to keep disposition records (ledgers, loose-leaf notebook, or file cards). Any one of these forms must contain information similar to that shown below if the sources are packaged in single-dose amounts (such as uptake capsules).

Lab no.	Patient's name	Date and hour	Number on hand	Number administered	Test performed	Results

As soon as a shipment of radioactivity is received, the shipment should be checked to ascertain whether everything that was ordered has been received. Immediately, information should be recorded as to date received, invoice number, and number of doses received. One of the labels attached to various inclusions in the package should be attached to a record sheet as proof of shipment. The packing slip is an NRC record and is filed chronologically. When the radiopharmaceutical is given, the patient's name, date of administration, number of doses on hand, number of administered, and type of test are recorded. The results can be recorded on completion of the test if desired. The latter sometimes serves as a quick reference should a question arise at a later date. At this point the record is complete until the next patient is considered. This process is continued until the sources are all used or outdated. If used, the record is complete. If outdated, the remaining sources are candidates for disposal. The number disposed of, the date of disposal, and the disposal method are recorded. The card is then filed for future reference and/or checked by the officials of the NRC. *Records should be kept on file for 2 years following disposal* in accordance with Title 10CFR30.51.

Multiple-dose disposition forms

In multiple-dose packaging of a radiopharmaceutical another form of record is used, as shown on the following page.

On receipt of an order from a radiopharmaceutical supplier, information is listed as before; the shipment is checked, receipt date and invoice number are noted, a label is attached to the use record, and the invoice is filed chronologically. On receipt of a request for a study, the patient's name and the date are recorded.

The first consideration is to determine how much activity is on hand. Should the time of use be something different than the precalibration date, the activity on hand is calculated by the following formula:

$$\text{Activity on hand} = \text{Original activity} \times \text{Decay factor}$$

The initial entry under volume should be identical to that on the label. Activity administered is predetermined depending on the patient and the desired study,

Lab no.	Patient's name	Date and hour	Activity on hand (μCi)*	Volume on hand (ml)	Activity administered (μCi)	Volume administered (ml)†	Activity remaining (μCi)	Volume remaining (ml)	Purpose of administration

*Activity remaining × Decay factor.
†Volume on hand × Activity administered ÷ Activity on hand.

and this predetermined amount of activity is entered in the space provided. The volume representing this predetermined activity must then be calculated. This is calculated by the following formula:

$$\text{Volume injected} = \frac{\text{Volume on hand} \times \text{Activity administered}}{\text{Activity on hand}}$$

After the activity and volume to be administered have been determined, the record is completed for this patient by subtracting activity administered from activity on hand to receive the activity remaining; the volume administered is subtracted from the volume on hand to determine the volume remaining.

A second request would be handled exactly the same way with the exception that the activity on hand would be calculated by the activity remaining from the first patient multiplied by the decay factor (which represents the time interval between the time the first source was used and the time the second source was to be used). The volume on hand for the second patient would be the same as the volume remaining from the first patient. This process is continued until the source is depleted or considered unusable. At that time the number of microcuries disposed of, date of disposal, and the disposal method are recorded on the record. The card is now completed and filed under the appropriate heading for future reference and/or NRC checking methods.

A system such as this covers every aspect of records to be kept by a nuclear medicine department regarding receipt and disposition of radiopharmaceuticals.

DISPOSAL

There are two philosophies concerning waste disposal: *concentrate and contain* or *dilute and disperse*. Because of the nature of most medical radioisotope departments and the quantity of radiopharmaceuticals used, the later philosophy is the usual maxim. Six methods are available to the licensee for the disposal of radioactive waste from a routine nuclear medicine department. They are: (1) sewer dilution, (2) incineration, (3) transfer to authorized recipient, (4) burial, (5) decay in storage, and (6) venting of radioactive gases. Regardless of the method used, *records must be maintained until their disposal is approved by the NRC.*

Sewer system

Radioactive wastes may be disposed of by any of several methods, depending on the quantity, concentration, type of radiation, and half-life. They may be flushed directly into the drain, emptied into an effluent pond or a retention basin to be held for decay, drained into hold-up tanks for decay and then flushed into the sewer, or put into special shielded containers for delivery to a chemical processing plant.

These alternatives have been listed in order of increasing radioactivity of the disposal products. Most waste can be disposed of by flushing it directly into the drain.

Title 10CFR20.303 states that no licensee shall discharge licensed material into a sanitary sewerage system unless (1) it is readily soluble or dispersible in water and (2) the quantity of any licensed or other radioactive material released into the system by the licensee in any 1 day does not exceed the larger of the following quantities:

1. Ten times the quantity listed in Appendix C of Title 10CFR20 (for example, iodine 131 = 1 μCi; therefore, 10 μCi of iodine 131 could be disposed of in a sanitary sewer system)

2. The quantity that, if diluted by the average daily quantity of sewerage released into the sewer by the licensee, will result in an average concentration equal to the limits specified in Appendix B, Table 1, Column 2 of Title 10CFR20 (for example, iodine 131 = 6 $\times$ 10^{-5} μCi/ml)

The average water flow for a hospital in the United States is about 1,000 liters per day per bed. Calculations for the disposal of iodine 131 for a 100-bed hospital would proceed as follows:

$$\text{Water flow} = 1{,}000 \text{ liters} \times 100 \text{ beds} \times 1 \text{ day} = 10^6 \times 10^2 \times 1$$
$$= 10^8 \text{ ml water flow}$$

Therefore:

$$6 \times 10^{-5} \ \mu\text{Ci/ml} \times 10^8 \text{ ml/day} = 6 \times 10^3 \ \mu\text{Ci/day}$$
$$= 6{,}000 \ \mu\text{Ci/day}$$
$$= 6 \text{ mCi/day}$$

Accordingly, a 100-bed institution could discard 6 mCi of iodine 131 into the sewer system in any 1 day.

The Code of Federal Regulations further states that the quantity of any licensed or other radioactive material released in any 1 month, if diluted by the average monthly quantity of water released by the licensee, will not result in an average concentration exceeding the limits specified in Appendix B, Table 1, Column 2 (6 $\times$ 10^{-5} of iodine 131). It has already been shown that sewerage flow is equal to 10^8 ml/day. Therefore for iodine 131 the monthly rate would be as follows:

$$6 \times 10^{-5} \ \mu\text{Ci/ml} \times 30 \times 10^8 \text{ ml/month} = 180 \times 10^3 \ \mu\text{Ci/month} = 180 \text{ mCi/month}$$

Accordingly, the total amount of iodine 131 discarded during any 1 month cannot exceed 180 mCi.

The Code of Federal Regulations further stipulates that the gross quantity of licensed or other radioactive material released into the sewerage system by the licensee cannot exceed 1 curie per year. This section of the regulations qualifies all the others. If 180 mCi were discarded per month as just calculated, this would be 2,160 mCi, or 2.16 Ci/year of iodine 131. Although the daily and monthly amounts have not been exceeded, the governing clause is 1 Ci/year. Furthermore, if it were desirable to dispose of 180 mCi in 1 day, the 180 mCi/month value would not be exceeded (providing nothing else was discarded during that month) but the 6 mCi/day value would be exceeded.

If it is necessary to dispose of a combination of radionuclides, the limit for each radionuclide is determined as follows. For each radionuclide in the combination the ratio between the quantity present and the limit for the nuclide as stated in Title 10CRF20 is determined. The sum of the ratios for all the radionuclides in the combination cannot exceed 1. For example, if a batch contains 2,000 μCi of gold 198 and 25,000 μCi of carbon 14, not more than 3,000 μCi of iodine 131 can be included. This value was derived as follows:

$$\frac{2,000\ \mu Ci\ ^{198}Au}{10,000\ \mu Ci} + \frac{25,000\ \mu Ci\ ^{14}C}{50,000\ \mu Ci} + \frac{3,000\ \mu Ci\ ^{131}I}{10,000\ \mu Ci} = 1*$$

These are all exaggerated examples to point out how *all* facets of the NRC regulations must be known and adhered to. A hospital should never discard 6 mCi of iodine 131 in 1 day.

A very important addendum to this regulation is "Excreta from individuals undergoing medical diagnosis or therapy with radioactive materials shall be exempt from any limitations contained in this section."

Incineration

According to Title 10CFR20.305, no licensee shall treat or dispose of licensed material by incineration except as specifically approved by the NRC. To obtain such approval, a special application is required that should include an analysis and evaluation of pertinent information as to the nature of the environment, usage of ground and surface waters in the general area, nature and location of other potentially affected facilities, and procedures to be observed to minimize the risk of unexpected or hazardous exposures.

The only basis by which an incinerator can be used without adherence to these regulations is to incinerate material that is equal to background radiation measured at contact with the Geiger-Mueller probe. The value generally accepted to be background or approaching background is 0.05 mr/hr, at which point the material can be treated as uncontaminated and incinerated in the usual manner.

Transfer to authorized recipient

Title 10CFR20.301 allows the transfer of radioactive wastes to an authorized recipient, thereby obviating many of the details of records regarding storage, disposal, and so on. Several companies offer this service. The Commission will not approve any application for a licensee to receive licensed material from other persons for disposal on land not owned by the federal government or by the state governments.

---

*The denominator in each ratio is obtained by multiplying the valve in Appendix C by 1,000 as stated in Title 10CFR20.

Burial

Another alternative for disposal of radioactive material is through the burial method. This method may be used provided the following regulations are observed:

1. The amount per burial does not exceed 1,000 times the amounts shown in Appendix C of Title 10CFR20. (For iodine 131, the value given is $10 \mu Ci$; therefore, 10 mCi of iodine 131 can be buried.)
2. The material is buried at a minimum depth of 4 feet.
3. Burials are spaced not less than 6 feet apart.
4. Burials are limited to 12 per year in any one area. Larger amounts may be approved on application to the NRC, supplying full details.

Decay in storage

One of the most practical approaches to the disposal of radioactive materials is that of decaying the material to background levels in a protected storage area. This is especially true with short-lived radionuclides such as ^{99m}Tc. The principle is simply to allow the radioactive material to decay through ten physical half-lives. At that time, it can be released into the sewer or subjected to incineration. Any source of radioactivity undergoing ten half-lives is essentially reduced to background radiation. (An exception to this is the molybdenum 99/technetium 99m generator, which should be allowed to decay for 25 half-lives because it has high activity to begin with.) For ^{99m}Tc with its 6-hour physical half-life, ten such time periods would be the 60 hours that lapses from 6 PM Friday evening to 6 AM Monday morning. This means that all ^{99m}Tc waste could be retained all week and all of it discarded in the regular trash on Monday morning. Medium-lived radionuclides (6 hours to 8 days) can be saved in one of two different storage cans behind lead bricks. The storage can is used for 3 months then sealed and allowed to decay while the second can is used for the second consecutive 3-month period. Following that period, the second storage can is sealed, the first can is emptied into the regular trash, and the cycle repeats itself for the next 3-month period. Long-lived radionuclides (8 days) would require decaying until they reach background levels on measurement or disposal by sewer dilution. Since there are so few of these long-lived radionuclides and their utilization rate is low, neither of these procedures is very space occupying or time consuming, respectively.

Venting to outside

In techniques using radioactive gases, such as Xenon-133, (where exhalation of radioactive gases is ancillary to the testing procedure, such gases must be either vented to the outside or contained through the use of activated charcoal traps. [Attention must also be directed to leakage from storage into the restricted area or the accidental release of xenon 133 by the patient during the clinical study.] Each method requires special considerations, separate and distinct from each other. Each will be treated separately.

I. Vent to the outside

Radioactive gases resulting from patient exhalation can be carried to the atmosphere through the use of face masks or mouthpieces connected through expandable tubing to the exhaust system. Since it is discharged directly into the atmosphere, some consideration must be given to the amount of radioactive gases thus released. 10 CFR 20 provides guidelines for determining the quantity of gas released into restricted areas and unrestricted areas through the use of its Appendix B, Tables I and II, respectively.

Title 10 of the Code of Federal Regulations Part 20.106(a), restricts the amount of radioactive gas in an unrestricted area to a concentration of $3 \times 10^{-7} \mu$Ci./ml. and in a restricted area to a concentration of $1 \times 10^{-5} \mu$Ci./ml. It is obvious that at the instant the patient exhales the 10mCi. of Xenon, this limit is exceeded. For this reason, 10 CFR 20.106(a) allows these concentrations to be averaged [according to the following format. In unrestricted areas, ventilation must be sufficient to maintain air concentrations less than $3 \times 10^{-7} \mu$Ci/ml *when averaged over a period of 1 year* and, in restricted areas, less than $1 \times 10^{-5} \mu$Ci/ml *when averaged over a 40-hour week*]. . . . One only has to know the ventilation rate of the exhaust hood, then to determine the amount of Xenon-133 able to be released each day; and therefore, the number of procedures that can be performed each work-day. A sample calculation is as follows:

Assumptions:
1. Hood discharges at rate of 1200 cfm.
2. Conversion factor to express ft³ in cm³ = 27,000
3. Assume exhaust hood to vent at roof.
[4. Assume roof to be an unrestricted area.]
5. Maximum concentration in effluent in unrestricted area is $3 \times 10^{-7} \mu$Ci/ml.
6. 100% of gases released to atmosphere via exhaust hood.

Calculation:
1. Air Flow (cfm) $\times$ V $\times$ F
   where, V = 10 CFR 20, Appendix B, Table II for Xe-133
   F = factor to convert ft³ to cm³
   1200cfm $\times$ 3 $\times$ 10^{-7} $\times$ 27,000 = 9.72 μCi/min.
2. Concentrations averaged over one year:

$$\frac{9.72 \ \mu\text{Ci.}}{\text{min.}} \times \frac{60 \ \text{min.}}{\text{hr.}} \times \frac{24 \ \text{hr.}}{\text{day}} \times \frac{365 \ \text{days}}{\text{year}} = 5,109 \ \text{mCi/year}$$

3. Yearly average extended to each workday:

$$\frac{5,109 \ \text{mCi.}}{\text{yr.}} \div \frac{260 \ \text{workdays}}{\text{yr.}} = 20 \ \text{mCi/workday}$$

4. Assuming a standard dose of 10mCi. per study, 2 studies could be performed each work day.

Other considerations:

A smaller hood ventilation rate would reduce the number of studies capable of being performed, at a proportional rate. The fan should be mounted at the roof level, rather than the hood level to prevent down drafts and eddy currents causing the Xenon to be released back into the room. The place where the Xenon is released at the roof level should be a minimum of [10 meters] . . . from the nearest *possible* point of reentry into the hospital, be it window, door, air intake vent, etc. The room in which the Xenon is used should have a negative pressure (more room exhaust than air intake) to prevent the Xenon from going into hall in the event of an accidental release into the imaging room. Since the Xenon has been known to "leak" from its source, it is important that the Xenon be stored in an area that is confined and capable of being easily evacuated; for these reasons, a fume hood, offers an excellent storage area for Xenon.

II. Xenon trap

Xenon traps utilizing activated charcoal filters are . . . commercially available. Since Xenon is an inert gas, there is no way to collect this gas by any chemical combination. Therefore, activated charcoal must be used. These systems are [said to remove] . . . up to . . . 95% of the Xenon in their pass through their filters, reducing the Xenon exhaust at the outlet to levels *less* than that allowed by 10 CFR 20. To insure that this is the case, the outlet can be attached to the exhaust hood, thereby directing whatever Xenon, if any, to the atmosphere. Some Xenon traps have a low level G-M tube constantly monitoring the exhaust, the response of which is designed to elicit an audible signal when the radioactivity reaches a pre-determined level. [Once traps have become saturated, they should be removed from the system and allowed to decay to background levels. A replacement charcoal filter should be used in the collection system.]

III. . . . Release [of Xenon into restricted area]

In the event that there is [leakage from the Xenon storage vessel or syringe or] an accidental release of Xenon in the imaging room, such as a patient's cough, or syringe leak, some provision must be made to handle the "spill". The fact that the room has a negative pressure helps to contain the "spill". [In order to keep radiation exposure ALARA,] all patients and personnel should be immediately removed from the room and the doors closed [for at least five complete room air exchanges]. . . .

[As already described,] the ventilation in restricted areas where ^{133}Xe is used and stored must be sufficient to maintain air concentrations less than $1 \times 10^{-5} \mu$Ci./ml. when averaged over a 40-hour week.

. . . Actual measurements of ^{133}Xe concentrations [can be taken or an evaluation of the situation is possible] . . . by means of calculations. If . . . the latter approach [is chosen], simplifying assumptions [may be made], *PROVIDING* they are reasonable [and] conservative. . . . The following procedures . . . [are] used to [exemplify the calculations of air] . . . concentration of ^{133}Xe in restricted areas:

1. Estimate the *maximum* amount of activity to be used per week (A).
2. Estimate the fraction of ^{133}Xe that is lost during use and storage (f).
3. Determine the ventilation rate in the area(s) of interest and calculate the volume of air available per week for dilution of the ^{133}Xe (V).
4. For restricted areas, Section 20.103 of 10 CFR Part 20 requires that:

$$\frac{A}{V} \times f \leq 1 \times 10^{-5} \ \mu\text{Ci/ml.}$$

Sample Problem

A nuclear medicine laboratory plans to use 10 mCi ^{133}Xe per patient and will perform a maximum of 10 studies per week. What ventilation rate is required to ensure compliance with Section 20.103 of 10 CFR Part 20?

a) Maximum activity used per week:

$$A = \frac{10 \text{ mCi}}{\text{patient}} \times \frac{10 \text{ patients}}{\text{week}} \times 1 \times 10^3 \frac{\mu\text{Ci}}{\text{mCi}} = 1 \times 10^5 \frac{\mu\text{Ci}}{\text{week}}$$

b) Assume a leakage rate of 25% (f).

c)
$$V = \frac{A \times f}{1 \times 10^{-5} \ \mu\text{Ci/ml}}$$

$$= \frac{1 \times 10^5 \ \mu\text{Ci/week} \times 0.25}{1 \times 10^{-5} \ \mu\text{Ci/ml}}$$

$$= 2.5 \times 10^9 \frac{\text{ml}}{\text{week}}$$

The required ventilation rate is

$$\frac{2.5 \times 10^9 \text{ ml/week}}{40 \text{ hrs/week}} \times \frac{1 \text{ cfm}}{1.7 \times 10^6 \text{ ml/hr[*]}} = 37 \text{ cfm}$$

The answer shows that, in order to meet the requirements of Section 20.103 of 10 CFR Part 20, the imaging room (RESTRICTED AREA) must have a ventilation rate of *at least* 37 cfm with no recirculation of air. Where practical, the ventilation rate should be greater than that shown necessary by the calculation in order to maintain the air concentration of ^{133}Xe as low as reasonably achievable in accordance with Section 20.1(c) of 10 CFR Part 20.

If the ventilation rate is inadequate to meet the requirements of Section 20.103, 10 CFR Part 20, methods of increasing ventilation or reducing the patient load [should be considered].

The following table gives the amount of ^{133}Xe that can be released per week without exceeding the permissible levels for ^{133}Xe in restricted areas.

Ventilation Rate (cfm)	Maximum ^{133}Xe released per 40 hour-week (mCi)
100	67.9
500	339.7
1000	679.4

The ALARA philosophy suggests that levels of some radioactive gases may require fume hoods to prevent buildup of ^{133}Xe or ^{131}I in the department. Also, in this way, a negative pressure can be created inside the nuclear medicine department. The face velocity of the fume hood should be at least 150 feet/min, measured no less than two times per year. It should exhaust no less than 10 m from the nearest point of intake back into the hospital.

ALARA addresses the use of ^{133}Xe gas specifically by suggesting the placement of 1.6-mm thick additional lead around the absorber cannister, oxygen bag, and waste receptacle in order to reduce radiation exposure to occupational personnel during the diagnostic study. Further, it suggests that an added shield of 3.2-

---

[*The value 1.7×10^6 is the conversion factor for ml/hr to cfm.]

mm thick lead be interposed between the ^{133}Xe dispenser and the camera for better diagnostic studies. Waste ^{133}Xe should be removed immediately following the study.

REGULATIONS FOR NUCLEAR MEDICINE LABORATORY PERSONNEL

Following are regulations that must be adhered to by all laboratory personnel.

1. Good housekeeping must be maintained at all times. The laboratory must be kept neat, glassware must be washed regularly, and waste or contaminated materials must not be allowed to accumulate.
2. No food may be eaten or stored in the radioisotope unit.
3. No smoking is allowed while handling radioactivity.
4. Protective outer garments such as laboratory coats and rubber gloves should be worn while handling radioactive materials.
5. All possible setups will be made on easily cleanable trays.
6. All trays and all other work surfaces will be covered with disposable absorbent paper.
7. All containers of radioactive materials must be labeled, stating the kind, quantity of isotope, dose of assay, and radiation symbol.
8. Some monitoring device, such as a film badge, should always be worn by occupational personnel while working in the unit. This should include a monitoring device for whole-body dose as well as dose to hands and forearms for personnel using a generator or preparing and injecting patient doses.
9. Pipetting by mouth is not allowed; an automatic pipette must always be used.
10. All work areas will be monitored regularly and results of surveys recorded.

Other points of the ALARA philosophy related to a diagnostic nuclear medicine department are as follows:

1. Nuclear medicine facilities:
   a. There should be sufficient space in the department so that the occupational personnel can be at least 1 m (preferably 2 m) from the patient when operating the equipment.
   b. There should be adequate space for stretcher patients. They emit radiation as high as 10 mr/hr from diagnostic doses of ^{99m}Tc.
   c. The doctor's and the technologists' offices should be near the nuclear medicine facilities but away from the storage area for isotopes.
2. Special waste receptacle for syringes
   a. The size of the receptacle should be sufficient to hold 1 week's supply of radioactive waste.
   b. The receptacle should have a removable pail with a lid.
   c. The pail and the lid should possess at least a 1-mm lead shield.
   d. Other radioactive waste cans also should be shielded.

    e. All radioactive waste cans should be placed near the area in which the waste is generated but away from a high occupancy area.

3. Hot sinks
    a. A sink in the department should be designated for waste only.
    b. Records should be kept as to the amount of radioactivity disposed.
    c. Records should also be kept of the total sewerage effluent.
    d. The sink should be connected directly to the main pipe.
    e. The water taps should be operable by foot, knee, or elbow.

4. Diagnostic nuclear medicine
    a. Generators should be stored in a separate area with an auxillary shield.
    b. Assay of ^{99m}Tc should be measured with the aliquot method, not the whole vial method, in order to reduce exposures.
    c. All doses should be measured prior to injection into a patient.
    d. Syringe shields should be used to dose patients.
    e. Vial shields should be used when dispensing aliquots of radioactivity.
    f. Tongs should be used to hold the vial for vial transfers.
    g. Vials should never be stored behind the bench shield, not without a vial shield.
    h. Radioactive "spills" should be cleaned up immediately.
    i. Areas in which radionuclides are used will be monitored at the end of each working day.

THERAPEUTIC USE OF RADIOPHARMACEUTICALS

Special precautions for patients treated with byproduct material listed in Groups IV or V, Schedule A, Section 35.100 of 10 CFR Part 35 are as follows:

    Method for preparation and administration of therapeutic doses of Iodine-131. Therapeutic doses of I-131 will be ordered from reputable suppliers and received precalibrated, ready for dispensing to patients. These materials will be stored until time for use in the isotope storage area behind sufficient shielding to reduce the radiation levels to 2.0mR/hr at a distance where occupational workers can conveniently stand. All liquid sources will be opened in a fume hood with the fan activated. Patients requiring therapeutic amounts of I-131 less than 30mCi will be dosed in the hot lab, held for 30 minutes for observation and sent home or to their room. Hospitalized patients receiving greater than 30mCi will be dosed in their rooms [if no special dosing room near the nuclear medicine department is available].

    Only patients treated with greater than 8mCi I-131* or 23mCi Au-198* who require hospitalization will be placed in a private room with a toilet. Attempts will be made to use a corner room in a low traffic section of hallway. Patients will use disposable items whenever possible (e.g., dishes, utensils, etc.). Surveys of the patient's room and surrounding areas will be conducted as soon as practicable after administration of the treatment dose. Exposure rates will be measured at the patient's bedside, three feet away and the entrance to the room. The Radiation Safety Office or his designate will then determine how long a person

*Table 2 of NCRP #37.

may remain at these positions and will post these times in the patient's chart and on his door. The results of daily surveys will be used to recalculate permitted times which will be posted on the patient's chart and on his door. (Refer to Item #19, Form A). Radiation levels in unrestricted areas will be maintained less than the limits specified in Section 20.105(b), 10 CFR Part 20. (i.e., 2mrems in any one hour or 100mrems in any seven consecutive days) Refer to . . . Form A.

All linens will be surveyed for contamination before being removed from the patient's room and will, if necessary, be held for decay. Disposable plates, cups, eating utensils, tissue, surgical dressings, and other similar waste items will be placed in a specially designated container. The material will be collected daily by the Radiation Safety Officer (or his designate), checked for contamination, and disposed of as normal or radioactive waste, as appropriate. Non-disposable items used for these patients will be held in plastic bags in the patient's room, and checked for contamination by the Radiation Safety Officer or his designate. Items may be returned for normal use, held for decay or decontaminated, as appropriate.

The form, Nursing Instructions for Patients Treated with Phosphorus-32, Gold-198, or Iodine-131, (. . . Form B) will be completed immediately after administration of the treatment dose. A copy will be posted in the patient's chart. Nurses should spend only that amount of time near the patient required for ordinary nursing care. Special restrictions may be noted on the precaution sheet in the patient's chart. Nurses should read these instructions before administering to the patients. Call the . . . [RSO] if you have any questions about the care of these patients. Visitors will be limited to those 18 years of age or over, unless other instructions are noted on the precautions sheet in the patient's chart. Patients must remain in bed while visitors are in the room and visitors should remain at least three feet from the patient. Radioactive patients are to be confined to their rooms except for special medical or nursing purposes approved by the . . . [RSO]. No nurse, visitor or attendant who is pregnant should be permitted in the room of a patient who has received a therapeutic amount of radioactivity until the patient no longer presents a radiation hazard. Female visitors should be asked whether they are pregnant. Attending personnel must wear rubber or disposable plastic gloves when handling urinals, bedpans, emesis basins or other containers having any material obtained from the body of the patient. Wash gloves before removing and then wash hands. The gloves must be left in the patient's room in the designated waste container. These gloves need not be sterile or surgical in type.

Therapy patients will be allowed to use the toilet facilities since human excreta is exempt from waste disposal considerations. The patient will be instructed, however, to flush the toilet, urinal or bed pan several times after use. If the nurse helps to collect the excreta, she should wear disposable gloves. Afterwards she should wash her hands with the gloves on and again after the gloves are removed. The gloves should be placed in the designated waste container for disposal by the . . . [RSO]. Vomiting within 24 hours after oral administration, urinary incontinence, or excessive sweating within the first 48 hours may result in contamination of linen and/or floor. If radioactive urine or feces is collected or spilled during collection, call the . . . [RSO]. Meanwhile, handle all contaminated material with disposable gloves and avoid spreading contamination. All vomitus must also be kept in the patient's room for disposal by the . . . [RSO]. Urine or feces need not be routinely saved, unless ordered on the chart. The same toilet should be used by the patient at all times and it

RADIATION SURVEY FORM

Room diagram

Film badges issued to:

	Time limit
Nurse @ bedside	min/hr
Visitor @ chair	min/hr
Pt. bed #	hrs
Pt. bed #	hrs
Pt. bed #	hrs
Pt. bed #	hrs

Name	Date	mrem

Certified by _____ Date/time_____

IMPORTANT: <u>THIS RECORD MUST BE PERMANENTLY MAINTAINED</u>

Form A

CALCULATIONS

Show line drawing of patient's and neighboring rooms on other side
of this form. Indicate location of patient and neighboring beds,
patient orientation, visitor's chair, hallways, doors, and outside
walls. Room must be a private one, preferably with two outside
walls and patient's feet oriented to outside wall. Use G-M (low
level) and ion (high level) chamber survey meter to determine
radiation levels. Record obtained values on drawing at location
of measured readings. Readings should be taken at (1) patient's
bedside, (2) visitor's chair, and (3) mid-bed on all neighboring
beds. Query for recently performed nuclear medicine procedures
if elevated readings are obtained.

Nurses- limited to 2.0mrems/hr (2.0 ÷ bedside reading) x 60 min/
hr = maximum minutes of bedside care each (but every)
hour.

Visitors- should be limited to 100mrems/total treatment time. If
visitor's chair mr/hr x total treatment time is greater
than 100mrems, limit visiting time as 100÷(total
treatment time x visitor's chair reading) x 60 min/
hr = maximum min/hr for each hour.

Neighboring
patients- should be limited to 100mrems. Readings taken at mid-
bed x total treatment time can usually be limited to
less than 100mrems either through distance or shielding. Neighboring patients should be transferred if
this is not possible when the total exposure approaches
100mrems.

Form A – cont'd

NURSING INSTRUCTIONS FOR PATIENTS TREATED WITH PHOSPHUS-32
GOLD-198, or IODINE-131

Patient's name _____

Room no. _____ Physician's name _____

Radioisotope administered _____

Date and time of administration _____

Dose received _____ Method of administration _____

Exposure rates in mr/hr

Date	3 feet from bed	10 feet from bed

(Comply with all check items)

_____1. Visiting time permitted _____
_____2. Visitors must remain_____from patient.
_____3. Patient may <u>not</u> leave room.
_____4. Visitors under 18 <u>not</u> permitted.
_____5. Pregnant visitors <u>not</u> permitted.
_____6. Film badges must be worn.
_____7. Use and complete the following tags:

      _____ door (see Form G)
      _____ bed (see Forms H, I, and J)
      _____ chart (see Forms H, I, and J)
      _____ wrist (see Form K)

_____8. Gloves must be worn while attending patient.
_____9. Patient must use disposable utensils.
_____10. All items must remain in room until OK'd by Radiation Safety.
_____11. Smoking is <u>not</u> permitted.
_____12. Do not release room to admitting until OK'd by Radiation Safety.
_____13. Other instructions.

In case of emergency, contact:

RSO_____ On/off duty telephone #_____ /_____

Form B

should be . . . [flushed well (3 times) after each use]. Utmost precautions must be taken to see that no urine or vomitus, is spilled on the floor or the bed. If any part of the patient's room is suspected to be contaminated, notify the . . . [RSO]. If a nurse, attendant or anyone else knows or suspects that his skin, or clothing, including shoes, is contaminated, notify the . . . [RSO] immediately. This person should remain in the patient's room and not walk about the hospital. If the hands become contaminated, wash immediately with soap and water. If a therapy patient should need emergency surgery or should die, notify the . . . [RSO] immediately. When the patient is discharged call the . . . [RSO] and request that the room be surveyed for contamination before remaking the room.

Surgical dressings should be changed only as directed by the physician. Gold-198 leaking from a puncture wound will stain the dressings dark red or purple. Such dressings should not be discarded but should be collected in plastic bags and turned over to the . . . [RSO]. Handle these dressings only with tongs or tweezers. Wear disposable gloves.

Disposable items should be used in the care of these patients, whenever possible. These items should be placed in the designated waste container. Contact the . . . [RSO] for proper disposal of the contents of the designated waste container. Disposable plates, cups, and eating utensils will be used by patients who are treated with Iodine-131. All clothes and bed linens used by the patient should be placed in the laundry bag provided and left in the patient's room to be checked by . . . the . . . [RSO]. All non-disposable items should be placed in a plastic bag and left in the patient's room to be checked by . . . [the RSO].

In most hospitals, deceased patients with large amounts of radionuclides will be encountered only rarely, since, in principle, radionuclide therapy is not given to moribund patients. If several days intervene between treatment and subsequent surgery or death, the radiation hazard is usually considerably reduced. In most hospitals, the number of patients receiving large internal doses of radionuclides in any one week is small. The need for emergency surgery would not be usual, nor would the death of one of these patients.[*]

The identification of a particular patient as radioactive is the responsibility of the physician in charge of the case. The radioactive patient shall be properly identified at all times. If a radioactive patient dies in the hospital, the physician who pronounces him dead should be responsible for attaching a radioactivity precautions tag to the body. The physician in charge of the case and the Radiation . . . [Safety] Officer shall be notified at once.

In general bodies containing less than 5mCi, need no precautions for any type of handling. Those containing between 5 and 30mCi may be buried or cremated with no preparation or embalmed according to standard injection procedures without special precautions. If the body is to be subjected to autopsy, the . . . [RSO] will designate any special precautions. The body containing more than 30mCi. can be buried or cremated with no preparation, but if embalming is to be carried out, it should be with the guidance of a . . . [RSO]. Among patients that die outside the hospital, the funeral director will seldom encounter bodies with hazardous exposure rates.

Preparation for burial or cremation without autopsy:

Consider first the cases in which no autopsy is to be performed and the body need not be opened. Embalming will be by the injection method, and the likelihood of contamination

---

[*Summary of information found in NCRP Report #37.]

of the embalmer is small. Nevertheless, even in these cases, rubber gloves shall be worn by all who are involved in the procedures in order to avoid the possibility of contamination by radioactive fluids from the body. The exposure rate at about 25cm. from the center of the radioactive material should be measured; if this is less than 0.25 R/h,* no further precautions are necessary as far as the gamma radiations are concerned. . . . Forms C and D will be completed.

Radioactive iodine, I-131, administered orally or intravenously; no autopsy:

The dose of I-131 administered in the treatment of thyroid disease rarely exceeds 100mCi. Within an hour after a patient has received this dose, measurements with an ionization chamber type survey meter may be expected to indicate a surface exposure rate over the abdomen on the order of 0.3 R/h. During the first 24 hours after administration of I-131, the blood and urine may contain considerable radioactivity. These fluids should accordingly be removed into closed systems . . . [or] flushed directly into the sewer, followed by an adequate volume of water.

The day after administration, the general distribution of radiation is greatly modified, both by urinary excretion of a large part of the radionuclide and by concentration of the remaining part in functioning thyroid tissue. At this time only radiation from these regions of iodine storage need be considered. Any region of high activity which is not to be removed, should be marked by the . . . [RSO] so that it can be avoided.

Any radionuclide injected interstitially or in seeds:
no autopsy:

Various colloidal radioactive preparations may be injected interstitially into tumors. Radon seeds, radioactive gold wires, radium wires, and other preparations may be implanted in limited regions. If the nuclide emits only beta rays, it is unlikely that there will be any appreciable external irradiation. If it is a gamma emitter, the active tissues may be extirpated or the region can be identified and avoided.

Body to be opened for surgery or autopsy:

The usual precautions for preventing the spread of an infectious material should aid in keeping the radioactive material localized. At autopsy the general principle is to remove the main source of radiation hazard as early as possible, without causing general contamination. At surgery this cannot usually be done, hence regions of high activity should be avoided or shielded. . . . Forms D and E will be completed.

As long as the body remains unopened, the radiation received by anyone near it, is due almost entirely to gamma rays. The change in emphasis when an operation or autopsy is to be performed is due to the possible exposure of the hands and face to relatively intense beta radiation. Beta radiation is readily absorbed by material interposed between its source and the operator. Even rubber gloves are useful in this regard. The gamma rays are not absorbed . . . by rubber gloves.

---

*Approximate activity that will produce an exposure rate of 0.25 R/hr at 25 cm is as follows: [198]Au, 70 mCi; ^{131}I, 70 mCi; ^{192}Ir, 30 mCi, [222]Rn, 20 mCi.

SPECIFIC INSTRUCTIONS TO REDUCE RADIATION EXPOSURE DURING EMBALMMENT
(To be filled out by Radiation Safety Officer and forwarded
to funeral director)

The following procedures should be implemented during the embalming
of _____.

( )   This body does not contain significant amounts of
      radioactive material. No special precautions are
      necessary if standard embalming procedures are
      employed.

      This body contains radioactive material. The following
      procedures should be observed:

   ( )   A closed system should be used to drain fluids.
         Use suction if necessary. Fluid can be disposed
         of via sewer, flush with copious amounts of
         water.

   ( )   Blood and urine should be removed via closed
         systems. Dispose via sewer with copious amounts
         of water.

   ( )   Other_____

         _____

         _____

                         Signed_____
                                Radiation Safety Officer

                         Date_____

Copy of this report is maintained in Radiation Safety Office files.

Form C

RADIATION HAZARD EVALUATION FORM
(to be filled out by Radiation Safety Officer for his/her use)

Name_____ Date and_____

Time of Death_____

Radioisotope_____

Amount administered_____

Route of administration_____

Amount present_____

Distribution within
    body   _____

_____

_____

_____

Indicate distances_____

Suggest ring badges if exposure
    0.25 r/hr @ 25 cm

See NCRP #37 p. 27.

Limit hand exposure to 1.5 rems

Date of survey_____

Instrument used_____

Signed_____
       Radiation Safety Officer

Date_____

Form D

SPECIFIC INSTRUCTIONS FOR AUTOPSY
(to be filled out by Radiation Safety Officer)

The following procedures should be followed if so indicated:

( ) Wear safety glasses.

( ) Wear plastic (nonabsorbant) gown.

( ) Cover floor with bench liner.

( ) Wear double thickness autopsy gloves.

( ) Wear whole body film badge.

( ) Wear ring badge.

( ) Remove the _____ area or tissue first before proceeding further. Identify it as radioactive.

( ) Leave the _____ area or tissue untouched until last.

( ) Cover the _____ area or tissue with shielding as provided.

( ) Use only long instruments--8 inches or greater.

( ) Fluids, blood, urine should be removed via closed system. Flush with copious amounts of water.

( ) Small specimens need/need not be handled with special precautions.

( ) Waste container needs to be provided for contaminated sponges, gowns, and instruments.

( ) Organs are to be kept in storage for _____ days before fixation.

Autopsy performed by _____ Patient name _____

Whole body or ringer badge no. _____ Exposure _____

Signed _____
        Radiation Safety Officer

Date _____

THIS REPORT MUST BE SAVED!

Form E

Any radionuclide in a body cavity which is to be opened:

The . . . [RSO] will evaluate the radiation hazard and suggest suitable procedures regarding the safety of personnel during the entire operation.

a. Autopsy —

As much body fluid as possible should be removed before the body is opened. The remaining radioactive material may be expected to be widely distributed over the surfaces of the cavity and of the organs within it. The use of bare hands will not be permitted because of the contamination of skin and nails that would result and the difficulty of complete removal of such contamination.

Monitoring the body after removal of the viscera may indicate a radiation level low enough so that subsequent procedures can be carried out without special precautions. Regions of high activity, if present, can be indicated and avoided or approached with precautions. If the removed organs are to be dissected immediately, each one should be monitored and treated in accordance with the findings. After desired small samples have been taken, the radioactive tissues that are to be retained should immediately be placed in appropriately shielded vessels for storage, or for disposal according to procedures approved by the Radiation . . . [Safety] Officer. Where adequate cold storage facilities are available, the organs may be stored for several days without significant alteration, or the viscera may be fixed. This would allow for the natural decay of the . . . [radioactivity] reducing possible exposure.

b. Emergency surgery —

If surgery must be carried out within a highly radioactive cavity, speed is desirable. Accordingly, an experienced surgeon should perform the operation. The surgeon and his assistants should wear gloves and glasses or goggles for the protection of the eyes from possible splashing of foreign material, as well as from beta radiation.

Radioactive iodine 131 orally or intravenously administered:

a. Autopsy —

Urine should be drained away and blood disposed of, if possible, in the same manner as if no autopsy were to be performed.

b. Surgery —

Precautions are essentially the same as for autopsy. During the first day after administration, the blood may be expected to contain considerable radioactivity, and care should be taken not to let it accumulate on gloves or gowns. After the first day, the circulating radioiodine has greatly decreased, and regions of high activity can be identified and usually avoided.

Interstitial implants and colloidal interstitial infiltration:

At surgery or autopsy, these regions can be readily identified, and avoided as far as possible. At autopsy, if the entire block of tissue containing the radionuclide can be removed readily, this should be done first. If only a sample of the treated region is to be taken, this part of the body should be avoided until the rest of the autopsy has been carried out.

Accident or injury during surgery or autopsy:

If an injury occurs during surgery or autopsy, where the rubber gloves are cut or torn, radioactivity may be introduced into the wound. In addition to ordinary treatment of the wound, the . . . [RSO] shall be consulted with regard to any possible radiation hazard.

Summary

In general, most procedures performed in nuclear medicine involve the use of Technetium 99m. Due to this radionuclide's short half-life, six hours, a period of 24 hours should reduce even the highest dose encountered in nuclear medicine to a safe level. Most other procedures generally encountered in nuclear medicine involving nuclides other than Technetium-99m require dose of 5mCi or less. As indicated in the opening paragraph, activities at this level require little or no special procedures. Those situations involving special precautions and procedures are generally limited to quantities of radioactivity introduced into the patient during therapy treatment. The . . . [RSO] should be consulted to establish proper precautions and procedures for each individual case.

Before a therapy patient's room is reassigned to another patient, the room will be surveyed for contamination (and decontaminated if necessary) and all radioactive waste and waste containers will be removed.

Instructions for Patient & Family — Patient will not be discharged until radioactivity reaches 30mCi. This will be determined by measuring the dose rate at time of administration from a distance of no less than 3 meters, allowing the patient to act as much like a point source as possible. Patient will be discharged when reading at identical location and circumstances reaches 30% of initial value.

(i) In the event that all persons in the household of the radioactive patient, and hence all those persons with whom the patient will have appreciable contact, are over the age of 45 years:
   • The patient should be instructed to remain at distances greater than 3 feet from other people, except for brief periods for necessary procedures.
   • Babies and young people (of ages less than 45 years) should not visit the patient, but if they do, the visits should be brief, and a distance of at least 9 feet from the patient should be maintained.

(ii) In the event that a person under the age of 45 years lives in the household of the patient:
   • Stricter precautions shall be observed than when all contacts are with persons over 45 years of age.
   • Children and persons under 45 years of age shall not be allowed in the same room, nor at a distance of less than 9 feet, for more than a few minutes a day. Observance of these conditions will insure that persons under 45 years of age will not be exposed to more than 0.5 R per year from the radioactive individual.
   • Other restrictions may be specified by the physician.

All restrictions will be removed when the activity reduces to a point that will result in no greater than 0.5 R to persons in the family from that point until total decay. For I-131, that will be the time where radioactivity in the thyroid gland reaches 8mCi.

INSTRUCTIONS FOR FAMILY OF RELEASED PATIENT

Name of patient_____
Name of hospital_____ Address_____ Tel. no._____
For further information contact_____ Tel. no._____

Please show this form to every physician consulted concerning the patient
  until_____
                  (date)

_____ was treated on_____, 19_____.
  (Name of patient)
with_____millicuries of_____in the form of_____.

NO SPECIAL RADIATION SAFETY PRECAUTIONS ARE NECESSARY AFTER_____.
                                                              (date)
UNTIL THAT DATE:

  Persons under 45 years of age should not remain closer than the following
  distances from the patient, for the time period indicated:
  _____ to_____
    (date)   (date)

    Permissible distance_____feet or more, for_____hours/week.
    (At other times remain farther than 6 feet).

    Note: During the above time, brief periods of closer contact
            (for example while shaking hands, or kissing the patient)
            are permissible.

  SPECIAL PRECAUTIONS:

    a) Spouse or other person caring for patient
        _____

        _____

    b) Children or pregnant women _____
        _____

        _____

    c) Sleeping arrangements _____
        _____

        _____

IF THE PATIENT IS TO BE HOSPITALIZED, OR IF DEATH SHOULD OCCUR, NOTIFY
THE FOLLOWING INDIVIDUAL(S) IMMEDIATELY: _____
                                         _____

  A COPY OF THIS FORM SHOULD BE KEPT WITH THE PATIENT'S RECORD.

Form F

or a reading of 1.8mR/hr @ 1 meter*. An effective half-life of six days will be used for this computation. For Au-198, those values will be 23 mCi or 5.3mR/hr @ 1 meter. An effective half-life of 65 hours will be used for this computation.

. . . Form F will be used for the purpose of informing all.

With respect to a radiopharmaceutical therapy program, the ALARA philosophy suggests the following:

1. A special room is desirable for the administration of the therapy source in order that the risk of contamination be reduced. This special room should be near the nuclear medicine department in order to reduce the transporting distance and thereby reduce exposure to personnel.

2. Patient's room may be used for administration of the therapy source provided the RSO is available to assist the administration and to monitor its progress. The RSO should also govern the transport of the material to the patient's room.

3. The therapy dose should be checked for accuracy prior to administration. If the dose should be ^{131}I in liquid form, then the source should be opened in a fume hood.

4. The nursing staff should be briefed and appropriate tags (Forms G to K) should be placed on the patient's chart, bed, and door and a wristband should be placed on the patient.

5. Contamination should be controlled by:
   a. Placing absorbent material over floors and furniture
   b. Using plastic mattress covers
   c. Covering the telephone with small plastic bags
   d. Covering door and toilet handles with small plastic bags
   e. Using disposable dishes, cups, and utensils

6. If collection of radioactive wastes is to be performed, they should be collected in wide-mouth waterproof plastic containers.

7. A large trash can should be made available for linens. These linens should be removed daily and monitored before removing to the laundry.

8. All waste will be removed from the patient's room by cart and taken to the decay bin, if necessary.

9. The patient's room should be resurveyed for missed areas prior to release for use by another patient.

Text continued on p. 330.

---

*Table 2 of NCRP Report #37.

———————————— HOSPITAL

RADIOACTIVITY

PRECAUTIONS

RADIONUCLIDE———— mCi ————
DATE————————————————

See Nursing Station for Instructions.

Tag is not to be removed until:

    1) Radioactive material is removed from patient, or

    2) Authorization is received from Radiation Protection Supervisor.

Signature————————————————
RADIATION PROTECTION SUPERVISOR

Form G. Tag to be placed on the foot of patient's bed or attached to door of patient's room. (From Precautions in the management of patients who have received therapeutic amounts of radionuclides NRCP Report No. 37, October 1970.)

_____HOSPITAL

PATIENT'S NAME_____ UNIT NUMBER_____

C A U T I O N

RADIOACTIVE MATERIAL

PERMANENT IMPLANT OR INTERNAL DOSE

Radionuclide_____mCi_____

Administered_____
                    (DATE)
Initial Exposure Rate at 1 Meter_____mR/h

   (SIGNATURE) _____

INSTRUCTIONS:

  Patient must remain in hospital until_____
                                    (DATE)
  "Radioactivity Precautions" tag may be removed_____
                                        (DATE)
  The Radiation Protection Office (Ext._____) must
    be notified before discharge or removal of patient.
  For further information call Radiation Protection Office.
  In case of an emergency, the telephone operator has a
    call list for use when the Radiation Protection Office
    is not open.

Date_____ Signature_____
                    RADIATION PROTECTION SUPERVISOR

Form H. Label for patient's chart for *permanent* implant or internal dose. (From Precautions in the management of patients who have received therapeutic amounts of radionuclides. NCRP Report No. 37, October 1970.)

---HOSPITAL

PATIENT'S NAME_____UNIT NUMBER_____

CAUTION

RADIOACTIVE MATERIAL

TEMPORARY IMPLANT

Radionuclide_____mCi_____

Inserted_____
             (DATE)

Initial Exposure Rate at 1 Meter_____mR/h

    (SIGNATURE)_____

To Be Removed _____
                  (DATE)

INSTRUCTIONS:

    Patient must remain in hospital until implant is removed.

    When implant is removed, "Radioactivity Precautions Tags" may also be removed.

    For further information call Radiation Protection Office (Ext_____)

    In case of emergency, the telephone operator has a call list for use when the Radiation Protection Office is not open.

Date_____ Signature_____

               RADIATION PROTECTION SUPERVISOR

Form I. Label for patient's chart for *temporary* implant. (From Precautions in the management of patients who have received therapeutic amounts of radionuclides, NCRP Report No. 37, October 1970.)

_____HOSPITAL

PATIENT'S NAME_____UNIT NUMBER_____

CAUTION

☢

PATIENT CONTAINS RADIOACTIVE MATERIAL

DO NOT REMOVE THIS LABEL UNTIL:

1) Radioactive material is removed from patient, or
2) Removal is authorized by Radiation
   Protection Supervisor (Ext._____).

VISITORS MUST CHECK WITH NURSING STATION
BEFORE GOING TO PATIENT.

Date_____ Signature_____

RADIATION PROTECTION SUPERVISOR

Form J. Label for cover of patient's chart. (From Precautions in the management of patients who have received therapeutic amounts of radionuclides, NCRP Report No. 37, October 1970.)

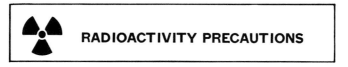

Form K. Wristband to be placed on patient. (From Precautions in the management of patients who have received therapeutic amounts of radionuclides, NCRP Report No. 37, October 1970.)

[SAFETY PRECAUTIONS IN THE] THERAPEUTIC USE OF SEALED SOURCES

Special procedures for patients treated with byproduct material listed in Group VI, Schedule A, Section 35.100 of 10 CFR Part 35, are as follows: . . .

Safety precautions in clinical applications

I. Transfer and Preparation of Sources.
   a. Forms will be used to record pre and post-use inventory. (. . . Form. . .[N])
   b. Sources will be dispensed with suitable protective devices and techniques, to include long forceps and TLD finger badges.
II. Application of Sources to the Patient.
   a. Distance, time, and when possible shielding, will be used to reduce radiation exposure to personnel attending the patient.
   b. Appropriate signs will be used to indicate levels of radiation exposure.
   c. Consideration will be given to the proximity of patients in adjoining rooms.
   d. A patient being treated with brachytherapy sources will wear suitable identification.
   e. Patient will not be allowed to leave his room unless accompanied by a hospital attendant.
   f. Persons who have short-lived sources which are not removable from their bodies will be allowed to leave the hospital provided precautions necessary to prevent other persons from receiving more than the permissible dose of radiation are observed.
III. Removal of Sources from Patient.
   a. Sources will be removed with same safety precautions as those used in their application.
   b. No linens, dressings, clothing or equipment will be removed from room until all sources are accounted for.
   c. Assurance of complete removal of all sources will be obtained using a G-M survey meter held in the treatment area of the patient.
   d. Should the patient die before brachytherapy is complete, the sources will be removed at once.
IV. Return of Sources to Storage.
   a. Following cleaning, sources will be returned immediately to their storage place.
   b. Post-use inventory forms will be completed to insure complete return of all sources to storage.
   c. Inventory of all sealed sources will be performed on a quarterly basis and recorded.

The form, Nursing Instructions for Patients Treated with Radioactive Sources, . . . [Form L], will be completed immediately after sources are implanted and placed in the patient's chart. Nurses will be instructed via . . . [Form M].

Nurses caring for brachytherapy patients will be assigned film badges. TLD finger badges will also be assigned to nurses who must provide extended personal care to the patient and to personnel handling sealed sources.

Sources will be transported from the storage site to place of use via [transport cart designed to reduce radiation levels to that consistent with Department of Transportation

NURSING INSTRUCTIONS FOR PATIENTS TREATED WITH
RADIOACTIVE SOURCES

Patient's name _____

Room number _____ Physician's name _____

Isotope activity_____

Date and time of administration _____

Date and time sources are to be removed _____ Isotope _____

Exposure rates in mr/hr

Bedside   3 feet from bed   10 feet from bed

_____

_____

_____

(Complete checked items)

_____ 1. Wear film badge.

_____ 2. Wear rubber gloves.

_____ 3. Place laundry in linen bag and save.

_____ 4. Housekeeping may not enter the room.

_____ 5. Patient may not have visitors.

_____ 6. No pregnant visitors.

_____ 7. No visitors under 18 years of age.

_____ 8. A dismissal survey must be performed <u>before</u> patient is discharged.

_____ 9. Patient must have a private room.

_____ 10. Other instructions.

RSO_____ , _____ / _____
              (Name)   on duty/off duty   telephone number

Form L

INSTRUCTIONS TO NURSES

1. Special restrictions may be noted on the precaution sheet in the patient's chart. Nurses should read these instructions before administering to the patient. Call the R.S.O. if you have any questions about the care of these patients.

2. Nurses should spend only the minimum necessary time near a patient for routine nursing care but must obtain and wear a film badge.

3. When a nurse receives an assignment to a therapy patient, a film or TLD badge should be obtained immediately from the R.S.O. The badge shall be worn only by the nurse to whom it is issued and shall not be exchanged between nurses.

4. Pregnant nurses should not be assigned to the personal care of these patients.

5. Never touch needles, capsules, or containers holding brachytherapy sources. If a source becomes dislodged, use long forceps and put it in the corner of the room or in the shielded container provided; contact the R.S.O.

6. Bed bath given by the nurse should be omitted while the sources are in place.

7. Perineal care is not given during gynecologic treatment; the perineal pad may be changed when necessary, unless orders to the contrary have been written.

8. Surgical dressings and bandages used to cover the area of needle insertion may be changed only by the attending physician or R.S.O. and MAY NOT BE DISCARDED until directed by the R.S.O. Dressings should be kept in a basin until checked by the R.S.O.

Special orders will be written for oral hygiene for patients with oral implants.

9. No special precautions are needed for sputum, urine, vomitus, stools, dishes, instruments, utensils, or bedding unless specifically ordered.

10. These patients must stay in bed unless orders to the contrary are written.

11. Visitors will be limited to those 18 years of age or over, unless other instructions are noted on the precaution sheet in the patient's chart.

12. Visitors should sit at least 3 feet from the patient and should remain no longer than the times specified on the form posted on the patient's door and in his chart.

13. No nurse, visitor, or attendant who is pregnant should be permitted in the room of a patient while brachytherapy sources are implanted in the patient. Female visitors should be asked whether they are pregnant.

14. Emergency procedures:

    a. If an implanted source becomes loose or separated from the patient
    <u>or</u>

Form M

b. If the patient dies <u>or</u>

c. If the patient requires emergency surgery, immediately call

_____. Phone no. (days)_____(nights)_____

15. At the conclusion of treatment, call the Radiation Safety Officer and request that the patient and room be surveyed to be sure all radioactive sources have been removed.

(DOT) regulations which is no greater than 200 mi/hr at the surface of the transport cart and no greater than 10 mi/hr at a distance of 3 feet.]

At the initiation of treatment, an inventory will be performed on all therapy sources to insure total accountability [and Usage Record (Form O) completed]. At the conclusion of treatment, another inventory will be performed to insure that all sources have been returned. . . . [(Form N)] In addition, a survey will be performed to ensure that all sources have been removed from the patient and that no sources remain in the patient's room or any other area occupied by the patient. At the same time, all radiation signs will be removed and all film and TLD badges assigned to nurses will be collected. . . . [Form O] will be used as a check-off procedure.

Surveys of the patient's room and surrounding areas will be conducted as soon as practicable after sources are implanted. Exposure rate measurements will be taken at the patient's bedside, three feet away and at the entrance to the room. The Radiation Safety Officer or his designate will then determine how long a person may remain at these positions and will post these times in the patient's chart. Refer to . . . [Form A]. Radiation levels in unrestricted areas will be maintained less than the limits specified in Section 20.105(b), 10 CFR Part 20. (i.e., 2mrems in any one hour or 100mrems in any seven consecutive days).

With respect to a sealed source therapy program, the ALARA philosophy suggests the following:

1. There should be a quarterly inventory of all sealed sources.
2. Sealed sources must be kept in a locked storage area with each brachytherapy source in a separate hole in the lead and with each hole identified as to the strength of the sealed sources.
3. A log must be stationed at the exit of the storage vault for recording the removal and return of sealed sources.
4. When there is more than one location in which to store these sealed sources, an inventory should be kept at a central office (such as the Radiation Safety Office) so as to not exceed the maximum limits of the NRC license.
5. The storage area should be included in the weekly survey of all storage/use areas for radioactive materials.
6. Doors to the storage area should be kept locked when not in use and posted with proper caution signs.
7. Any areas near the storage area exceeding 0.2mr/hr should be posted with proper caution signs.
8. The Radiation Safety Office should be alerted immediately if all sources are not returned.

RECEIPT/SHIPMENT RECORD
RADIATION SOURCE THERAPY APPLICATIONS

Patient_____ ID no _____ RM_____

Pretreatment inventory

                                                    Subtotal

_____ sources of _____ mg _____

_____ sources of _____ mg _____

_____ sources of _____ mg _____

_____ sources of _____ mg _____

Applicator(s)_____Total_____ mg

Posttreatment inventory

_____ sources of_____ mg _____

_____ sources of_____ mg _____

_____ sources of_____ mg _____

_____ sources of_____ mg _____

Applicator(s)_____ Total _____mg

Comments:

Certified by _____   Date_____

IMPORTANT: THIS RECORD MUST BE PERMANENTLY MAINTAINED

Form N

RADIATION THERAPY SOURCE USAGE RECORD

Patient_____ ID no _____ Rm _____

Ordering physician_____

Applicator(s) used_____ Sources_____

mr/hr at 1 m from applicator (not after loading)_____ mr/hr_____

Date and time of insertion   AM/PM

	Yes	See comments
Lead aprons not worn during insertion?	( )	( )
X-ray techs informed prior to obtaining localizing films?	( )	( )
Recovery room nurses instructed to use time/distance?	( )	( )
Patient assigned private room?	( )	( )
Film badges issued to nursing personnel?	( )	( )
Safety instruction given to nurses?	( )	( )
Safety procedures placed in patient's chart?	( )	( )
Caution sign placed on patient's chart?	( )	( )
Caution signs placed on patient's room door?	( )	( )
Nursing care rotated?	( )	( )
Known pregnant nurses not attending patient?	( )	( )
Pregnant visitors prohibited?	( )	( )
Visitors under 18 prohibited?	( )	( )
Safety survey performed and recorded?	( )	( )
Limits of nursing care time posted?	( )	( )
Removal notice posted in patient's chart prior to removal of all posted signs?	( )	( )
All signs removed?	( )	( )
Room surveyed and background radiation levels present?	( )	( )

Date/time of removal_____ AM/PM _____

Applicator_____ Sources_____

Comments:

Certified by _____ Date_____

IMPORTANT: THIS RECORD MUST BE PERMANENTLY MAINTAINED

Form O

BIBLIOGRAPHY

Blahd, W. H.: Nuclear medicine, New York, 1965, McGraw-Hill Book Co.

Brodsky, A.: Principles and practices for keeping occupational radiation exposures at medical institutions as low as reasonably achievable, Washington, D.C., 1977, Office of Standard Development, United States Nuclear Regulatory Commission.

Goodwin, P. N., and Rao, D. V.: The physics of nuclear medicine, Springfield, Ill., 1977, Charles C Thomas, Publisher.

Johns, H. E.: The physics of radiology, ed. 2, revised edition, Springfield, Ill., 1964, Charles C Thomas, Publisher.

Precautions in the management of patients who have received therapeutic amounts of radionuclides, NCRP Report No. 37, October 1970.

Rollo, F. D.: Nuclear medicine physics, instrumentation, and agents, St. Louis, 1977, The C. V. Mosby Co.

Shapiro, J.: Radiation protection, Cambridge, Mass., 1972, Harvard University Press.

Title 10. Code of Federal Regulations, Part 20. Washington, D.C., United States Nuclear Regulatory Commission.

PART TWO

CLINICAL NUCLEAR MEDICINE

14 Surface anatomy

There is no doubt that an accurate description of the site and size of the various internal organs would be much easier with the use of known and fixed reference points or landmarks. Although soft tissue landmarks (such as the nipple and umbilicus) have been commonly used, their positions are affected by various factors such as age, sex, pregnancy, and intra-abdominal and pelvic tumors. In contrast, bony landmarks are fixed; they can be easily recognized on x-ray films and enable accurate superimposition of a radioisotope photoscan on the corresponding radiograph (Fig. 14-1).

Some of the main bony landmarks in the head are the nasion, inion, mastoid process, and mandible. The nasion is the depression at the root of the nose; the inion, or external occipital protuberance, is the midline bony prominence situated on the back of the skull at the junction of the head and neck. The mastoid process is the bony projection behind the ear that points downward and forward.

Passing the finger along the midline from the mandible downward, one encounters the hyoid bone, thyroid cartilage, cricoid cartilage, and trachea in that order (see Fig. 18-1).

Two of the major landmarks in the neck are muscles, the sternocleidomastoid and trapezius. The sternocleidomastoid, as its name implies, extends from the mastoid process to the upper part of the sternum and clavicle. The trapezius forms the upper border of the shoulder and slopes upward from the point of the shoulder toward the back of the head and medially toward the midline of the back. The neck can therefore be divided into two main triangles—the anterior and the posterior. The anterior triangle is bounded anteriorly by the midline, posteriorly, by the anterior border of the sternocleidomastoid, and upward by the lower border of the body of the mandible. The boundaries of the posterior triangle are the posterior margin of the sternocleidomastoid, by the anterior margin of the trapezius, and by the middle third of the clavicle downward.

The clavicles, the sternum, and the ribs (with the intercostal spaces) form the main landmarks over the front of the chest. The suprasternal or jugular notch lies at the upper border of the manubrium sterni, between the sternal attachments of both sternocleidomastoid muscles. About 2 inches (5 cm) along the midsternal line is a transverse ridge at the junction of the manubrium with the body of the sternum (Fig. 14-2). This ridge is called the *sternal angle* (angle of Louis or Ludwig's angle) and lies opposite the sternochondral junction of the second rib. Therefore

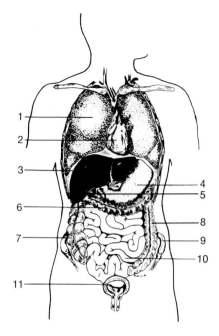

Fig. 14-1. Soft tissue organs of the body.

1. Lung
2. Heart
3. Liver

4. Stomach
5. Gallbladder
6. Transverse colon

7. Ascending colon
8. Descending colon
9. Iliac crest

10. Small bowel
11. Bladder

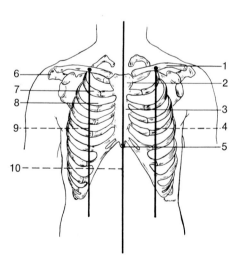

Fig. 14-2. Anatomic landmarks of the thorax.

1. Clavicle
2. Manubrium sterni
3. Sternum

4. Midclavicular line
5. Xiphoid
6. Acromion

7. Second rib
8. Second intercostal space
9. Midclavicular line
10. Midline

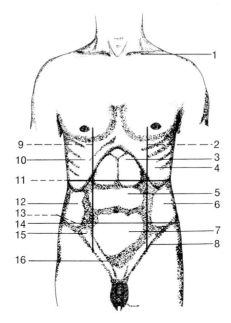

Fig. 14-3. Anatomic landmarks of the anterior thorax and abdomen.

1. Clavicle
2. Left lateral line
3. Epigastrium
4. Left hypochondrium
5. Umbilical region
6. Left lumbar region
7. Hypogastrium or suprapubic region
8. Left iliac region
9. Right lateral line
10. Right hypochrondrium
11. Transpyloric plane
12. Right lumbar region
13. Transtubercular plane
14. Anterior superior iliac spine
15. Right iliac region
16. Inguinal ligament

the second rib is the most easily and accurately identifiable one and the one from which other ribs can be recognized. The second intercostal space is the one immediately below this rib. The lowest part of the sternum is called the *xiphoid process*. It varies in shape and is usually cartilaginous. Parallel to the midsternal line and passing through the middle of the clavicle is the midclavicular line, which forms an important line of orientation over the front of the chest.

On each side of the chest the hollow of the armpit, or axilla, is limited by two muscular folds, the anterior and posterior axillary folds. Halfway between these folds the midaxillary line is drawn to serve as a landmark.

On the back, the furrow down the midline corresponds to the tips of the spinous processes of the vertebrae.

For descriptive purposes the abdomen is divided into nine regions by two horizontal and two sagittal planes (Fig. 14-3). The transpyloric plane lies halfway between the suprasternal notch and the upper margin of the symphysis pubis, which is situated at the lowest part of the front of the abdomen. This plane cuts through the pylorus, the tip of the ninth costal cartilage, and the lower border of the first lumbar vertebra. The transtubercular plane joins the highest points on the iliac crests as identified on both sides of the body and passes through the body of the fifth lumbar vertebra. The two sagittal planes are drawn parallel to the midline from the midinguinal point. This point lies halfway between the symphysis pubis and the anterior superior iliac spine, which is the anterior end of the iliac crest. These regions, from top to bottom, are the epigastric, the umbilical, and the hypogastric (suprapubic) regions in the middle. On both sides of these areas the hypochondriac, lumbar, and iliac (inguinal) regions are situated. The abdomen may also be subdivided by means of two planes drawn at right angles giving four quadrants. These planes are a midsagittal and a transverse plane passing through the umbilicus. However, the position of the umbilicus is affected by so many factors that this subdivision is inaccurate.

BIBLIOGRAPHY

Brash, J. C., and Jamieson, E. B.: Cunningham's manual of practical anatomy, Oxford, 1945, Oxford University Press.

Dawson, H. L.: Basic human anatomy, New York, 1974, Appleton-Century-Crofts.

Johnston, T. B., and Whillis, J.: Gray's anatomy, London, 1944, Longmans, Green and Company.

15 Hematology

CONSTITUENTS OF BLOOD

Blood is a part of the main transport system of the body that delivers oxygen, nutrients, hormones, and antibodies to the tissues. It also receives waste products, including carbon dioxide from the cells, and transports them to the organs involved in their subsequent elimination from the body. Blood makes up approximately 7% to 8% of the total body weight and consists of a fluid fraction (plasma) and formed elements that can be differentiated into red cells (erythrocytes), white cells (leukocytes), and platelets (thrombocytes). Since the specific gravity of these formed elements is greater than that of the plasma, the cells tend to settle if allowed to stand, provided clotting has been prevented by the addition of an anticoagulant. The rate of this separation can be augmented by centrifugation.

Because of the abundance of red cells (5,000,000/mm³) in relation to the leukocytes (8,000/mm³), together with the relatively small size of the platelets, most of the volume of the formed sediment can be attributed to the erythrocytes. The volume of the packed erythrocytes expressed as percentage of the blood sample used is called the *hematocrit*. Normally it averages 45%. Therefore the supernatant plasma expressed as percent of the blood sample (plasmacrit) would be 55%.

In contrast, if the blood is allowed to clot and the clot is removed, the remaining straw-colored fluid is called *serum*. This serum differs from the plasma mainly in that it contains no fibrinogen.

Plasma. The plasma is a complex, watery fluid that contains various ions as well as inorganic and organic molecules. Its main solid constituent is represented by the plasma proteins, which average 7.5 gm/100 ml. These are usually divided into albumin, 4.8%; globulin, 2.3%; and fibrinogen, 0.3%. Because of the impermeability of the capillary walls to the plasma proteins, these latter exert an osmotic force across this membrane of about 25 mm Hg, which tends to pull water into the capillaries. Another function of the plasma proteins is their help in maintaining the constancy of the blood reaction. Furthermore, some of the proteins that have been isolated from the globulin fraction have specific functions, such as transport of hormones, blood clotting, and development of resistance to infections.

The albumin fraction together with the proteins concerned in blood clotting are manufactured in the liver. The globulins, including the fibrinogen, are formed by the reticuloendothelial system, plasma cells, and lymphoid nodules.

The formation, function, and fate of each of the formed elements of the blood differ.

Red blood cells. The red cells are circular, nonnucleated, biconcave discs that are manufactured by the red bone marrow situated in the vertebrae, sternum, ribs, and bones of the skull and pelvis. Because of their hemoglobin content, the red cells form an efficient oxygen-carrying system. Furthermore, the hemoglobin plays an essential role in carbon dioxide transport and in regulation of the blood pH. The average hemoglobin content of the blood in adults is 15 gm/100 ml. In man the red cells usually survive for about 120 days. Thereafter, they are destroyed by the reticuloendothelial system, and the hemoglobin is released. The iron and globin are split off, leaving bilirubin. The iron is reused in the synthesis of new hemoglobin.

White blood cells. The white blood cells, or leukocytes, are nucleated cells that can be differentiated into three main types: granulocytes (polymorphonuclear leukocytes), lymphocytes, and monocytes. The granulocytes are normally formed in the red bone marrow and survive for less than 2 weeks. They can be further subdivided into neutrophils (50% to 70%), eosinophils (1% to 4%), and basophils (0% to 1%). Their main function is to combat infections, and they are destroyed in the spleen and other parts of the reticuloendothelial system.

The lymphocytes are formed chiefly in the lymphoid tissues of the body and to a lesser extend in the bone marrow. They form from 20% to 40% of the total number of white cells and live from 2 to 200 days. The lymphocytes are essential for the development of immunity.

The monocytes form from 2% to 8% of the leukocytes. Their main site of origin is in the lymphoid tissues; a few originate in the bone marrow. Monocytes are phagocytic and play a major role in the production of antibodies.

Platelets. The blood platelets are small, nonnucleated granulated bodies formed in the red bone marrow. Their number averages 200,000/mm³, and they survive for about 10 days in the bloodstream. Their main function is the provision of support for the endothelium of injured vessels and formation of a hemostatic plug; they also participate in the processes of blood coagulation and clot retraction.

BLOOD VOLUME DETERMINATION

Although nonradioactive methods are available for estimation of blood volume, these techniques are tedious and require meticulous care in their performance. This is mainly because these methods depend on the determination of the concentration of a dye (such as Evans blue) after its intravenous administration. Since the determinations are performed by colorimetry, the readings are affected by turbidity caused by high blood fat content, by the presence of abnormal pigments in the blood, and/or hemolysis. Also, these tests cannot be repeated at frequent intervals. Most of these drawbacks have been obviated with the introduction of radioisotopic techniques for blood volume determination.

Radioactive tracers used for volume measurements must be nontoxic and completely safe for parenteral administration. Furthermore, they should mix rapidly and uniformly with the diluting fluid and remain for a reasonable time interval. In addition, these tracers must be easily detected and quantitated in high dilutions. These criteria are fulfilled to a great extent by most of the radioactive tracers utilized for determination of blood volume.

Ideally, accurate measurement of the circulating blood volume should be performed by simultaneous determinations of the volume of both blood components — plasma and blood cells. Therefore two radioactive tracers of different energies are used to enable their differentiation by means of pulse height analysis with the aid of a gamma ray spectrometer. As an example, ^{125}I human serum albumin together with ^{51}Cr-tagged erythrocytes can be used to measure plasma and red cell volume, respectively. However, this procedure necessitates the use of dual tracers and specific equipment, together with time-consuming and tedious calculations to correct the ^{125}I measurements for contributions from ^{51}Cr. For the sake of simplicity and expedience a single tracer is used for determination of the volume of either the plasma or red cells using the principle of dilution. According to this principle:

$$Q = V \times C$$
$$V = \frac{Q}{C}$$

Q = Total quantity of tracer
V = Diluting volume
C = Tracer concentration in diluting fluid

Since the volume of one of the blood components has been determined, the total blood volume can be calculated with the aid of the hematocrit:

$$\text{Total blood volume} = \frac{\text{Plasma volume}}{\text{Plasmacrit}} = \frac{\text{Red cell volume}}{\text{Hematocrit}}$$

Consequently, the volume of the other blood component is obtained by subtraction.

However, it should be remembered that the average whole-body hematocrit is roughly 92% of the venous blood hematocrit. This discrepancy in hematocrit values occurs because of the difference in the hematocrits of blood obtained from different size vessels, as well as from different organs. In addition, during hematocrit determination, some of the plasma is trapped with the cells, which introduces an error of 2% to 4% in the obtained value. To account for both sources of errors, the hematocrit is multiplied by a correction factor equal to 0.90 (0.92 × 0.98) to give a corrected hematocrit that is to be used in the calculations.

Plasma volume determination

Several radioactive tracers have been used for estimation of the plasma volume All of them depend on the ability of the radioactive tag to attach itself to the plasma proteins.

Radioiodinated ¹³¹I human serum albumin (RISA or ¹³¹IHSA). Radioiodinated human serum albumin is the tracer most commonly used for plasma volume determination. A venous blood sample is obtained to estimate the background radioactivity in the plasma. The test dose of RISA (5 to 30 μCi) is then transferred into a volumetric container and diluted up to 1,000 ml to act as a standard. An exactly equal amount of tracer is injected into one of the patient's antecubital veins, using the same syringe and taking care to inject the full amount intravenously. After 15 minutes a blood sample is withdrawn from the patient's other arm in a heparinized syringe. The hematocrit is determined and the plasma separated by centrifugation. Radioactivity in equal volumes of the standard and plasma is measured in a scintillation well counter for an equal time. The background is subtracted to give the net counting rate of the plasma. The plasma volume is calculated according to the following equation:

$$\text{Plasma volume (liters)} = \frac{\text{Counting rate of standard}}{\text{Net counting rate of plasma}}$$

Since the volume of the plasma and plasmacrit is known, the total blood volume can be calculated, and by subtraction the red cell volume is obtained.

In addition to technical factors, the main source of error in this technique is the leakage of the tracer from the vascular compartment. The rate of this loss averages about 10% per hour, which makes it negligible within the 15 minutes of the test. However, for increased accuracy, multiple blood sampling is used with backward extrapolation to calculate the plasma counts and subsequently the plasma volume at zero time.

The plasma volume in normal individuals has been found to be 43 ml/kg of body weight with this method.

¹²⁵I human serum albumin. ¹²⁵I human serum albumin is used for plasma volume determination, particularly when simultaneous estimation of the red cell volume is done with ⁵¹Cr-tagged sodium chromate. The ¹²⁵I is a pure but weak gamma emitter, with a longer half-life (60 days) than ¹³¹I (8.1 days). Its main disadvantage is its low counting efficiency with ordinary counting equipment.

⁹⁹ᵐTc-labeled human serum albumin. The same general principles as previously stated are still applicable for plasma volume determination. The highest labeling efficiency (above 90%) is achieved with 25% human serum albumin (salt poor). A commercial kit for the electrolytic preparation of ⁹⁹ᵐTc HSA has been introduced. However, rigorous quality check of this radiopharmaceutical must be carried out before it is used.

⁵¹Cr-tagged chromic chloride. ⁵¹Cr-tagged chromic chloride is a trivalent salt. When injected intravenously, about 98% labels the plasma proteins and the remainder becomes attached to the red cells. Therefore this radioactive compound can be used for plasma volume determination if a correction factor is applied for the amount of radionuclide that is attached to the erythrocytes. In calculating the result, only 98% of the standard (administered dose) is taken into consideration, to avoid overestimation of the plasma volume. The main disadvantage of this technique is the larger radiation dose delivered to the patient.

Red cell volume determination

Determination of the red cell volume depends on the use of labeled erythrocytes as the tracer. Such labeling can be done either in vitro or in vivo by means of various radioactive agents.

Sodium chromate (^{51}Cr). Radiochromate is the most commonly utilized radioactive tagging agent for the red cells in clinical use. It is a hexavalent compound that can easily penetrate the red cell membrane and appears to be reduced to the trivalent form that establishes a firm tag with the betachain hemoglobin. Tagging is done in vitro. For this purpose an anticoagulated blood sample (10 ml) is obtained from the patient and transferred into a sterile container to mix with 50 μCi of radiochromate. The mixture is left at room temperature for 15 minutes if ACD solution is used or for 60 minutes if the anticoagulant is heparin. The radiochromate should not be added to the ACD solution before use, since ACD is going to reduce the chromate and hinder the tagging process. Most of the radiochromate enters the cells, but a small portion (10% to 20%) is left in the plasma. To remove this free radiochromate, the red cells are washed three times and then resuspended in normal saline. An easier and less time-consuming alternative is to add 100 mg ascorbic acid (vitamin C) to the mixture to reduce the unbound radiochromate and thus prevent it from tagging any other erythrocytes when reinjected into the patient.

An accurately measured volume (m) of this tagged mixture is kept as a standard, and an exactly equal amount (m) is injected intravenously into the patient. After 15 to 30 minutes a venous blood sample is withdrawn from the patient's other arm. The hematocrit of this blood sample (Hct_{pt}), as well as that of the standard (Hct_s), is determined. Finally, the radioactive content of 1 ml of the whole blood and plasma of the standard (B_s and Pl_s) and that of the venous blood sample (B_{pt} and Pl_{pt}) is estimated in a scintillation well counter.

According to the principle of dilution, the diluting volume (V)—which in this particular situation is the red cell volume—can be calculated by dividing the amount of radioactivity injected (Q) by the concentration of the radioactivity (C). If washing is used, Q is going to equal m $\times$ B_s. However, in case washing is not performed, which is more common, the radioactivity in the plasma has to be calculated and subtracted from the radioactivity in the corresponding blood sample. Radioactivity in the plasma contained in 1 ml of the tagged blood (standard) equals radioactivity in 1 ml of this plasma (Pl_s) times the plasmacrit. Therefore the amount of radioactivity injected and contained in the red cells can be calculated from the following equation:

$$Q = m[B_s - (Pl_s \times plasmacrit_s)]$$

On the same assumptions, radioactivity in the red cells contained in 1 ml of the withdrawn blood sample equals $B_{pt} - (Pl_{pt} \times plasmacrit_{pt})$. Dividing this last value by the hematocrit gives the radioactivity per unit volume of red cells or, in other words, the concentration of radioactivity (c).

By substituting for the values of Q and C in the original equation of dilution:

$$V = \frac{Q}{C}$$

$$V = \frac{m \, [B_s - (Pl_s \times plasmacrit_s)]}{\dfrac{B_{pt} - (Pl_{pt} \times plasmacrit_{pt})}{Hct_{pt}}}$$

$$V = \frac{m \, [B_s - (Pl_s \times plasmacrit_s)] \times Hct_{pt}}{B_{pt} - (Pl_{pt} \times plasmacrit_{pt})}$$

The red cell volume as estimated by this technique in normal male subjects averages 28 ml per kilogram of body weight. Although chromium is not a normal constituent of the red cells, its binding with the cell components is very firm. Thus its elution is slow. Any released ^{51}Cr is not reusable for further labeling of other red cells. In addition, the physical characteristics of ^{51}Cr are very suitable for counting and external monitoring.

The disadvantages of this method are mainly technical, such as errors encountered by the occurrence of extravasation during the intravenous injection of the tagged cells, the lack of tagging as a result of the presence of reducing agents in the blood, formation of clots in the standard, and hemolysis of the tagged cells. Some of these drawbacks can be avoided by using labeled cells from fresh blood bank O (Rh −), preferably filtered blood and without washing.

Technetium 99m. Because of its favorable physical characteristics, ^{99m}Tc has been suggested as a red cell label. However, the labeling achieved by incubation of erythrocytes with ^{99m}Tc is not stable. More dependable labeling is produced in the presence of the reducing stannous ion. Lower labeling yields are encountered when the stannous chloride is added after ^{99m}Tc as well as in the presence of the plasma or carrier ^{99}Tc. In contrast, consistent higher yields (95%) are obtained with pretreatment of the red cells with the stannous ion before the addition of the radiopharmaceutical. Nevertheless, because of the probable damage to the red cells by the labeling procedure and the marked variability in the stability of the ^{99m}Tc-labeled erythrocytes among individual patients, this radionuclide is not widely used for red cell volume determination.

Sodium phosphate (^{32}P). ^{32}P-labeled sodium phosphate can be used to tag red cells in vitro to estimate the red cell volume. The same technique as with the radiochromate is used. However, only 20% to 30% of the radiophosphorus becomes fixed to the erythrocytes. Therefore washing is essential. Elution occurs at the rate of about 6% per hour. Furthermore, ^{32}P is a beta emitter, which makes its counting efficiency inferior to that of radiochromate.

Iron^{59}. ^{59}Fe, when injected in vivo, becomes incorporated in the hemoglobin during the process of red cell production. Although it can be used for the determination of red cell volume, it needs a compatible donor for the preparation of the labeled cells.

. . .

As previously mentioned, the most accurate method for determination of total blood volume is the simultaneous estimation of the volume of both plasma and red cells. An easier, less time consuming, and sufficiently accurate technique is determination of the red cell volume by radiochromate, with subsequent calculation of the total blood volume with the aid of the hematocrit. The easiest but the least accurate method of determining the total blood volume is the use of radioiodinated human serum albumin. The same procedure as that described under the plasma volume determination is followed, except that radioactivity in the whole blood, rather than in the plasma alone, is measured and used in the calculation. Under such circumstances the main sources of error are the lack of uniform mixing and the difference between the average whole-body hematocrit and that determined from a blood sample withdrawn from a relatively large vein such as the antecubital.

With the introduction of automated blood volume measuring devices, errors caused by pipetting and dilution are eliminated. In addition, the time consumed is much less. But for the sake of accuracy the resultant dilution volume should be corrected for the difference between the body and venous hematocrits.

Using radioisotopic techniques, the average values for red cell volume (RCV), plasma volume (PV), and total blood volume (TBV) expressed in milliliters per kilogram of body weight in normal adults are as follows:

	Male	*Female*
RCV	28	24
PV	44	42
TBV	72	66

Clinical indications for blood volume determination

Under certain circumstances, alteration might occur in the total amount of cells or plasma or both without a corresponding change in these blood constituents in a given unit of volume. Therefore neither blood counts nor hematocrit determination, both of which are expressed per unit volume, can detect or accurately quantitate such changes. However, such changes are easily diagnosed and quantitated by means of blood volume determinations. This is why blood volume determinations are advisable after acute blood loss, whether early or late, and after extensive burns. False results caused by compensatory mechanisms can therefore be avoided. Blood volume should be determined preoperatively in patients of the extreme age groups (children and the elderly) before any major surgery. In this way any volume deficit that would adversely affect the result of surgery can be detected and treated. Postoperatively, the best guide for transfusion therapy regarding the type and amount required is estimation of the volume of both cells and plasma. In addition, the most reliable measure for the degree of anemia, especially in the presence of a change in the plasma volume, is red cell volume determination.

RED CELL SURVIVAL

Red cell survival is measured by following a given group of erythrocytes to determine the time required for their elimination from the circulation. To make this possible, the specified erythrocytes should be easily identifiable from the remainder of the red cells by a label or tag. The tag may be either incorporated during the process of formation of the red cells (selective or cohort labeling) or introduced into a heterogenous group of erythrocytes that happen by mere chance to be present in the circulation at the time of tagging (random labeling).

Selective labeling

Selective labeling is usually done with glycine ^{14}C, glycine ^{15}N, glycine ^{3}H, ^{59}Fe, or ^{75}Se selenomethionine. The tagged cells are of the same age and are followed for their full life-span until they are eliminated from the circulation. This necessitates a long period of observation that might extend for more than 4 months. Furthermore, these radionuclides are expensive, and special preparation and specific equipment are required for counting the radionuclides used. However, this technique can easily differentiate between finite and random destruction of the red cells. Another advantage is the relative insensitivity of the test to concomitant shifts in the red cell volume during the period of the study.

Random labeling

Random labeling is easier than selective labeling and can be performed using radioactive as well as nonradioactive techniques. Since the tagged cells are of different ages, they are eliminated from the circulating blood at different times, making identification of the end point of elimination difficult. Therefore the red cell survival time is calculated from the percent of surviving tagged erythrocytes as determined at periodic time intervals. However, because of the inaccuracy of determinations encountered during the latter part of the study when the percent of surviving tagged erythrocytes is rather low, it is preferable to rely on the results of the first 3 weeks and to express the survival in terms of the time required for elimination of 50% of the tagged erythrocytes (survival half-life). Since the survival is computed from the percent of surviving tagged cells as determined per unit volume, wide fluctuations in the blood volume would undoubtedly invalidate this result. Another disadvantage of the random labeling technique is the inability to differentiate a short finite life-span from random destruction of the red cells.

Ashby's differential agglutination technique. Ashby's differential agglutination technique is a method of measuring the survival time of transfused, but immunologically identifiable, erythrocytes that have been obtained from a donor. The surviving donor cells are counted following agglutination or hemolysis of the patient's erythrocytes by appropriate antisera. Thus it is not possible to study the survival of the red cells of a specified subject in his own circulation. Furthermore, this technique suffers from the inherent errors in cell counting together with the hazards of transfusion, since a rather large volume from the donor's blood is administered.

Sodium chromate. The disadvantages associated with Ashby's method are completely obviated by tagging the erythrocytes with sodium chromate (^{51}Cr).

The tagged cells are reinjected into the patient, and a blood sample is obtained after 30 minutes for blood volume determination. A heparinized blood sample is withdrawn after 24 hours. Thereafter, samples are obtained every third day for a period of 3 to 4 weeks. To abolish the effect of physical decay, all the samples are counted in a scintillation counter at the same time after the final sample is collected. Radioactivity per milliliter of red cells is estimated as previously described under red cell volume determination and is plotted as a function of time on linear and semilogarithmic graph paper, starting with the 24-hour sample to avoid errors caused by loss of radioactivity (5% to 10%) during the first 24 hours. The data are made to fit a straight line on the suitable type of graph paper (linear or semilogarithmic). From this line of best fit the blood radioactivity disappearance half-time is calculated (Fig. 15-1).

The disappearance half-time (T_{50}) represents the time after injection of the labeled erythrocytes at which blood radioactivity has fallen to 50% of its initial value. In normal subjects it averages 25 to 35 days, which is much shorter than expected. A major part of the difference is attributed to elution of the ^{51}Cr from

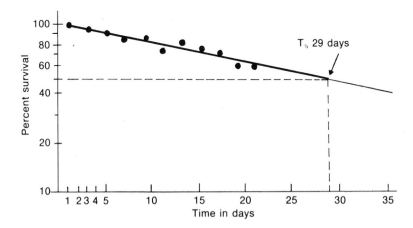

Fig. 15-1. Radiochromate-tagged red cell survival in a normal subject plotted on semilogarithmic scale. Level of radioactivity at 24 hours is considered 100%. The blood radioactivity disappearance half-time (T_{50}) is 29 days.

the intact surviving cells (roughly 1% per day). To apply a fixed correction factor to account for such an error is rather inaccurate because of the unpredictable variability in the rate of ^{51}Cr elution. Therefore the estimated or apparent red cell survival half-time is used.

For better accuracy, the radioactivity measurements are corrected for ^{51}Cr elution using a correction factor dependent on the date of sample collection and obtainable from specific tables. The resultant values are plotted on linear and semilogarithmic graph paper to obtain the line of best fit. The reciprocal of the slope of this line equals the mean red cell life-span, which can be defined as the mean survival time of all circulating erythrocytes. If the data fit a line on semilogarithmic paper, the mean red cell life-span can be calculated by multiplying the half-time of the fitted line times 1.44.

At the end of the study the red cell volume is determined again to exclude any gross change in the blood volume that might invalidate the obtained result.

If the red cell survival half-time is found to be shorter than normal, the test may be repeated by injecting the patient's cells into a normal recipient or by injecting normal erythrocytes into the patient or both. This is done to determine whether the cause of this decreased survival is corpuscular or extracorpuscular in nature or both. Further helpful information is obtained by periodic measurement of the radioactivity over the precordium, liver, and spleen at the same time the blood samples are withdrawn.

External monitoring is performed by a collimated scintillation detector, with the clinician taking care to use exactly the same detector placement every time. The pattern of behavior of the counting rates recorded over the liver and spleen in relation to those recorded over the heart is determined in a trial to identify the site of red cell destruction. The spleen sequestration index is calculated by estimating the percentage increment in the spleen/precordium radioactivity ratio from zero time to T_{50} blood radiochromium. In the meantime, the spleen/liver radioactivity ratio is determined at T_{50} ^{51}CR.

Diisopropyl (^{32}P) fluorophosphate. The radioactive diisopropyl fluorophosphate is less effective than sodium chromate in labeling the red cells, whether used in vitro (5% to 10%) or in vivo (25% to 40%), but it is much easier to use. It binds irreversibly with the red cells and does not damage them. There is no elution of the radionuclide after the first few days, which makes the determination of red cell survival more accurate and true. However, ^{32}P, which acts as the radioactive label, is a beta emitter; moreover, diisopropyl fluorophosphate labels the leukocytes and platelets, together with the red cells. Consequently, the preparation for counting the radioactivity is not easy. In addition, external monitoring of the radioactivity accumulating in the different organs cannot be performed.

Clinical applications

Measurement of red cell survival is invaluable in the study of cases of unexplained anemia, especially the hemolytic type. Further help can be obtained from determination of the nature of the defect causing the shortened red cell survival, whether the cause is intrinsic in the cells or extracorpuscular in origin or both. Also, investigation of the site of red cell sequestration helps in the choice of the proper line of treatment. For example, with exaggerated splenic sequestration of the tagged erythrocytes, as evidenced by a splenic sequestration index exceeding 100 and by a spleen/liver radioactivity ratio determined at T_{50} ^{51}Cr greater than 2.5, splenectomy usually proves beneficial.

WHITE CELL SURVIVAL

Leukokinetics and survival studies have been mainly concerned with the neutrophil granulocytes and lymphocytes. For this purpose many radionuclides were investigated. ^{32}P phosphate and ^{3}H thymidine can be incorporated into the deoxyribonucleic acid (DNA) of cells before their division, at which time DNA synthesis is taking place. ^{32}P diisopropyl fluorophosphate is another radionuclide used for labeling the granulocytes. The labeled granulocytes have to be separated from the other blood cells to enable measurement of blood granulocyte radioactivity. With these in vivo labeling techniques, some of the precursors are labeled. Therefore the curve of blood granulocyte radioactivity reflects the turnover from the precursors to the circulating granulocyte rather than the life-span of the mature cell.

In vitro labeling of granulocytes can be performed with ^{32}P diisopropyl fluorophosphate, ^{51}Cr sodium chromate, ^{99m}Tc sulfur colloid, or ^{111}In chelated with 8-hydroxyquinoline (oxine), which is considered an efficient leukocyte-labeling agent. Labeling with ^{99m}Tc sulfur colloid is accomplished by phagocytosis of the radiocolloid and is enhanced in the presence of normal serum. After an early and rapid loss of radioactivity, the disappearance curve of the labeled leukocytes is an exponential function, with a half-time of 6 hours and a mean time of 9 hours.

In the case of lymphocytes, the cells are isolated, purified, and labeled with ^{51}Cr sodium chromate, ^{3}H thymide, ^{67}Ga, ^{197}Hg, or ^{99m}Tc. The labeling efficiency with ^{99m}Tc can be increased by reduction with stannous chloride.

PLATELET SURVIVAL

Because of the important functions of platelets in the hemostatic and coagulation mechanisms of the blood, study of platelet integrity, function, and life-span is important. In this respect, radioactive techniques are much simpler and more reliable.

Various tracers have been used such as ^{32}P orthophosphate, ^{14}C 5-hydroxytryptamine, ^{35}S sulfate, ^{32}P diisopropyl fluorophosphate, and ^{51}Cr sodium chromate. Out of these, only the latter two radionuclides are widely accepted, ^{32}P diisopropyl fluorophosphate as an in vivo label and ^{51}Cr sodium chromate for in vitro labeling of the platelets. For counting purposes as well as for in vitro labeling the platelets are separated from the other blood cells by differential centrifugation. In the radiochromate technique a better labeled-platelet yield is obtained by use of an ACD anticoagulant solution with a higher citrate concentration and a low pH.

With the use of these radioisotopic methods the platelet life-span has proved to be 8 to 11 days in normal subjects.

With the introduction of ^{51}Cr sodium chromate as a label for the platelets, external monitoring has become possible and is used to determine sites of platelet sequestration, especially in cases of thrombocytopenic purpura.

IRON METABOLISM AND FERROKINETICS

Although radionuclide techniques have provided valuable information concerning the proper understanding of iron metabolism, such techniques are still far from being routine laboratory clinical tests. This is generally because of the complexity of the factors involved in the regulation of iron metabolism.

The total body iron content, which averages 4.5 grams (2 to 6 grams), tends to remain fixed within narrow limits. Therefore the amount lost must be matched by absorption. Apart from blood loss, iron is lost through desquamation of cells from the skin and intestinal mucosa, cells discharged in body secretions, falling hair, and cut nails. Traces are excreted through the urine and bile. Normally this loss ranges from 0.5 to 1.5 mg of iron per day. Since only about 10% of food iron is absorbed, the daily dietary iron intake should be from 10 to 15 mg to maintain a steady state. Foods known to be rich in iron are liver, meat, eggs, peas, lentils, and leafy vegetables. Favored by the acid medium in the stomach, the dietary iron complexes are broken down and ultimately reduced to the absorbable ferrous form. Absorption takes place mainly in the duodenum. The rate and degree of absorption depend on the state of iron stores, the degree of hemopoietic activity, and the dietary iron intake. The absorbed iron is transported through the plasma by a beta globulin called *transferrin*. Normally, only about one third of transferrin is saturated with iron. The plasma iron concentration, which averages 100 mg/ 100 ml, represents the result of iron delivery to the circulating blood by absorption, hemoglobin breakdown, and release from the iron stores against iron removal by hemoglobin synthesis, cell metabolism, excretion, and deposition in the iron stores.

The available radionuclide techniques provide information about measurement of iron absorption as well as determination of the rate of disappearance of radioiron from plasma and its subsequent distribution in the body.

Measurement of iron absorption. After a night's fast, 10 μCi of ^{59}Fe ferrous citrate in a ferrous sulfate carrier (5 mg of iron) are administered orally to the patient. The total fecal radioactivity during the next 5 to 10 days is computed as percentage of the oral dose. Care must be taken to use identical geometry during each counting.

The main sources of error in this technique are encountered during the collection and counting of the stool samples. These drawbacks are easily overcome by the use of whole-body counting. The percentage of radioiron retention is calculated by comparing whole-body radioactivity recorded at 4 hours and at 14 days after the oral administration of the tracer dose. Normally the amount of radioiron absorbed ranges between 5% and 15% of the orally administered dose.

Plasma iron disappearance. For this test, about 10 μCi of ^{59}Fe ferrous citrate are injected intravenously into the patient. The radioactive ferrous citrate is used as is or bound to transferrin by incubation with fresh plasma for 30 minutes. Serial blood samples are collected for a period of 2 hours. Radioactivity per unit volume of plasma is estimated and plotted on semilogarithmic paper against time to calculate the time required for half the radioactivity to disappear from the plasma.

Normally the plasma radioiron disappearance half-time ($T_{1/2}$) averages 90 minutes, the range being 60 to 120 minutes. It is considered as a rough index of erythropoietic activity. It is shortened in iron-deficiency anemia, polycythemia vera, and hemolytic anemia. In contrast, it is lengthened in hypoplastic anemias. Thus determination of radioiron disappearance half-time may be used to distinguish a hemolytic from a hypoplastic process. Furthermore, this disappearance half-time has proved a valuable index of prognosis in cases of polycythemia vera and hypoplastic anemias.

Plasma iron turnover rate. From the plasma radioiron disappearance half-time, together with the plasma volume and the level of serum iron as determined by the available chemical methods, *the plasma iron turnover rate* (PITR) can be calculated as follows:

$$\text{PITR} = \frac{0.693}{T_{1/2}(\text{hr})} \times \text{Serum iron (mg/ml)} \times \text{Plasma volume (ml)} \times 24$$

The normal plasma iron turnover rate ranges between 20 and 42 mg/day (average 37 mg/day) and can be used as an index of total erythropoietic activity.

Red cell iron turnover rate and utilization. For this test a blood sample is obtained 15 minutes after the intravenous injection of the plasma-bound iron complex. Thereafter, blood samples are collected every third day for 2 weeks. Radioactivity per unit volume of the hemolyzed blood is determined and expressed as a percentage of the radioactivity present in the first sample (obtained 15 minutes after the dose was given) to determine the maximum red cell uptake of radioiron.

Normally, more than 80% of the injected radioiron is incorporated in the newly formed erythrocytes and appears in the circulating blood within 10 days.

From the maximum red cell uptake of radioiron (MC) and the plasma iron turnover rate (PITR), the red cell iron turnover rate (RCITR) can be calculated:

$$\text{RCITR} = \text{PITR} \times \frac{\text{MC}}{100}$$

In normal subjects the RCITR averages 29 mg/day, with a range from 20 to 40 mg/day, and indicates the effectiveness of red cell production.

From the red cell iron turnover rate the fraction of red cell iron renewal per day, as well as the mean red cell life-span, can be calculated.

In vivo distribution and movement of radioiron. After the intravenous injection of the radioiron complex, external counting is performed periodically and simultaneously over the precordium, sacrum, spleen, and liver over a period of 2 weeks.

Normally, within the first few hours after the injection of the tracer dose, the counting rate over the precordium, which represents the blood radioactivity, diminishes. Consequently, the counting rates over the spleen and liver decrease. In contrast, radioactivity over the sacrum, which represents the bone marrow radioactivity, increases and remains at a peak for about 2 days before it rapidly diminishes. In the meantime, precordial radioactivity increases to reach a maximum within 7 to 10 days, which denotes the appearance of radioactivity within the newly formed erythrocytes in the circulating blood. A similar, but much less pronounced, increase in the counting rate is noticed over the liver and spleen.

A significant increase in the splenic counting rate, which exceeds the original level of radioactivity as measured after radioiron injection, denotes splenic sequestration of red cells. If radioactivity over the liver or spleen behaves in a similar way to that over the sacrum, extramedullary erythropoiesis is suggested.

The main indication for ferrokinetic studies is the investigation of obscure hematologic disorders. In this respect, simultaneous studies with ^{51}Cr (for red cell survival) and ^{59}Fe (for ferrokinetics) using pulse height analysis would be of great help.

VITAMIN B$_{12}$ ABSORPTION

Vitamin B$_{12}$ is a very potent, cobalt-containing dietary factor available in many foods of animal origin, such as liver, kidney, muscle, milk, and eggs. It plays a major role in the synthesis of nucleic acid and therefore is particularly important in the process of cell maturation. Consequently, the first cells to suffer from its deficiency are the rapidly dividing cells, such as those of the bone marrow and gastrointestinal tract. The proper absorption of the small amounts of vitamin B$_{12}$ available in the daily food intake depends on the adequate secretion of intrinsic factor by the glands of the body of the stomach. The vitamin B$_{12}$-intrinsic factor complex thus formed is mainly absorbed in the terminal ileum. After absorption, vitamin B$_{12}$ is carried by the blood, bound to the plasma proteins. It goes to the liver, which serves as its main storage depot. It stays in the liver for months or even years and is slowly released to carry out its normal cellular metabolic functions. Vitamin B$_{12}$ is generally excreted through the urine, but any that is not absorbed in the ileum is excreted in the stool.

The presence of a cobalt atom in each molecule of vitamin B$_{12}$ made it possible to synthesize a radioactive cobalt-labeled vitamin B$_{12}$. The radionuclides used are ^{57}Co, ^{58}Co, and ^{60}Co. The long half-life of ^{60}Co (5.26 years) has made its use limited. Although ^{57}Co has a longer half-life (270 days) than ^{58}Co (71.3 days), ^{57}Co is preferred because of its better counting efficiency and the absence of beta radiation, with consequent reduction in the radiation dose delivered to the patient.

Absorption of vitamin B_{12} can be studied by one or more of the following tests: fecal excretion, plasma radioactivity, hepatic uptake, urinary excretion, or whole-body radioactivity. Since many of the patients to be tested have already received other radionuclides for diagnostic purposes, it is advisable to obtain control samples of stools, plasma, or urine before giving the test dose of radioactive vitamin B_{12} in every case. The usual dose of radioactive vitamin B_{12} is 0.5 μCi, which is given orally with half a glass of water on an empty stomach. A light breakfast is given after approximately 2 hours. The remainder of the procedure depends on the type of test to be performed.

Fecal excretion method. All stools of the patient are collected for at least 72 hours. The net amount of radioactivity in all the stools is counted and expressed as percentage of the administered dose. This represents the amount of radioactive vitamin B_{12} that was not absorbed. Therefore the remainder should be the amount absorbed.

To overcome the necessity of complete stool collection, a nonabsorbable stool marker is given orally with the test dose of radioactive vitamin B_{12}. The fraction of the marker excreted in the collected stool is used to correct the level of radioactivity recovered in these stool specimens for the effect of incomplete collection.

Normally the stools contain from 30% to 70% of the administered dose. With defective absorption the amount of radioactivity recovered in the stool is higher than these normal values.

Using this technique, erroneous results might be obtained because of contamination of the stools with urine during their collection or incomplete stool collection or both. This, together with the unpleasant task of dealing with fecal matter and the time consumed, have limited the use of the fecal excretion method.

Level of plasma radioactivity. Approximately 8 to 10 hours after the oral administration of the tagged vitamin, plasma radioactivity reaches its peak level. Accordingly, a blood sample of about 10 ml is obtained at that time. Radioactivity in 5 ml of the plasma is estimated in a scintillation well counter, and the background count is subtracted to give the net counting rate. The obtained figure is multiplied by 200 to give the net radioactivity per liter of plasma. Similarly, the net counting rate of 1% of the test dose dissolved into 10 ml of water is estimated and designated as the standard. Dividing the net plasma radioactivity by the counting rate of the standard gives the percentage of dose per liter of plasma.

Normally the level of plasma radioactivity ranges between 0.25% and 2.54% of the administered dose per liter of plasma. However, because of some overlap between the low normal and abnormal results, values between 0.25% and 0.50% should be considered suspicious.

This plasma radioactivity measurement method serves as an adjunct to the other quantitative vitamin B_{12} absorption studies. Its main advantages are that it requires minimum cooperation from the patient and nurses, and errors caused by loss of samples are avoided. The test is completed on the same day it is given, and there is no need to inject nonradioactive vitamin B_{12}, which might affect any subsequent studies. However, because of the low counting rate, extreme caution must be given to the preparation and counting of the plasma. In addition, the counting time should be reasonably long, and the use of pulse height analysis is advisable.

Hepatic uptake test. Five days after the oral ingestion of the tracer dose of radioactive vitamin B_{12}, the subject is given a laxative to clear his alimentary tract of any remaining radioactive material. Two days later, radioactivity accumulating in four different areas over the liver, left iliac fossa, and thighs is measured by means of a collimated scintillation detector. The mean of the counts over the thighs is considered as body background. This is subtracted from the average counting rates over both the liver and left iliac fossa. The ratio between the net hepatic counting rate and that over the iliac fossa is then calculated.

In normal subjects the ratio between the counts over the liver and those over the left iliac fossa should be at least $2.5:1$.

The avoidance of excreta collection is the main advantage of this technique. On the other hand, the time required for completion of the test and the fact that it is a qualitative rather than a quantitative test are its main disadvantages. In a trial to make this test quantitative the hepatic counting rate recorded after the oral radioactive test dose is compared to the increase in the hepatic counts produced by the intravenous injection of a known amount of radioactive vitamin B_{12}.

Urine radioactivity (Schilling test). This method is the most commonly applied one. For this test the patient is given nonradioactive vitamin B_{12}, which will reach and block the specific binding sites before the absorbed radioactive vitamin B_{12} can arrive at them. Consequently, the absorbed unbound radioactive vitamin is excreted with the urine. To achieve this purpose, 1,000 μg of stable vitamin B_{12} are injected within 2 hours after the oral administration of the tracer dose. The urine is collected for the next 24 hours, and its radioactivity is estimated and expressed as a percentage of the administered oral dose. Urine should have been collected from the patient the day before the test. This urine is diluted with water up to 1 or 2 liters in a volumetric container. The radioactivity in this urine is measured on top of a well counter and is considered as background. Exactly the same is done to the urine collected after the test dose is given and to the test dose itself. The background is subtracted to give the net counting rate. Finally, the result is obtained by dividing the urine radioactivity by that of the tracer dose and multiplying times 100 to express it as a percentage.

The percent of dose that is absorbed and consequently recovered in the urine by flushing with stable vitamin B_{12} is normally 7% or more.

The main sources of error in this test lie in the collection of urine and measurement of its radioactivity. Furthermore, the result can be affected by renal disease and previous administration of large amounts of vitamin B_{12}. The possible effects of the flushing dose of stable vitamin B_{12} on subsequent studies, as well as on the course of the disease and the hematologic picture of the patient under investigation, should be considered.

Whole-body radioactivity method. The patient's radioactivity is measured before and after the administration of the $^{57}Co\ B_{12}$ to give the net counting rate that corresponds to 100% retention of the tracer dose. The measurement is repeated after 1 week to allow for excretion of the nonabsorbed portion of the test dose. Consequently, the retained activity that represents the absorbed portion is calculated as percentage of the administered dose. Normally it ranges between 30% and 80% of the test dose.

This technique obviates the need for excreta collection with all its drawbacks. However, the necessary equipment is expensive.

· · ·

Although most workers use one of the procedures just discussed to test vitamin B_{12} absorption, a combination of two of these methods using the same oral tracer dose would definitely give more accurate information.

If the obtained result indicates impaired absorption of vitamin B_{12}, the test should be repeated after about 1 week, using 30 mg of intrinsic factor together with the radioactive tracer dose. This delay is suggested to avoid inhibition of radioactive vitamin B_{12} absorption in the repeat study by the parenteral flushing dose applied in the first test. However, Grames and co-workers have shown that the amount of vitamin B_{12} injected as a flushing dose does not produce significant absorption inhibition of orally ingested vitamin B_{12}. Accordingly, they suggest that serial Schilling tests could be performed not only on alternate days but also on consecutive days. However, this is not valid with renal insufficiency.

Normalization of the result after the addition of intrinsic factor denotes that the impaired absorption of vitamin B_{12} is caused by lack of adequate secretion of intrinsic factor. This is seen after gastrectomy and in cases of pernicious anemia and gastric carcinoma.

If the result of the absorption test remains within the abnormal range, the cause should be looked for in the intestine. In some cases the basic defect is competition for vitamin B_{12} by intestinal parasites or by microorganisms, as in the blind loop syndrome, intestinal strictures, and diverticulosis. Defective absorption in the remaining cases can be explained on the basis of a quantitative or qualitative diminution or both in the intestinal absorptive surface as seen after extensive intestinal resections, regional enteritis, tropical sprue, celiac disease, and idiopathic steatorrhea.

To circumvent the problems of sequential testing, an absorption ratio of free vitamin B_{12} to intrinsic factor-bound vitamin B_{12} is determined following the simultaneous administration of free and intrinsic factor-bound vitamin B_{12}; each being labeled with a different radioisotope of cobalt. Measurement of this absorption ratio can be done on stools, urine, and blood, or the measurement may be of whole-body radioactivity.

Clinical indications

The main clinical application of radioactive vitamin B_{12} absorption studies is in the differential diagnosis of megaloblastic anemias. The test has proved most useful in the detection of cases of pernicious anemia in spite of previous therapy. Other indications for these vitamin B_{12} absorption tests are the investigation of the intestinal malabsorption syndrome and the study of patients with neurologic disorders, particularly peripheral neuropathy.

BIBLIOGRAPHY

Abdel-Razzak, M., Kenawy, M., and Fahmy T.: The absorption and hepatic uptake of orally ingested radioactive cyanocobalamine in diabetes mellitus, J. Egypt. Med. Assoc. 46:471-475, 1963.

Britton, C. J. C.: Whitby and Britton disorders of the blood, ed. 10, London, 1969, J & A Churchill Ltd.

Callahan, R. J., McKusick, K. A., Lamson, M., Castronovo, F. P., and Postpaid, M. S.: Technetium-99m-human serum albumin; evaluation of a commercially produced kit, J. Nucl. Med. 17:47-49, 1976.

Ducasson, D., Arnaud, D., Bardy, A., Beydon, J., Hegesippe, M., and Baqney, C.: A new stannous agent kit for labelling red blood cells with ^{99m}Tc and its clinical applications, Br. J. Radiol. 49:344-347, 1976.

Fish, M. B., Pollycove, M., Wallerstein, R. O., Cheng, K. K., and Tono, M.: Simultaneous measurement of free and intrinsic factor (IF) bound vitamin B_{12} (B_{12}) absorption; absolute quantitation with incomplete stool collection and rapid relative measurement using plasma B_{12}(IF): B_{12} absorption ratio, J. Nucl. Med. 14:568-575, 1973.

Glass, G. B. J., Boyd, L. J., Gellin, G. A., and Stephanson, L.: Uptake of radioactive vitamin B_{12} by the liver in humans; test for measurement of intestinal absorption of vitamin B_{12} and intrinsic activity, Arch. Biochem. Biophys. 51:251-257, 1954.

Grames, G. M., Reiswig, R., Jansen, C., and Herber, R.: Feasibility of consecutive-day Schilling tests, J. Nucl. Med. 15:949-952, 1974.

Macpherson, A. I. S., Richmond, J., and Stuart, A. E.: The spleen, Springfield, Ill., 1973, Charles C Thomas, Publisher.

McAfee, J. G., and Thakur, M. L.: Survey of radioactive agents for in vitro labelling of phagocytic leukocytes. 1. Soluble agents, J. Nucl. Med. 17:480-487, 1976.

Mitchell, T. G., Spencer, R. P., and King, E. R.: The use of radioisotopes in diagnostic hematologic procedures. III. Simultaneous Cr^{51} and Fe^{59} studies, Am. J. Clin. Pathol. 28:461-468, 1957.

Nelp, W. B., McAfee, J. G., and Wagner, H. N.: Single measurement of plasma radioactive vitamin B_{12} as a test for pernicious anemia, J. Lab. Clin. Med. 61:158-165, 1963.

Pollycove, M.: Absorption, elimination and excretion of orally administered vitamin B_{12} in normal subjects and in patients with pernicious anemia, N. Engl. J. Med. 255:207-212, 1956.

Razzak, M. A., and Ata, A. A.: The absorption and hepatic uptake of orally ingested radioactive vitamin B_{12} in hepato-splenic bilharziasis, J. Trop. Med. Hyg. 66:319-321, 1963.

Razzak, M. A.: The gastric motility and absorption of orally ingested radioactive vitamin B_{12} in pellagra, Z. Tropenmed. Parsitol. 15:208-211, 1964.

Ryo, U. Y., Mohammadzadeh, A. S., Siddiqui, A., Colombetti, L. G., and Pinsky, S. M.: Evaluation of labelling procedures and in vivo stability of ^{99m}Tc-red blood cells, J. Nucl. Med. 17:133-136, 1976.

Schilling, R. F.: Intrinsic factor studies. II. The effect of gastric juice in the urinary excretion of radioactivity after the oral administration of radioactive vitamin B_{12}, J. Lab. Clin. Med. 42:860-866, 1953.

Silberstein, E. B.: Causes of abnormalities reported in nuclear medicine testing, J. Nucl. Med. 17:229-232, 1976.

Spencer, R. P., and Pearson, H. A.: Radionuclide studies of the spleen, Cleveland, Ohio 1975, CRC Press, Inc.

Smith, T. D., and Richards, P.: A simple kit for the preparation of ^{99m}Tc-labeled red blood cells, J. Nucl. Med. 17:126-132, 1976.

Thakur, L. M., Lavender, J. P., Arnot, R. N., Silvester, D. J., and Segal, A. W.: Indium-111-labeled autologous leukocytes in man, J. Nucl. Med. 18:1012-1019, 1977.

16 Spleen

ANATOMY AND PHYSIOLOGY

The spleen is a soft, friable, highly vascular organ situated principally in the left hypochondrium behind the stomach and in close relation with the left leaflet of the diaphragm. It lies in the shelter of the ninth, tenth, and eleventh ribs, with its long axis parallel to them. Its medial end is approximately 2 inches from the midline in the back at the level of the eleventh dorsal vertebra, whereas its lateral end reaches the midaxillary line in the ninth intercostal space (Figs. 21-1, *A* and *B*, and 24-1, *A* and *C*).

In normal adults the spleen measures nearly 5 inches (12 cm) in length, 3 inches (7 cm) in breadth, and 1½ inches (4 cm) in thickness. It weighs about 200 gm, but tends to diminish in size and weight with advancing age.

The blood vessels and nerves supplying the spleen enter and leave the organ along a fissure on its visceral surface, called the *hilum*. At the hilum the fibroelastic capsule that covers the spleen is prolonged inward around the vessels in the form of sheaths. From these sheaths and to a lesser extent from the capsule, small fibrous bands or trabeculae are given off and constitute the framework of the spleen. The arteries branch repeatedly with the trabeculae and ultimately give off branches that leave the trabeculae to enter the pulp of the organ. As a support, these arterial branches are ensheathed with condensed reticular tissue that is heavily infiltrated with lymphocytes. From time to time, this sheath with its lymphocytic infiltration expands to form lymph nodules or follicles. These nodules represent the white pulp and appear as islands of irregular gray areas scattered throughout the red pulp, which constitutes the remainder of the organ. The red pulp is made of a framework of reticular fibers accompanied by fixed macrophages and reticular cells. This framework is permeated by pathways termed *venous sinusoids*. In the meshes of the reticular framework, lymphocytes, free macrophages, and elements from the circulating blood are encountered. The arteries that emerge from the lymph nodules (white pulp) into the surrounding red pulp ultimately terminate in tufts or penicilli of minute arteries. According to the closed theory of intrasplenic circulation, these arterioles open directly into the venous sinusoids. According to the open theory, the arterioles open into the meshes between the venous sinusoids and blood returns to the sinusoids by way of apertures in their walls. Having reached the sinusoids by whichever route, the blood is drained by the red pulp veins, which coalesce to form veins of the

363

trabeculae. These latter unite to give approximately six branches that emerge at the hilum and ultimately form the splenic vein, which is the largest radicle of the portal vein.

Functions

As a blood-forming organ, the normal adult spleen is chiefly involved in the production of lymphocytes and monocytes. However, under certain conditions of bone marrow stress or disease the spleen can become the site of extensive extramedullary erythropoiesis.

On the other hand, because of its unique type of circulation, the spleen functions as an organ of red blood cell destruction. The intrasplenic circulation permits separation of plasma from cells and allows stasis in either the sinusoids or pulp spaces. This arrangement enables phagocytosis and lytic factors to work more effectively on the senescent and abnormal red cells, leading ultimately to their destruction.

The iron derived from the destruction of aged erythrocytes, as well as from those cells that did not meet the minimum body standards, is conserved and made available by the splenic macrophages for further erythropoiesis.

Because of its large content of lymphoid and reticuloendothelial cells, the spleen plays a major role in the immunologic reactions and defense mechanisms of the body.

RADIONUCLIDE SCANNING

There is no doubt that successful visualization of an organ by radionuclide scanning depends on the selective deposition of a gamma-emitting radionuclide in that organ, which produces a higher concentration of radioactivity relative to the surrounding structures. Consequently, splenic scanning can be achieved by the use of radioactively tagged erythrocytes that have been treated or altered to promote their rapid and selective trapping by the functional splenic tissue.

Alteration of the red cells can be induced by physical factors, chemical agents, or the application of antibodies.

A completely different approach to this problem of radionuclide scanning of the spleen depends on labeling of the reticuloendothelial cells with radiocolloids tagged with short-lived radionuclides such as ^{99m}Tc and ^{113m}In.

Coating with incomplete anti-D antibodies

Although coating with incomplete anti-D antibodies was the method used to obtain the first clinically usable scans for the human spleen, this technique cannot be applied in patients with D-negative blood grouping, and it necessitates serologic typing of the patient's blood. In this technique the red cells are labeled with radiochromate.

Heat-treated ^{51}Cr-tagged red cells

The red cells are tagged with 200 to 300 μCi of ^{51}Cr-labeled sodium chromate. The anticoagulant used is ACD (acid citrate dextrose solution) rather than heparin, which was shown to stabilize the cells against alteration. After tagging either the cells are washed or ascorbic acid is added, and the mixture is heated in a water bath at 50° C for a period of time that varies from 20 to 60 minutes, depending on the apparatus used for heating–whether hot air oven or water bath. This step is critical, since raising the temperature or increasing the duration of heating as well as using a higher concentration of ACD results in excessive damage to the erythrocytes (Fig. 16-1), with fewer cells accumulating in the spleen and more appearing in the liver. The heated cells are left to cool to room temperature prior to their reinjection into the patient from whom they were withdrawn. Scanning is performed at least 1 hour later (Fig. 16-2).

The main disadvantages of this technique of splenic scanning are the extreme care needed in the control of the technical factors involved in the preparation of the altered erythrocytes and the time consumed in this procedure. However, this technique remains the best for searching for accessory spleens and evaluating patients with suspected asplenia and polysplenia. Specific splenic imaging can also be of great help in patients with suspected splenic laceration or trauma.

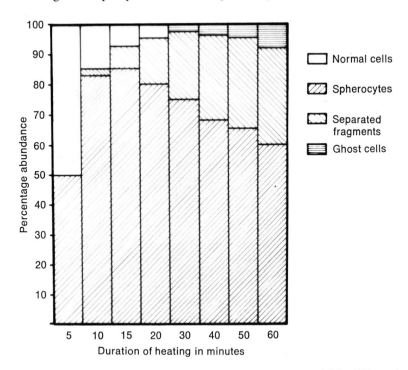

Fig. 16-1. Changes observed in the red cells on heating in a water bath at 50° C for different durations. The concentration of ACD is 1 ml for every 3 ml of blood.

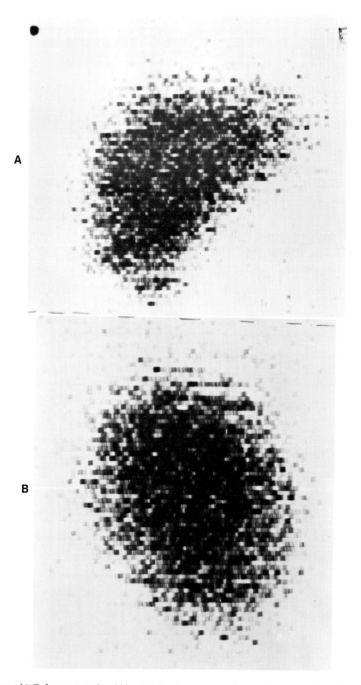

Fig. 16-2. Normal ^{51}Cr heat-treated red blood cell spleen scan series. **A,** Posterior view of the spleen. **B,** Lateral view of the spleen. These two views are necessary to correctly estimate the size of the spleen.

Additional information about the spleen can be obtained by studying the disappearance of heat-treated ^{51}Cr-tagged red cells from the circulation. For this purpose, serial blood samples are withdrawn from the patient's other arm over a period of 30 minutes. Radioactivity per unit volume from each sample is determined and plotted against time on semilogarithmic paper to calculate the disappearance half-time of radioactivity from the circulation. To obviate the discomfort caused by frequent blood sampling, the radioactivity disappearance half-time can be calculated from the radioactivity clearance curve monitored by a collimated-scintillation detector placed over the manubrium sterni or from the splenic radioactivity build-up tracing. To identify the abnormalities, the range for normal subjects should be determined using the specific method chosen for radioactivity monitoring and preparation of the tagged altered red cells. This is necessary because of the wide variability in the results reported by various groups of workers using different techniques. Disappearance half-times that are shorter than normal denote exaggerated splenic trapping of heat-treated tagged red cells. In 20 normal subjects examined with the splenic radioactivity build-up method, the disappearance half-time of tagged erythrocytes treated with both heat and excess ACD was found to range between 3.5 and 10.3 minutes, with an average of 6.1 $\pm$ 2.1 minutes (mean, $\pm$ 1 SD).

Application of chemical agents

N-Ethylmaleimide. This substance can be used for alteration of the red cells to promote their sequestration by the spleen. However, since it is a sulfhydryl inhibitor, the degree of damage to the erythrocytes cannot be controlled because of the variability in the concentration of the sulfhydryl-containing enzymes in the red cells of different individuals.

MHP [197]Hg. I-mercuri-2-hydroxypropane labeled with [197]Hg is able to tag red cells and causes only moderate damage to the cells.

Three hundred microcuries of MHP [197]Hg are placed in a sterile vacutainer. Since the specific activity is known, the weight of the stable MHP present in this amount of radionuclide is calculated. A sufficient volume of blood is withdrawn from the patient and added to the MHP [197]Hg in the vacutainer to provide 1 ml of packed red cells for each microgram of MHP. The contents are allowed to mix well for a few minutes, then the labeled blood is reinjected into the patient; scanning is performed after 1 hour.

The main advantages of this technique are its simplicity and the shorter time involved to complete the test. The use of a radioactive compound with high specific activity and accurate calculations is essential to avoid any possibility of toxic reactions. However, because of the renal accumulation of radioactivity in the absence of a spleen, this method cannot be used in the search for accessory spleens, since they can be hidden by radioactivity in the left kidney.

Excess ACD. Excess ACD whether alone (Table 16-1) or in combination with

Table 16-1. Effect of variation in the concentration of ACD on the morphologic changes occurring in the red cells on heating at 50°C for 15 minutes in a water bath

Cell type	ACD to blood ratio		
	1:3	1.5:2.5	2:2
Unaffected cells	7	—	—
Spherocytes	85	70	57
Fragments	8	30	36
Ghost cells	—	—	7

stable sodium chromate can be used to denature ^{51}Cr-labeled red cells as a prerequisite for splenic scanning.

Excess Sn (II) ion. This is the least effective method for damaging the red cells.

COMBINED EFFECT OF PHYSICAL AND CHEMICAL AGENTS

In order to cut down the time needed for the preparation of thermally damaged erythrocytes, the effect of heat is combined with a chemical agent, namely excess ACD. Heating in a water bath at 50° C in the presence of ACD in the ratio of 1 ml ACD for every 3 ml blood leads, after 15 minutes, to the production of spherocytes averaging 85% of the heat-treated red cell population.

With the recent availability of efficient methods of labeling red cells with ^{99m}Tc pertechnetate and in order to obtain better counting statistics, the red cells can be tagged with technetium 99m before being damaged to augment their uptake by the spleen.

Radiocolloids

During scintillation scanning of the liver using colloids labeled with short-lived radionuclides such as ^{99m}Tc and ^{113m}In, the spleen is usually visualized. This method of splenic scanning lacks specificity but has the advantage of being simpler and reasonably reliable. The quality of the scan pictures obtained is excellent because of the high counting rate and good counting statistics allowable with short-lived radionuclides (Fig 16-3). The major drawback of this method is the inability to differentiate the spleen from the left lobe of the liver, especially in the left lateral view. For this purpose, angulated views such as left anterior oblique can be quite helpful in separating these organs from each other in the scan image. Furthermore, colloid scintigraphy is not a completely reliable indicator of lymphomatous involvement of the spleen. On the other hand, the radiation dose delivered to the patient during this procedure is rather low.

·   ·   ·

Splenic scanning can be performed from either the anterior or posterior approach. An added lateral view can sometimes be of great value. In the accurate

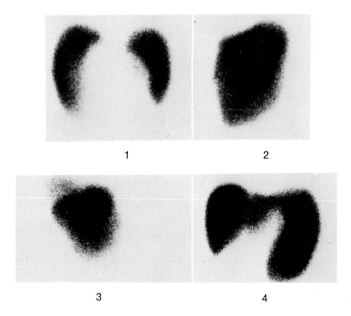

1   2

3   4

Fig. 16-3. Liver spleen scans done with ^{99m}Tc sulfur colloid showing a grossly enlarged spleen in a patient with chronic myeloid leukemia. **1,** Posterior; **2,** left lateral; **3,** right lateral; **4,** anterior.

interpretation of the obtained picture the scan is superimposed on a plain x-ray film of the left half of the abdomen. Proper superimposition is obtained through the use of fixed landmarks, such as the left fifth intercostal space in the midclavicular plane, xiphisternum, and top of the iliac crest.

In interpretation, the first points to be checked are the site, size, and shape of the organ. The spleen lies immediately underneath the diaphragm. In the posterior view, it appears oval with an oblique long axis in 65% of cases and with a transverse long axis in another 15%. In the remaining 20%, the spleen is rounded or globular. In the same view, the average measurements of the spleen are 10.5 cm in length (range 7.5 to 13.0) and 7.0 cm in breadth (range 6.0 to 11.0). By planimetry the surface area of the scan picture ranges between 35 and 90 cm². In the lateral view, the spleen appears larger than the picture obtained through the posterior approach by an average of 40%. The distribution of radioactivity throughout the spleen is almost homogeneous, with less density towards the periphery. Since the distribution of radioactivity represents the functioning splenic tissue, areas of destroyed function such as tumors, cysts, abscesses, and infarcts should appear as regions with little or no radioactivity (Fig. 16-4).

The main clinical indication for splenic scanning is to detect the presence of functioning splenic tissue and provide information about its quantitative assessment. This is of great help in the differential diagnosis of a shadow or mass in the left upper abdomen. Furthermore, the presence of accessory spleens could be detected and intrasplenic space-occupying lesions delineated.

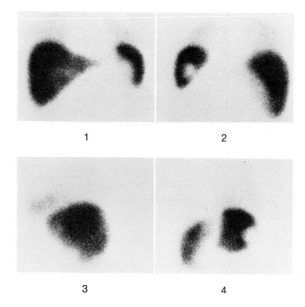

Fig. 16-4. Liver spleen scans done with ^{99m}Tc-labeled sulfur colloid showing a splenic space-occupying lesion caused by metastatic malignant melanoma.

BIBLIOGRAPHY

Fischer, J., and Wolf, R.: Resultats de l'application clinique de la scintigraphie de la rate dans 500 cas. Possibilites et limites, Medical Radioisotope Scanning (Proc. Symp. Athens 1964), 337-353, IAEA, Vienna 1964.

Hassaballa, N. A.: Evaluation of splenic activity by means of partially damaged tagged red cells, thesis (Clinical Pathology), 1974.

Holzbach, R. T., Shipley, R. E., Clark, R. E., and Chudzik, E. B.: Influence of spleen size and portal pressure on erythrocyte sequestration, J. Clin. Invest. **43**:1125-1135, 1964.

Johnson, P. M., Herion, J. C., and Mooring, S. K.: Scintillation scanning of the normal human spleen utilizing sensitized radioactive erythrocytes, Radiology **74**:99-101, 1960.

Kimber, R. J., and Lander, H.: The effect of heat on human red cell morphology, fragility and subsequent survival in vivo, J. Lab. Clin. Med. **64**:922-933, 1964.

Larson, S. M., Tuell, S. H., Moores, K. D., and Nelp, W. B.: Dimensions of the normal adult spleen scan and prediction of spleen weight, J. Nucl. Med. **12**:123-126, 1971.

Razzak, M. A., and Hassaballa, N. A.: Splenic radionuclide scanning and sequestration of thermally altered erythrocytes in hepatosplenic schistosomiasis, Tropenmed. Parasitol. **27**:343-348, 1976.

Razzak, M. A., and Sodee, D. B.: Radioisotope scanning as an aid in the diagnosis of splenic cysts, Nucl. Med. **7**:59-64, 1968.

Razzak, M. A., Ziada, G., and Hassaballa, N. A.: Radionuclide scanning of the spleen. Technical modification, normal variants and dimensions, Strahlentherapie **152**:52-56,1976.

Sharma, S. M., Patel, M. C., Ramanathan, R. D., and Ganatra, R. D.: A new technique to denature red cells for spleen scanning, J. Nucl. Med. **11**:228-232, 1970.

Wagner, H. N., Razzak, M. A., Gaertner, R. A., Caine, W. P., and Feagin, O. T.: Removal of erythrocytes from the circulation, Arch. Intern. Med. **110**:90-97, 1962.

Wagner, H. N., Weiner, I. M., McAfee, J. G., and Martinez, J.: 1-mercuri-2-hydroxypropane (MHP); A new pharmaceutical for visualization of the spleen by radioisotope scanning, Arch. Intern. Med. **113**:696-701, 1964.

Winkelman, J. W., Wagner, H. N., McAfee, J. G., and Mozley, J. M.: Visualization of the spleen in man by radioisotope scanning, Radiology **75**:465-466, 1960.

17 Bone

Inorganic materials make up 45% of the constituents of bone. These materials include calcium, phosphate, and magnesium. Organic materials make up 30%, and water constitutes 25% of bone weight. Calcium makes up about 15% of the weight of fresh osseous tissue. Bone calcium exists in two forms, calcium carbonate and tricalcium phosphate; the ratio of calcium to phosphate is approximately 2.2:1.

There are two types of ossification—intramembranous and intracartilaginous (endochondral). The cranial vault, maxilla, and mandible are formed through ossification of membranes. The bones of the limbs, trunk, and base of the skull are transformed from cartilage to bone by both forms of ossification. It has been shown that calcium and phosphorus are first laid down in the epiphysis of developing bone and later move to the shaft, or diaphysis. Growth occurs at both ends of the bone. The cells involved in ossification are called *osteoblasts;* cells that deossify bone are called *osteoclasts.* Through the combined action of the osteoblasts and osteoclasts, complete replacement of calcified cartilage results in adult bone.

Hormones control bone formation and bone breakdown. Primarily parathormone, which is elaborated to the parathyroid gland, and thyrocalcitonin, which is produced by the thyroid gland, have roles in bone formation and destruction.

ANATOMY (Figs. 17-1 and 17-2)

The anatomy of bone has become of increasing importance in the technology and practice of nuclear medicine. With the introduction of excellent bone-seeking radionuclides and improvement of instrumentation, a complete knowledge of the gross anatomy and microanatomy of bone is needed by all in this field. Because of the complexity of the 206 bones of the skeleton, the student is referred to basic anatomy textbooks such as *Gray's Anatomy* or to the chapter on the skeleton in *Structure and Function in Man* by Jacob and Francone. Illustrations included in this text will introduce the student to the important skeletal structures visualized in bone scanning and imaging.

PHYSIOLOGY

The skeleton is composed primarily of collagen, cartilage, and osteoid tissues. Collagen is firm and pliable, cartilage is hard and resilient, and mineralized osteoid is hard and rigid. *Collagen* is made up of reticulum, elastin, and ground sub-

371

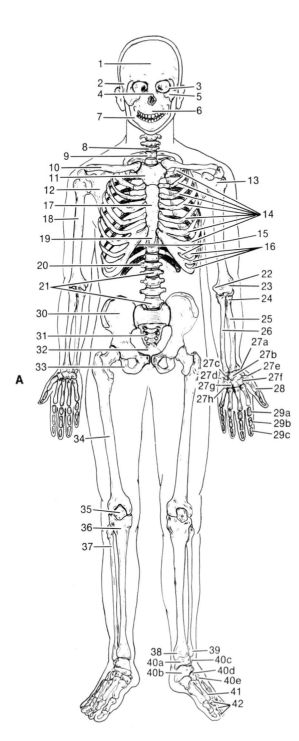

Fig. 17-1. A, Anterior skeleton.

1. Frontal bone
2. Temporal bone
3. Orbit
4. Nasal bone
5. Zygomatic bone
6. Maxilla
7. Mandible
8. Seventh cervical vertebra
9. Thoracic vertebra I
10. Clavicle
11. Manubrium of sternum
12. Shoulder blade
13. Head of humerus
14. True ribs
15. Kidneys
16. False ribs
17. Body of sternum
18. Humerus
19. Xiphoid process
20. Transverse process
21. Lumbar vertebrae
22. Medial condyle of humerus
23. Lateral epicondyle of humerus
24. Capitulum of radius
25. Radius
26. Ulna
27. Carpal bones
    a. Scaphoid bone of hand
    b. Lunate bone
    c. Triangular bone
    d. Pisiform bone
    e. Trapezium
    f. Trapezoid
    g. Capitate bone
    h. Hamate bone
28. Metacarpal bones
29. Finger bones
    a. Proximal phalanx
    b. Middle phalanx
    c. Distal phalanx
30. Iliac bone
31. Sacrum
32. Bladder
33. Ischium
34. Femur
35. Patella
36. Tibia
37. Fibula
38. Medial malleolus
39. Lateral malleolus
40. Tarsal bones
    a. Talus
    b. Navicular bone
    c. Calcaneus
    d. Cuneiform bones I to III
    e. Cuboid bone
41. Metatarsal bones
42. Phalanges of toes

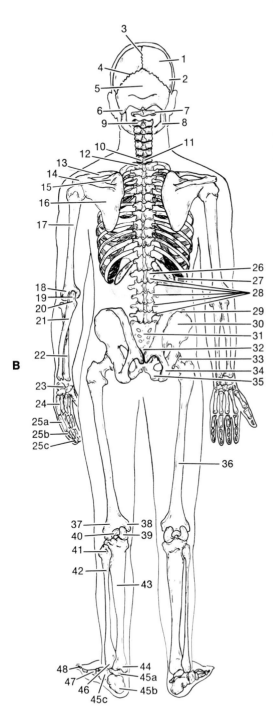

Fig. 17-1. B, Posterior skeleton.

1. Parietal bone
2. Temporal bone
3. Sagittal suture
4. Lambdoidal suture
5. Occipital bone
6. Mastoid process
7. Atlas
8. Mandible
9. Axis, or second cervical vertebra
10. Seventh cervical vertebra
11. Spinous process
12. Thoracic vertebra I
13. Clavicle
14. Acromion
15. Spine of scapula
16. Scapula, or shoulder blade
17. Humerus
18. Lateral epicondyle of humerus
19. Olecranon
20. Head of radius
21. Ulna
22. Radius
23. Carpal bones
24. Metacarpal bones
25. Finger bones
   a. Proximal phalanx
   b. Middle phalanx
   c. Distal phalanx
26. Transverse process
27. Kidneys
28. Lumbar vertebrae
29. Iliac crest
30. Upper part of ilium
31. Sacrum
32. Bladder
33. Head of femur
34. Ischium
35. Pubic bone
36. Femur
37. Lateral epicondyle of femur
38. Medial epicondyle of femur
39. Medial condyle of femur
40. Lateral condyle of femur
41. Head of fibula
42. Fibula
43. Tibia
44. Medial malleolus
45. Tarsal bones
   a. Talus
   b. Calcaneus
   c. Cuboid bone
46. Lateral malleolus
47. Metatarsal bones
48. Phalanges of toe —
conform to those of hand

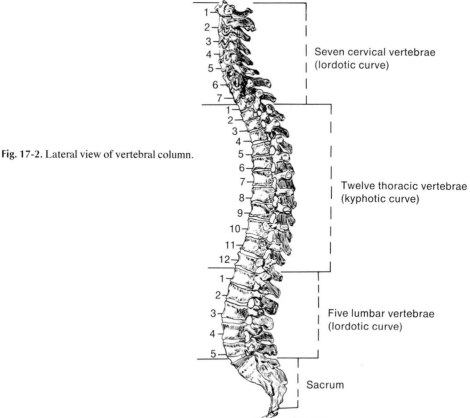

Fig. 17-2. Lateral view of vertebral column.

Seven cervical vertebrae (lordotic curve)

Twelve thoracic vertebrae (kyphotic curve)

Five lumbar vertebrae (lordotic curve)

Sacrum

Coccyx

stance. This latter compound substance selectively protects and supplies the parenchymal cells it supports. Therefore it becomes an important water-binding agent and plays an *ion-exchange resin* role important in mineral metabolism of bone. *Cartilage* is made up of collagen fibrils and elastin and ground substance. Hyalin cartilage is found in relation to bone growth and joint surfaces. *Osteoid* is morphologically identical to collagen. Its differential features are its osteoblasts and the advent of mineralization.

Bone, like every other tissue, is dynamic and is being remodeled throughout life. The histophysiologic resolution of old bone and replacement with new bone is called *internal remodeling of bone.* This requires continuous development of new generations of differentiating cells. Bone morphogenesis is the process of differentiation and organization of progenitor cells, into cartilage or woven bone, and then reabsorption and replacement of woven bone with a lamellar bone and bone marrow. Bone morphogenesis is the function of the biochemical components of the organic matrix of bone, collectively referred to as *bone morphogenic property.*

This property consists of a protein (BMP), support fibrous protein (collagen), and a proteinase (BMPase) that degrades BMP.

The fact that bone is constantly renewed and regenerated in the adult is evidence that embryonic morphogenesis persists throughout life. Morphogenesis in bone is demonstrated as mesenchymal cells proliferate and differentiate into osteoprogenitor cells, eventually reassembling as osteoblasts and forming new bone and finally interacting with perivascular connective tissue cell populations to develop bone marrow.

FORMATION

Periosteal tissue (the covering of bone) is differentiated into two layers. The cells of the inner layer that lie in contact with bone or cartilage become separated by a homogenous substance called *osteoid,* which is laid down by cells called *osteoblasts.* The osteoblasts in their elaboration of osteoid become surrounded by osteoid and shrink to compact cells with pyknotic nuclei within their cell spaces, the lacunae, and are known as *osteocytes.* Successive layers of bone are laid down in concentric circles, and each layer is called a *lamina* (Fig. 17-3). Thus compact bone is formed. This manner of bone production is known as intramembranous ossification. Almost all the long and flat bones are formed by this method, and worn-out bone is replaced in the same manner. Thus this form of bone accounts for the bulk of the skeletal tissue.

MINERALIZATION

Bone mineral exists in an apatite crystal form. Ions are arranged in units, and units are shared by contiguous units in a lattice arrangement much like interior walls of buildings are shared by adjacent rooms. The formula for bone salt is best represented by a hydroxyapatite:

$$3 \ Ca_3 \ (PO_4)_2 \ \cdot \ Ca \ (OH)_2$$

Other ions in trace amounts are Na^+, Mg^{++}, K^+, Cl^-, and F^-.

There is a continuous interchange of ions between the crystal lattice and the fluid that bathes it. Thus bone is a dynamic system in constant flux. Because of the unit structure of the crystalline component of bone, it has an immense surface area, approximating 100 acres in man.

The factors involved in bone mineralization are still not well understood. The osteoblastic cells elaborate alkaline phosphatase, which plays a role in formation of ground substance but does not enhance mineralization. However, the osteocytes continue to elaborate phosphatase, although buried in a calcified intercellular substance that maintains a high phosphate ion concentration in the tissue fluid in the canaliculi, which prevents the ionic concentration from falling to a point where bone salt would go back into solution. The osteocyte may also resorb surrounding bone in a process termed *osteoclytic osteolysis.*

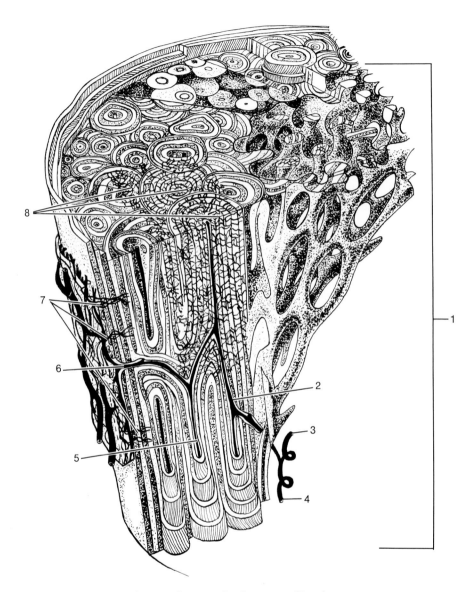

Fig. 17-3. Cross-sectional anatomy of long bone.
1. Medullary cavity
2. Haversian canal
3. Ascending medullary artery
4. Descending medullary artery
5. Arterioles derived from medullary artery
6. Anastomosis
7. Periosteal arteries
8. Haversian system

NORMAL LYSIS

The stress stimulus is the most important factor in the modeling and remodeling of bone. Modeling of bones is completely the result of reorientation of lamellae into haversian systems (Fig. 17-3) laid down in lines of mechanical stress. Stress may be a matter of pressure or tension. The osteoclast is the cell that primarily causes deossification, the disappearance of bone organic matrix and its mineral content. Apparently the osteoclast disintegrates osteoid first, thus releasing the mineral content. Actually alteration of blood supply, mechanical trauma, parathyroid hormone, and vitamin D are also involved in bone destruction.

FACTORS IN METABOLISM

Of the body calcium, 99% is in the skeleton, and less than 1% is in the extracellular fluid, organelles, and membranes. This latter 1% is under the physiologic control of the endocrine systems and transport mechanisms. Most calcium is in the structural calcium in the skeleton. Calcium is ingested in the diet and absorbed from the gut. It is continuously lost from the body through renal excretion, which is relatively fixed in most humans, fecal loss, and sweat.

If losses of calcium are smaller than that absorbed, then excess calcium can be deposited in the skeleton. If losses of calcium from the body are greater than that absorbed, then calcium must be mobilized from the skeleton to maintain the homeostatic concentration in the extracellular fluid necessary for life. Vitamin D is the primary governing factor in the gut absorption of calcium and in large doses enhances the exchange of calcium from bone into serum. Mobilization of calcium is influenced by various endocrine glands. Growth hormone controls longitudinal growth of bone; linear growth is accompanied by remodeling of bone, removal of calcium from formed bone, and redeposition in new epiphyseal areas. Thyroid hormone increases both bone formation and, to a greater degree, bone reabsorption rates. Adrenocortical hormones inhibit bone formation to a greater extent than bone reabsorption. Parathyroid hormones influence bone reabsorption, bone remodeling, and increased bone turnover. Finally, calcitonin, a hormone secreted by cells found in the thyroid, reduces bone turnover, lowering serum calcium. The net effect of all the hormone systems is on the deposition or removal of calcium to and from the skeleton, which provides the homeostatic concentration of calcium in extracellular fluid.

CIRCULATION (Fig. 17-3)

The bone nutrient arterial system consists of branches of the nutrient artery and the metaphyseal arteries in anastomosis with each other to become the medullary blood supply. The periosteal arterial system is a component of the arterial system that supplies the surrounding muscles. Three fourths or more of the compactum is supplied with blood by the medullary system; therefore, the blood flow through bone is normally centrifugal from medulla to periosteum. In animal research it has been shown that if the nutrient system is blocked, the periosteal system is able to reverse the usual flow and convey blood supply to the compactum. Bone is well supplied with nutrients because no bone cell is more than 0.10 mm away from a capillary. Bone is permeated by a system of tiny canals (canaliculi) that extend from one lacuna to another and extend to a bony surface where the capillary is situated. These canals are actually the remnants of the cytoplasmic connecting process of osteoblasts. As osteoid and calcified bone are formed, these processes are retracted, leaving the canals (canaliculi) in their place. Tissue fluid originating from the capillary fills the canaliculi and lacunae. Thus metabolites are brought to the osteocyte, and waste is carried away. This fluid bathes the crystalline component of bone, and ion exchanges are made between this component and the extracellular fluid.

BONE MARROW

While bone formation is extending from ossification centers toward each end of the fetal cartilaginous bone model, the periosteum continues to add bone to the sides of the model. As the periphery becomes stronger, the cancellous bone in its central portion is no longer necessary for support, so this bone dissolves and leaves a cavity called the *marrow cavity*. In the fetus the marrow of most bones is red marrow, which derives its color from the vast numbers of red blood cells in various stages of production. During the growth period the marrow of most bones becomes yellow or filled with large quantities of fat. In the adult, red marrow is found only in the bones of the vault of the skull, flat bones, bodies of the vertebrae, cancellous bone of some of the short bones, and at the ends of long bones. Under conditions in which increased red blood cell production is needed, yellow marrow becomes reconverted to red marrow. In red bone marrow multipotential stem cells called the *primitive reticular cell* and the *endothelial cell* differentiate into the erythrocytic, myelocytic, and megakaryocytic series of cells that generate the adult red blood cell, the granular leukocyte, and the platelet. The vascular supply of bone marrow is derived from the nutrient artery. The arterioles divide into capillaries, and the latter run into sinusoids. Sinuses form a system of vessels running from the periphery toward a central longitudinal vein. Hemopoietic tissue lies between the sinuses. Capillaries stemming from marrow arterioles enter the haversian canals to supply endosteal parts of the diaphyseal bone. The blood flow of bone marrow is 0.5 ml/gm/min, as compared to liver blood flow, which is 0.56 ml/gm/min and may be altered by physiologic demand.

RADIONUCLIDES IN STUDY OF BONE

The metabolism of bone has been studied by the use of radioisotopes of calcium. Calcium 47, which is a gamma emitter, has been used in the study of bone metabolism; however, the high energy of its gamma ray requires extremely heavy shielding. Therefore the use of this radionuclide is limited.

Radioisotopes of strontium, which mimic calcium metabolism, have been used in the study of normal and abnormal bone physiology. The useful isotopes of strontium are ^{85}Sr and ^{87m}Sr. These radionuclides came into extensive use because bone has to be decalcified by approximately 50% before decreased density can be visualized on radiographs. Therefore lesions have usually been existent for some time and have destroyed a great deal of bone before standard radiographs become positive. In abnormalities of bone, it was found that the radionuclides ^{85}Sr and ^{87m}Sr could be statistically counted with any standard detector or imaged at a very

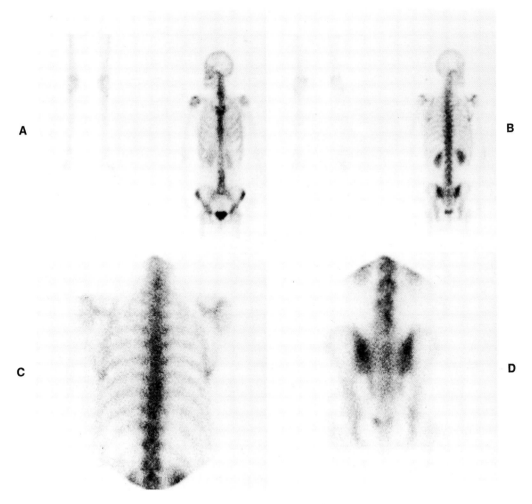

Fig. 17-4. Normal bone images performed 2 hours after administration of a 20-mCi dose of pyrophosphate. **A,** Anterior whole-body image. **B,** Posterior whole-body image. **C,** Spot image of cervical-thoracic spine, ribs, and scapulae. **D,** Spot image of lumbar spine and pelvis.

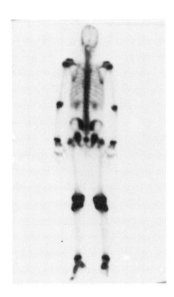

Fig. 17-5. Posterior whole-body polyphosphate ⁹⁹ᵐTc bone study. Normal images in 14-year-old patient showing the normal increased concentration seen in new bone formation.

early stage of the disease process. The increased deposition of these radionuclides is strongly linked to osteoblastic activity and new bone formation.

Since these radionuclides are found in areas of new bone formation, there is increased strontium deposition in the normal areas of new bone growth (the epiphyseal ends of the long bones).

One hour after the injection of radioactive strontium, most of the strontium deposition has taken place in bone. Strontium is excreted both by the kidney and the large bowel; therefore, these two organ systems will interfere with bone counting and imaging for a period of time. Most of extraskeletal strontium has been excreted from the body within 72 hours. This is usually aided somewhat by the clinician by giving the patient cleansing enemas for several days after the administration of strontium.

Fluorine 18 also has been found useful in bone imaging. This radionuclide is primarily accumulated by the exchangeable portion of bone, the apatite crystalline structure. Its concentration by bone is secondary to ion exchange with the volume of bone apatite crystal surface available and blood flow to bone.

Technetium 99m-labeled diphosphonate and pyrophosphate have become the primary bone imaging agents because of their bone-seeking qualities, the imaging efficiency of technetium 99m, and the ability to administer multimillicurie quantities based on the short effective half-lives of these compounds. Their bone concentration mechanisms are similar to fluorine 18, and, in addition, there is selective binding affinity of ⁹⁹ᵐTc pyrophosphate by immature *collagen*. These

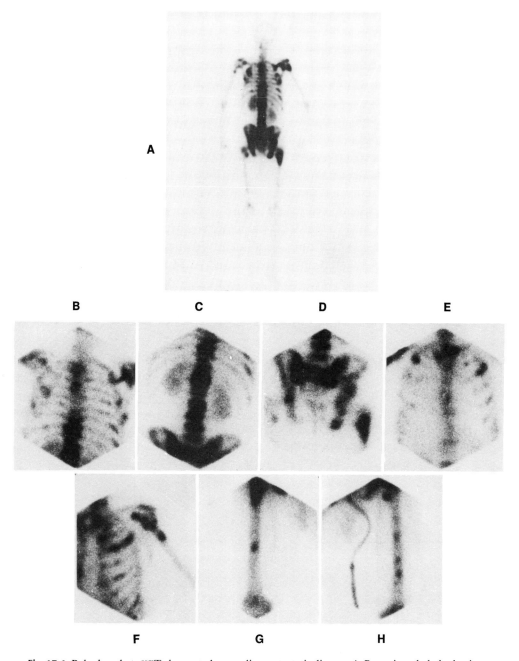

Fig. 17-6. Polyphosphate ^{99m}Tc bone study revealing metastatic disease. **A,** Posterior whole-body view. **B,** Posterior cervical-thoracic region. **C,** Thoracic-lumbar region. **D,** Pelvis and upper femurs. **E,** Anterior chest. **F,** Anterior oblique view of left chest wall and humerus. **G,** Right femur. **H,** Left femur; urinary catheter in field of view. Note on femur views that the abnormal concentrations appear to be extending from the medullary portion of bone.

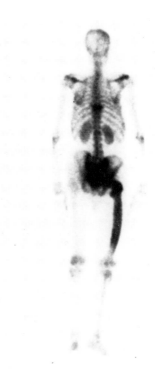

Fig. 17-7. Posterior whole-body polyphosphate ^{99m}Tc image. Study reveals Paget's disease involving skull, thoracic vertebrae, and right femur.

radionuclides are primarily excreted by the kidney, with approximately 50% of the injected dose concentrated by bony tissue.

The radionuclide bone survey is frequently employed in the search for breast, prostatic, and lung metastatic carcinoma sites in bone. These carcinomas have a predilection to spread to bone, and 30% or more of these patients will have metastatic disease to bone at the time of diagnosis. The radionuclide bone survey is also a sensitive indicator of primary bone tumors, osteomyelitis, arthritis, metabolic bone disease, and fractures (Figs. 17-4 to 17-7). An accompanying radiograph may aid in the diagnosis of abnormal deposition.

Because of the diagnostic sensitivity of bone imaging, this procedure is gaining wide acceptance in the physician's search for possible metastatic disease to bone and in the primary evaluation of bone and joint pathology previously evaluated only by radiographic or biopsy techniques.

BIBLIOGRAPHY

Aegerter, E., and Kirkpatrick, J.: Orthopedic disease, Philadelphia, 1968, W. B. Saunders Co.

Freeman, L. M., and Blaufax, M. D., editors: Seminars in nuclear medicine. Benign bone disorders,

New York, 1976, Grune & Stratton, Inc., vol. VI, no. 1.

Jones, A. E., and Johnston, G. S.: Bone imaging. In Potchen, E. J., editor: Current concepts in radiology, St. Louis, 1977, The C. V. Mosby Co., pp. 193-216.

Kaye, M., Silverton, S., and Rosenthall, L.: Technetium-99^m pyrophosphate: studies in vivo and in vitro, J. Nucl. Med. **16:**40, 1975.

Lutwak, L., Singer, F. R., and Urist, M. R.: Current concepts of bone metabolism, Ann. Intern. Med. **80:**630, 1974.

Rhinelander, F. W.: Circulation in bone. In Bourne, G., editor: Biochemistry and physiology of bone, ed. 2, New York, 1972, Academic Press, Inc., vol. II.

Whaler, J. P., Krook, L., and Nunez, E. A.: Some metabolic considerations in bone disease. In Potchen, E. J., editor: Current concepts in radiology, St. Louis, 1977, The C. V. Mosby Co., pp. 143-192.

GENERAL BIBLIOGRAPHY

Ashkar, F. S., Miale, A., and Smoak, W.: A general guide to nuclear medicine, Springfield, Ill., 1975, Charles C Thomas, Publisher.

Best, C., and Taylor, N. B.: Physiological basis of medical practice, ed. 10, Baltimore, 1979, The Williams & Wilkins Co.

Blahd, W. H.: Nuclear medicine, ed. 2, New York, 1971, McGraw-Hill Book Co.

Deland, F. H., and Wagner, H. N.: Atlas of nuclear medicine, Philadelphia, 1969, W. B. Saunders Co., vol. 1.

Freeman, L. M., and Blaufax, M. D.: Physicians desk reference for radiology and nuclear medicine, Oradell, N.J., 1977-1978, Medical Economics Co.

Freeman, L. M., and Johnson, P. M.: Clinical scintillation scanning, New York, 1975, Grune & Stratton, Inc.

Grant, J. C. B., and Basmajian, J. V.: A method of anatomy, ed. 7, Baltimore, 1965, The Williams & Wilkins Co.

Gross, C. M.: Gray's anatomy of the human body, ed. 28, Philadelphia, 1966, Lea & Febiger.

Guyton, A. C.: Textbook of medical physiology, ed. 3, Philadelphia, 1966, W. B. Saunders Co.

Ham, A. W.: Histology, Philadelphia, 1957, J. B. Lippincott Co.

Holvey, D. N.: The Merck manual of diagnosis and therapy, ed. 12, Rahway, N.J., 1972, Merck Sharp & Dohme Research Lab.

Jacob, S. W., and Francone, C. A.: Structure and function in man, ed. 2, Philadelphia, 1970, W. B. Saunders Co.

Maynard, C. D.: Clinical nuclear medicine, Philadelphia, 1969, Lea & Febiger.

Powsner, E. R., and Raeside, D. E.: Diagnostic nuclear medicine, New York, 1971, Grune & Stratton, Inc.

Rhodes, B. A., editor: Quality control in nuclear medicine: radiopharmaceuticals, instrumentation, and in vitro assays, St. Louis, 1977, The C. V. Mosby Co.

Shtassel, P.: Speak to me in nuclear medicine, New York, 1976, Harper & Row, Publishers.

Silver, S.: Radioactive nuclides in medicine & biology — medicine, Philadelphia, 1968, Lea & Febiger.

Wagner, H. N.: Principles of nuclear medicine, Philadelphia, 1968, W. B. Saunders Co.

Wagner, H. N.: Nuclear medicine, New York, 1975, HP Publishing, Co.

18 Thyroid

The thyroid is an endocrine organ, and thyroid hormones have a direct effect on the body's metabolism. The thyroid's function is under the direct control of the anterior pituitary gland, which secretes thyroid-stimulating hormone (TSH). The output of thyroid-stimulating hormone is directly related to the secretion of thyrotropin-releasing hormone (TRH) by the hypothalamus. The relationship between TRH, TSH, and thyroxine is called the *hypothalamic pituitary thyroid axis.*

ANATOMY AND PHYSIOLOGY

During embryonic development the thyroid is derived from the ventral wall of the primitive pharynx (Figs. 18-1 and 18-2). This median outgrowth migrates downward, and at its lower end it bifurcates to form the isthmus and lateral lobes of the thyroid. In some cases the thyroid does not progress down into the neck but remains at the base of the tongue. Thyroid tissue may also continue down into the mediastinum and thus become substernal. However, the thyroid is usually found between the thyroid cartilage and the suprasternal notch. The isthmus is astride the trachea with one lobe on either side of the trachea. In many cases there is a slight extension of thyroid tissue from the lobes or from the isthmus or both. This is normal thyroid tissue that lines the tract the thyroid follows down into the neck. This tissue is called the *pyramidal lobe.*

Thyroid tissue is composed of cuboidal epithelial cells arranged in single layers around spherical spaces called *follicles.* In the human fetus the thyroid becomes functional during the third month of gestation.

The thyroid's blood supply arises from the superior and inferior thyroid arteries; the blood flow to the thyroid, as well as its capillary bed, is profuse.

Normally, control of thyroid activity is exerted by the thyroid thyrotropic hormone (TSH), which is secreted by the anterior pituitary. The normal weight of the human thyroid is from 20 to 35 gm, and the usual normal adult thyroid gland is barely palpable, if at all. The thyroid gland's primary function is to synthesize, store, and secrete the thyroid hormones.

The thyroid extracts iodide from the blood supply (I⁻) and converts iodide to iodine (I^2), which is utilized in the synthesis of thyroid hormone.

Iodine and thyroid hormone metabolism

The hypothalamus regulates the pituitary secretion of thyrotropic hormone (TSH) by secreting a thyroid factor (thyrotropin-releasing factor) into the portal

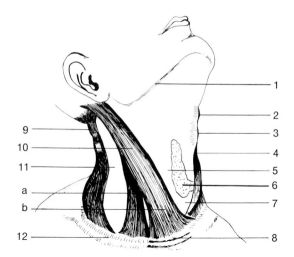

Fig. 18-1. Anatomy of the neck region.

1. Mandible
2. Hyoid bone
3. Thyroid cartilage
4. Cricoid cartilage
5. Anterior triangle

6. Thyroid gland —
   right lobe
7. Suprasternal
   notch
8. Sternum

9. Trapezius
10. Sternocleidomastoid
   muscle
   a. Sternal head
   b. Clavicular head

11. Posterior triangle
12. Clavicle

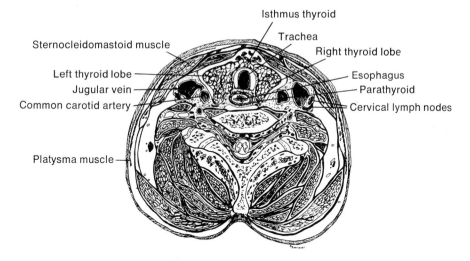

Fig. 18-2. Transverse section through the seventh cervical vertebra.

vessels of the pituitary stalk (Fig. 18-3). Cells of the anterior pituitary secrete TSH, which has four distinct effects on the thyroid gland. There is a reciprocal relationship between TSH output and the serum and/or tissue levels of the free thyroid hormone. It is not known whether the level of thyroid hormone acts primarily through its effect on the hypothalamus or on the pituitary. It is possible that the feedback mechanism of the thyroid pituitary axis operates at both levels.

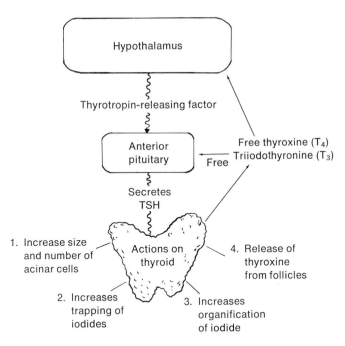

Fig. 18-3. Iodine and thyroid hormone metabolism.

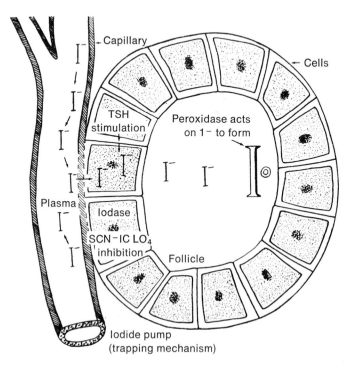

Fig. 18-4. I⁻(iodide) thyroidal trapping mechanism and conversion of I^- to I^2 ($I^\bullet$).

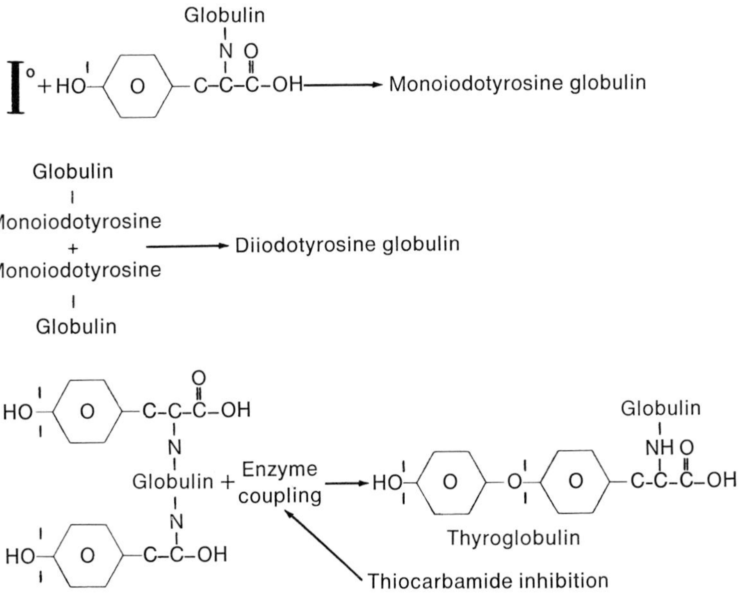

Fig. 18-5. Thyroid hormonal synthesis.

The ability of the thyroid gland to concentrate iodide is found in the thyroid epithelial cells (Fig. 18-4). The iodide-concentrating mechanism of the thyroid gland is referred to as the *iodide trap,* or *iodide pump.* This mechanism may concentrate iodide to 25 times that of the plasma level or in some abnormal instances may increase this concentration to 500 times that of the plasma concentration. The iodide pump is so efficient that tagged iodine has been found in the colloid (which is on the other side of the epithelial cell) as early as 2 minutes after iodide was injected intravenously. The next step that iodide takes in the course of biosynthesis of thyroid hormone is the formation of iodinated amino acids. This is also an extremely rapid process and takes place in the colloid at the surface of the thyroid epithelial cells (at the cell colloid interface). At this stage it is thought that the iodide is oxidized to iodine, which in turn reacts with the tyrosyl residues of the protein chain of tyroglobulin to form monoiodotyrosine globulin (Fig. 18-5).

Further iodination leads to the formation of diiodotyrosine globulin, and subsequent coupling of the two iodinated tyrosyl groups will form the tetraiodinated compound thyroxine, still attached to the globulin moiety. If one monoiodotyrosyl molecule couples with a diiodotyrosyl molecule, triiodothyronine globulin is formed. These compounds are then stored in the thyroid follicle in the form of thyroglobulins. Active proteolytic enzymes release thyroxine and triiodothyronine from thyroglobulin. This process is probably intracellular, since small fragments of colloid appear as droplets in thyroid epithelial cells. Free thyroxine (T_4) and triiodothyronine (T_3) are then released into the venous drainage of the thyroid gland (Fig. 18-6).

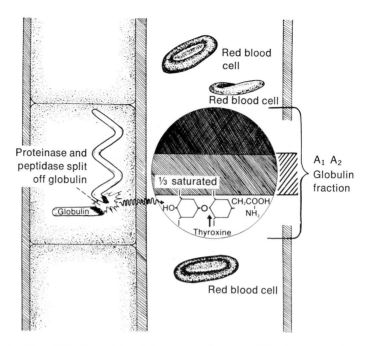

Fig. 18-6. Thyroidal release of thyroid hormone and method of blood transport of hormone.

The thyroid gland has a remarkable affinity for iodide; although the gland constitutes only 0.05% of the total body weight, the normal gland contains half the body's entire iodine content.

Iodine turnover in the human

The most commonly used radioactive forms of iodine are ^{123}I and ^{131}I, which act exactly like stable [127]I in the body. Therefore very small amounts of ^{123}I and ^{131}I may be introduced into the body to trace the role of stable iodine in metabolic pathways.

Since iodine is distributed in all areas of the body, there are several iodine "compartments"; these include the intracellular, extracellular, thyroid, and extrathyroidal compartments. There are also extrathyroidal iodide spaces and intrathyroidal and extrathyroidal organic iodine compartments. The terminology in this section should not be too difficult, and this portion of the chapter should be studied in detail. With the understanding of the iodide and iodine compartments, the student will be able to predict the results of almost all the radioactive iodine studies, as well as the chemical iodine studies that will be discussed later in this chapter.

Iodine metabolism in the body has been roughly divided into a three-compartment model. Compartment I is the extrathyroidal iodide pool that receives its io-

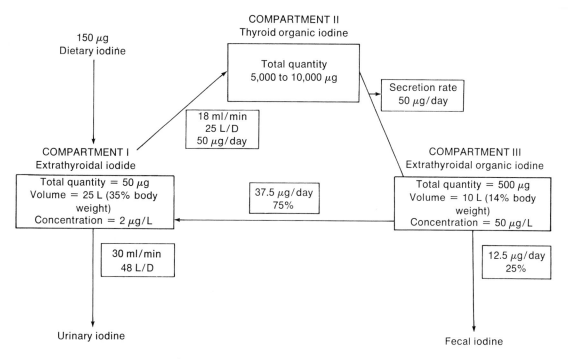

Fig. 18-7. Iodine and iodide body compartments.

dide from both the diet and the extrathyroidal deiodinization or removal of iodine from secreted thyroid hormone. Iodide is removed from this pool by thyroid accumulation and renal excretion. Compartment II is the thyroidal organic iodine pool from which hormonal iodine is secreted into Compartment III, the extrathyroidal organic iodine pool. Iodine is transported from Compartment III by removal of iodide from the organic thyroid hormone (which reenters Compartment I) and by fecal excretion in an organic form (Fig. 18-7).

Compartment I—extrathyroidal iodide pool. Approximately 150 to 300 μg of dietary iodide are normally ingested by the human daily. For purposes of this discussion, an ingested amount of 150 μg will be used.

Iodine is absorbed by the gastrointestinal tract, largely by the stomach mucosa, in the first 15 to 30 minutes after ingestion and thus enters the extrathyroidal pool. This pool is approximately 25 liters in volume (35% of the total body weight). Therefore at any period in time approximately 50 μg (or 2 μg/liter) of iodide should be found in this pool. As mentioned previously, iodide leaves this pool by two routes: (1) by entering the thyroid organic iodine pool and (2) by renal excretion. The kidneys have a rather fixed rate of excretion of iodide and will clear approximately 40 ml of plasma of iodide per minute; in a 24-hour period, approximately 48 liters of the extrathyroidal iodide pool is cleared of iodide.

Compartment II—thyroid organic iodine pool. The thyroid actively extracts iodide from the extrathyroidal iodide pool, converting the iodide into thyroid organic iodine. The thyroid normally contains 5,000 to 10,000 μg of thyroid organic iodine. The thyroid normally extracts iodide from 18 ml of plasma per minute (50 μg of iodide are extracted from the plasma per 24-hour period). The thyroid then clears approximately 25 liters of the extrathyroidal iodide pool of iodide per 24 hours. The thyroid organic iodine pool, as can be seen by the quantity of iodine extracted, contains a rather static quantity as compared to Compartment I. The majority of the thyroid organic iodine compartment is composed of the central follicular storage of thyroid hormone, which is the static moiety of this compartment. The dynamic portion of the compartment is the external follicular areas, which are close to the thyroidal cells. These are the areas where most of the synthesis and release of thyroid hormone takes place. The thyroid organic iodine pool actively secretes thyroid hormone into the extrathyroidal organic iodine compartment (Compartment III). The secretion rate of thyroid hormones is approximately 50 μg per 24-hour period.

Compartment III—extrathyroidal organic iodine pool. The extrathyroidal organic pool contains approximately 500 μg of iodine, which are distributed in a 10-liter space (about 14% of the body weight). By measurement the organic iodine in this pool is approximately 50 μg per liter; the extrathyroidal organic iodine pool is known as the protein-bound iodine pool. The extrathyroidal organic iodine pool is decreased in a 24-hour period by approximately 50μg, primarily because of thyroxine degradation. Approximately 25% of the iodine freed by thyroxine degradation is excreted in the feces. The remainder returns to the extrathyroidal iodide space.

Special clinical note. With this introductory understanding of the quantities of iodine in the various spaces, the reader will be able to recognize that if Lugol's solution, which contains 130,000 μg of iodine per milliliter (a 1,000-day supply of the iodine requirements), is introduced into the body, any study using an infinitesimal tracer dose of radioactive iodide will be invalidated. Another commonly used pharmaceutical, potassium iodide, contains 800,000 μg of iodine (a 20-year supply of the iodine requirements) in 1 ml. Obviously, the iodide pool would be greatly increased, and its specific activity would be reduced to exceedingly low levels. If the stable iodine uptake of the thyroid remains unchanged, the tracer radioactive iodide would be taken up in reduced amounts, since radioactive iodide is being used to measure the percentage of the iodine pool that is being trapped by the thyroid. If the total amount of iodide trapped in Compartment I is to be measured, it must be of normal size for these measurements to be of any value. If substances in which iodine is bound to an organic nucleus (such as compounds employed for urography, cholecystography, and opacification studies) are introduced into the bloodstream or intracavitary spaces, the tracer iodine studies will be influenced. In their original state these compounds would not influence thyroid function because the iodine is not ionized. However, these compounds undergo degradation when introduced into the body, and the iodine that is freed enters the iodide pool. The compounds can then disturb tracer studies for months or even years.

TESTS FOR ASSESSING TURNOVER OR RELEASE OF THYROIDAL IODINE
Thyroid accumulation of iodine (thyroid uptake of iodine)

The radioactive estimation of iodine accumulation by the thyroid is a dynamic study, which is directly related to the flow of iodide from Compartment I to Compartment II and the flow of organic iodine from Compartment II to Compartment III. Iodide leaves the extrathyroidal pool and enters the thyroid cell through an active metabolic process (the thyroid trapping mechanism) and thus enters the thyroid organic iodine pool and is involved in thyroxine synthesis. The thyroid clearance of iodide from the extrathyroidal pool is usually measured soon after ^{131}I or ^{123}I administration, and appropriate corrections for the extrathyroidal neck radioactivity are essential. Under normal circumstances the clearance of circulating thyroid is unidirectional, with iodide being actively transported into the gland so rapidly that the efflux of trapped iodide from the gland into the circulation is not appreciable. As mentioned previously, iodide is almost instantaneously organified; therefore, the accumulation of iodide is almost always the same as the thyroid rate of binding iodide.

The thyroid uptake of radioiodine should be done at varying time periods — from 2 to 24 hours after administration of the tracer dose. Normal values for euthyroid, hypothyroid, and hyperthyroid subjects should be individually established and correlated with the results obtained by other workers in the same geographic area.

Any gross increase or decrease in the iodide pool will invalidate the thyroid uptake measurement as a diagnostic entity. It must also be understood that in approximately 20% of the hyperthyroid patients, the secretion rate of organically bound iodine (thyroid hormones) is greatly increased. Therefore the iodide uptake, if it is done later than 6 hours after ingestion of iodide, will be falsely low. Likewise, earlier uptakes are more likely to be abnormal in hypothyroid patients because slow trapping of radioactive iodine in hypothyroidism will make the uptake closer to normal at 24 hours than at the shorter time period. Therefore it is strongly recommended that 2-hour and 24-hour uptakes be completed on every patient; in questionable cases, a 6-hour uptake should be obtained.

Radioiodide thyroid uptakes in today's medical practice are not as useful in the diagnosis of thyroid diseases as they were in the past because of multiplicity, ease of performance, and specificity of the thyroid in vitro tests in the prediction of thyroid status. [131]I delivers approximately 1 rad to the thyroid for each microcurie of ^{131}I administered to the patient, assuming a 15% thyroid accumulation. The radiation dose to the thyroid with uptake and imaging doses of ^{131}I is, in today's practice, not recommended. [123]I, which delivers approximately one hundredth the radiation dose of ^{131}I, is the recommended radioiodide. However, this cyclotron-produced nuclide is approximately 500 times the cost of [131]I. There is a small group of patients in whom iodide uptakes aid in diagnosis and therapy. Iodide uptakes are useful in patients with hyperthyroidism in which ^{131}I therapy is indicated and in patients with a defect in organification, that is, subacute thyroiditis, congenital organification defect, and chronic lymphocytic thyroiditis. Uptakes in this group of patients should be performed with [123]I.

Direct measurement of radioactive iodide release

If serial counts are taken after the accumulation of radioactive iodide by the thyroid gland, a direct measurement of organically bound radioactive iodide release may be obtained. So that the study will not be obscured by reaccumulation of radioactive iodide, the function of the patient's thyroid is blocked with an antithyroid agent. After this is done, the curve of thyroid counts will indicate the release of a constant fraction of thyroidal radioactive iodide per unit time. When corrected for physical decay of the isotope, the observations indicate a rate of turnover of accumulated radioactive iodide, which is accelerated in thyroid hyperfunction.

In vitro studies of thyroid function

Thyroxine is bound primarily in the globulin portion of plasma. However, three proteins that carry thyroxine have been identified: (1) thyroxine-binding prealbumin, which on electrophoresis has a mobility greater than that of serum albumin, (2) serum albumin, and (3) thyroxine-binding globulin, which on electrophoresis has a mobility intermediate between α_1 and α_2 globulin. Approximately 10% of thyroxine is associated with thyroxine-binding prealbumin; T_3 is bound primarily to thyroid-binding globulin and secondarily to serum albumin. However, it has been shown that the association is much looser than the corresponding thyroxine-protein complex. T_3 is not bound to thyroxine-binding prealbumin.

Thyroxine-binding globulin, which is the most important of the binding site for thyroxine, has a normal binding capacity ranging from 16 to 24 μg/100 ml. Thyroxine-binding globulin has a molecular weight of 59,000 and is probably a glycoprotein. Thyroxine-binding globulin is normally one-third saturated with thyroid hormone. The concentration of free thyroxine in normal human plasma is 0.01% to 0.04% of the total plasma thyroxine concentration and therefore is extremely difficult to measure by conventional chemical measurement.

SPECIAL PROCEDURES IN STUDY OF THYROID FUNCTION
In vitro tests of thyroid function

In clinical medicine many nonradioactive tests of thyroid function are used routinely. Therefore the student must have a general understanding of these tests and what the specific tests measure.

Protein-bound iodine. The protein-bound iodine test (Table 18-1) is simply a measure of the protein precipitable iodine or the organified iodine in the serum. This test measures the amount of T_4, T_3, iodinated dyes, thyroglobulin, and iodo-

Table 18-1. Factors that may increase or decrease T_3 uptake and protein-bound iodine values

Factor	Protein-bound iodine	T_3 uptake
Hyperthyroidism	Increased	Increased
Hypothyroidism	Decreased	Decreased
Inorganic iodides	Increased	No change
Contrast media containing iodine	Increased	No change
Estrogens (including oral contraceptives and pregnancy)	Increased	Decreased
Acidosis	No change	Increased
Cancer	No change	Increased
Subacute thyroiditis	Increased	Increased

protein in the blood. It therefore is an indirect study of organified iodide in the form of thyroid hormone. However, any iodine contamination will invalidate this particular study. The protein-bound iodine can be improved on slightly by a butanol extraction, which will remove the thyroglobulin, iodoprotein, and free iodide. However, even with the use of butanol extraction, contrast media such as iodinated dyes cannot be removed, and the studies will be invalidated.

Radioactive in vitro tests of thyroid function. Many procedures have been developed to assess the state of the thyroid hormone plasma protein interaction. The in vitro uptakes generally reflect a portion of hormone in serum that is free. Because of the intense binding of T_4 by plasma proteins, in vitro uptake values for labeled T_4 are usually quite low. Greater ease in counting is obtained when labeled T_3 is employed. The weaker binding of T_3 results in higher uptake values; therefore, T_3 is more practical than T_4 in in vitro testing.

Hamolsky and Freedberg developed the first in vitro tests of thyroid function. It was shown that if triiodothyronine labeled with ^{131}I was incubated with whole blood and the erythrocytes were then separated and washed, diagnosis could be drawn from the percent of the original labeled T_3 that remained fixed to the red blood cells. That is, the more saturated the binding protein is with thyroxine, the greater the quantity of the added radioactive T_3 available for absorption on the red cell. The T_3 in vitro test has been changed with replacement of the red cell by anion exchange resins; however, the basic principles are relatively the same. In hyperthyroidism the binding sites are more filled, and therefore a greater proportion of the added radioactive T_3 will be found unbound to the serum protein. In hypothyroidism the binding sites are not saturated and therefore the added radioactive T_3 will be bound to the available binding sites. Thus the results of the in vitro uptake studies will be relatively diagnostic. A large amount of unbound T_3 will occur in patients with hyperthyroidism, and decreased amounts will be found in patients with hypothyroidism. Values are greatly influenced by changes in the activity in the binding proteins as well as by changes in hormonal concentrations. For instance, estrogens increase the amount of binding sites available; therefore a greater amount of the added radioactive T_3 will be found on the binding sites, which will invalidate the test. It has also been found that this particular in vitro test is relatively accurate in the diagnosis of hyperthyroidism and relatively in-accurate for diagnosing hypothyroidism.

Measurement of T_4 by binding displacement. The method for measuring T_4 by binding displacement depends on the ability of increments of stable T_4 to progres-sively displace ^{125}I-labeled T_4 from thyroid-binding globulin. Ethanol, which dena-tures thyroxine-binding globulin (TBG), is added, releasing thyroxine into the serum. After centrifugation a sample of the supernatant that contains free T_4 is obtained, the ethanol is evaporated, and a known quantity of TBG with ^{125}I-labeled T_4 is added. The combination is incubated with a resin sponge. Since the stable T_4 will displace the labeled T_4 on TBG, it is then possible to calculate the amount of T_4 in the patient's serum using a standard curve of known concentra-tions of T_4. By knowing the total amount of thyroxine in the patient's blood, we have a better estimation of the patient's metabolic status. However, this test measures total thyroxine content that is effected by the quantity of binding globulin and, therefore, may not correlate with the true metabolic status.

Measurement of T_4 by RIA. Measurement of total serum thyroxine (bound and free) by radioimmunoassay obviates the separation of T_4 from its binding proteins, which was necessary in competitive binding assay and which induced a source of error in the measurement of T_4. The precision and reproducibility of the RIA method are comparable to competitive binding assay; however, the greater sensi-tivity of RIA allows for measurement of T_4 over a larger range.

Thyroxine is the predominant hormone secreted by the normal thyroid gland. In circulation 99.96% of T_4 is bound to thyroxine-binding proteins, the major pro-tein being thyroxine-binding globulin (TBG). A dynamic equilibrium exists be-tween the bound and free T_4, with only the free moiety being metabolically active.

Free thyroxine index (FT_4-T_7). Neither the T_3 uptake test nor T_4 test alone gives totally adequate information about the patient's thyroid status. To compensate for the inability of either test alone to adequately reflect thyroid status, the test results are multiplied to yield a calculated numerical value (free thyroxine index, or FTI) that reflects more accurately the thyroid status than either test alone. It has been found that this calculated numerical value approximates clinically the measured level of free thyroxine in approximately 96% of patients studied.

When the T_3 uptake test and T_4 test results are both outside the normal ranges but in the opposite direction, the FTI is normal and the patient is euthyroid. When both tests are abnormal in the same direction, the FTI is also abnormal and the patient is hypothyroid or hyperthyroid. A high T_3 uptake test combined with a low T_4 level would indicate a low TBG level, and a low T_3 uptake test combined with a high T_4 level would indicate a high TBG level.

Those diseases associated with elevated T_3 secretions (T_3 toxicosis or subclin-ical hypothyroidism) obviously will need further evaluation for correct diagnosis.

Free thyroxine concentration measurements. The concentration of free thyrox-ine and free triiodothyronine in serum is measured by enriching serum with a very low concentration of ^{125}I-labeled T_4 and ^{125}I-labeled T_3 to determine the proportion of endogenous hormone that is free to cross a semipermeable membrane. These small quantities of free hormones may also be measured by radioimmunoassay. Normally, the proportion of free thyroxine in serum is no more than approximately 0.01% to 0.04% of the total amount of thyroxine and 0.23% to 0.47% of the total amount of triiodothyronine. Obviously, increased concentration of the thyroid hormones in serum is found in hyperthyroidism, but high values may also be obtained if there is decreased binding by the binding proteins.

Measurement of T_3 by RIA. In the circulation, T_4 is present in concentration approximately 50 times higher (μg/100ml) than T_3 (ng/100ml). Therefore, the assay of T_3 concentration was not practical until the radioimmunoassay of T_3 became available. T_3 at the peripheral tissue level possesses several times greater potency than T_4. T_3 is cleared from the blood much more rapidly than T_4 and approximately two thirds of the T_3 measured at any time is obtained from the peripheral tissue conversion from T_4. The thyroid, economically, when under stress, will also produce and secrete T_3 in preference to T_4. Therefore, T_3 is, for all practical purposes, the primary metabolically active thyroid hormone.

T_3 measurements are useful in establishing the diagnosis of T_3 toxicosis. This is a hyperthyroid state in which the serum T_4 level is in the normal range, however, the T_3 level has become elevated. This is seen in early Graves' hyperthyroidism and frequently in Plummer's Disease (autonomous nodule). In assessing thyroid residual function after administration of TRH or TSH, a normal mean increase in T_3 levels in 105% whereas the T_4 levels increase 41% during the same period of time. Therefore, in the hypothyroid patient or the patient with low thyroid reserve, the T_3 measurement (unless the thyroid gland is grossly damaged) will be in the normal range.

Medications affecting the T_3 and T_4 tests. Following is a partial list of drugs that can affect the T_3 and T_4 tests. Knowledge of administration of medications to the patient is essential for correct interpretation of test results.

Drugs that elevate T_3 test results

Salicylates
Warfarin (Coumadin) derivatives
Phenytoin
Halofenate
Heparin
Liotrix
Anabolic steroids
Phenylbutazone
Thyroid
TSH
Androgens
Penicillin

Drugs that decrease T_3 test results

Estrogens
Diazepam
Chlordiazepoxide
Lithium
Methimazole
Propylthiouracil
Iodides
Thiazide diuretics
Perphenazine
Clofibrate
Epinephrine

Drugs that elevate T₄ test results

Estrogens	TSH
Thyroid	Sulfamethoxazole
Levodopa	

Drugs that decrease T₄ test results

Salicylates	Ethionamide
Chlorpromazine	Heparin
Chlorpropamide	Iodides
Cholestyramine	Triiodothyronine (T₃)
Adrenocorticotropic	Lithium
hormone (ACTH)	Antithyroid drugs
Prednisone	Reserpine
Dinitrophenol	Sulfonamides
Phenytoin	Tolbutamide

Measurement of TSH by RIA. The secretion of thyrotropin-stimulating hormone (TSH) regulates the circulating thyroid hormone concentration whose free component at the cell level in turn regulates TSH secretion. TSH secretion is also regulated by the hypothalamic factor known as the thyrotropin-releasing hormone (TRH). TSH radioimmunoassay measurements of TSH in plasma or serum are valuable in assessing quantitatively the role of TSH in the maintenance of thyroid secretion and the affect of thyroid hormones on its secretion. With the availability of injectable synthetic TRH, the TSH assay has gained prominence as a diagnostic test in various thyroid disorders. Plasma TSH concentrations are low or undetectable in hyperthyroidism and are elevated in hypothyroidism or low thyroid reserve states. The TSH level is of great utility in managing the thyroid replacement therapy of hypothyroid patients.

TRH test. After the administration (intravenous) of synthetic TRH, TSH levels remain unchanged in patients with hyperthyroidism and hypopituitarism. TSH levels rise moderately in normal patients and slowly in patients with hypothalamic lesions, and there is an exaggerated response in patients with hypothyroidism of primary thyroid etiology.

The TRH test is valuable in:

1. Confirming the diagnosis of primary hypothyroidism or incipient primary hypothyroidism (low thyroid reserve)
2. Differentiating primary and secondary hypothyroidism
3. Differentiating pituitary and hypothalmic causes of hypothyroidism
4. Establishing the diagnosis of pituitary TSH suppression by thyroid hormones

DISEASES OF THYROID

To understand why the physician should want so many tests to study a small 20- to 35-gm organ, the student will have to understand both the importance of the thyroid gland to the body's metabolism and how diseases that affect the thyroid can have far-reaching metabolic effects in the human body. It is obvious that since there are so many tests to study the thyroid, no single test will give the clinician a definitive answer as to the thyroid status of the patient. The thyroid uptake test is used only to study how much radioiodine is found in the thyroid gland at given time intervals. The in vitro T_3 test is an indirect study of the thyroid hormone–binding proteins, and even the direct assessment of free thyroxine may lead to an erroneous diagnosis if the patient's thyroid hormone–binding proteins are abnormal in quantity or quality. Therefore a discussion of all the ramifications of the results of these tests, as well as a discussion of thyroid diseases, is necessary.

Hyperthyroidism

An excess of free thyroid hormone has a direct effect on the metabolic rate of the patient. Therefore with an excess of free thyroid hormone the patient becomes hypermetabolic. Hyperthyroidism is a relatively common disease and may be roughly broken down into two distinct entities: (1) Graves' disease and (2) Plummer's disease. The following outline gives the symptoms and the pathophysiology for each.

> Graves' disease
>> Signs and symptoms
>>> Diffuse thyroid enlargement (goiter)
>>> Hypermetabolism
>>> Exophthalmopathy
>>> Dermopathy (pretibial myxedema)
>> Pathophysiology
>>> Semiautonomous thyroid tissue (may still be responsive to TSH)
>>> Long-acting thyroid substance (LATS)
>>> Absent plasma levels of TSH
>>> Increased serum levels of thyroxine, triiodothyronine
>> Etiology—unknown
> Plummer's disease
>> Signs and symptoms
>>> Nodular thyroid enlargement
>>> Hypermetabolism
>> Pathophysiology
>>> Autonomous nodularity (normal areas of thyroid tissue may persist)
>>> Absent levels of TSH
>>> Increased serum levels of thyroxine, triiodothyronine
>> Etiology—unknown

Graves' disease. Graves' disease is usually characterized by diffuse, smooth thyroid enlargement and hypermetabolism. The majority of patients with Graves' disease will have exophthalmopathy and dermopathy. The dermopathy usually takes the form of pretibial myxedema, which is a pale, nonpitting swelling in the tibial areas.

Generally the patient will have increased serum levels of thyroxine and decreased plasma levels of TSH. In the majority of cases, long-acting thyroid stimulator substance (LATS) may be found. LATS has been found to be a 7S gamma globulin; therefore, it is probably an antibody. Thus this form of hyperthyroidism may have an immunologic basis. It has been shown that LATS does stimulate the human thyroid. However, LATS probably has no relationship to the ophthalmopathy of Graves' disease. The thyroid tissue of Graves' disease appears to be stimulated by LATS and in the early stages of the disease may be further stimulated by TSH. However, in hyperthyroid Graves' disease, endogenous TSH release is suppressed by the high tissue levels of free T_3 and T_4.

Graves' disease is of uncertain etiology, and approximately 50% of the patients with this disease may have spontaneous remissions. This disease occurs in persons of all age groups. Although classically patients have obvious signs of hypermetabolism, there are many in the younger as well as in the elderly groups who have few, if any, signs of hypermetabolism. Graves' disease is extremely protean. Classically, the patient with Graves' disease will have extreme nervousness, fatigue, weight loss, proximal muscle wasting, protrusion of the eyes, heat intolerance, and a wasting-away of the nail beds. Many of the patients will have pretibial myxedema.

The majority of patients with hypermetabolic Graves' disease are treated with therapy doses of radioactive iodide. Younger patients may be treated with antithyroid drugs (propylthiouracil, Tapazole); however, approximately 50% of these patients go on to develop recurrent Graves' disease. Surgery may be utilized (subtotal thyroidectomy); however, there may be surgical morbidity and possibly recurrence of Graves' disease. The only true contraindications of radioiodide therapy are in pregnant women and nursing mothers.

Plummer's disease. Patients with Plummer's disease may be hypermetabolic and have solitary or multiple nodules in the thyroid. These nodules are autonomous and are not under pituitary control. Decreased serum levels of TSH and increased levels of T_3 and possibly T_4 are found when the patient is hyperthyroid.

The etiology of Plummer's disease is unknown. Since Plummer's disease is a nodular autonomous disease, the therapy of this particular form of hyperthyroidism is different from that for Graves' disease. Patients with Plummer's disease do not have circulating LATS; therefore, this form of hyperthyroidism is different from that of Graves' disease.

Hypothyroidism

The signs and symptoms of hypothyroidism are all related to hypometabolism, which is caused by decreased tissue levels of thyroid hormone. In all patients except those with pituitary failure, increased serum levels of TSH and decreased serum levels of thyroxine are found. Following is an outline of the symptoms, pathophysiology, and etiologies of hypothyroidism.

Signs and symptoms
Hypometabolism

Pathophysiology
    Increased serum TSH level in all except pituitary failure
    Decreased serum levels of thyroxine, triiodothyronine
Etiology
    Iodine deficiency
    Iatrogenic
        Iodine 131 therapy
        Antithyroid therapy
        Surgery
    Inborn error of metabolism (trapping iodide through secretion of thyroxine)
    Inflammatory (thyroiditis)
        Bacterial
        Viral
        Autoimmune

The etiologies of hypothyroidism are varied. Many cases of hypothyroidism in children are of the inherited enzyme defect type. In the baby and child, hypothyroidism is severe. The baby born hypothyroid is called a *cretin* and has a very definite lethargic appearance, potbelly, and enlargement of the tongue. Physical and mental growth and development are severely retarded.

Hypothyroidism in the adult may be secondary to iodine deficiency. However, since iodized salt is used throughout the world, iodine deficiency is much less common than it was formerly. There is a large group of patients who have inborn errors of metabolism. These adults have a very slow onset of hypothyroidism, and the defect may be found anywhere from the trapping of iodide through the secretion of thyroid hormone. The patient with an inborn error of metabolism of thyroid hormone production usually has an enlarged thyroid (a goiter), and the patient with pituitary failure will have no palpable thyroid.

Another major cause of hypothyroidism is inflammatory disease of the thyroid (thyroiditis). The inflammatory process may be bacterial, viral, or autoimmune. Autoimmune disease is being recognized more frequently. In patients with autoimmune thyroiditis, there is a process of immunization against the body's own protein (in this case protein derived from the thyroid) and the body's reaction causes the thyroiditis.

Hypothyroidism may also occur secondary to ^{131}I therapy or to medical therapy of hyperthyroidism. It may also be caused by surgical ablation of the thyroid. A rare cause of hypothyroidism is pituitary failure or insufficient secretion of thyrotropine-releasing factor by the hypothalamus.

True myxedema, which is the end stage of hypothyroidism, is fairly easy for the physician to recognize. However, the lesser forms of hypothyroidism are much more difficult to recognize. The classic myxedematous patient is extremely pale, has puffy facies and obvious fluid retention, and is lethargic. Few studies are necessary to make a diagnosis. However, other signs of hypometabolism, such as excessive tiredness, fatigability, and irritability, are common signs and symptoms of anxiety. Therefore, there is always a large group of patients under study for possible hypometabolism. If hypothyroidism is proved, exogenous thyroid replacement therapy is indicated, regardless of the cause of the hypometabolism.

The adequacy of the thyroid replacement therapy is monitored by following the blood levels of TSH (RIA). The TSH (RIA) level that is elevated in hypothyroidism will fall into the normal range when the patient is on adequate thyroid replacement.

THYROID SCANNING WITH RADIONUCLIDES

Imaging and/or scanning of the thyroid is performed (1) to estimate the site, size, and shape of the thyroid gland, (2) to define visually whether all or part of the thyroid is functional and/or nonfunctional, or for both reasons. A combination of both purposes is usually involved when the physician sends the patient for a thyroid scan, after an abnormality in the thyroid gland has been palpated. The various disease states associated with an enlargement of the thyroid gland are as follows:

1. Decreased iodine intake
2. Goitrogenic agents
3. Familial goiter (usually produced by intrathyroidal organification defects)
4. Hashimoto's struma, chronic thyroiditis, lymphadenoid goiter, autoimmune thyroiditis
5. Subacute thyroiditis
6. Graves' disease
7. Autonomous nodular thyroid disease (Plummer's disease)
8. Carcinoma

The relationships involved in the pituitary thyroid axis explain why many of the disease states listed would increase the size of the thyroid by interfering with the usual thyroid pituitary relationships. For example, if there were a decreased intake of iodine by the patient, there would be an increased output by the pituitary

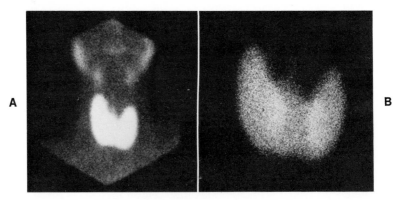

Fig. 18-8. Abnormal pinhole thyroid image 20 minutes after 10-mCi dose of ^{99m}Tc pertechnetate. Diagnosis: Graves' disease. A, Image encompasses mandibular-neck region. There is gross increased concentration of nuclide as compared to the salivary gland in a markedly enlarged thyroid gland. B, Pinhole image of the thyroid reveals marked increase in the size of the gland. The intensity was decreased to visualize evenness of distribution.

of thyroid-stimulating hormone, and this would cause physical enlargement of the thyroid gland. In familial goiter a similar process takes place because of various biochemical defects in the thyroid; there is decreased output of thyroxine and an increased stimulation of thyroid-stimulating hormone. In chronic thyroiditis the gland enlarges partially because of its decreased output of thyroxine, but also because of growth of replacement tissue caused by the destruction of the thyroid gland. It is obvious that cancer would cause disruption of the thyroid gland and enlargement of all or part of the area palpated as thyroid tissue. It is also true that various thyroid carcinomas will metabolize iodine when they metastasize. Therefore metastatic disease of the thyroid can sometimes be evaluated by radioiodine scanning.

In Graves' disease and Plummer's disease, enlargement of the thyroid gland is not under thyroid-stimulating hormone control (Fig. 18-8).

Radionuclides used in thyroid scanning and imaging

The most common radiopharmaceuticals used in thyroid scanning are ^{99m}Tc (in the form of pertechnetate), ^{131}I, ^{125}I, and ^{123}I. Pertechnetate localizes in the iodide-trapping mechanism of the acinar cell and therefore does not give information about organification, storage, or hormone release functions of the thyroid gland, which the iodide radionuclides demonstrate.

Radiopharmaceutical parameters

The differences between ^{99m}Tc pertechnetate imaging and that of ^{123}I (or other iodide radionuclides) are very important in diagnosis (Fig. 18-9). ^{99m}Tc pertechnetate localizes in the acinar cell of the thyroid and iodide radionuclides are organified in the thyroid follicle. In destructive diseases of the thyroid functional unit

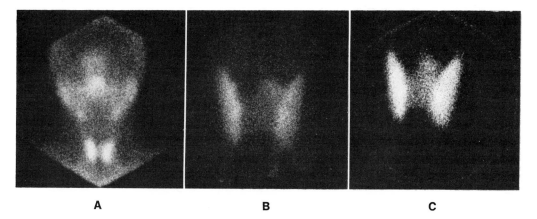

A   **B**   **C**

Fig. 18-9. Abnormal pinhole thyroid images 20 minutes after 10-mCi dose of ^{99m}Tc pertechnetate and 6 hours after 200-μCi dose of ^{123}I. **A,** Image encompasses mandibular-neck region. **B,** Image reveals enlargement of the pyramidal lobe with normal distribution in both lobes. **C,** ^{123}I image 6 hours after dose reveals normal distribution in both lobes and the enlarged pyramidal lobe.

(such as carcinoma), organification is lost; however, the acinar cell may still retain its iodide accumulation ability—pertechnetate localization. Therefore, a carcinoma may have ^{99m}Tc pertechnetate localization and be visualized as "functional" tissue. Approximately 4% of carcinomas do accumulate ^{99m}Tc pertechnetate. Therefore, when a nodule accumulates ^{99m}Tc pertechnetate the image should be repeated with an iodide radionuclide. All intrathyroidal carcinomas are "cold" (nonfunctional) on radioiodide imaging. Conversely a nodule that is cold with ^{99m}Tc pertechnetate will be predictably cold on radioiodide imaging.

The recommended iodide nuclide for imaging is ^{123}I since the radiation dose absorbed by the thyroid when ^{123}I is used is approximately one hundredth that of ^{131}I for the appropriate imaging dose of the two radioiodide nuclides.

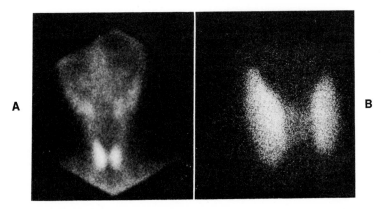

Fig. 18-10. Normal pinhole thyroid image 20 minutes after 10-mCi dose of ^{99m}Tc pertechnetate. **A,** Image encompasses mandibular-neck region. Note the thyroid concentration of technetium is greater than the salivary gland accumulation. This is equivalent to a normal 24-hour radioiodine uptake. **B,** Pinhole image of the thyroid reveals even concentration of nuclide throughout both lobes of the thyroid.

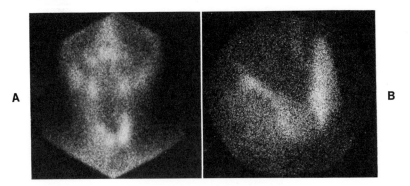

Fig. 18-11. Abnormal pinhole thyroid image 20 minutes after 10-mCi dose of ^{99m}Tc pertechnetate. Diagnosis: papillary carcinoma. **A,** Image encompasses mandibular-neck region. There is markedly decreased concentration in the right lobe of the thyroid. **B,** There is a large 3 × 4 cm cold nodule compressing functional right lobe tissue across the midline. By palpation this area was hard.

Normal thyroid image

Normal thyroid images (Fig. 18-10) have an even distribution of the radioisotope throughout the area of the thyroid gland. The isthmus is so thin that it is poorly delineated on most thyroid images; however, the lobes can be visualized well. With today's instrumentation, the pyramidal lobe is seen frequently, and, since the embryologic as well as the adult anatomy of the thyroid is understood, tissue that could be found at the base of the tongue will be picked up on a thyroid scan, as would a thyroid in the mediastinum, where it is occasionally found. Aberrant thyroid tissue is found infrequently; however, aberrant thyroid tissue can be found both in the neck and in the abdomen. The thyroid tissue in the abdomen is usually found in female patients where it is associated with the ovaries.

Imaging of abnormal thyroid

All thyroids that are imaged should be palpated before, during, and after the procedure so that the radionuclide localization of the scan can be correlated with what is palpated by the referring and consulting physician.

Nonfunctioning areas of the thyroid are called *cold* areas; functioning areas are called *hot* areas. With an understanding of collimation, the student can readily see that the same problems encountered in imaging other organs are present in thyroid scanning. If an area is either hot or cold, there is little difficulty in performing the study. However, if there is functioning tissue between a cold area and the detector or in the field of resolution of the detector, there are no longer black and white guidelines. Therefore the thyroid, as well as other organs, should be imaged in various positions to clearly delineate whether a palpable mass is nonfunctioning or has some functional tissue residing in the area.

Cold nodule. It has been found through long experience that 25% of the cold nodules (Fig. 18-11) are malignant. Therefore physicians place much emphasis on the patient who is found to have a solitary nodule by palpation. It is also known that when there are multiple cold nodules in the thyroid, as well as multiple areas of nodularity, the incidence of malignancy decreases sharply. The cold nodules may be thyroid adenomas, cysts, degenerated areas, areas of hemorrhage, or areas of lymphoid infiltration. A cold nodule in the thyroid may also be caused by metastatic disease from another primary site.

Recently it has been shown that there is an increased incidence of thyroid carcinoma in patients who have received radiation therapy to the head and neck region. In the second quarter of this century, inflammatory diseases (tonsillitis, ear infections, acne) and benign problems (enlarged thymus) were treated with external radiation. In this decade it has been recognized that the risk of thyroid carcinoma increased many fold in this group of patients and increases with time. This group is now being screened with thyroid imaging to determine which patients should have surgical exploration (those with nonfunctional thyroid nodules) and which should have thyroid suppressive therapy with exogenous thyroid medication. The at risk population that has had external radiation to the head and neck

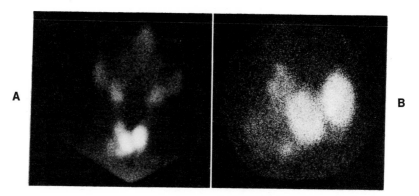

Fig. 18-12. Abnormal pinhole thyroid image 20 minutes after 10-mCi dose of ^{99m}Tc pertechnetate. Diagnosis: Graves' disease superimposed on Hashimoto's disease. **A,** Image encompasses mandibular-neck region. There is marked increased concentration in multiple nodules relative to the concentration in the salivary glands, which would be the equivalent of an elevated ^{131}I 24-hour thyroid uptake. The ^{131}I 24-hour uptake was 54%. **B,** Pinhole image of the thyroid reveals multiple hot nodules in the left and right lobes with hypofunctional nodules primarily in the right lobe.

should be followed on a regular basis for their lifetime with repalpation of the thyroid and neck region.

Hot nodule. Hot nodules are almost always benign. The hot nodule has significance when it leads to the diagnosis of autonomous nodular thyroid disease, as in Plummer's disease.

Thyroid imaging of a hot nodule is interesting because the patient usually has a solitary palpable nodule that is found on scan to be hyperfunctional, and the remainder of the gland is nonfunctional. In these patients the thyroid hormone put out out by the autonomous nodule is enought to shut off the normal pituitary thyroid relationship. The amount of thyroid hormone put out by the autonomous nodule may be enough to make the patient hyperthyroid. However, the patient may be found to be euthyroid or hypothyroid.

Mixed lesions in thyroid (Fig. 18-12). It is obvious that there can be all gradations of abnormality in the thyroid, which will cause varying degrees in concentration of the radionuclide. When the diagnostician has gained experience, he or she may be able to infer certain diagnoses by palpatory findings in relation to the differing concentrations of the radionuclide on the thyroid scan. However, a definitive diagnosis is usually made only by biopsy and by pathologic examination.

ULTRASONOGRAPHY OF THE THYROID GLAND

Gray scale thyroid ultrasonography differentiates a cystic from a solid mass in the thyroid. Since in both cases the radionuclide image will demonstrate a cold, space-occupying lesion, ultrasound evaluation would be the next step in noninvasive investigation. Ultrasound waves pass through cystic lesions with ease, and in partially solid or solid lesions, sound waves will be reflected and/or attenuated. A thyroid cyst is almost always benign and therefore can be aspirated or treated surgically in a conservative manner (Fig. 18-13).

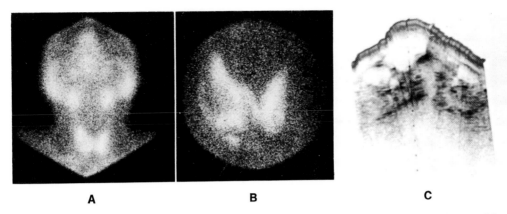

| **A** | **B** | **C** |

Fig. 18-13. Abnormal pinhole thyroid image 20 minutes after 10-mCi dose of ^{99m}Tc pertechnetate. Diagnosis: benign cysts. **A**, Image encompasses mandibular-neck region. There is an irregularity in concentration of nuclide in lateral right lobe. **B**, Pinhole image reveals a 2.5-cm palpable cold nodule in the lateral right lobe with irregular concentration of nuclide in the inferior right lobe and inferolateral left lobe. **C**, B-mode gray scale ultrasound evaluation utilizing a MHZ transducer. The lesion is to the left (images are displayed as if viewed from the feet) on this sagittal section of the neck. Note that the lesion is 2.5 cm in diameter (marker through lesion) and is sonolucent (no internal echoes) and that tissue behind the lesion has increased echogenicity (increased sound transmission through a cystic lesion). This patient had benign cysts of the thyroid.

SPECIAL STUDIES OF THYROID FUNCTION AND SCANNING

Thyroid stimulation tests and suppression tests have been developed to help the diagnostician come to a definitive diagnosis. Since the introduction of TSH (RIA) and TRH tests, these tests are infrequently used. The methodology of the best-known tests follows.

I. Suppression tests
    A. Werner's suppression test
    B. Modified suppression test
        1. A baseline 24-hour RAIU is performed.
        2. Triiodothyronine, 75 μg, q.i.d., is given for 2 days, followed by 25 μg q.i.d. on days 3 and 4.
        3. Residual activity is measured; repeat 24-hour RAIU between days 3 and 4.
        4. If inadequate suppression is induced, T_3 is continued through day 8.
        5. Residual activity is measured, and a third 24-hour RAIU is given between days 8 and 9.
II. Stimulation test (TSH)
    A. Use
        1. Differentiation of primary thyroid failure from hypothyroidism associated with pituitary hyposecretion
        2. Diagnosis of type of myxedema (primary or pituitary)
    B. Procedure
        1. A baseline 24-hour RAIU and a T_3 (RIA) and T_4 are performed.
        2. Thyrotropin, 5 units, is given intramuscularly.
        3. Twenty-four hours after the thyrotropin injection and following a count of residual activity in the gland, a second injection of TSH is administered, followed by a tracer dose of ^{131}I, and a 24-hour RAIU is completed the following day (48 hours after injection of TSH).

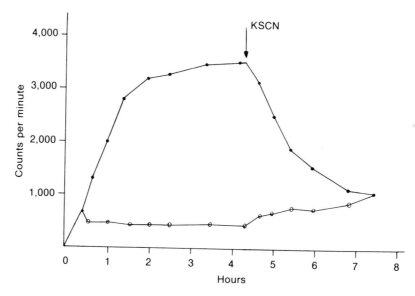

Fig. 18-14. Potassium thiocyanate (KSCN) release test revealing a defect in organification of iodide.

    4. A second PBI is obtained 48 hours after the TSH injection.

    5. T_3 (RIA) and T_4 (RIA) are obtained.

III. Stimulation test (TRH)

    A. Basal levels of T_3 (RIA) and TSH (RIA) are established.

    B. TRH, 400 μg, is administered intravenously through indwelling catheter.

    C. T_3 (RIA) and TSH (RIA) concentrations are measured at 10, 20, 30, 60, 120, and 180 minutes.

    Both the stimulating and the suppression tests will give physiologic information and may also give anatomic information to the physician. In the case of TSH stimulation, the physician may want to see whether there is tissue in the neck that cannot be palpated or whether nonfunctional tissue as seen on an initial scan is still nonfunctional tissue after administration of TSH. The suppression study is generally used by a physician to identify autonomous thyroid tissue, which is found in both Graves' disease and Plummer's disease. It is used particularly for scanning a patient with a nodular thyroid, when the physician would like to know whether a nodule can be suppressed or not.

    The TRH test is a very sensitive method of establishing pituitary (TSH) integrity and judging the ability of the thyroid to produce and release triiodothyronine. Failure to elevate the T_3 level more than 23% is a better indication of early thyroid failure than the TSH stimulation test.

    The physician may have a basic interest in intrathyroidal biochemical disturbances, such as may be found in congenital goiters. One test that is used to define one aspect of this disease process is the potassium thiocyanate discharge study, which is illustrated in Fig. 18-14. Since potassium thiocynate blocks the iodide-trapping mechanism, if the patient has any defect in organification, nonorganified iodide will return through the cell wall back into the patient's vascular system.

Finally, the ^{99m}Tc pertechnetate thyroid accumulation test may be used to evaluate thyroid function. Since pertechnetate lodges in the iodide-trapping mechanism, the 20-minute concentration of ^{99m}Tc pertechnetate in the thyroid has been shown to correlate with thyroid function. Because only approximately 4% of the administered dose is found in the thyroid, this test is best done with the scintillation camera with some computer capability.

BIBLIOGRAPHY

Astwood, E., and Cassidy, C.: Clinical endocrinology, New York, 1968, Grune & Stratton, Inc., vol. 2.

Beeson, P. B., and McDermott, W.: Cecil-Lobe textbook in medicine, ed. 12, Philadelphia, 1967, W. B. Saunders Co.

Brown, J., and others: Thyroid physiology in health and disease, Ann. Intern. Med. **81**:68-81, 1974.

Deland, F. H., and Wagner, H. N.: Atlas of nuclear medicine. R. E. S. Liver, spleen and thyroid, Philadelphia, 1972, W. B. Saunders Co. vol. 3.

Hollander, C. S., and others: Clinical and laboratory observations in cases of triiodothyronine toxicosis confirmed by radioimmunoassay, Lancet **1**:609-611, 1972.

Marsden, P., and others: Hormonal pattern of relapse in hyperthyroidism, Lancet L (7913): 944-949, 1975.

Stock, J. M., Surks, M. I., and Oppenheimer, J. H.: Replacement dosage of L-Thyroxine in hypothyroidism: a re-evaluation, N. Engl. J. Med. **290** (10): 529-533, 1974.

Werner, R. H.: Textbook of endocrinology, ed. 4, Philadelphia, 1968, W. B. Saunders Co.

GENERAL BIBLIOGRAPHY

Ashkar, F. S., Miale, A., and Smoak, W.: A general guide to nuclear medicine, Springfield, Ill., 1975, Charles C Thomas, Publisher.

Best, C., and Taylor, N. B.: Physiological basis of medical practice, ed. 10, Baltimore, 1979, The Williams & Wilkins Co.

Blahd, W. H.: Nuclear medicine, ed. 2, New York, 1971, McGraw-Hill Book Co.

Deland, F. H., and Wagner, H. N.: Atlas of nuclear medicine, Philadelphia, 1969, W. B. Saunders Co., vol. 1.

Freeman, L. M., and Blaufax, M. D.: Physicians desk reference for radiology and nuclear medicine, Oradell, N. J., 1977-1978, Medical Economics Co.

Freeman, L. M., and Johnson, P. M.: Clinical scintillation scanning, New York, 1975, Grune & Stratton, Inc.

Grant, J. C. B., and Basmajian, J. V.: A method of anatomy, ed. 7, Baltimore, 1965, The Williams & Wilkins Co.

Gross, C. M.: Gray's anatomy of the human body, ed. 28, Philadelphia, 1966, Lea & Febiger.

Guyton, A. C.: Textbook of medical physiology, ed. 3, Philadelphia, 1966, W. B. Saunders Co.

Ham, A. W.: Histology, Philadelphia, 1957, J. B. Lippincott Co.

Holvey, D. N.: The Merck manual of diagnosis and therapy, ed. 12, Rahway, N.J., 1972, Merck Sharp & Dohme Research Lab.

Jacob, S. W., and Francone, C. A.: Structure and function in man, ed. 2, Philadelphia, 1970, W. B. Saunders Co.

Maynard, C. D.: Clinical nuclear medicine, Philadelphia, 1969, Lea & Febiger.

Powsner, E. R., and Raiside, D. E.: Diagnostic nuclear medicine, New York, 1971, Grune & Stratton, Inc.

Rhodes, B. A., editor: Quality control in nuclear medicine: radiopharmaceuticals, instrumentation, and in vitro assays, St. Louis, 1977, The C. V. Mosby Co.

Shtassel, P.: Speak to me in nuclear medicine, New York, 1976, Harper & Row, Publishers.

Silver, S.: Radioactive nuclides in medicine & biology — medicine, Philadelphia, 1968, Lea & Febiger.

Wagner, H. N.: Principles of nuclear medicine, Philadelphia, 1968, W. B. Saunders Co.

Wagner, H. N.: Nuclear medicine, New York, 1975, HP Publishing, Co.

19 Brain

ANATOMY AND PHYSIOLOGY

The nervous system together with the endocrine system controls the functions of the body. The nervous system controls the rapid activities of the body, which include muscular contraction, perception of changing visual events, and the secretion rates of endocrine glands. The nervous system is the computer of the body; it receives thousands of bits of information from the internal and external environments and integrates all of them to determine the response to be made by the body. The nervous system is usually described as having a sensory division and a motor division. The cerebral cortex integrates the body's higher functions; most of the cerebral cortex is located in the cerebral hemispheres.

Cerebral hemispheres

The twin cerebral hemispheres, which make up a large portion of the brain, are separated by the longitudinal cerebral fissure (Fig. 19-1). The falx cerebri, an extension of the dura mater, projects into the longitudinal cerebral fissure. The cerebral hemispheres have dorsolateral, medial, and basal surfaces, which contain many grooves or furrows known as *fissures* and *sulci*. The part of the brain that lies between the grooves is known as *convolutions*, or *gyri*. The cerebral hemispheres are divided into four lobes: frontal, parietal, occipital, and temporal. The lateral cerebral fissure (fissure of Sylvius) separates the temporal from the frontal lobe. The central sulcus (fissure of Rolando) separates the frontal lobe from the parietal lobe; the parietal occipital fissure passes along the medial surface of the posterior portion of the cerebral hemisphere dividing the parietal from the occipital lobe. The cerebral cortex has an area of approximately 220,000 mm^2, and not more than one third of this area lies on the free surface or crown of the convolutions. The total number of the nerve cells in the human cerebral cortex has been estimated at between 7×10^9 and 14×10^9. There are approximately 200 million nerve fibers that are received from and projected to the lower levels of the nervous system. Many times this number of fibers associates the cells within the cortex.

Functions. The functions of the four lobes can be grossly subdivided as follows. The posterior portion of the frontal lobe, the so-called prefrontal cortex of man, affects the motor system. This posterior portion is called the *motor cortex*, and it controls discrete voluntary movements of skeletal muscles. (The right side

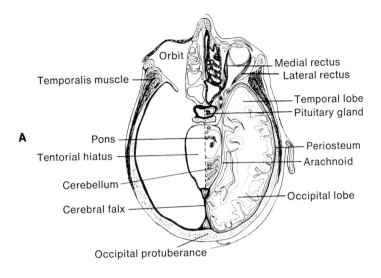

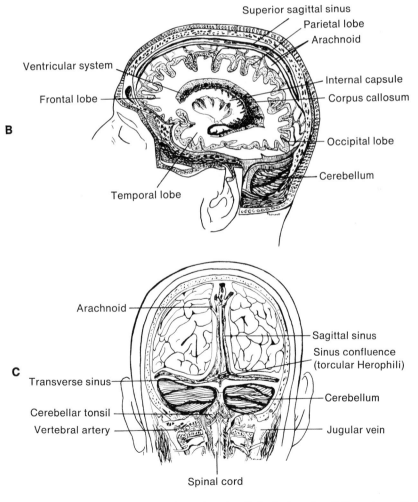

Fig. 19-1. Cerebral hemispheres. **A,** Horizontal section. **B,** Sagittal section. **C,** Posterior section.

of the motor cortex controls the left side of the body and vice versa.) The parietal lobe receives the somatic sensory messages, and separate parts of the body are represented in a pattern closely resembling that of the adjacent motor cortex. The parietal lobe is also the part of the brain that receives sensations of stereoperception and can discriminate between differences in weight, texture, and position. The temporal lobe contains the cortical representation for hearing and is necessary to recognize and organize language. The occipital lobe's function is entirely related to vision. The nerve fibers that emanate or end in the cerebral cortex cross in the brain stem; therefore, lesions of the left cerebral cortex are recognized peripherally in the opposite extremities.

Basal ganglia

The basal ganglia are masses of gray matter situated deep within the cerebral hemispheres. These ganglia exert important regulating and controlling influences on motor integration, in addition to relaying messages to the cerebral cortex. This area of the brain may also inhibit somatic reactions initiated by the cerebral cortex.

Thalamus and hypothalamus

The thalamus is a large ovoid gray mass located on either side of the third ventricle. It is crucial for the perception of some types of sensations. The hypothalamus lies below or ventral to the thalamus and forms a floor and part of the inferior and lateral walls of the third ventricle. This small area of the brain has diversified activities. The hypothalamus has a stimulatory control over many of the hormonal activities of the pituitary gland.

Cerebellum

The cerebellum is located in the posterior fossa of the skull behind the pons and medulla and is separated from the overlying cerebrum by an extension of the dura mater, the tentorium cerebri. The surface of the cerebellum, as does the surface of the cerebrum, has many sulci in furrows. The cerebellum is composed of a small, unpaired medium portion of the vermis and two large lateral masses, the cerebellar hemispheres.

Functions. The cerebellum controls individual orientation in space and the antigravity muscles of the body. The nerve fibers that emanate from and end on one side of the cerebellum control that same side of the body (ipsilateral control).

Medulla oblongata

The medulla oblongata is a pyramid-shaped portion of the brain stem located between the spinal cord and the pons. The dorsal portion of the upper half forms the floor of the body of the fourth ventricle. The majority of the so-called cranial nerves have their primary nuclei in this portion of the brain. The cranial nerves are listed in Table 19-1. Since most of them have very specific functions, they can be easily learned and remembered and are useful in the localization of neurologic lesions in patients.

Spinal cord

The spinal cord, which traverses the vertebral column, consists of 31 symmetrically arranged pairs of spinal nerves, each derived from the spinal cord by two roots, a sensory root and a motor root. The nerves can be divided topographically into eight cervical pairs, 12 thoracic pairs, five lumbar pairs, five sacral pairs,

Table 19-1. Cranial nerves

Nerve	*Component*	*Course*	*Peripheral termination*
Abducens	Somatic motor	Under pons, into orbit	Rectus lateralis
Accessory	Branchial motor	Side of neck	Sternocleidomastoid
Facial	Branchial motor	Temporal bone, side of face	Muscles of expression, hyoid elevators
	Visceral motor	1. Greater superficial petrosal to sphenopalatine ganglion	Glands of nose, palate; lacrimal gland
		2. Chorda tympani to submaxillary ganglion	Submaxillary and sublingual glands
Glossopharyngeal	Branchial motor	Jugular foramen side of pharynx	Superior constrictor, stylopharyngeus muscles
	Visceral motor	Lesser superficial petrosal, to optic ganglion, to auriculotemporal nerve	Parotid gland
Hypoglossal	Somatic motor	Side of tongue	Muscles of tongue
Oculomotor	Somatic motor	Orbit	Rectus superior, inferior, medial; obliquus inferior; levator palpebrae muscles
Olfactory		Through roof of nasal cavity	Olfactory epithelium
Optic	Special somatic sensory	Orbit, to optic chiasm, to optic tracts	Bipolar cells of retina; rods and cones
Trigeminal	Branchial motor	With mandibular branch	Muscles of mastication
	General somatic sensory	Ophthalmic, maxillary, mandibular branches	Face, nose, mouth
Trochlear	Somatic motor	Orbit	Obliquus superior muscle
Vagus	Branchial motor	Recurrent and external branch of superior laryngeal nerve	Pharyngeal and laryngeal muscles
	Visceral motor	Along carotid artery, esophagus, stomach	Viscera of thorax and abdomen
	Visceral sensory	With motor	Viscera of thorax and abdomen
	General somatic sensory	Auricular branch	Pinna of ear
Vestibular	Special somatic sensory	Internal acoustic meatus	Cristae of semicircular canals, maculae of utricle and saccule
Cochlear	Special somatic sensory	Internal acoustic meatus	Organ of Corti

and one coccygeal pair. Each nerve contains several kinds of fibers. The motor fibers originate in large cells in the anterior gray column of the spinal cord. These form the ventral root and pass to the skeletal muscles. Sensory fibers originate in unipolar cells in the spinal ganglia within the ventricles.

Ventricle system

The ventricular system is a communicating system of four cavities, or ventricles.

Lateral ventricles. Each of the two lateral ventricles has an anterior horn and a posterior horn. The anterior horn is embedded in the frontal lobe, and the posterior horn extends into the occipital lobe. The inferior horn traverses the temporal lobe. Cerebrospinal fluid, which bathes the brain, is manufactured in the choroid plexus, which is found on the interior of the lateral ventricles as a vascular fringe-like process of cellular material projecting into the ventricular cavity. It is covered by an epithelial layer of cells.

Third ventricle. The third ventricle is a vertical cleft between the two lateral ventricles.

Fourth ventricle. The fourth ventricle is a cavity that traverses the pons and medulla oblongata and is bordered dorsally by the cerebellum. The cerebrospinal fluid bathes the entire brain and the spinal cord. It is reabsorbed by the arachnoid—a tissue that covers the surface of the brain.

BRAIN CIRCULATION

Studies of the extent and quantity of arterial flow to the brain are important, since the brain is very sensitive to oxygen deprivation.

Arterial circulation

Arterial blood is delivered to the brain through the twined internal carotid arteries and the vertebral artery. The internal carotid artery primarily branches into the anterior cerebral artery and the middle cerebral artery and the posterior cerebral artery is filled by the basilar artery. There is communication between the blood delivered by the internal carotid artery and that delivered by the vertebral arteries in the communicating circle of Willis at the base of the brain.

Venous circulation

The venous drainage of the brain is primarily through the dural sinuses, which are vascular channels lying within the dura. The superficial cortical veins drain largely into the medial superior longitudinal sinus. The two major cortical veins are the great veins of Trolard and the smaller anastomotic vein of Labbe, which drains caudally into the transverse sinus. Other important internal venous drainage veins are the internal cerebral vein, the great vein of Galen, and the inferior sagittal sinus, all of which flow into the straight sinus. The straight sinus drains caudally into the junction (torcular Herophili) of the superior sagittal sinus and the lateral sinuses. The lateral sinuses drain primarily into the internal jugular vein.

Pathophysiology of cerebral circulation

The brain has great need of oxygen. It has been shown that brain metabolism accounts for approximately 8% of the total oxygen consumption of the body. Oxygen is used primarily for the oxidation of glucose; in the brain, carbohydrate metabolism is a chief source of energy. In man the brain contains approximately 7-ml total oxygen, which at normal rates of use would last approximately 10 seconds. Therefore the central nervous system tissues cannot withstand an oxygen deficit for longer than a few minutes.

The oxygen supply of the brain is maintained primarily by controls on cerebral circulation. The most important of these are systemic blood pressure, certain vasomotor receptors (such as the carotid sinus receptor), and the aortic receptor. Vasomotor centers in the reflex regulation of blood flow depend on cortical sensitivity to both blood pressure and metabolic changes.

Each internal carotid artery supplies the cerebral hemisphere on its respective side of the body, and the basilar artery carries blood to the posterior fossa. The circle of Willis functions as an anastomotic pathway whereby, if an internal carotid artery is occluded, a pressure of about half of normal blood flow can be maintained through collateral blood vessels.

Blood-brain barrier

In the central nervous system of an adult, all cellular processes and vascular elements are closely packed; there is little or no extracellular space. The capillaries are completely invested by glial or neural processes, so there is no perivascular space. In the immature cerebrospinal central nervous system, glial development is incomplete; neurons may contact capillary surfaces, and there is direct neuron-to-neuron contact. There may also be space between cells and around capillaries.

In the immature central nervous system there is permeability to certain dyes, such as ferricyanide or blood bilirubin. Radioactive phosphorus enters more readily and in greater amounts in the brains of the newborn, since the central nervous system is incompletely developed. With complete glial investment, a blood-brain barrier develops that hinders the free passage of many metabolites into the brain, thus protecting the brain from variations of blood composition and from entry of any toxic compound.

Simple expansion of the intracellular volume of water of the brain cells will cause the breakdown in this blood-brain barrier. Other disease states that influence the brain will also influence the breakdown of this protective blood-brain barrier. Inflammations involving the brain, brain tumors, or simple anoxia can also cause a breakdown in this protective barrier. Whether this barrier is intact or broken is most important in radionuclide diagnosis of disease states.

NONRADIOACTIVE STUDIES OF BRAIN PATHOPHYSIOLOGY
Cerebrospinal fluid tests

Examination of the cerebrospinal fluid for pressure, protein, sugar, cell count, cultures, serologic tests, and cytologic analysis is usually helpful in the diagnosis of intracranial tumor. The incidence of abnormalities varies with the stage of the disease and the site and nature of the neoplasm. With slowly growing neoplasms the intracranial pressure will remain normal until late in the illness. Many tumors cause a significant elevation of the protein level in the cerebrospinal fluid. With slowly growing tumors the protein may be normal, despite the presence of a huge mass. The lumbar puncture is contraindicated for critically ill patients with clinical signs of increased intracerebral pressure. However, the hazard is minimal if the patients do not have clinical signs of incipient herniation of the temporal lobe or of the cerebellar tonsils through the foramen magnum.

Electroencephalography

The electroencephalograph (EEG) is a method of studying the electrical brain wave pattern. Persons with epilepsy or seizures will have an abnormal EEG. The electrical discharges will be essentially synchronous discharges, interspersed with nonspecific patterns of high amplitude spikes and flow waves. Flow wave discharges localized in one region may suggest a focal cerebral lesion. In other types of epilepsy such as petit mal (absence attack), which usually consists of a loss of consciousness for a short time, the electroencephalographic record reveals a slow rhythmic spike and wave discharge. The electroencephalograph has been used in screening for possible brain tumors. Focal changes, particularly a slowing in frequency of the record, are indications of neoplasm in the cerebral hemispheres. Rapidly growing tumors are more likely to evoke focal changes than are slowly progressive tumors; with the latter the record may be entirely normal. The EEG is often normal with posterior fossa neoplasms.

Radiographic contrast studies

Pneumoencephalography by the lumbar route (the introduction of air into the cerebrospinal fluid), ventriculography, and arteriography are of importance in the diagnosis and localization of brain tumors. Pneumoencephalography delineates the ventricular system and the subarachnoid space. It may reveal the presence of a mass lesion by displacement of the ventricles or invasion of the ventricular system. In ventriculography, air is injected through burr holes in the skull directly into the lateral cerebral ventricles. Cerebral angiography by way of the carotid, vertebral, or brachial arteries may reveal the vascular patterns of the tumor, since the main arterial tree of the cerebrum may be displaced by the tumor or contrast media may stain the tumor. All the radiographic contrast studies are special procedures and merit special handling techniques of the patient by specialized personnel.

The pneumoencephalography studies are best suited to small midline lesions, and the arteriography techniques are limited if a space-occupying lesion has not disrupted the normal arterial tree.

Echoencephalography

Transmission of ultrasonic energy through the head and recording of the returning echoes can determine the displacement of midline structures. For tumors or other lesions that will cause a shift of the intracerebral structures, this test is a useful screening device.

RADIONUCLIDE LOCALIZATION OF BRAIN PATHOLOGY

Brain imaging using radionuclides was introduced in the late 1940s and early 1950s. Since that time this technique has become a well-established technique for the screening of suspected neuropathology. The popularity of brain scanning or brain imaging as a screening technique is based on the fact that localization of neuropathology on the basis of altered function is difficult. Such localization is difficult because localization of function is not fully understood and localizing clinical signs may be produced by involvement of structures remote from the original lesion. Based on the previously discussed neurology, it can be readily understood that signs and symptoms of cerebrovascular disease may be diffuse. The medical procedures mentioned previously to localize neuropathology have serious limitations when compared to radionuclide localization. Electroencephalography and echoencephalography are innocuous procedures, but many lesions may be missed with these two screening modalities. Radiographic contrast studies as performed today are not harmless, since they necessitate the intra-arterial injection of contrast media. All these procedures have known morbidity. Therefore, because brain scanning and imaging are safe procedures, they have earned a place in the medical armamentarium.

Radionuclides used in brain scanning and imaging

A major reason for the passage of radionuclides into abnormal areas of the brain is the breakdown of the so-called blood-brain barrier. Obviously, there are many disease states that will influence the blood-brain barrier and will increase permeability to substances not normally found in the cerebral cells. True proof of this localization has awaited the increasing use of the electron microscope and microautoradiography techniques. These improved qualitative and quantitative techniques will open the way for further improvements in this field.

Radioiodinated human serum albumin (RHISA). Radioactive albumin injected intravenously diffuses slowly into brain tumors but not into normal brain cells. The blood level remains high, since labeled albumin is not excreted and is catabolized at a slow rate. Persistence of a high level of radioactivity in the blood enhances diffusion of the albumin into tumors or abnormal tissue or both; however, it decreases the so-called target (tumor)-to-nontarget (normal brain) ratio. It has been shown that radioiodinated albumin is transferred into the capillary endothelium of tumors by pinocytosis and that the degree of pinocytotic activity is increased in neoplastic cells. (Pinocytosis is the process by which particles, molecules, or ions are engaged by the cytoplasmic membrane of the cell, which creates a vesicle including them. The vesicle is then pinched off from the cell surface, and it travels into the intracytoplasmic compartment. Here the vesicles may release their contents or remain as cell components, or they may extrude the contents from the cell. Therefore the uptake of RHISA is explained by high pinocytotic activity of the tumor cells.) Twenty-four hours after the injection of radioactive albumin, 59% of the radioactivity of the tumor is found in the tumor cell, 25% is intravascular, and 16% is interstitial. All the radioactivity in the tumor is protein bound. Radioactive albumin has been utilized for brain work since 1953. However, because of the initial concentration of labeled albumin in the vasculature, scanning or imaging has to be delayed for at least 24 hours. Also, because ^{131}I is used, some of the high energies of iodine penetrate commercial collimators, which impairs spatial imaging.

Although it has been reported that albumin-bound substances have a greater tumor-to-normal brain ratio than other substances, investigators have been able to quantitatively demonstrate in vitro that the radioactive mercurial nuclides have twice the uptake in abnormal tissue as compared to radioactive albumin.

[131]I albumin has also been utilized intrathecally. It has been introduced into the ventricular system to aid in the diagnosis of brain tumor, internal hydrocephalus, and cerebrospinal fluid rhinorrhea. The leaking site may be found with apparent ease using this technique.

Radioactive mercury chlormerodrin. Chlormerodrin is a mercurial diuretic that is rapidly excreted by the kidneys after intravenous injection. It therefore decreases the blood level much more rapidly than RHISA.[203]Hg chlormerodrin was first used for brain scanning; however, [197]Hg chlormerodrin is now preferred, since [203]Hg causes irradiation of the kidneys. [197]Hg chlormerodrin has a blood clearance half-life from 1 to 3 hours. It has been shown through microautoradiography of tumors that radioactive mercury is deposited on or in abnormal tumor cells. By the use of quantitative counting it has been shown that the majority of the radioactive mercury ions are concentrated in tumor cells. It has also been shown that radioactive mercury localizes in nearly all areas of cerebral pathology.

Technetium 99m pertechnetate. Technetium 99m pertechnetate has an ionic extracellular distribution pattern; however, it remains mainly in blood pools for 5 to 15 minutes after intravenous injection. Technetium 99m has become the primary imaging nuclide because it has a half-life of 6 hours, emits monoenergetic gamma rays at 140 kev, and is easily collimated. One of the main screening defects of the pertechnetate is that it localizes in the choroid plexus. The choroid accumulation at times makes the interpretation of this area difficult. Preadministration of perchlorate or utilization of ^{99m}Tc DTPA or ^{99m}Tc glucoheptonate eliminates the choroid plexus concentration of technetium.

Positron emitters and other generator-produced radionuclides. The positron emitters such as arsenic 74 and rubidium 84 are primarily found in the intracellular spaces and are characterized by a rapid rate of diffusion into brain tumor. However, cyclotron facilities are needed for their production.

CEREBRAL PERFUSION STUDIES (Fig. 19-2)

With the development of the sensitive high-resolution scintillation camera systems, the dynamic study of the passage of a radioactive bolus through the brain is now an integral part of nuclear medicine. With the use of stop-flow photography, magnetic tape systems, or video tape systems, the arterial capillary and venous phase of a radioactive bolus may be imaged.

The cerebral perfusion study is usually performed with a multimillicurie intravenous dose of technetium 99m or a ^{99m}Tc-labeled compound.

The anterior position is the usual dynamic flow position. Flow can be visualized in the common carotid, internal carotid, and external carotid arteries, the circle of Willis, and the anterior, middle, and posterior cerebral artery regions. The second phase is the capillary flush phase, which ends with visualization of the large venous drainage veins of the brain.

With this technique the presence or absence of the larger cerebral arteries and the capillary perfusion regions can be established. Putting this dynamic flow information together with following static brain imaging information can help establish the proper diagnosis in almost all cases of cerebral pathology.

BRAIN SCANNING AND IMAGING

The routine positions used in brain scanning or imaging are illustrated in Fig. 19-4.

Accurate positioning is more important in nuclear medicine than in radiology. In nuclear medicine the physician does not have the bony landmarks portrayed on the scan; therefore the technician must place markers on the scan that accurately denote the landmarks.

Delayed brain imaging will primarily portray the venous mixing phase of the radionuclide and will also portray abnormal accumulation of the radionuclide in brain tissue. Thus normal and abnormal architecture of the brain can be inferred from a brain image or scan.

CLINICAL INDICATIONS FOR CEREBRAL PERFUSION STUDIES AND BRAIN SCANNING

Brain tumors and other neuropathology. One of the fundamental reasons for employing delayed brain imaging as a screening study is to localize a brain tumor (Figs. 19-5 and 19-6). Brain tumors account for approximately 3% of all neo-

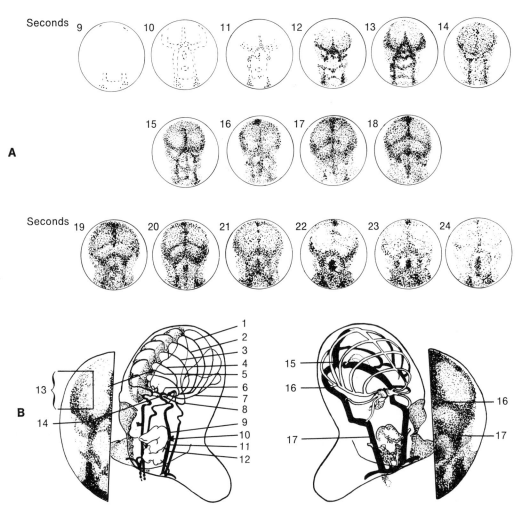

Fig. 19-2. A, Cerebral perfusion stop-time frames. **B,** Cerebral perfusion—arterial phase/venous phase. (From Brucer, M.: Cerebral perfusion, St. Louis, 1974, Mallinckrodt, Inc.)

1. Posterior parietal artery
2. Anterior parietal artery
3. Rolandic artery
4. Prerolandic artery
5. Anterior cerebral artery
6. Middle cerebral stem
7. Inferior division, middle cerebral artery
8. Posterior cerebral artery
9. Internal carotid artery
10. External carotid artery
11. Bifurcation
12. Common carotid artery
13. Divisions of middle cerebral artery
14. Stem of middle cerebral artery
15. Torcula
16. Transverse sinus
17. Internal jugular vein

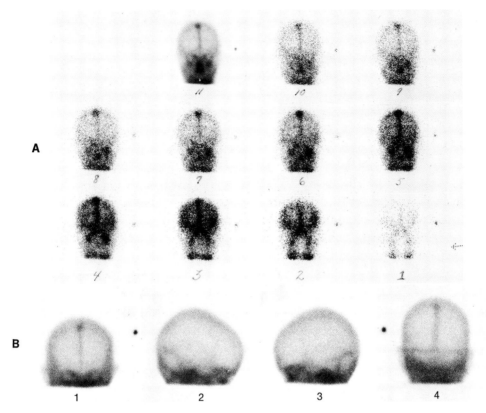

Fig. 19-3. A, Normal cerebral perfusion study after injection of 20 mCi of ^{99m}Tc DTPA. *1,* Early arterial phase showing carotid arteries and anterior and middle cerebral arteries. *2,* Continuation of arterial phase. *3,* Capillary venous phase. *4* to *10,* Venous phase. *11,* Static image, primarily to show that position was correct. **B,** Static images performed 2 hours after dose. *1,* Anterior view. *2,* Right lateral view. *3,* Left lateral view. *4,* Reverse Towne's view.

plasms and occur in all age groups. Metastatic brain tumors, however, are now recognized with increasing frequency, since brain imaging is more widely used. In metastatic disease there are usually multiple sites, whereas primary tumors usually occur singly (Figs. 19-7 and 19-8).

Positive cerebral perfusion studies and brain images are related to the amount of neovascularity in the abnormal brain tissue. Therefore in certain cases early images are negative, whereas delayed images are positive. In such disease states, because of the decreased vascularity of the lesion, it takes longer to obtain sufficient concentration of radioactivity in the area to visualize the abnormality. Metastatic brain disease, infarcts, inflammatory disease, and intracerebral hemorrhage have decreased vascularity. Therefore both early and delayed imaging or scanning using several radiopharmaceuticals may be indicated.

Cerebrovascular diseases. Abnormalities of the circulation of the brain may

Text continued on p. 424.

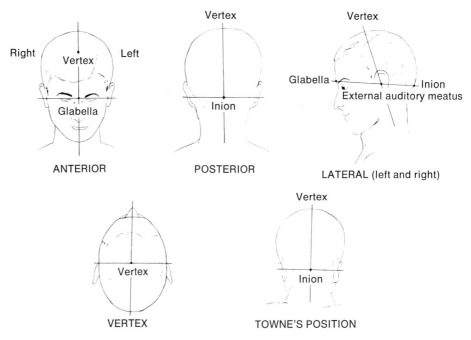

Fig. 19-4. Nuclear medicine brain scanning positions. *Anterior position,* The patient is in a supine position; his head is elevated, and his chin is tucked down until a horizontal line passes through the external auditory meatus and the outer canthus of the eye; the midsagittal line is perpendicular to this line. *Posterior position,* The patient is in a prone position. The chest is elevated, and the chin is tucked down as in anterior view. The chin is tucked toward the chest so that a horizontal line will pass through the external auditory meatus and the outer canthus of the eye and the midsagittal line forms a perpendicular with the horizontal line. *Lateral position,* With patient on his side, his head is positioned so that a line drawn from vertex to external auditory meatus superimposes an identical line on the other side of the head. The chin should be brought toward the chest until a horizontal line can be drawn from the glabella to the inion. *Vertex position,* The patient is sitting; midsagittal and coronal lines are drawn crossing at the vertex. Of all positions, this is the least useful. *Towne's position,* The patient is positioned as for a posterior view; however, greater angulation of approximately 10 to 30 degrees is obtained by pulling the chin toward the chest to allow the straight sinus to be tipped out of view so that the cerebellum (posterior fossa) can be observed without background interference.

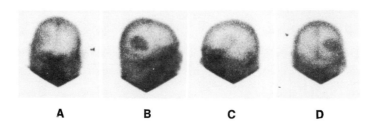

Fig. 19-5. Brain images, after 20-mCi dose of ^{99m}Tc DTPA administered intravenously. **A,** Anterior view. **B,** Right lateral view. **C,** Left lateral view. **D,** Posterior view. Images reveal 4 × 3 cm increased concentration of nuclide extending close to midline with apparent central necrosis in posterior parietal occipital region. Pathology: astrocytoma, Grade III.

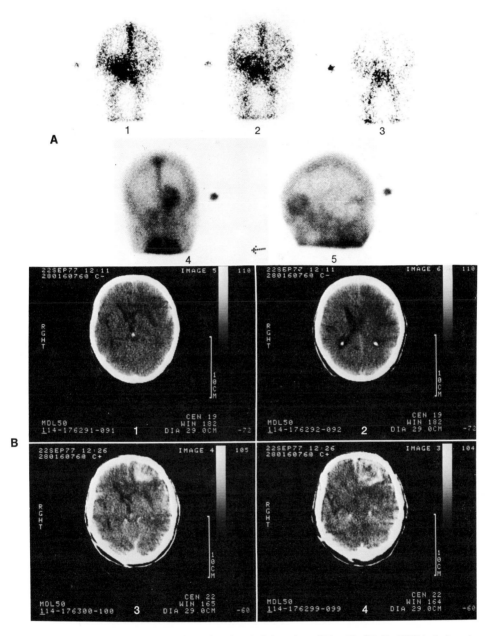

Fig. 19-6. A, Brain images performed following the administration of 20 mCi of ^{99m}Tc DTPA. *1,* Arterial phase of carotid-cerebral study revealing early increased arterialization of a left hemispheric lesion. *2,* Capillary phase reveals marked capillary blush of left hemispheric lesion. *3,* Venous phase of study. *4,* Anterior static view performed 2 hours after dose reveals a large space-occupying lesion with a central region of decreased concentration. *5,* Left lateral view reveals the lesion to be in the left frontal lobe. **B,** CT study. *1* and *2,* No injection of contrast material. Large poorly demarcated area of low density in left frontal temporal region with significant displacement of midline structures and compression of left frontal horn. *3* and *4,* Following injection of contrast material there is mottled contrast enhancement in the left frontal temporal region. Final diagnosis: astrocytoma Gr IV. (CT images courtesy Drs. Sachs, Ross and Associates, Beachwood, Ohio.)

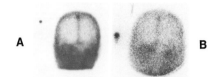

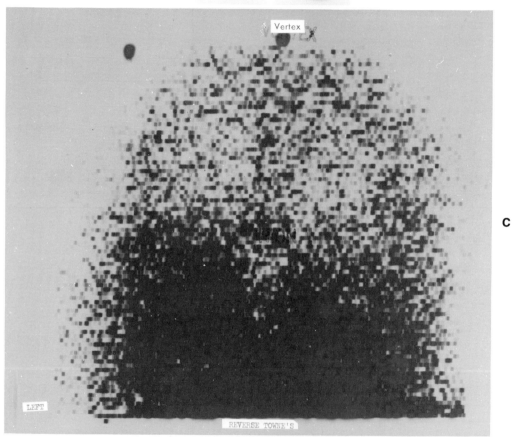

Fig. 19-7. A, Brain image 2 hours after administration of ^{99m}Tc DTPA, intravenously, reverse Towne's position. Separate 2-cm lesions can be seen in each cerebellar hemisphere. **B,** Four-hour delayed brain image, reverse Towne's position (^{99m}Tc DTPA, intravenous). Lesions are larger than suspected on 2-hour view, and there is increased concentration relative to the venous sinuses. **C,** Six-hour delayed brain scan, reverse Towne's position (^{197}Hg chlormerodrin, intravenous). Mottled distribution and increased concentration of large lesions almost completely replace the cerebellum. Diagnosis: metastatic breast carcinoma.

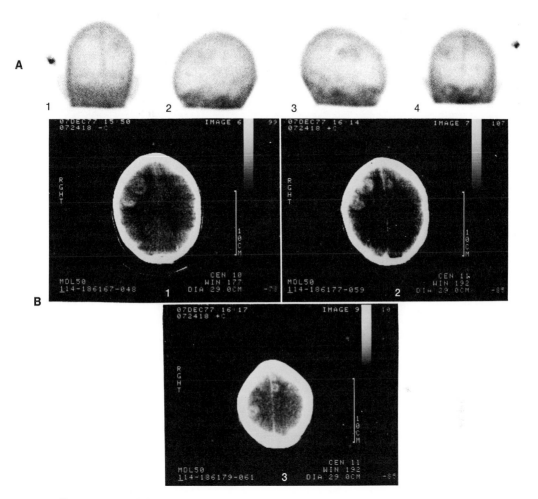

Fig. 19-8. A, Brain images performed 2 hours after 20-mCi dose of ⁹⁹ᵐTc DTPA. *1,* Reverse Towne's view. Large area of increased concentration in right parietal region. *2,* Left lateral and, *3,* right lateral views reveal nodular areas of increased concentration throughout the brain. *4,* Anterior view reveals large right hemispheric lesion as seen on reverse Towne's view. Several small areas of increased concentration in left hemisphere. Image diagnosis: multiple sites of metastatic disease. **B,** CT study. *1,* No contrast injected. At level 6 there are two large areas of increased density representing microcalcifications in metastatic lesions. *2* and *3,* Following the injection of contrast material there is contrast enhancement of the metastatic lesions demonstrated on image *1* without contrast injection. There are also numerous other contrast enhancing metastases in other parts of the brain. There is edema around several of the large metastases. (CT images courtesy Drs. Sachs, Ross and Associates, Beachwood, Ohio.)

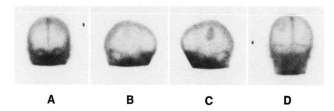

A   **B**   **C**   **D**

Fig. 19-9. Brain images performed 2 weeks after left cerebral insult. **A,** Anterior view. **B,** Right lateral view. **C,** Left lateral view. **D,** Reverse Towne's view. Images reveal left parietal 3 × 3.5 cm well-demarcated increased concentration of nuclide with an area of central decrease. Diagnosis: cerebral infarction.

result from decreased oxygen content in the brain, subdural hematoma, occlusion of one of the intracerebral or extracerebral perfusion arteries, emboli to the brain, hemorrhage from one of the cerebral vessels, and cerebral contusion. These defects in cerebral blood flow will be visualized on the cerebral perfusion study as an absence or decrease in blood flow in the affected region. Positive brain scans may be obtained when there is hemorrhage into surrounding brain tissue and infarction (death of tissue).

Obviously, small cerebral thromboses or small areas of embolization may not cause gross defects in the blood-brain barrier because of the collateral circulation of the brain. However, for reasons that are difficult to define, approximately half the patients with clinical vascular occlusions will develop a positive brain scan over a period of as long as 3 weeks after the insult (Fig. 19-9). These lesions can usually be differentiated by interpreter experience, but in some instances further radiographic techniques must be employed.

With knowledge of the arterial tree of the brain it is sometimes possible to tell whether the abnormality on the brain scan has been caused by a specific vessel that is occluded. Nearly half the large vascular occlusions occur in the middle cerebral artery. It has also been found that in most of the patients who have vascular accidents that produce abnormal brain scans, there is gradual clearing of part or all of the abnormality over a period of weeks. In brain tumors this change is not seen; the count rate in the area of the brain tumor over a period of weeks will increase as the size of the lesion increases.

STUDIES OF CEREBROSPINAL FLUID

Certain conditions may be studied with injection of radionuclides into the spinal fluid (Figs. 19-10 and 19-11). Congenital abnormalities, hemorrhages, infections, or tumor may involve the cerebrospinal space and cause total or subtotal blocks that can be easily studied. The intrathecal injection of ^{131}I albumin, ^{99m}Tc albumin, ^{169}Yb DTPA, or ^{111}In DTPA has been used to study the ventricular system, brain tumor, internal hydrocephalus, and cerebral rhinorrhea. The latter is a sequel to skull fracture. With a basilar skull fracture, cerebrospinal fluid will

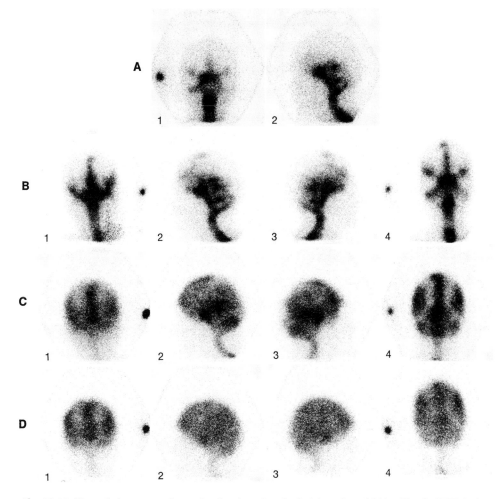

Fig. 19-10. Normal cisternography study after intrathecal administration of 900 μCi ^{111}In DTPA. **A,** Image 3 hours after injection. Progression of nuclide into the basilar cisterns; absent visualization of ventricles. **B,** Image 6½ hours after injection reveals early penetration of the foramina, with nuclide beginning to flow over cerebral hemispheres anteriorly. *1,* Anterior; *2,* left; *3,* right; *4,* posterior. **C,** Image 24 hours and, **D,** 48 hours after injection reveals normal distribution of nuclide over both cerebral hemispheres. *1,* Anterior; *2,* left; *3,* right; *4,* posterior.

leak through the bony tables into the nasal region. This may be visualized on multiple views after the injection of the radionuclide into the cerebrospinal fluid as a leak of radioactivity into the nasal region.

CEREBRAL CIRCULATION TIME AND CEREBRAL BLOOD FLOW

Cerebral circulation time and blood flow are not unlike the dynamic function and flow studies of other organs of the body. In studying the cerebral circulation

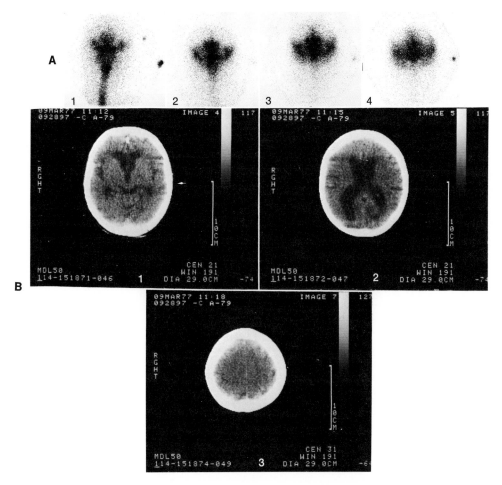

Fig. 19-11. A, Cisternography performed after intrathecal administration of 1 mCi of ¹¹¹In DTPA. *1,* Image 2.5 hours after dose. Progression of cerebrospinal fluid flow into the basilar cisterns and early penetration of the lateral ventricle. *2,* Image 5 hours after dose. Excellent demonstration of lateral ventricles. *3,* Image 26 hours after dose. Almost no flow over the hemispheres. *4,* Image 48 hours after dose. Markedly delayed progression over hemispheres. Diagnosis: communicating low-pressure hydrocephalus. **B,** CT images. *1, 2,* and *3,* CT without contrast demonstrates markedly enlarged ventricles with no displacement. There is some prominence of the Sylvian fissure but no deepening of the convexity sulci. The differential diagnosis is communicating hydrocephalus; rule out changes secondary to significant cortical cerebral atrophy. (CT images courtesy Drs. Sachs, Ross and Associates, Beachwood, Ohio.)

time, a nondiffusible radionuclide, such as ^{131}I albumin, is injected intravenously and its course through the brain measured with appropriate instrumentation. Diffusible tracers are used for the measurement of total cerebral blood flow. The most common diffusible tracers are the inert gases, such as krypton 79 and xenon 133.

These techniques are applicable in very few medical centers. However, there is much interest in the possible screening reliability of these procedures in cerebrovascular disease.

SUMMARY

Radionuclide cerebral perfusion and brain imaging are accepted screening procedures that are now widely used by all medical specialties. These procedures as performed today have no patient morbidity, and patients with the earliest of neurologic symptoms or behavior disorders may be studied. Therefore correctable neurosurgical lesions may be inferred at a stage in their development for which greater cure rates are possible.

Computerized axial tomography (CT) of the head is becoming the primary anatomic imaging procedure for studying patients with suspected brain pathology; however, radionuclide imaging will give physiologic information not visualized with CT. The combination of these modalities will screen the majority of patients with neuropathology correctly and will obviate unnecessary invasive neuroradiologic procedures.

BIBLIOGRAPHY

Brucer, M: Cerebral perfusion, St. Louis, 1975, Mallinckrodt, Inc.

Buell, U., and others: Computerized transaxial tomography and cerebral serial scintigraphy in intracranial tumors. Rates of detection and tumor-type identification: concise communication, J. Nucl. Med. **19**: 476-479, 1978.

Chandler, W., and Shuck, L. D.: Abnormal technetium 99m pertechnetate imaging following stannous pyrophosphate bone imaging, J. Nucl. Med. **16**:518, 1975.

DeBlanc, H. J., and Sorenson, J. A.: Noninvasive brain imaging computed tomography and radionuclides, New York, 1975, Society of Nuclear Medicine.

DeLand, F. H.: Cerebral radionuclide angiography, Philadelphia, 1976, W. B. Saunders Co.

James, A. E., and others: Some basic considerations of cerebrospinal fluid physiology as reflected by CSF imaging studies. In Potchen, E. J., editor: Current concepts in radiology, St. Louis, 1977, The C. V. Mosby Co., vol. III.

Khentigan, A., and others: Effects of prior administration of Sn (II) complexes used in nuclear medicine on in vivo distribution of subsequently administered Tc 99m pertechnetate and Tc 99m compounds, J. Nucl. Med. **16**:541, 1975.

Rollo, F. D., and others: Comparative evaluation of 99mTcGH, 99mTcO$_4$ and 99mTc DTPA as brain imaging agents, Radiology **123**:379-383, 1977.

Sargent, T., and others: A potential new brain scanning agent: 4-Br 77-2, 5-dimethoxyphenylisopropylamine (4-Br-DPIA), J. Nucl. Med. **16**: 243, 1975.

Walker, A. G.: Effect of Tc 99m Sn bone agents on subsequent pertechnetate brain scans, J. Nucl. Med. **16**:579, 1975.

Waxman, A. D., and others: Technetium 99m glucoheptonate as a brain scanning agent. Critical comparison with pertechnetate, J. Nucl. Med. **17**:345-348, 1976.

Waxman, A. D., and others: Steroid-induced suppression of gallium uptake in tumor of the central nervous system: concise communication. J. Nucl. Med. **19**: 480-482, 1978.

GENERAL BIBLIOGRAPHY

Ashkar, F. S., Miale, A., and Smoak, W.: A general guide to nuclear medicine, Springfield, Ill., 1975, Charles C Thomas, Publisher.

Best, C., and Taylor, N. B.: Physiological basis of medical practice, ed. 10, Baltimore, 1979, The Williams & Wilkins Co.

Blahd, W. H.: Nuclear medicine, ed. 2, New York, 1971, McGraw-Hill Book Co.

Deland, F. H., and Wagner, H. N.: Atlas of nuclear medicine, Philadelphia, 1969, W. B. Saunders Co., vol. 1.

Freeman, L. M., and Blaufax, M. D.: Physicians desk reference for radiology and nuclear medicine, Oradell, N.J., 1977-1978, Medical Economics Co.

Freeman, L. M., and Johnson, P. M.: Clinical scintillation scanning, New York, 1975, Grune & Stratton, Inc.

Grant, J. C. B, and Basmajian, J. V.: A method of anatomy, ed. 7, Baltimore, 1965, The Williams & Wilkins Co.

Gross, C. M.: Gray's anatomy of the human body, ed. 28, Philadelphia, 1966, Lea & Febiger.

Guyton, A. C.: Textbook of medical physiology, ed. 3., Philadelphia, 1966, W. B. Saunders Co.

Ham, A. W.: Histology, Philadelphia, 1957, J. B. Lippincott Co.

Holvey, D. N.: The Merck manual of diagnosis and therapy, ed. 12, Rahway, N. J., 1972, Merck Sharp & Dohme Research Lab.

Jacob, S. W., and Francone, C. A.: Structure and function in man, ed. 2, Philadelphia, 1970, W. B. Saunders Co.

Maynard, C. D.: Clinical nuclear medicine, Philadelphia, 1969, Lea & Febiger.

Powsner, E. R., and Raeside, D. E.: Diagnostic nuclear medicine, New York, 1971, Grune & Stratton, Inc.

Rhodes, B. A., editor: Quality control in nuclear medicine: radiopharmaceuticals, instrumentation, and in vitro assays, St. Louis, 1977, The C. V. Mosby Co.

Shtassel, P.: Speak to me in nuclear medicine, New York, 1976, Harper & Row, Publishers.

Silver, S.: Radioactive nuclides in medicine & biology — medicine, Philadelphia, 1968, Lea & Febiger.

Wagner, H. N.: Principles of nuclear medicine, Philadelphia, 1968, W. B. Saunders Co.

Wagner, H. N.: Nuclear medicine, New York, 1975, HP Publishing, Co.

20 Gastrointestinal system

Foods, minerals, vitamins, and fluids enter the body by mouth, which represents the upper end of the gastrointestinal tract. In the mouth, chewing breaks down the large food particles and mixes the food with the secretions of the three pairs of salivary glands (parotid, submaxillary, and sublingual) that open into the oral cavity. By virtue of its lubricating action the saliva facilitates swallowing and keeps the mouth moist and clean. The salivary enzyme, ptyalin, begins the process of starch digestion. The lubricated food is then propelled through the pharynx, down the esophagus, and into the stomach.

In the stomach, food is stored and mixed with the gastric secretions that contain hydrochloric acid, mucus, pepsin, lipase, and intrinsic factor. In the presence of acidity, pepsin breaks down the proteins into polypeptides. The gastric lipase plays a minor role in the digestion of fats. Mucus is protective for the gastric mucosa, whereas the intrinsic factor is needed for the absorption of dietary vitamin B_{12}. The partially digested food is released from the stomach at a controlled steady rate into the duodenum, the first portion of the small intestine. The rate of gastric emptying depends on the nature of the stomach contents. It is most rapid with carbohydrates and slowest with fats.

The small intestine measures about 280 cm (roughly 3 yards) and can be divided into the duodenum, jejunum, and ileum. In the lumen of the small intestine the contents are mixed with the intestinal secretions, pancreatic juice, and bile. The pancreatic and intestinal enzymes complete the breakdown of the partially digested foodstuffs. The proteins are ultimately broken down into amino acids, carbohydrates into simple sugars, and fats into glycerides and fatty acids. These final products of digestion are then absorbed from the small intestine into the blood and lymph. The proper absorption of fats and fat-soluble substances requires the presence of bile. What remains after the process of absorption is driven from the ileum into the large intestine, or colon.

In the colon, absorption of water and minerals converts the contents into semisolid feces. The colonic contents are propelled from the ascending colon through the transverse, descending, and sigmoid colons into the rectum. The colon normally contains large numbers of bacteria. Some of these are beneficial, whereas others are possibly harmful.

From the rectum the fecal matter is expelled through the anal orifice, which represents the lower end of the gastrointestinal tract.

RADIONUCLIDE SCANNING OF
SALIVARY GLANDS

Taking advantage of the pertechnetate-concentrating ability of the salivary glands, radionuclide scanning of these glands is performed after the intravenous injection of 1.5 to 3.0 mCi of ^{99m}Tc pertechnetate.

To facilitate interpretation, an anterior and two lateral views are obtained with landmarks over the angle of the mandible, chin, and external auditory meatus. Normally, the parotid gland is larger than the submaxillary gland and the distribution of radioactivity is homogenous.

Radionuclide scanning is indicated to detect any displacement of the normal salivary gland tissue by pathologic processes such as tumors, cysts, and fibrosis. Another indication for radiosialography is evaluation of salivary glandular function by sequential scintiphotographs obtained with the aid of a gamma camera.

FAT ABSORPTION STUDIES

Dietary fat is ingested as neutral fat or triglycerides, which are made of three molecules of fatty acids attached to one molecule of glycerol. In the duodenum the neutral fat is rapidly emulsified by the bile and hydrolysed by the exocrine pancreatic lipase. This results in a progressive loss of a fatty acid molecule from the triglyceride to form diglycerides, then monoglycerides, and ultimately free fatty acids and glycerol. These mixed products of digestion, together with the bile, form an emulsion that passes from the lumen of the small intestine into its cells. Fatty acids with less than 10 carbon atoms (short chain) are directly absorbed into the portal blood. Long-chain fatty acids (with 16 carbon atoms or more), together with the lower glycerides (di and mono), are resynthesized within the intestinal cells into newer forms of triglycerides that finally pass into the lymph. After absorption a portion of the fat is oxidized by the tissues to yield energy, CO_2, and water. Another fraction is used in building the structure of tissues and some hormones. What remains is stored as neutral fat in the fat depots.

The normal individual can almost fully digest and absorb up to 150 gm of fat per day. Therefore fecal fat, which normally amounts to less than 7.5 gm per day, represents a small amount of unabsorbed exogenous fat, together with a relatively larger portion of endogenous origin. This latter portion is derived from fat secreted into the intestinal lumen by way of the bile, together with fat of the desquamated epithelial cells and fat synthesized by the intestinal bacteria.

With malabsorption, there is an abnormal increase in the fat content of the stools, or steatorrhea. The abnormality can be suspected by inspection of the stools and verified by microscopic examination. A more accurate diagnosis is obtained by chemical determination of the fecal fat. The absorption of less than 90% of dietary fat (100 gm of fat per day) indicates defective absorption. Similarly, a fat content of over 30% by weight of a single dried stool specimen is indicative of malabsorption.

To obviate the technical difficulties of fecal fat determination by chemical methods, together with the time involved in the metabolic balance studies, radioactive tracer techniques were introduced. Labeled fats such as ^{131}I triolein and ^{14}C tripalmitate, as well as labeled fatty acids (^{131}I oleic acid) are used.

Radioiodinated triolein test. After an overnight fast, the patient is given 25 to 50 μCi of ^{131}I triolein in the form of an emulsion, together with the calculated dose of nonradioactive carrier fat (1 ml/kg body weight), taking care to avoid the intake of absorption-modifying agents such as dextrose and casein. The uptake of free ^{131}I by the thyroid gland is blocked by the oral administration of 10 to 20 drops of Lugol's solution. Serial blood samples are withdrawn 4, 5, and 6 hours after administration, and all the stools passed are collected for at least 72 hours. Net radioactivity per unit volume of the blood sample is determined in a scintillation well counter and expressed as percentage of the administered dose in the total circulating blood volume. This requires knowledge of the total blood volume, which may be predicted from the height or weight of the patient or both. Radioactivity in the total amount of the collected stools is determined on top of a scintillation counter and expressed as percentage of administered dose, taking care to use identical geometry in counting the stools and tracer dose. In addition, contamination of the stools with urine during their collection should be strictly avoided to prevent urinary radioactivity from invalidating the results. A further precaution is the use of a radiopharmaceutical with reasonable chemical purity and stability of its radioactive label. The iodine tag, which is rather stable in vitro, is relatively unstable in the gut and blood. Therefore, in order to avoid errors caused by measurement of free radioiodine included in the test meal as well as that caused by degradation hydrolysis, it is better to measure the plasma lipid iodine radioactivity rather than whole blood radioactivity. Measured radioactivity is then expressed as percentage of tracer dose in total plasma volume.

With the fecal collection method the upper limit for fecal radioactivity in normal subjects is 7% of the dose if the collection period is at least 72 hours.

With blood sampling, the lowest limit for the sum of radioactivity in the three samples withdrawn 4, 5, and 6 hours after administration of the dose in normal subjects is 23% of the dose in the total blood volume. In the same time interval (4 to 6 hours after dose) the plasma lipid radioactivity should exceed 3% of the administered dose in normal subjects.

Although tracer techniques used for detection of fat malabsorption are easy to perform, they suffer from lack of accuracy and sensitivity, especially when not done properly. The accuracy of these methods bears a linear relationship to the severity of the absorption defect. The false-negative and false-positive results are not few. Most false-negative results are encountered in patients with minimal malabsorption. Blood sampling is less reliable than the fecal collection technique. A combination of both gives the best results and differentiates borderline cases into truly abnormal and normal. Another disadvantage of the radioiodinated triolein test is its inability to quantitate the fat malabsorption.

Radioiodinated oleic acid. The procedure and results of the radioiodinated oleic acid test are similar to those of ^{131}I triolein.

It was thought that since fats require prior digestion by the pancreatic lipase before being absorbed whereas fatty acids do not, testing for the absorption of both fats and fatty acids would distinguish between steatorrhea caused by pancreatic insufficiency from that caused by intestinal disease. However, these hopes did not materialize when this combined testing was applied in clinical practice.

To avoid the effect of variability in intestinal absorption from day to day, both the labeled fat (^{131}I triolein) and fatty acid (^{125}I oleic acid) are administered simultaneously to the fasting subject, together with a carrier of 1 ml fat per kg body weight. Heparinized blood samples are withdrawn at the specified times, and the plasma is separated. The stools are collected. All samples are counted for the presence of both radioisotopes (^{131}I and ^{125}I), and the counts contributed by ^{131}I in the ^{125}I channel should be eliminated. Therefore a spectrometer is absolutely necessary.

Radiocarbon-labeled fat. Unlike iodine, carbon is a normal constituent of the fat molecule. Therefore ^{14}C-labeled fat should be a better tracer for the study of fat metabolism than the radioiodinated form.

After the oral administration of 5 to 20 μCi of ^{14}C tripalmitate, the stools are collected for at least 72 hours. Fecal radioactivity is determined and expressed as percentage of the administered dose.

The results of this technique show much better correlation with chemical fecal fat determination than those obtained by the radioiodinated fat studies. However, measurement of ^{14}C radioactivity is difficult and time consuming and necessitates specific equipment.

To obviate some of these difficulties, an index of fat absorption can be obtained by determining the maximum specific activity of Co_2 in the expired air collected 3, 4, and 5 hours after administration of the dose. Radioactivity in the collected samples is measured in a liquid scintillation counter.

Although the technique is rather simple, various pathophysiologic conditions related to lymphatic flow and the metabolic state of the patient to be studied limit the use of this test for the study of fat absorption. Furthermore, this test is a measure of fat utilization rather than its gastrointestinal absorption.

TESTS FOR PROTEIN ABSORPTION

Proteins have a complex molecular structure. They are made up of amino acids. These amino acids enter the structure of every cell in the body. Therefore they are needed for the maintenance of cellular integrity and for building up new tissues. In addition, they provide raw material for the manufacture of certain secretions, both exocrine and endocrine in nature. The maintenance of normal concentrations of plasma proteins and hemoglobin depends on the presence of an adequate supply of amino acids. Proteins containing amino acids in the proportions needed by the body to fulfill these functions are called *grade I*, or *first-class, proteins*. These are mostly of animal origin. Proteins that contain different proportions of amino acids and/or lack some of the essential amino acids that cannot be manufactured by the body are called *grade II*, or *second-class, proteins*. Most of these are of plant origin.

Digestion of proteins begins in the stomach and ends in the small intestine with the release of the constituent amino acids. These free amino acids cross the cell of the intestinal mucosa to enter the portal blood. About 10% of the ingested protein enters the colon and is eventually passed in the stools.

Malabsorption of proteins can be diagnosed by the presence of excessive numbers of striated muscle fibers in the stools as detected by microscopic examination. A more accurate index of protein absorption can be obtained by the chemical determination of fecal nitrogen. The normal excretion of nitrogen in the stools of a person on a well-balanced diet varies between 1 and 1.5 gm of nitrogen per day, corresponding to about 10 gm of protein. Protein absorption can also be studied by radioactive-labeled proteins.

Radioiodinated protein absorption test. Either casein or serum albumin labeled with ^{131}I is used. Others have used tritium-labeled proteins. The stools are collected for 72 hours. Fecal radioactivity is measured and expressed as percentage of the orally administered dose of the labeled protein.

Normally, less than 5% of the ingested radioactivity is recovered in the fecal specimen. The main advantage of the technique is its technical simplicity. However, from the point of view of accuracy the chemical determination of fecal nitrogen is still the more reliable index of protein absorption.

The main sources of error in the radioisotopic protein studies are the deiodination that occurs during hydrolysis when ^{131}I-labeled protein is used and the recycling of labeled endogenous protein into the gastrointestinal tract if tritium-labeled proteins are used.

CARBOHYDRATE ABSORPTION STUDIES

Carbohydrates are the cheapest source of calories and represent more than 50% of most diets. They are ingested in the form of large molecular polysaccharides, disaccharides, and smaller amounts of free sugars. The polysaccharides are hydrolysed primarily by the amylase enzyme of the salivary glands and to a greater extent by that of the pancreas with the production of glucose and disaccharides. The disaccharides are further hydrolysed by the intestinal enzymes into monosaccharides. Almost all these simple sugars are absorbed from the upper small intestine into the portal blood.

Consequently, carbohydrate absorption can be studied by following the blood concentration of a sugar after its oral administration. In this respect the glucose tolerance technique is the most commonly used method. It is easy to perform and readily available in most chemical laboratories.

Since the chemical methods are easy and accurate, there appears to be no need for a radioactive technique for the study of carbohydrate absorption.

ASSESSMENT OF GASTROINTESTINAL BLOOD LOSS

The presence of blood in the stool indicates a break somewhere in the gastrointestinal mucosa. With relatively large amounts of blood, the color of the stools is changed. Red blood is almost always caused by bleeding from the lower large bowel; blood that has passed through the intestine becomes darker and gives the stools a tarry color. If the amount of blood is insufficient to cause a change in fecal color, certain tests must be applied for the detection of this occult blood. In this respect, microscopic examination of the stools is not very helpful. The chemical methods (guiac, benzidine) are much more adequate. They depend on color change of an indicator in the presence of an added source of oxygen and a peroxidase catalyst. What makes these tests positive in the presence of blood is the peroxidase found in the heme portion of the hemoglobin. However, the fact that other fecal constituents such as meat fibers, pus, and plants contain peroxidase makes these chemical tests nonspecific. In contrast, the radionuclide techniques are more specific and offer an accurate estimate of the amount of blood loss.

Radiochromium method. In the radiochromium method an anticoagulated blood sample is withdrawn from the patient, and the red cells are tagged with ^{51}Cr sodium chromate as described on p. 349. After the reinjection of the labeled erythrocytes into the patient, the stools are collected for the next 72 hours. Blood samples are obtained 15 minutes after the injection of the tagged cells and at the end of the test period. Radioactivity in the stools is measured on top of a scintillation counter. Using identical geometry and equal counting time, radioactivity in the blood samples is measured to calculate the average net counting rate per milliliter of blood. The amount of gastrointestinal blood loss is determined by dividing the net counting rate of the collected stools by that present in 1 ml of blood.

Normally, the amount of blood lost in the stools never exceeds 3 ml per day. In this regard, slow intestinal transit can lead to a false-negative result or to underestimation of the amount of blood lost. To minimize the effect of this problem, the start of stool collection should be delayed either empirically to day 3 after tracer dose administration or until the appearance in the stool of a nonabsorbable marker given orally at the same time with the injection of the ^{51}Cr-tagged red cells. Another precaution worth mentioning is to avoid contamination of the stools with urine during collection because of the fact that released ^{51}Cr is excreted with the urine. For the same reason, this method cannot be used for estimation of blood loss through the urinary tract. The amount of urinary blood loss can be determined following the intravenous injection of ^{59}Fe ferrous sulfate since the urinary excretion of radioiron is insignificant under normal circumstances.

The main use of this test is the detection and estimation of blood loss through the gastrointestinal tract, which has been known to be the underlying cause in some cases of unexplained anemia.

Diagnosis of Meckel's diverticulum

Meckel's diverticulum is a small evagination of the intestine resulting from persistance of the proximal end of the fetal vitelline or omphalomesenteric duct. It is usually located on the antimesenteric border of the ileum within a meter of the ileocecal valve. It is more common in males and generally asymptomatic. In 20% of the cases, the diverticulum contains heterotopic mucosa that may be gastric, pancreatic, duodenal, jejunal, or colonic.

The clinical importance of Meckel's diverticulum lies entirely in its many complications, the most serious and common being ulceration and hemorrhage, which occur more frequently in children and young adults. Gastrointestinal bleeding associated with Meckel's diverticulum is caused by involvement of the heterotopic mucosa, which is usually gastric.

The diagnosis of Meckel's diverticulum proved to be very difficult even with the aid of barium contrast radiography and selective arteriography. ^{99m}Tc pertechnetate abdominal scanning has been reasonably successful in the preoperative detection of this abnormality, especially if the condition is complicated by bleeding.

Following the intravenous injection of 2 to 5 mCi of ^{99m}Tc pertechnetate, sequential scans of the abdomen are performed in the anterior projection over the next 30 to 45 minutes. Imaging may be done with a rectilinear scanner or scintillation camera. Visualization of the stomach is an essential component of a successful study. Lateral views are sometimes helpful to exclude false-positive results caused by renal shadows.

In view of the fact that ^{99m}Tc pertechnetate is concentrated in the gastric mucosa, the diagnostic usefulness of abdominal pertechnetate scintigraphy in the detection of Meckel's diverticulum depends on the presence of ectopic functioning gastric tissue in the diverticulum. Accordingly, false-negative results are expected in the absence of functioning gastric mucosa or if the ectopic gastric tissue present is below the detection capability of the equipment used. On the other hand, false-positive results have been reported, especially with small bowel obstruction, intussusception, hydronephrosis, and arteriovenous malformation.

ASSESSMENT OF PROTEIN LOSS THROUGH GASTROINTESTINAL TRACT

Under normal circumstances, a significant proportion of the daily breakdown (catabolism) of plasma albumin and probably other plasma proteins occurs by exudation into the gastrointestinal tract, where they are subsequently digested and reabsorbed. To maintain a state of equilibrium, albumin is manufactured by the liver at a rate equal to its catabolism. With the exudation of abnormally large amounts of proteins into the gastrointestinal tract, the ability of the liver to synthesize albumin is exceeded. This results in diminution of the concentration of the plasma proteins with the production of generalized or localized edema.

Excessive loss of albumin has been shown to occur in the stomach in giant hypertrophic gastritis, diffuse ulceration of the stomach, and gastric carcinoma.

An increased loss of albumin from the intestine has been observed in regional enteritis, ulcerative colitis, celiac disease, intestinal lymphangiectasia, and carcinoma. Extraintestinal disorders such as nephrosis, hepatic cirrhosis, constrictive pericarditis, and congestive heart failure can also lead to excessive protein loss through the gastrointestinal tract.

Since the protein leaking through the gastrointestinal tract is liable to digestion by the proteolytic enzymes and reabsorption, the level of fecal nitrogen is not affected. Consequently, chemical methods would not be suitable for the detection of these cases of protein-losing gastroenteropathy. However, the diagnosis of this phenomenon can be easily and accurately done by means of radionuclide techniques.

Radioiodinated human serum albumin. The earliest evidence for excessive protein loss through the gastrointestinal tract was obtained by recovering injected ^{131}I-labeled human serum albumin from gastric aspirates in patients with giant hypertrophic gastritis. However, because of the technical difficulties of intubation, this approach cannot be applied for the detection of enteric protein loss in routine clinical practice. Furthermore, the leaking protein is liable to digestion by the proteolytic enzymes with the production of amino acids and ^{131}I, both of which are reabsorbed. Also, ^{131}I is secreted in the saliva and gastric juice, leading to false elevation in the fecal radioactivity.

To prevent iodine reabsorption, an ion exchange resin (Amberlite IRA-400) is given orally (5 gm every 4 to 6 hours) to bind the radioiodine freed during the breakdown of the leaking labeled albumin. The radioactivity thus bound is excreted with the resin in the stools. However, the problem of secretion of ^{131}I in the salivary and gastric secretions has not been solved.

Another source of error is that a fraction of the radioiodine might be reabsorbed before being bound by the resin. Furthermore, part of the ^{131}I originally bound to the resin might be lost during its passage through the intestine.

The most accepted method employing radioiodinated albumin depends on following the daily levels of plasma, urinary, and fecal radioactivity over a period of at least 2 weeks after the intravenous injection of 30 to 100 μCi of ^{131}I-labeled human serum albumin. From the obtained values, the plasma volume, total exchangeable body albumin, half-life of ^{131}I-labeled albumin, and albumin turnover are calculated. Lugol's solution is administered to block the uptake of ^{131}I by the thyroid gland, whereas radioiodine reabsorption is prevented by the resin. The information obtained about protein metabolism by means of this technique is extensive and very valuable. However, collection of the stools and urine over such a prolonged period, together with the tedious calculations involved, makes the application of this technique for clinical use impractical.

Radioiodinated polyvinylpyrrolidone (PVP). The patient's stools are collected for 96 hours after intravenous injection of 10 to 25 μCi of ^{131}I-labeled PVP. Fecal radioactivity is measured and expressed as percentage of the administered dose, and care is taken to use identical geometry during counting. Normally, the level of radioactivity in the 96-hour stool does not exceed 1.5% of the injected dose.

The main advantages of PVP are its resistance to proteolytic enzymes and its relatively poor absorption. However, this substance is not a natural plasma constituent but a synthetic polymer with a spectrum of different molecular weights. Therefore it cannot reflect the true picture of protein metabolism. The survival of PVP in the blood is shorter than that of plasma proteins. It is rapidly cleared by the reticuloendothelial system and excreted by the kidneys. Consequently, the fecal excretion of radioiodinated PVP cannot be used as a quantitative measure of protein loss through the gastrointestinal tract but is a very useful simple screening test.

Radiochromium human serum albumin. The dose applied is 30 to 50 μCi of ^{51}Cr-labeled albumin. Normal subjects excrete less than 0.7% of the intravenously administered dose in stools collected over a period of 96 hours.

In this technique there is neither salivary secretion nor intestinal reabsorption of radioactivity. However, since ^{51}Cr is gradually eluted from the albumin, this technique cannot be used for determination of albumin turnover.

To quantitate the gastrointestinal protein loss, fecal radioactivity is expressed as number of milliliters of plasma lost through the intestine per day. This is obtained by dividing radioactivity in the 24-hour stool by the counting rate of 1 ml of plasma of the same day. Normally, 5 to 25 ml of plasma are cleared from their albumin into the gastrointestinal tract on each day.

This technique not only detects protein leakage through the gastrointestinal tract but also offers a quantitative measure of the amount lost.

Radioiron dextran. In contrast to ^{131}I- and ^{51}Cr-labeled compounds, the label of ^{59}Fe dextran is not excreted in urine. This obviates a major source of error, the contamination of the collected stools with radioactive urine.

As explained in the ^{51}Cr-labeled albumin technique, the gastrointestinal protein loss is quantitated by calculation of the gastrointestinal ^{59}Fe clearance. This is achieved by relating the fecal ^{59}Fe excretion to the mean ^{59}Fe concentration in the plasma.

BIBLIOGRAPHY

Beeson, P. B., and McDermott, W.: Textbook of medicine, Philadelphia, 1967, W. B. Saunders Co.

Berquist, T. H., Nolan, N. G., Stephens, D. H., and Carlson, H. C.: Specificity of ^{99m}Tc-pertechnetate in scintigraphic diagnosis of Meckel's diverticulum; review of 100 cases, J. Nucl. Med. 17:465-469, 1976.

Braunstein, P., and Song, C. S.: The uses and limitations of radioisotopes in the investigation of gastrointestinal diseases, Am. J. Dig. Dis. 20:53-90, 1975.

Chafetz, N., Taylor, A., Schleif, A., Verba, J., and Hooser, C. W.: A potential error in the quantitation of fecal blood loss, J. Nucl. Med. 17:1053-1054, 1976.

Chaudhuri, T. K.: Can ^{99m}Tc-pertechnetate be used to assess the secretion of gastric acid in pernicious anemia? J. Nucl. Med. 18:121-122, 1977.

Ganong, W. F.: Review of medical physiology, Los Altos, Calif. 1967, Lange Medical Publications.

Gordon, R. S., Jr.: Exudative enteropathy. Abnormal permeability of the gastrointestinal tract demonstrable with labelled polyvinylpyrrolidone, Lancet **276**:325-326, 1959.

Jeejeebhoy, K. N., and Coghill, N. F.: The measurement of gastrointestinal protein loss by a new method, Gut **2**: 123-130, 1961.

Mahmood, A.: Blood loss caused by helmenthic infections, Trans. R. Soc. Trop. Med. Hyg. **60**:766-769, 1966.

Marsden, D. S., and Priebe, C. J.: Preliminary appraisal of present ^{99m}Tc-pertechnetate techniques for detecting ectopic gastric mucosa, Radiology **113**: 459-460, 1974.

Palmer, E. D.: Clinical gastroenterology, New York, 1957, Hoeber-Harper.

Razzak, M.A.: The application of nuclear medicine technology in schistosomiasis. In Compiled review on schistosomiasis, The National Information and Documentation Centre, Egypt, 1976, pp. 203-213.

Razzak, M. A., and Sodee, D. B.: Radioisotope photoscanning of the salivary glands, Am. J. Gastroenterol. **49**:503-505, 1968.

Silberstein, E. B.: Causes of abnormalities reported in nuclear medicine testing, J. Nucl. Med. **17**:229-232, 1976.

Sodeman, W. A., and Sodeman, W. A., Jr.: Pathologic physiology: mechanisms of disease, Philadelphia, 1967, W. B. Saunders Co.

Sterling, K.: The turnover rate of serum albumin in man as measured by ^{131}I-tagged albumin, J. Clin. Invest. **30**:1228-1237, 1951.

Spencer, R. P., Koons, C. R., Maxfield, W. S., and King, E. R.: Clinical diagnostic studies of the gastrointestinal tract utilizing radioisotopes, South. Med. J. **51**:1374-1377, 1958.

Turner, D. A.: The absorption, transport and deposition of fat, Am. J. Dig. Dis. **3**:594-540, 682-708, 1958.

Wagner, H. N., Jr.: Radioactive pharmaceuticals, Clin. Pharmacol. Ther. **4**:351-370, 1963.

Wilson, J. P., Wenzel, W. W., and Campbell, J. B.: Technitium scans in the detection of gastrointestinal hemorrhage: preoperative diagnosis of enteric duplication in an infant. J.A.M.A. **237**:265-266, 1977.

Wine, C. R., Nahrwold, D. L., Rose, R. C., and Miller, K. L.: Effect of histamine on technetium-99m excretion by gastric mucosa, Surgery **80**:591-594, 1976.

21 Liver

ANATOMY AND PHYSIOLOGY

The liver is the largest solid organ in the body, weighing almost 3 pounds (1.5 kg) in the adult. It occupies the right hypochondrium and part of the epigastric area, extending into the left hypochondrium and downward into the right lumbar region. It lies directly under the diaphragm and is sheltered in its greater part by the ribs (Figs. 14-1, 21-1, and 24-1, *B*).

The liver consists of two main lobes, the right much larger than the left. On the medial portion of the right lobe are two lesser segments called the *caudate* and *quadrate* lobes. They are separated on the inferior or visceral surface of the liver by a deep, short fissure called the *porta hepatis*. Through the porta most of the blood vessels, nerves, and lymphatics as well as the hepatic bile ducts enter and leave the organ.

The liver has a dual blood supply. The portal vein brings venous blood from the intestine and spleen. It normally accounts for 65% to 75% of the total flow. The remainder is delivered by the hepatic artery, which supplies the liver with arterial blood. Both vessels enter the liver through the porta hepatis. In the liver the portal venous and hepatic arterial bloods mix at different levels in the hepatic sinusoids. Blood is then drained by way of the central hepatic veins into the hepatic veins, which emerge from the back of the liver and enter into the inferior vena cava.

Most of the lymphatic vessels of the liver terminate in a small group of glands around the porta hepatis. Others pierce the diaphragm to end in the mediastinal glands, and the remainder accompany the inferior vena cava to terminate in glands around it in the thorax.

On the surface of the body the outline of the liver can be simulated by a triangle. The upper border of the liver corresponds to a line drawn from a point slightly medial to the left midclavicular line at the upper border of the sixth rib, crossing the midline at the junction of the body of the sternum and the xiphoid process, and ending at the level of the fifth rib in the right midclavicular line. The lateral border extends from this point downward and outward to meet the seventh rib at the side of the chest and continues downward to about ½ inch (1cm) below the costal margin. The lower border can be indicated by a line drawn ½ inch (1 cm) below the costal margin to the right ninth costal cartilage, then obliquely upward to cross the midline at the transpyloric plane and meet the left eighth costal cartilage.

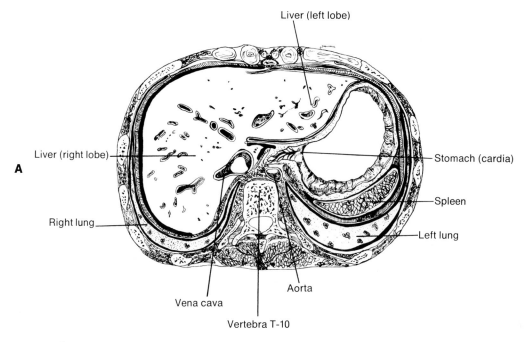

Liver (left lobe)

Liver (right lobe)

A

Stomach (cardia)

Spleen

Right lung

Left lung

Vena cava

Aorta

Vertebra T-10

Fig. 21-1. Transverse sections through the abdomen to demonstrate the relative positions of the internal organs. **A,** At the level of the tenth thoracic vertebra. **B,** At the level of the twelfth thoracic vertebra. **C,** At the level of the third lumbar vertebra.

From there it extends with a slight downward convexity to end at the beginning of the first line.

Structure and function

The liver is covered by a connective tissue capsule that dips at the porta hepatis, where it grows deep and branches into the substance of the organ, providing it with internal support.

For descriptive purposes, the liver can be compared to a sponge. Its main substance suggests anastomosing plates one cell thick or sheets of polyhedral parenchymal hepatic cells. Between the adjacent rows of hepatic cells of the same plate are tiny passageways called *bile canaliculi,* or *capillaries.* The irregularly disposed cavities between the cell plates represent the sinusoids. These sinusoids are lined by a very thin layer of endothelial cells. Some of these are flat, whereas the others bulge with raylike extensions that gave them the name *stellate cells* (also called *Kupffer cells*). Pervading the liver and running in variable directions are two separate systems of pipelines: the portal tracts or canals and the hepatic central canals. The portal tracts contain a portal vein radicle, hepatic arteriole, and bile duct. The central hepatic canals contain radicles of the hepatic veins.

Because of its intermediate position in the circulation between the intestines and the heart, the liver serves as a receiving depot, storehouse, and chemical fac-

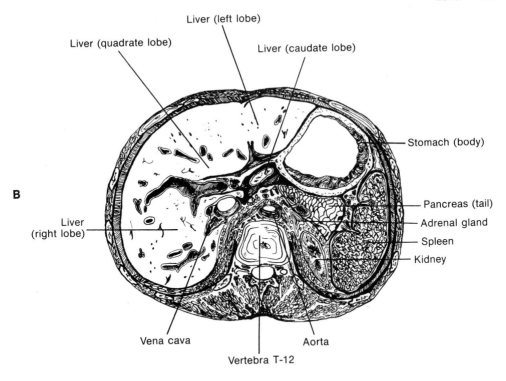

Liver (left lobe)

Liver (quadrate lobe)

Liver (caudate lobe)

Stomach (body)

B

Liver
(right lobe)

Pancreas (tail)

Adrenal gland

Spleen

Kidney

Vena cava

Aorta

Vertebra T-12

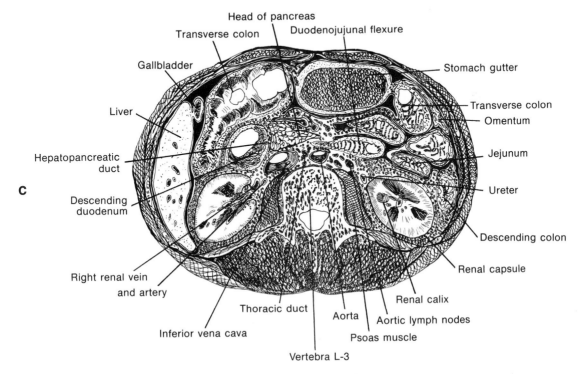

Head of pancreas

Transverse colon

Duodenojujunal flexure

Gallbladder

Stomach gutter

Liver

Transverse colon

Omentum

Hepatopancreatic
duct

Jejunum

C

Ureter

Descending
duodenum

Right renal vein
and artery

Descending colon

Renal capsule

Renal calix

Thoracic duct

Aorta

Aortic lymph nodes

Inferior vena cava

Psoas muscle

Vertebra L-3

Fig. 21-1, cont'd. For legend see opposite page.

tory. Through the portal vein it receives all the absorbed products of digestion from the intestines with the exception of some fats. In the liver these absorbed materials are metabolized by the polygonal parenchymal cells and prepared either for storage or for use by the various tissues of the body. These parenchymal cells also function in the formation and secretion of bile as well as the excretion of exogenous substances, particularly dyes such as rose bengal, sulfobromophthalein (BSP), and fluorescein. As a storage organ the liver deals with glycogen, fats, proteins, vitamins, and other substances needed for blood formation and regeneration. In synthesis the liver is active in the anabolic formation of glycogen, serum lipids, ketone bodies, plasma proteins, and some of the enzymes. In addition, the liver has a detoxicating action by which endogenous or exogenous harmful substances are made innocuous. Furthermore, the liver plays a major role in the metabolism of blood pigments.

As part of the reticuloendothelial system, Kupffer cells participate in production of antibodies, blood pigment breakdown, and phagocytosis (engulfing of microorganisms, cell fragments, foreign particles, and colloidal suspensions).

The excretory system of the liver begins with the biliary canaliculi, which lie between the hepatic parenchymal cells and communicate with the ducts in the portal canals. In the porta hepatis the ducts from the different lobes of the liver fuse to form the *common hepatic duct*. The common hepatic duct, after receiving the *cystic duct* from the gallbladder, continues as the *common bile duct*; it opens into the duodenum either by a common orifice with the pancreatic duct or separately.

The *gallbladder* can be considered as a side arm to the biliary system. Its main functions are concentration and storage of the biliary secretion during the intervals between meals. Expulsion of the bile from the gallbladder into the duodenum occurs through gallbladder contractions, accompanied by relaxation of the sphincter of Oddi surrounding the end of the common bile duct. The chief components of bile are bile salts, bile pigments, cholesterol, lecithin, fats, and various inorganic salts. With the exception of bile salts, biliary constituents are excretory products. Bile salts are needed for the proper digestion and absorption of fats and related substances such as fat-soluble vitamins.

RADIONUCLIDE EVALUATION

The introduction of improved radiopharmaceuticals and the availability of sensitive equipment have made it possible to use radionuclide techniques for the study of the hemodynamic pattern, function, and morphology of the liver.

According to their nature, radioactive nuclides used for hepatic evaluation can be classified into two main groups. The first group is represented by radionuclides that are picked up by the phagocytic Kupffer cells. These radiopharmaceuticals are usually colloidal suspensions such as ^{32}P chromic phosphate, ^{198}Au colloidal gold, denatured or microaggregated ^{131}I serum albumin, ^{99m}Tc-labeled sulfur colloid and ^{99m}Tc-tagged calcium phytate. The second group consists of soluble dyes and substances that are removed from the circulation mainly by the hepatic parenchymal polygonal cells, such as ^{131}I rose bengal, ^{35}S sulfobromophthalein, ^{123}I rose bengal, ^{99m}Tc penicillamine, ^{99m}Tc pyridoxylideneglutamate, ^{99m}Tc-N-(2,6-dimethylphenylcarbamoylmethyl) iminodiacetic acid, and ^{99m}Tc-N-(2,6-diethylacetanilide) iminodiacetic acid.

Determination of hepatic blood flow and liver function

If a substance that is removable solely by a single organ is injected intravenously, its disappearance from the circulating blood will depend on the blood flow carrying this substance to the particular organ, together with the state of function of the cells responsible for its removal. Thus with diminution in the blood flow to the organ, the disappearance of the substance is less rapid, which also means that the time taken for removal from the circulation is longer. The same result can be caused by a decrease in the functional ability of the cells responsible for removal of the test substance.

In the liver the situation is complicated by the presence of two types of cells, each of which is responsible for the removal of materials of specific nature. The parenchymal cells remove dyes, whereas the Kupffer cells remove colloids. Therefore each case much be considered separately.

When colloid particles of certain size are injected intravenously, their removal from the circulation should depend on the amount of blood filtered by the liver, together with the phagocytic activity of Kupffer cells. However, if the number of particles entering the liver is kept low in relation to the number of receptor sites, these particles should be totally phagocytized in a single passage through the liver. Consequently, the rate of removal of the colloid from the blood is no longer affected by the phagocytic activity of Kupffer cells, which is more than enough, but is dependent only on the amount of liver blood flow. Such limitation is easily achieved in clinical practice if the concentration of particles is kept below a certain critical level. This is helped to a great extent by the fact that with inflammation, damage, or exhaustive use of Kupffer cells, the disabled cells are rapidly discharged and replaced by a new generation of phagocytic cells; the phagocytic receptor sites are thus kept in abundance at all times. Therefore if the rate of disappearance of colloid particles from the circulating blood could be determined, it would represent an index of the liver blood flow.

These assumptions do not hold true in the case of dyes that are removed from the circulation by the hepatic parenchymal cells, presumably through a process of active transport. Their removal is followed by a brief phase of intracellular storage of the dye before its ultimate secretion into the bile. Therefore the rate of removal of these dyes from the circulating blood depends on both the liver blood flow and the functional capacity of the hepatic parenchymal cells.

Estimation of blood flow. Determination of the rate of disappearance of colloid particles from the circulation reveals the state of blood flow in the liver. However, the size of these particles is critical if they are to be extracted in a single passage through the liver. If they are too large, they are caught in the pulmonary bed, the first vascular bed encountered by substances injected intravenously. If the particles are too small, they pass through the liver without being picked up by the Kupffer cells.

Various radiocolloids have been tried, but none of them has proved to be completely satisfactory. ^{32}P chromic phosphate, apart from being difficult to prepare in uniformly sized particles, is a beta emitter and therefore cannot be monitored externally. Similarly, the preparation of denatured albumin tagged with ^{131}I is complicated and rather uncertain. The most commonly used radiopharmaceutical for determination of the hepatic blood flow is colloidal gold particles tagged with the gamma-emitting radionuclide ^{198}Au. This radiocolloid is easy to prepare and widely available. However, because its particles vary in size, some of the particles pass through the liver without being extracted by the Kupffer cells. Nevertheless, colloidal gold is better than ^{99m}Tc-labeled sulfur colloid in this determination since it is a more uniform and reproducible colloid with a stable label.

To determine the disappearance rate of radiogold from the circulation, 20 to 40 μCi of colloidal gold (^{198}Au) is injected intravenously. The level of radioactivity in the circulating blood is followed either by serial blood sampling or, more easily, by external monitoring.

For external monitoring a collimated scintillation detector is either centered over the temple or placed over the thigh. The information collected is counted by a rate meter with a time constant of 3 seconds and drawn on a stripchart recorder moving at a rate of $^3/_4$ inch per minute. When the information thus obtained is drawn on a semilogarithmic scale, the disappearance of radiogold from the circulation appears to be a complex exponential function of time, being made of an early rapid phase and a later slow phase. This time variation is a result of the varied sizes of the colloid particles, which result in different disappearance rates. To correct for the effect of the smaller particles, which are not removed by the liver and which cause the slower phase, the tail of the curve is extrapolated back to zero time and subtracted from the original reading (Fig. 21-2). The resulting values are plotted on a semilogarithmic scale, and the time taken for the disappearance of half the radioactivity is determined. This is called the *disappearance,* or *clearance,* half-time ($T_{1/2}$). The disappearance rate constant (K) is obtained by dividing 0.693 (natural log of 2) by the disappearance half-time. The disappearance rate constant represents the fraction of total blood volume that is cleared of the colloid by the liver per unit time, that is, the liver blood flow as a fraction of the total blood volume. Therefore the hepatic blood flow can be calculated by multiplying K times the blood volume.

The disappearance half-time of radiogold can also be determined from the hepatic uptake curve as obtained by a collimated scintillation detector placed over the right eighth intercostal space in the midaxillary plane. The obtained readings

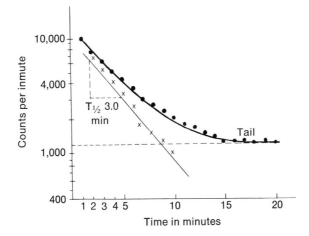

Fig. 21-2. Determination of the disappearance half-time of radiogold from the circulation by means of a detector placed over the temple. The tail of the curve is extrapolated and subtracted from the original readings.

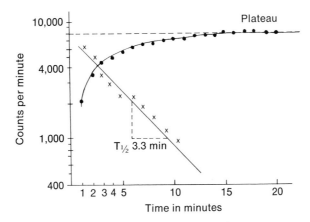

Fig. 21-3. Determination of the disappearance half-time of radiogold by the hepatic uptake technique. The recorded values are subtracted from the level of plateau activity.

are subtracted from the level of plateau activity, and the resultant values are plotted on a semilogarithmic scale against time to enable calculation of the disappearance half-time (Fig. 21-3). From this value, the disappearance rate constant is calculated and liver blood flow is determined.

Theoretically the hepatic counting rate represents a complex combination of hepatic accumulation of radioactivity versus blood disappearance occurring simultaneously in the field of the detector; however, in reality the level of the decreasing blood radioactivity in relation to the hepatic uptake (especially at the later time intervals) is too low to exert any significant effect. Therefore it can be ignored during the calculations.

The main advantage of the hepatic uptake technique is that it offers a direct measurement of the hepatic uptake of radioactivity without being affected by the extrahepatic removal of the radiocolloid particles. In addition, the increasing counting rate recorded with time makes it possible to use rather small tracer doses of the radiocolloid, with minimal statistical fluctuations in the obtained values.

Assessment of parenchymal cell function. Because ^{131}I rose bengal is representative of the group of dyes, the rate of its disappearance from the circulation should depend on both the liver blood flow and the functional capacity of the hepatic parenchymal polygonal cells. Therefore, slower removal of the dye from the circulation, as evidenced by prolongation in the disappearance half-time, can be caused by either diminished liver blood flow or impaired parenchymal cell function or both.

The source of the prolonged removal time can easily be identified by the subsequent determination of the liver blood flow by the radiogold method. If the liver blood flow is normal, then the fault is in the parenchymal cells. However, if the hepatic blood flow is diminished, the answer depends on the degree of abnormality, whether it can totally explain the prolongation in the disappearance half-time of rose bengal, denoting simply affection of the hepatic blood flow, or whether it cannot explain the obtained result, indicating diminution in the hepatic blood flow, together with parenchymal cell dysfunction.

The test itself is performed by the consecutive determination of the disappearance half-times of rose bengal and radioactive colloidal gold. This can be done by external monitoring of either tracer disappearance from the blood or, better, accumulation of tracers in the liver. The dosage used is 20 to 30 μCi of each, beginning with ^{131}I rose bengal, followed approximately 30 minutes later with radiogold. The various possible combinations of results and their interpretation are shown in Table 21-1.

Another test for evaluation of parenchymal cell function depends on estimation of the amount of ^{131}I rose bengal accumulating in the liver per unit of time and

Table 21-1. Combinations of results of test for parenchymal cell function

Test	*Condition*	$T_{1/2}$ *gold*	$T_{1/2}$ *rose bengal*	$\dfrac{T_{1/2}\ gold}{T_{1/2}\ rose\ bengal}$
Liver blood flow	Normal	3	6	0.50
Parenchymal cell	Normal	(2.0 to 4.3)	(4.0 to 8.0)	(0.40 to 0.70)
Liver blood flow	Normal	3	9	0.33
Parenchymal cell	Impaired			
Liver blood flow	Diminished	6	12	0.50
Parenchymal cell	Normal			
Liver blood flow	Diminished	8	30	0.27
Parenchymal cell	Impaired			

expressing it as a fraction of the hepatic blood pool. The hepatic blood pool (not blood flow) is estimated by recording the counting rate over the liver by means of a strip chart recorder after the intravenous injection of 10 μCi of radioiodinated serum albumin. This is followed by the intravenous administration of an exactly equal dose (10 μCi) of radioactive rose bengal; the hepatic counting rate is recorded with respect to time. This enables calculation of the amount of activity caused by radioactive rose bengal accumulating in the liver per unit of time. This is then expressed as percentage of the counting rate caused by the hepatic blood pool.

The sensitivity of this test can be enhanced by the simultaneous injection of BSP (2.5 mg/kg) with the radioactive rose bengal. The BSP acts as a stress to the liver cells and thus helps differentiate borderline normal and abnormal cases.

Under these specifications, the lowest value for normal is 10.5%. Lower values are indicative of impaired parenchymal cell function.

The two radioactive liver function tests just discussed have the advantage of demonstrating the functional capacity of the parenchymal cells separately from the state of the hepatic blood flow. In contrast, the result of the chemical BSP test (the most commonly used liver function test in cases without jaundice) is affected by both the liver blood flow and the parenchymal cell function. Consequently, an abnormal BSP test does not necessarily indicate impaired parenchymal cell function as it usually thought.

Patency of biliary system

Normally rose bengal is extracted from the blood by the hepatic parenchymal cells, where is stays for a short time before being secreted with the bile into the duodenum. Therefore after the intravenous injection of a tracer dose of ^{131}I rose bengal, radioactivity should be detectable by a collimated scintillation detector centered over the intestine. (Care should be taken to avoid having the liver in the field of the detector.) In cases of biliary obstruction, there is no significant rise above background radioactivity in 1 hour after the injection. More valuable information can be obtained if this test is performed concomitantly with radionuclide photoscanning of the liver.

The value of the radioactive rose bengal test as an aid in distinguishing medical from surgical causes of jaundice has been enhanced with the introduction of rapid organ imaging devices, such as the scintillation camera, and the development of pharmaceuticals labeled with radionuclides having short physical half-lives. The availability of these devices has made the dynamic visualization of biliary kinetics not only possible but also practical. Serial scintiphotographs obtained with the gamma camera after the intravenous administration of labeled rose bengal or ^{99m}Tc-N-(2,6 diethylacetanilide) iminodiacetic acid enable the assessment of the rate and magnitude of the hepatic uptake of the radioactive dye, as well as its mode of excretion into the biliary tree and intestine (Fig. 21-4).

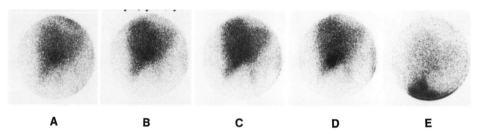

A　　　　**B**　　　　**C**　　　　**D**　　　　**E**

Fig. 21-4. Sequential ^{131}I rose bengal scintiphotographs demonstrate the normal time relationship of dye transport through the biliary system and its release from the gallbladder into the intestine. **A,** Exposure up to 7 minutes after rose bengal administration shows the even distribution of radioactivity throughout the liver. Gradual filling of the gallbladder and clearing of the liver parenchyma are well illustrated in **B, C,** and **D,** obtained at 29 to 33 minutes, 37 to 41 minutes, and 53 to 57 minutes after dose administration, respectively. Evidence of gastrointestinal excretion of the dye is seen in these same exposures. **E,** Emptying of the gallbladder is shown 4 hours after rose bengal administration. In this study the level of blood radioactivity was 21,673 cpm and 7,131 cpm at 5 and 20 minutes after dose administration, respectively. Accordingly, ^{131}I rose bengal blood retention is $7,131/21,673 = 33\%$.

Clinical applications

The previously described radionuclide techniques are indicated in the evaluation of hepatic disorders, irrespective of the presence or absence of jaundice. They are most commonly used in the study of hepatic cirrhosis, parasitic affection of the liver, jaundice, postnecrotic scarring, or any diffuse affection of the liver.

RADIONUCLIDE SCANNING

Liver scanning may be carried out by means of the rectilinear scanner or the gamma camera. The latter offers the advantages of speed and ability to take multiple pictures in a short time, especially if short-lived radionuclides are used.

Since successful visualization of an organ depends on the selective deposition of a gamma-emitting radionclude in that organ, any of the previously mentioned labeled colloids or dyes can be used for radionuclide scanning of the liver. However, each one has advantages and drawbacks.

^{131}**I rose bengal.** Radioiodinated rose bengal is extracted from the blood by the hepatic parenchymal cells and rapidly secreted with the bile. This particular behavior is the source of both its advantages and its disadvantages.

Because of its rapid secretion with the bile, the biologic half-life of ^{131}I rose bengal is very short, resulting in marked diminution of the radiation dose delivered to the liver and to the patient as a whole. In addition, the appearance of radioactivity in the region of the bowel can be taken as an indication of biliary patency.

On the other hand, the secretion of radioiodinated rose bengal with the bile into the gallbladder might mask any lesion in the area of the bed of the gallbladder.

Furthermore, the level of hepatic radioactivity changes over the period of scanning; this definitely affects the quality of the scan picture obtained.

In an attempt to solve the difficulties outlined in the previous paragraph, scanning is started from below to hit the area of the gallbladder before the radioactivity-containing bile reaches this region. Another method is to inject some nonradioactive rose bengal with the tagged material to slow down its excretion and stabilize the counting rate. There is still one main problem without solution. It depends on the fact that ^{131}I rose bengal is extracted from the circulation by the hepatic parenchymal cells. When there is parenchymal cell dysfunction, the hepatic counting rate is low, with wide statistical fluctuations, resulting in a poor scan picture. Allowing more time for the hepatic uptake process to increase the counting rate does not overcome this difficulty, since it is counteracted by the occurrence of secretion, which tends to decrease the level of radioactivity over the liver.

Usually 150 μCi of ^{131}I rose bengal is used. At least two views, anterior and right lateral, are obtained. Then the area to the left of the umbilicus is scanned. Appearance of radioactivity in this area in the scan picture indicates biliary patency. If patency is not verified, scanning is repeated after 24 hours. Absence of radioactivity in the bowel without significant change in the hepatic counting rate indicates complete biliary obstruction. With partial biliary obstruction there is progressive diminution in the hepatic counting rate, accompanied by increased visualization of radioactivity in the region of the intestine.

Accordingly, the main indication for hepatic scanning with ^{131}I rose bengal is the study of cases with possible biliary obstruction. Radioactive rose bengal is also used to verify the diagnosis of focal defects seen in hepatic scans performed after the administration of colloidal particles. If both scan pictures have the same appearance, the defect should represent a true focal lesion. On the other hand, focal defects encountered in hepatic scans performed with colloidal particles and not confirmed in the rose bengal scan picture should point to a diffuse disease of the liver such as cirrhosis, since damage to Kupffer cells does not parallel that to parenchymal cells.

The physical characteristics of the radionuclide, ^{131}I, used to label rose bengal are not optimal for imaging, especially with the relatively thin crystal of the scintillation camera. As an alternative, ^{123}I, with its shorter physical half-life (13 hours) and lower energy, can be used for labeling to obtain better quality pictures because of the higher counting rates allowable with the high dosage of the radionuclide (2 mCi). However, this radionuclide is expensive. In this connection, a technetium-labeled agent is preferable because of the excellent physical characteristics of ^{99m}Tc for imaging as well as its ready availability.

^{99m}Tc **pyridoxylideneglutamate.** This compound has the advantage of being rapidly excreted through the biliary tree, with marked accumulation in the gallbladder and intestine. However, the gallbladder is not consistently visualized in all normal subjects, and the biliary concentration of this material is always lower than that of rose bengal. A further disadvantage is the time consumed in the preparation of this radiopharmaceutical.

[99m]Tc-N-(2,6-diethylacetanilide) **iminodiacetic acid.** This radiopharmaceutical exhibits most of the characteristics required in an ideal agent for hepatobiliary scintigraphy, such as rapid extraction and fast transit through the hepatic polygonal cells, high biliary concentration, little absorption from the intestine, minimal concentration in the urinary tract, high labeling yield with ^{99m}Tc, and availability as a sterile nontoxic kit. Following the intravenous injection of 5 to 8 mCi of this radiopharmaceutical, radioactivity disappearance from the blood is a biphasic exponential function of time, starting with an early rapid component and ending with a much slower phase. The gallbladder is usually visualized in normal patients, especially when fasting. In contrast, the gallbladder is not seen in patients having jaundice. Careful interpretation of properly performed sequential scintiphotography might enable differentiation of these cases. Thus, in patients with complete biliary obstruction, as well as in most cases of severe hepatocellular disease, no radioactivity is detected in the duodenum; whereas, with incomplete obstruction, the duodenum is usually visualized somewhat later than normal. Another diagnostic clue that can prove very helpful is the visualization of the distended extrahepatic bile ducts in patients with incomplete obstruction of the hepatobiliary ducts. This phenomenon is never seen in either complete obstruction or in severe hepatocellular damage. The demonstration of the distended biliary tree could be easily achieved with greater accuracy with ultrasonography and/or computerized transaxial tomography.

[198]**Au colloidal gold.** Colloidal gold particles are picked up by the phagocytic Kupffer cells, where they stay until they are discharged with the cells. Therefore, the biologic half-life of radiogold depends mainly on its physical half-life, which is 2.7 days. This makes the radiation dose delivered by radiogold administration for hepatic scanning higher than that caused by radioiodinated rose bengal. Nevertheless, it is definitely much lower than the permissible levels. The persistence of radiogold particles in the Kupffer cells can be considered an advantage from another point of view. Thus in cases in which the uptake of radiogold is impaired by vascular affections leading to a low hepatic counting rate, the level of radioactivity can be increased simply by allowing a longer time interval between the injection of the radiogold particles and the scanning procedure. In this connection it should be remembered that, in contrast to labeled dyes, the hepatic uptake of radiocolloids is not affected by the functional capacity of the parenchymal cells of the liver. Therefore, a reasonable hepatic uptake of the radiogold colloid can be obtained even with marked hepatic parenchymal cell dysfunction. Further advantages of radiogold are its easy preparation and its widespread commercial availability. To these we may add the reasonable suitability of radiogold for the estimation of the hepatic blood flow.

Scanning of the liver is performed after the intravenous injection of about 150

μCi of ¹⁹⁸Au colloidal gold. It is preferable to start the scanning procedure 2 to 4 hours after injection to allow enough time for the hepatic counting rate to be reasonable and stable, especially in patients with hepatovascular impairment. At least two views, anterior and right lateral, should be obtained (Fig. 21-5).

⁹⁹ᵐTc-labeled sulfur colloid. As is true of radiogold, the biologic half-life of technetium sulfur colloid depends mainly on its physical half-life, which is short (6 hours); the radiation dose is therefore rather low. For this reason and because technetium is low in energy, a relatively large dose (2 to 4 mCi) can be used, with the production of a higher counting rate and good counting statistics allowing greater diagnostic accuracy. Consequently, the time needed for scanning of the liver is shortened. However, because of the low energy of technetium and its short penetration, deep-seated lesions are easily missed. Furthermore, sometimes it is difficult to delineate the left lobe of the liver from the spleen, which is visualized even in normal individuals. To overcome these difficulties, more views are performed, and this undoubtedly involves more time when a single crystal rectilinear scanner is used. This problem can be easily solved by the use of a stationary imaging device (Fig. 21-6).

Because of its short shelf half-life, technetium sulfur colloid shipments should be frequent; otherwise, the colloid has to be prepared on location and this necessitates good quality control measures to ensure producing a colloid of uniform size, batch after batch. This fact limits the widespread use of technetium sulfur colloid for the routine radionuclide scanning of the liver in distant small hospitals.

In addition, because of the wide range in the size of its particles, ⁹⁹ᵐTc-labeled sulfur colloid cannot be used for the determination of the hepatic blood flow with reasonable accuracy. Variability in the particle size distribution and its subsequent organ uptake are primarily dependent on the technical factors involved in the preparation of this radiocolloid. The larger particles that are formed, especially in the

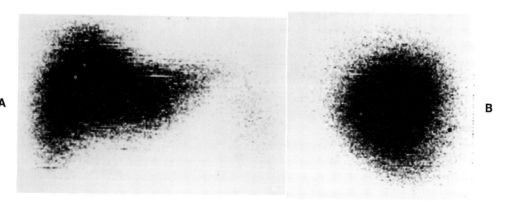

A   **B**

Fig. 21-5. Normal liver scan done with colloidal ¹⁹⁸Au. **A,** Anterior view. **B,** Right lateral view. Note the rather even distribution of radioactivity in the right lobe with less radiogold in the thinner left lobe. The spleen is barely visible.

presence of excess aluminum, are trapped in the lung capillaries. Another reason for the increased lung activity encountered in some of the cases during hepatic scintigraphy with ^{99m}Tc-labeled sulfur colloid might be increase in circulatory macrophages noticed in some pathologic states such as prolonged hepatic disease and Hodgkin's disease.

^{113m}In colloid. The major advantage of ^{113m}In is its short half-life (1.7 hours), as well as its availability from a parent (^{113}Sn) with a sufficiently long half-life of 118 days. This abolishes the difficulties encountered by distant users, especially in the developing countries.

The dose needed for hepatic scanning is the same as that of ^{99m}Tc sulfur colloid (2 to 4 mCi). Similarly, the spleen is usually visualized in the obtained scan picture.

Denatured human serum albumin and microaggregated albumin colloid tagged with ^{131}I. Particles of denatured human serum albumin and microaggregated albumin tagged with ^{131}I differ from those of other colloids in being metabolized after their capture by the phagocytic Kupffer cells. This behavior makes the radiation dose delivered to the liver lower than that caused by the other radiocolloids. However, the preparation of such particles with uniform size has not yet become standardized on a commercial basis.

Usually 500 μCi of the radioactive material are used, and at least two views are obtained.

^{99m}Tc phytate. ^{99m}Tc phytate is a stannous complex of inositol hexaphosphoric acid. After its intravenous injection, the phytate forms an insoluble microcolloid in vivo by chelating blood calcium. The colloidal calcium phytate has uniform size particles that undergo reticuloendothelial localization by phagocytosis predominately in the hepatic Kupffer cells. The degree of splenic accumulation is similar to that observed with colloidal gold and much less than with sulfur colloid. Accordingly, the spleen is not visualized in normal subjects.

Scanning is usually started about 20 minutes after the intravenous injection of 1 to 4 mCi of the radiopharmaceutical.

Interpretation of hepatic scans

In the interpretation of the scan pictures obtained, the size, site, and shape of the liver are to be considered. This is facilitated by the application of some fixed reference points on the scan picture. The reference points suggested are the xiphisternum in the midline, the fifth intercostal space, and the costal margin in the midclavicular planes of both sides. Further help is achieved by the superimposition of the scan picture on a plain x-ray film of the abdomen. Normally the liver lies immediately underneath the diaphragm and extends slightly below the costal margin in the right midclavicular plane. Because of its pliability, marked variation in the scintigraphic appearance of the liver has been noticed even among normal subjects. The other points to be considered are the distribution of radioactivity all over the liver and the visualization of the spleen. Usually the distribution of radioactivity is more or less homogeneous (Fig. 21-6), with density maximal in the center of the right lobe and decreasing gradually towards the periphery. Sometimes the extreme lateral end of the left lobe and the lower part of the right lobe are not quite apparent. Furthermore, because of their relative thinness, they may manifest areas of diminished concentration of radioactivity. Defects and irregularities along the margins are occasionally seen and explained by pressure effects of surrounding organs and by movements of the liver during respiration. Apart from these, diminished concentration of radioactivity whether localized or diffuse should be considered abnormal. In this connection it should always be remembered that radionuclide scans are diagnostic of morphology rather than pathology. Thus a localized area of diminished or absent concentration of radioactivity is diagnostic of a space-occupying lesion and can be produced by a variety of causes, such as tumor (whether primary or metastatic), pseudotumor of cirrhosis, abscess, or cyst (Fig. 21-7). In this connection, focal defects in the region of the porta hepatis must be interpreted with extreme caution. To increase the specificity of hepatic scintiscanning, one can resort to dynamic sequential imaging or use radionuclides with high uptake in tumor tissue, such as ^{67}Ga citrate, or those remaining exclusively intravascular to get blood pool images. Diffuse irregular deposition of radioactivity or mottling is seen with metastatic disease (Fig. 21-8) as well as with diffuse parenchymatous hepatic involvement, as in hepatitis, fibrosis, amyloidosis, and cirrhosis (Fig. 21-9). Consequently, the obtained scan should be interpreted in relationship to the history, physical findings, and other laboratory tests. Further help can be obtained from ultrasonography and computerized transaxial tomography.

Visualization of the spleen is a remote possibility in radiogold and phytate scans of the liver in normal subjects because of the low splenic uptake of colloidal particles. However, in cases of cirrhosis, in which the hepatic uptake is slow and diminished, the splenic uptake of radiocolloid is high enough to permit its visualization. In more advanced cases of cirrhosis the radioactivity is also seen in the bone marrow, especially that of the vertebral column. In contrast, during scintigraphy of the liver, whether ^{99m}Tc-labeled sulfur colloid or [113m]In colloid is used,

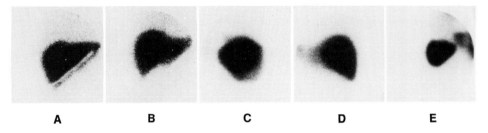

A   **B**   **C**   **D**   **E**

Fig. 21-6. Normal liver and spleen images. A, Anterior view with costal marker. B, Anterior view. C, Right lateral view. D, Posterior liver view. E, Posterior spleen view.

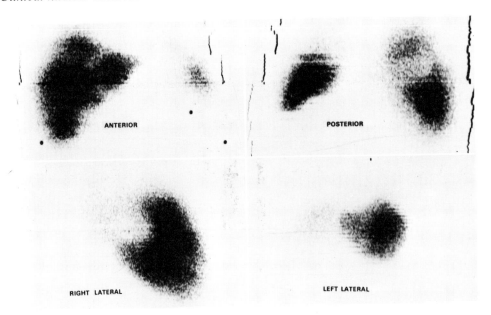

Fig. 21-7. 99mTc-labeled sulfur colloid liver spleen scan showing space-occupying lesion in the postero-superior aspect of the right lobe of the liver.

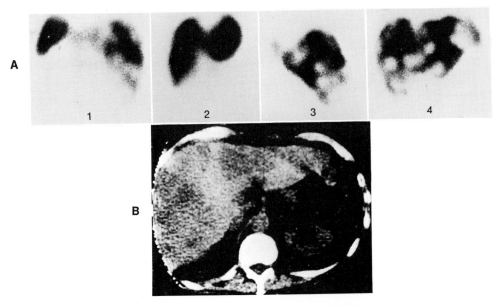

Fig. 21-8. A, 99mTc-labeled sulfur colloid liver spleen scan series showing multiple space-occupying lesions caused by metastatic deposits. *1*, Posterior; *2*, left lateral; *3*, right lateral; *4*, anterior. **B,** Computerized transaxial tomography of the same patient to demonstrate the degree of liver involvement.

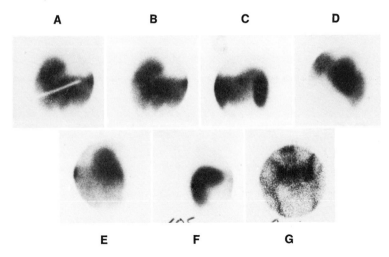

Fig. 21-9. Liver scan series. **A,** Anterior view with costal marker. **B,** Anterior view showing an abnormal hepatic contour with enlargement of accessory lobes and left lobe. The distribution of radioactivity throughout the liver is patchy. **C,** Anterior view to illustrate diminution in radionuclide concentration in the left lobe of the liver and good visualization of the spleen. **D,** Right lateral view. **E,** Posterior view of the liver. **F,** View of posterior spleen showing increased concentration of nuclide. **G,** Pelvic view showing expansion of bone marrow space into femurs. This patient had advanced nutritional (Laennec's) cirrhosis.

the spleen is regularly seen, to the extent that it may be difficult to differentiate from the left lobe of the liver. In cirrhosis, a higher amount of the radiocolloid accumulates in the spleen and to a lesser extent in the bone marrow (Fig. 21-9). This splenic shift of radiocolloid is also seen in other disease states such as polycythemia, extramedullary erythropoiesis, Hodgkin's disease, and congestive heart failure.

For quantitative analysis of liver scan data obtained with the aid of the gamma camera and rectilinear scanner, computer processing has been used with success.

The diagnostic accuracy of hepatic scintiscanning is roughly 75%. The false-negative results are caused by lesions smaller than the resolving power of the system used or by the presence of a good deal of overlying normal tissue. On the other hand, false-positive results are explained by the presence of overlying objects interferring with the detection of radioactivity or by the occurrence of anatomic variants and pressure effects from the adjacent structures.

Clinical applications

The main indication for radionuclide scanning of the liver is the demonstration of space-occupying lesions, especially metastatic deposits. In addition, accurate information about the size, shape, and site of the liver is obtained. This information may prove very helpful in the differential diagnosis of pain or mass in the right upper quadrant of the abdomen as well as in the detection of subdiaphragmatic

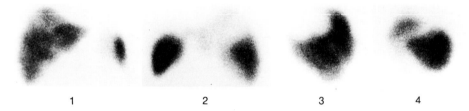

1   2   3   4

Fig. 21-10. Follow-up scans of the patient shown in Fig. 21-7 showing an increase in the size of the lesion. *1*, Anterior; *2*, posterior; *3*, right lateral; *4*, left lateral.

abscess. The diagnosis of this latter condition can be reached with greater accuracy by means of combined radionuclide scanning of the liver and lungs. A special indication is the use of ^{131}I rose bengal or ^{99m}Tc-N-(2,6-diethylacetanilide) iminodiacetic acid for the evaluation of biliary patency. Furthermore, hepatic scanning can be used for the evaluation of diffuse parenchymal disease of the liver without any danger or discomfort to the patient. Similarly, a follow-up of patients suffering from hepatic disorders can be obtained by a nontraumatic technique (Fig. 21-10).

BIBLIOGRAPHY

Akisada, M., and Miyamae, T.: Dynamic and scintigraphic studies of diffuse hepatic diseases using ^{99m}Tc-Sn-Phytate (Comparative analysis with ^{198}Au-colloid), Radioisotopes **24**:626-632, 1975.

Christie, J. H., MacIntyre, W. J., Crespo, G. G., and Koch-Weser, D.: Radioisotope scanning in hepatic cirrhosis, Radiology **81**:455-469, 1963.

Gomez-Crespo, G., MacIntyre, W. J., and Christie, J. H.: A comparison of ^{131}I rose bengal and colloidal ^{198}Au in liver scanning, Am. J. Roentgenol. Rad. Ther. Nucl. Med. **88**:296-303, 1962.

Iio, M., Kameda, H., and Ueda, H.: The study on hepatic blood flow determination by ^{198}Au colloid using deviced recording method. Jpn. Heart J. **1**: 17-36, 1960.

Larson, S. M., and Nelp, W. B.: Radiopharmacology of a simplified technetium-99m-colloid preparation for photoscanning, J. Nucl. Med. **7**:817-826, 1966.

Lunia, S., Parthasarathy, K. L., Bakshi, S., and Bender, M.: An evaluation of ^{99m}Tc-sulfur colloid liver scintiscans and their usefulness in a metastatic workup: a review of 1424 studies, J. Nucl. Med. **16**:62-65, 1975.

McClelland, R. R.: Focal porta hepatis scintiscan defects: what is their significance? J. Nucl. Med. **16**: 1007-1012, 1975.

Mustafa, A., Razzak, M. A., Mahfouz, M., and Guirgis, B.: Radioisotope photoscanning of the liver in bilharzial hepatic fibrosis, J. Nucl. Med. **7**:909-916, 1966.

Nagler, W., Bender, M., and Blau, M.: Radioisotope photoscanning of the liver, Gastroenterology **44**: 36-43, 1963.

Razzak, M. A.: The use of radioactive isotopes to study the hemodynamic pattern, function and morphology of the liver in hepatosplenic bilharziasis (Schistosomiasis), J. Nucl. Med. **5**:125-133, 1964.

Razzak, M. A.: Amoebic liver abscess, Tropenmed. Parasitol. **16**:284-291, 1965.

Razzak, M. A.: Assessment of the liver in bilharziasis by means of a modified radioactive rose bengal test, Am. J. Trop. Med. Hyg. **15**:37-42, 1966.

Razzak, M. A., and Wagner, H. N.: Measurement of hepatic blood flow by colloidal gold clearance, J. Appl. Physiol. **16**:1133-1138, 1961.

Ronai, P. M., Baker, R. J., Bellen, J. L., Collins, P. J., Anderson, P. J., and Lander, H.: Technetium-99m pyridoxylideneglutamate: a new hepatobiliary radiopharmaceutical. II. Clinical aspects. J. Nucl. Med. **16**:728-738, 1975.

Ryan, J., Cooper, M., Loberg, M., Harvey, E., and Sikorski, S.: Technetium-99m-labeled N-(2,6-dimethylphenyl carbamoylmethyl) imino-diacetic acid (Tc-99m HIDA): a new radiopharmaceutical for hepatobiliary imaging studies, J. Nucl. Med. **18**: 997-1002, 1977.

Serafini, A. N., Smoak, W. M., Hupf, H. B., Beaver, J. E., Holder, J., and Gilson, A. J.: Iodine-123-rose bengal: an improved hepatobiliary agent, J. Nucl. Med. **16**:629-632, 1975.

Silberstein, E. B.: Causes of abnormalities reported in nuclear medicine testing, J. Nucl. Med. **17**:229-232, 1976.

Stadalink, R. C., DeNardo, S. J., DeNardo, G. L., and Raventos, A.: Critical evaluation of hepatic scintigraphy for neoplastic tumors of the liver, J. Nucl. Med. **16**:595-601, 1975.

Taplin, G. V., Meredith, O. M., and Kade, H.: The radioactive ^{131}I tagged rose bengal uptake excretion test for liver function using external gamma ray scintillation counting technique, J. Lab. Clin. Med. **45**:665-678, 1955.

Taylor, R. D., Anderson, P. M., Winston, M. A., and Blahd, W. H.: Diagnosis of hepatic hemangioma using multiple-radionuclide and ultrasound techniques, J. Nucl. Med. **17**:362-364, 1976.

Wagner, H. N., McAfee, J. G., and Mozley, J. M.: Diagnosis of liver disease by radioisotope scanning, Arch. Intern. Med. **107**: 324-334, 1961.

Wistow, B. W., Sburamanian, G., VanHeertum, R. L., Henderson, R. W., Gagne, G. M., Hall, R. C., and McAfee, J. G.: An evaluation of ^{99m}Tc labeled hepatobiliary agents, J. Nucl. Med. **18**: 455-461, 1977.

Yeh, E., Pohlmann, G. P., and Meade, R. C.: Liver-heart imaging in evaluating hepatic focal defect, J. Nucl. Med. **16**:896-898, 1975.

22 Pancreas

ANATOMY AND PHYSIOLOGY

The pancreas has both an exocrine (external) and an endocrine (internal) function. It is approximately 5 to 6 inches in length, and it extends obliquely upward from the duodenum behind the stomach and across the posterior abdominal wall to the spleen at the level of the first and second lumbar vertebrae. The pancreas lies within the concavity of the duodenum to which it is attached by blood vessels, pancreatic ducts, and loose connective tissue. The adult pancreas is divided into a head, neck, body, and tail. The head is flattened dorsally and ventrally. The body of the pancreas is extremely thin; the tail thickens out slightly and is the pointed tonguelike left end of the gland that lies in contact with the spleen.

The primary exocrine function of the pancreas is mediated through the acinar cells, where the pancreatic enzymes are manufactured. The pancreatic enzymes and juices are carried through a ductal system, which empties into the duodenum through a primary duct and an accessory duct. The endocrine function of the pancreas is the manufacture of insulin in the islets of Langerhans found throughout the pancreas.

The pancreas is made up of alveoli, which resemble the salivary gland in their general arrangement and design. The part of the pancreas involved in its exocrine function is made up chiefly of groups of cells forming acini, which tend to be spherical. Groups of acini form primary lobules, and numerous adjacent primary lobules form a secondary lobule. Therefore the pancreatic tissue proper is composed of acinar cells, islet cells, and ductal cells. The acinar cells are large and have well-developed nuclei and abundant grandular cytoplasm. The granules, called *zymogen granules*, vary in number and position in the cell, depending on the state of activity of the gland.

The pancreas receives an abundant nerve supply from both the vagi and splanchnic nerves. The pancreas secretes a colorless, odorless, alkaline fluid of low viscosity through its ductal system. The pancreatic juice has a high bicarbonate content. Secretin is an endogenous hormone secreted by the duodenal mucosa. This hormone has a direct effect on the ductal cell and does not alter the output of enzymes from the gland. Pancreozymin, which is also an endogenous hormone secreted by the duodenal mucosa, does not stimulate the flow of juice but sharply increases enzyme concentration. Vagal stimulation, when superimposed on secretin-stimulated flow, also increases enzyme output. The protein content or the enzyme content of pancreatic juice varies between 0.1% and 0.3%. The enzymes of the pancreas are capable of digesting all three types of foodstuff; therefore, pancreatic juice is proteolytic, amylolytic, and lipolytic. The main proteolytic enzymes secreted from the pancreas are trypsinogen, chymotrypsinogen, peptidase, and carboxypeptidase. The lipolytic enzymes are lipase, phospholipase A, and phospholipase B. The amylolytic enzyme is pancreatic amylase.

Amino acid requirements for enzyme synthesis

It has been found that ten amino acids are required for maximum exocrine enzyme synthesis. These amino acids are tryptophan, arginine, threonine, valine, tyrosine, lysine, leucine, histadine, isoleucine, and phenylalanine. The only essential amino acid present in the crystalline enzymes that is not required for maximum synthesis is methionine. This amino acid is present in smaller amounts in the enzymes than any of the other amino acids. Presumably, the levels of free methionine in the tissue can satisfy the small demands for this amino acid for protein synthesis.

Pancreatic enzyme synthesis

Pancreatic enzymes removed from their site of synthesis in the pancreatic acinar cell are transported through a series of cell compartments and finally stored intracellularly in the zymogen granules. This transport has been studied and has been found to take approximately 45 minutes to 1 hour. The enzymes remain in storage in the zymogen granule. There is still controversy as to whether there is intermittent or continuous pancreatic secretion in humans.

SPECIAL PROCEDURES IN STUDY OF PANCREATIC FUNCTION—IN VITRO TESTING
Nonradioactive tests

Pancreatic exocrine insufficiency may be caused by a number of diseases. Since the pancreas is the principal source of lipase used for the digestion of fats, any decrease in the amount of lipase secreted will result in maldigestion of fats and will cause steatorrhea. Digestion is not affected as seriously as it would be if there were a defect in the output of proteolytic enzymes of the pancreas since there are other proteolytic enzymes found in the intestine. However, one of the clinical manifestations of pancreatic insufficiency is an excess of fat excreted in the feces.

Fecal fat excretion. Fecal fat excretion may be chemically measured. Normal individuals on an average diet seldom excrete more than 6 to 7 gm of fat in the feces in a 24-hour period.

Secretin and pancreozymin tests of function. Secretin, pancreozymin, or the combination may be injected into patients. The secretion of the pancreatic tree is collected by intubation. A double-lumen tube is passed through the patient's nose or mouth into the stomach and duodenum, one lumen opening into the stomach for draining gastric juice and the other into the duodenum for collection of the pancreatic and duodenal secretions. Samples from the duodenum are collected every 10 to 20 minutes. Depending on the type of study performed, secretin or pancreozymin is injected, and the duodenal contents are collected over a period of time. Volume, pH, bicarbonate, and enzyme determinations are then made on the collected samples.

In diseases of the pancreas associated with destruction of the secreting parenchyma the flow rate of the pancreas is decreased below 1 to 2 ml/kg of body weight for a 30-minute period. The bicarbonate content is decreased in inflammatory disease of the pancreas below 90 mEq/liter. It has been found that the addition of pancreozymin to the standard secretion test does not significantly improve the diagnostic accuracy of the procedure. The secretin test has been found to be of limited usefulness in the diagnosis of acute pancreatitis, and its chief usefulness has been in the determination of chronic pancreatitis. In pancreatic carcinoma the volume flow is depressed if the carcinoma is in the head. The amount of depression depends on the size and extent of the pancreatic duct obstruction. The secretin test has limited usefulness in patients with carcinoma of the body or tail of the pancreas. However, many of the pancreatic carcinomas of the head may be inferred by a carefully performed secretin test.

Ultrasound pancreatic evaluation. Ultrasound (gray-scale, real time) is of primary importance in pancreatic visualization. The pancreas can be visualized by ultrasound imaging in the majority of patients and abnormalities defined. Acute pancreatitis, pancreatic carcinoma, and pancreatic cysts may usually be inferred by ultrasonic evaluation. X-ray computed tomography (CT) has also been used to visualize the pancreas; however, this technique is more successful in the moderately obese patient in whom there is a fat plane surrounding the pancreas.

Radionuclide pancreatic studies

Fecal fat may be quantitated chemically; however, the fecal measurement is somewhat tedious. In 1949 it was found that following the ingestion of ^{131}I triolein, there was a characteristic fat tolerance blood curve, as well as fecal excretion of the labeled fat in 72 to 96 hours. The latter was found to be a more reliable indicator of the total absorption of the labeled fat.

The normal blood values were 10% or more of the administered dose of the radioactive material in the average of the fourth-, fifth-, and sixth-hour blood samples (or a peak blood radioactivity of 9% or more using a total blood volume radioactivity based on the anticipated volume of 3,000 ml per square meter of body surface). The fecal fat results are usually interpreted over the 72- to 96-hour period; the upper limit of normal is 7% of the ingested dose. Obviously, any disease that would lower the lipase content of the pancreatic secretion should give an abnormal result.

However, the triolein test has been found to be most unreliable as a predictor of malabsorption. In 1963 it was found that the commercially available radioiodinated triolein was contaminated with many free fatty acids and other substances. However, even with purified ^{131}I triolein, the most reliable test (the 96-hour stool collection) still does not exclude the presence of steatorrhea.

Iodine 131-labeled oleic acid test. By the combined use of a neutral fat, ^{131}I triolein, and a radioiodinated fatty acid (^{131}I oleic acid), early studies indicated that in pancreatic insufficiency the radioiodinated fatty acid was absorbed normally, whereas the labeled neutral fat was absorbed poorly. Of course, in malabsorption it was found that the absorption of both substances was depressed. However, through the years it has been shown that the ^{131}I oleic acid absorption is extremely unpredictable.

Carbon 14-labeled fats. Recently ^{14}C-labeled fats have been introduced into medicine to help estimate pancreatic insufficiency or malabsorption of the small bowel. The ^{14}C-labeled fat on absorption is monitored as the ^{14}C is expired as labeled carbon dioxide. These studies are still in the experimental stage at the present time.

PANCREATIC IMAGING WITH [75]SE SELENOMETHIONINE

In 1949 it was found that tagged methionine localized within the pancreas. In 1962 Blau and Bender reestablished this fact when they employed ^{75}Se selenomethionine for visualization of the pancreas. Of all the organs that have been imaged successfully with a gamma ray imaging device, the pancreas is undoubtedly one of the most difficult organs to picture successfully.

A review of the transverse section anatomic drawings in Fig. 21-1, *B* and *C*, shows that the pancreas is a deep-seated organ, normally 5 inches or more away from the abdominal wall. This 3½-ounce organ is also surrounded by a number of large organs of the abdomen. These points will be stressed in the following discussion.

Physiopharmacology

The physiopharmacology of ^{75}Se selenomethionine is complicated. Methionine is a basic amino acid important to all organ metabolism. The normal circulating volume of methionine is approximately 100 μg. Approximately 50% of the methionine is taken up by muscle, and the remainder of the methionine is distributed in the other large organs. Approximately 4% of the injected ^{75}Se selenomethionine is found in the pancreas 1 hour after injection. Twelve percent is found in the liver, 2.5% in the lung, and 1.5% in the kidney. On a per gram basis, the intestine has one tenth as much selenomethionine per gram as the pancreas. Obviously, the amount of radioactivity found in the organs surrounding the pancreas makes the imaging of this organ more difficult, for example, than the imaging of the thyroid gland with [131]I. It has been found that none of the proposed procedures to increase the amount of ^{75}Se selenomethionine in the pancreas was useful in investigations on animals.

Clinical considerations

Position of patient. In reviewing Fig. 21-1, *B*, the reader will note that in the anterior view the left lobe of the liver overshadows the tail of the pancreas; with slight enlargement of the right lobe of the liver, the head of the pancreas will be overshadowed. The student will also note that if the left side of the patient is elevated, the liver is thrown upward and the pancreas may be visualized from the anterior view. This is the pancreatic scanning position.

Rectilinear scanning (Fig. 22-1). Since by animal investigation it has been shown that the peak uptake of ^{75}Se selenomethionine is between 30 minutes and 2 hours, the rectilinear scan is begun immediately after the dose is given. The head of the pancreas is always found below the porta hepatis; therefore, if the rectilinear crystal is placed over the umbilicus and moved diagonally toward the porta hepatis, the first organ that the crystal will pass over is the head of the pancreas.

Rectilinear

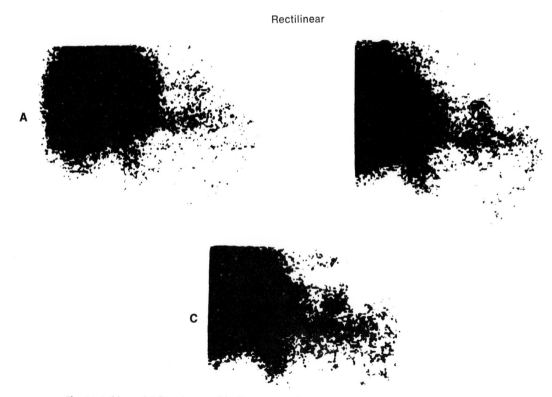

Fig. 22-1. Normal ^{75}Se selenomethionine pancreatic scans performed 10 minutes (**A**), 1 hour and 10 minutes (**B**), and 2 hours and 10 minutes (**C**) after administration of dose.

Since the head of the pancreas measures about 2 cm in diameter, there will be a slight counting drop as the probe passes over the head and into the edge of the right lobe of the liver. Thus the pancreas may be localized without difficulty. In rectilinear scanning a crystal larger than 3 by 2 inches must be used, since the pancreas is usually more than 5 inches away from the abdominal wall. Therefore the collimator focal depth must be 5 inches or more to put the pancreas into the correct focal plane. Other rectilinear techniques include the use of twin 5-inch probes and subtraction techniques.

Camera imaging techniques (Fig. 22-2). Immediately after injection of seleno-methionine, the pancreas can be visualized. The pancreas lies just below the porta hepatis with the tail running toward the hilum of the spleen. Technetium sulfur colloid is administered to the patient and the liver and spleen positioned on the persistence scope so that the pancreas will be visualized at approximately the center of the camera scintillation crystal. This is done through patient positioning and proper rotation of the camera head. We have found that the peak concentration of selenomethionine over the pancreas is 1 minute after injection. The majority of

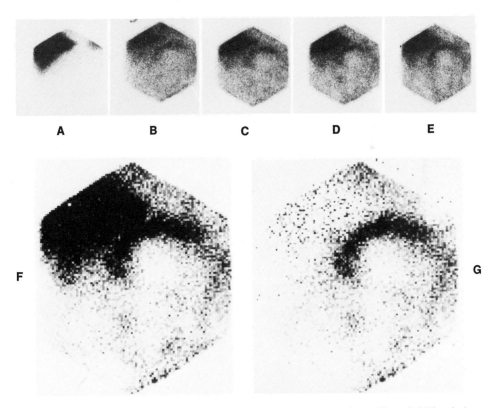

Fig. 22-2. Normal ^{75}Se selenomethionine pancreatic images. **A,** Technetium sulfur colloid liver/spleen image. **B** to **E,** Ten-minute sequential pancreatic images with selenomethionine. **F,** Selenomethionine 40-minute playback without subtraction. **G,** Selenomethionine 40-minute playback with subtraction.

blood background is cleared at 20 minutes after administration; therefore, the best background-to-target ratio is at this time. Two 20-minute consecutive pancreatic images are done, and through the data processor, a play-back 40-minute statistical pancreatic image is obtained, utilizing the core memory of the data processor. The liver and spleen images are then subtracted from the field for better visualization of the pancreas. Employing the data processor, the number of counts obtained over the pancreatic head and tail are quantitated, and concentration curves are generated that further aid in diagnosis.

Clinical applications

The pancreas in the human has many different shapes. As will be understood by a review of the anatomy of the pancreas, the head of the pancreas has greater activity than the tail; the body is very thin and is visualized very poorly in pancreatic imaging.

The normal pancreas is obviously the easiest to visualize, and once the normal

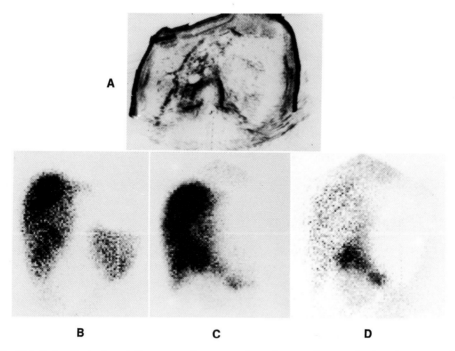

Fig. 22-3. Patient had a large left upper quadrant mass that subsequently proved to be a large necrotic renal cell carcinoma. **A,** Sagittal-view ultrasound revealing the liver to be compressed laterally by a large left-sided mass. Because of distortion caused by the mass, the pancreatic body and tail could not be identified. **B,** Anterior technetium sulfur colloid liver/spleen image reveals extrinsic compression of the liver and caudal displacement of the spleen. **C,** Forty-minute accumulated abdominal image following the injection of selenomethionine revealing caudal displacement of the pancreatic body and tail. The pancreatic head is difficult to differentiate from the liver. **D,** Computer subtraction image reveals normal pancreatic tissue displaced by the left abdominal mass.

variants of pancreatic shape are understood, the imaging and interpretation of the normal pancreas may be done without difficulty (Figs. 22-1 and 22-2).

Inflammatory disease of the pancreas, such as pancreatitis, is difficult to infer with pancreatic imaging because even with inflammatory disease there may be a normal counting rate over the pancreas. Conversely, a decreased counting rate from the pancreatic bed may be caused by many technical factors, such as tissue absorption, scatter, or positioning of the rectilinear focusing collimator at the wrong focal depth.

In carcinoma of the pancreas there is decreased metabolism of methionine by the carcinoma. Therefore pancreatic carcinoma may be inferred by pancreatic imaging. Again, correct differentiation of a small area of abnormality can be done using the rectilinear scanner only if the focusing collimator is focused at the correct depth. Camera studies are better than rectilinear studies of the pancreas with a saving of patient study time.

Based on clinical experience with pancreatic imaging, patients suspected of having pancreatic disease should first undergo ultrasound pancreatic evaluation or CT abdominal evaluation. If the pancreas cannot be identified by these techniques, the radionuclide pancreatic series is usually successful in visualization of the normal pancreas (Fig. 22-3).

BIBLIOGRAPHY

Aschkar, F., and Miale, A.: The gastroinestinal system. In Aschkar, F., editor: Practical nuclear medicine, New York, 1974, Medcom Press, pp. 63-80.

de Reuck, A. V. S., and Cameron, M. P.: The exocrine pancreas—normal and abnormal functions, Boston, 1961, Little, Brown & Co.

Filly, R.: Pancreatic ultrasonography. In Norman, D., Korobkin, M., and Newton, T. H.: Computed tomography 1977, St. Louis, 1977, The C. V. Mosby Co., pp. 113-120.

Sodee, D. B.: Pancreas: imaging. In Rothfeld, B., editor: Nuclear medicine—endocrinology, Philadelphia, 1978, J. B. Lippincott Co.

Stanley, R.: CT of the pancreas. In Norman, D., Korobkin, M., and Newton, T. H.: Computed Tomography 1977, St. Louis, 1977, The C. V. Mosby Co., pp. 121-128.

Taylor, K.: Atlas of gray scale ultrasonography, Edinburgh, 1978, Churchill Livingstone, pp. 131-169.

Weill, F. S.: Ultrasonography of digestive disease, St. Louis, 1978, The C. V. Mosby Co.

GENERAL BIBLIOGRAPHY

Ashkar, F. S., Miale, A., and Smoak, W.: A general guide to nuclear medicine, Springfield, Ill., 1975, Charles C Thomas, Publisher.

Best, C., and Taylor, N. B.: Physiological basis of medical practice, ed. 10, Baltimore, 1979, The Williams & Wilkins Co.

Blahd, W. H.: Nuclear medicine, ed. 2, New York, 1971, McGraw-Hill Book Co.

Deland, F. H., and Wagner, H. N.: Atlas of nuclear medicine, Philadelphia, 1969, W. B. Saunders Co., vol. 1.

Freeman, L. M., and Blaufax, M. D.: Physicians desk reference for radiology and nuclear medicine, Oradell, N.J., 1977-1978, Medical Economics Co.

Freeman, L. M., and Johnson, P. M.: Clinical scintillation scanning, New York, 1975, Grune & Stratton, Inc.

Grant, J. C. B., and Basmajian, J. V.: A method of anatomy, ed. 7, Baltimore, 1965, The Williams & Wilkins Co.

Gross, C. M.: Gray's anatomy of the human body, ed. 28, Phildelphia, 1966, Lea & Febiger.

Guyton, A. C.: Textbook of medical physiology, ed. 3., Phildelphia, 1966, W. B. Saunders Co.

Ham, A. W.: Histology, Philadelphia, 1957, J. B. Lippincott Co.

Holvey, D. N.: The Merck manual of diagnosis and therapy, ed. 12, Rahway, N.J., 1972, Merck Sharp & Dohme Research Lab.

Jacob, S. W., and Francone, C. A.: Structure and function in man, ed. 2, Philadelphia, 1970, W. B. Saunders Co.

Maynard, C. D.: Clinical nuclear medicine, Philadelphia, 1969, Lea & Febiger.

Powsner, E. R., and Raeside, D. E.: Diagnostic nuclear medicine, New York, 1971, Grune & Stratton, Inc.

Rhodes, B. A., editor: Quality control in nuclear medicine: radiopharmaceuticals, instrumentation, and in vitro assays, St. Louis, 1977, The C. V. Mosby Co.

Shtassel, P.: Speak to me in nuclear medicine, New York, 1976, Harper & Row, Publishers.

Silver, S.: Radioactive nuclides in medicine & biology—medicine, Philadelphia, 1968, Lea & Febiger.

Wagner, H. N.: Principles of nuclear medicine, Philadelphia, 1968, W. B. Saunders Co.

Wagner, H. N.: Nuclear medicine, New York, 1975, HP Publishing, Co.

23 Cardiovascular system

The cardiovascular, or circulatory, system is the chief transport system in the body. It delivers oxygen and nutrients to the tissues and carries carbon dioxide and other waste products to the lungs and kidneys for elimination from the body. It carries the protective substances that can help in the combat of noxious agents and distributes chemicals and hormones to regulate cell function.

As the word cardiovascular implies, this system consists of the heart (cor) which pumps a complex fluid called blood carrying the materials just mentioned into a closed system of tubes, or blood vessels. These vessels are differentiated into arteries (which carry the blood from the heart to the different tissues of the body), capillaries (where the interchange of gases, food, and waste occurs), and veins (which return the blood from the tissues back to the heart).

The heart is a hollow, muscular organ that lies between the lungs behind the body of the sternum and the adjoining parts of the rib cage, projecting farther to the left than to the right of the median plane. Normally, it measures 12 cm (about 5 inches) from base to apex and 9 cm (roughly 3½ inches) traversely at its broadest part. When projected on the anterior chest wall, the outline of the normal heart can be simulated by an irregular quadrangular area. Its upper border, or base, corresponds to a line drawn from the lower border of the second left costal cartilage 4 cm (1½ inches) from the median plane to the upper border of the third right costal cartilage 2 cm (roughly 1 inch) from the middle line. From there, the right border extends down to the sixth right cartilage 1 cm (about ½ inch) from its junction with the sternum. The lower border is represented by a line drawn from the last point to the apex beat, which normally lies in the fifth left intercostal space 9 cm (3½ inches) from the median plane. A line joining the cardiac apex with the left end of the upper border represents the left border of the heart.

The heart, together with the roots of the great vessels, is enclosed in a fibroserous sac called the *pericardium*. The external layer is fibrous, whereas the internal is a closed, invaginated, two-layered serous sac. The serous pericardium is made of an inner visceral layer and an outer parietal layer separated by a thin film of fluid to lessen the friction between these two surfaces as they move during the cardiac cycle of contraction (systole) and relaxation (diastole). Under abnormal conditions, excess fluid accumulates in the serous pericardial sac and is called *pericardial effusion.*

The heart itself is divided into four chambers, which are lined with endothelium or *endocardium*. Two of these chambers—the right and left atria—receive blood from the great veins and expel it into the distributing chambers, the right and left ventricles. Since they have to pump the blood for a short distance in the face of minor resistance, the atria have thin walls of cardiac muscle, or *myocardium*. The distributing chambers, or ventricles, have thicker walls of myocardium, the thickness being more marked in the left ventricle. Each atrium communicates freely with its corresponding ventricle, whereas the right and left chambers are completely separated from one another by partitions called *interatrial* and *interventricular* septa. To prevent the backflow of blood, each atrioventricular communication is guarded by a *valve* (the tricuspid on the right and mitral on the left). Similarly, the backflow from the great vessels into the corresponding ventricles is prevented by the presence of the semilunar valves on the origins of the pulmonary artery and aorta.

With each heartbeat, blood is pumped by the left ventricle into a large artery (the aorta) and is distributed by way of its numerous branches to all tissues and organs of the body with the exception of the lungs. The deoxygenated blood carrying the waste products returns to the right atrium by means of the superior vena cava from the head, neck, and upper limbs and by the inferior vena cava from the trunk and lower limbs. This constitutes the *greater or systemic circulation*.

The deoxygenated blood passes from the right atrium into the right ventricle, which expels it through the pulmonary artery to the lungs for its fresh supply of oxygen. The oxygenated blood, which has lost some of its carbon dioxide, returns by way of the pulmonary veins to the left atrium and on to the left ventricle. The passage of blood from the right ventricle through the lungs to the left atrium is called the *lesser,* or *pulmonary, circulation*.

The rhythmic contraction of the heart is called *heartbeat*. Normally, the heart beats 70 to 80 times per minute. The heartbeat originates in a specialized tissue in the wall of the right atrium called the *sinoauricular node* (SA node). From there, the wave of excitation spreads throughout the muscles of both atria, which respond by contraction. The impulse is picked up by another mass of nodal tissue, called the *auriculoventricular node* (AV node), and is relayed by a specialized conducting bundle to the ventricles, which respond and contract. During ventricular contractions, blood is forced into the aorta. The amount of blood pumped per unit time is designated as cardiac output. The expelled blood moves the blood in the vessels forward and sets a pressure wave that travels down the arteries. The pressure wave expands the arterial wall as it travels and is felt as the pulse. It must be noted that the rate at which the pulse wave travels is completely independent of the velocity of the blood flow.

After the onset of ventricular systole, the aortic semilunar valve opens. Blood passes into the aorta and the large arteries. The pressure rises smoothly to a maximum (systolic blood pressure) and normally measures 120 mm Hg. As the blood passes onward into the arterioles and the ventricles relax during ventricular diastole, with no more blood being driven into the aorta, the pressure drops to a minimum (diastolic pressure). This usually amounts to 80 mm Hg. The arterial pressure is usually written as systolic over diastolic (120/80 mm Hg). As we proceed down the arterial tree, the vessels decrease in caliber and the blood pressure falls, with diminution in the difference between systolic and diastolic levels. In the medium-size arteries the degree of blood pressure fall is slight. In contrast, the blood pressure falls rapidly in the small arteries and arterioles. In the arterioles the average pressure is approximately 40 mm Hg.

By a process of repeated divisions and ramifications, the arterioles open into a closely meshed network of microscopic vessels (capillaries) that have semipermeable walls, which allow movement of water and solutes. This movement is governed by diffusion and filtration. Because they are in higher concentration in the blood, oxygen and glucose diffuse outward into the tissue spaces. Carbon dioxide, because it is in higher concentration in the tissues, moves inward. The rate and direction of filtration depend on the net result of the intracapillary pressure driving outward and the osmotic pressure of the plasma proteins, together with the pressure in the tissue spaces working in the opposite direction. With a more or less steady osmotic pressure of plasma proteins (25 mm Hg) and an interstitial pressure of 1 to 2 mm Hg, the main determining factor in filtration is the capillary pressure. At the arteriolar end the capillary pressure is 35 mm Hg. Therefore, the net result is a driving force that moves the fluid and electrolytes outward into the tissue spaces. At the venular end where the capillary pressure averages 15 mm Hg, the net result is a pulling force that draws water and electrolytes from the tissue fluids back into the bloodstream. The excess fluid that does not return by this route is drained by the lymphatics and is carried back into the blood. The exchange that takes place across the capillary membrane results in a continuous turnover and removal of tissue fluids.

After passing through the capillaries, blood is collected by a series of minute vessels called *venules*. These unite with one another to form veins that ultimately form two main venous trunks (the superior and inferior vanae cavae), which open in the right atrium. Proceeding along the venous system toward the heart, the caliber of the vessels increases, and the pressure diminishes. In the venules the pressure is about 15 mm Hg, whereas in the large veins outside the chest it averages 5 mm Hg, or 6 ml of water. The pressure in the great veins at the entrance in the right atrium amounts to 4 ml of water and fluctuates with respiration and cardiac contractions. In this connection it should be noted that the negative intrathoracic pressure with its fluctuations during respiration aids the venous return to a great extent. This return is further aided by contractions of the skeletal muscles, which squeeze the veins and move the blood toward the heart.

DETERMINATION OF CARDIAC OUTPUT

Cardiac output can be defined as the effective volume of blood expelled by either ventricle per unit time. It is usually expressed as milliliters or liters per minute. The output of either ventricle per beat is called the *stroke volume*. Consequently, the cardiac output would be equal to the stroke volume times the heart rate.

If the concentration of oxygen in the blood going to the lungs is 14% and that in the outflowing blood is 19%, then each 100 ml of blood has gained 5 ml of oxygen (or each liter of blood has absorbed 50 ml of oxygen) as it passed through the lungs. If the individual has consumed 250 ml of oxygen from the alveolar air per minute, then the amount of blood that has passed across the alveoli during this minute in order to absorb this amount of oxygen should be 250/50, or 5 liters. This is actually the pulmonary blood flow, the right ventricular output, or, simply, the cardiac output, according to the Fick principle.

The oxygen consumption can be estimated by a spirometer. The oxygen concentration should be determined in an arterial blood sample as well as in venous blood. The arterial blood is obtained by arterial puncture, whereas the venous sample is collected through cardiac catheterization from the right ventricle or pulmonary artery. Although this method is accurate, the technical requirements make it impractical for routine clinical use.

A completely different approach to this problem of determination of the cardiac output depends on the application of the indicator dilution principles. In a static system (Fig. 23-1) in which an indicator is mixed with a certain volume of fluid, the relationship between the amount of indicator *(I)*, its concentration *(C)*, and the volume of fluid present *(V)* is exemplified by the following equation:

$$I = C \times V$$

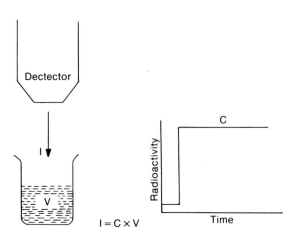

Fig. 23-1. Indicator dilution in a static system: *I*, indicator; *C*, concentration; *V*, volume.

In a dynamic system represented by a receptacle having an inlet and an outlet (Fig. 23-2), in which the indicator is injected as a bolus of highly concentrated material through the inlet, application of the principle of dilution imples certain changes. With sampling along the outlet, the volume of dilution (V), or the amount of fluid flowing during the time interval taken by the dilution process, can be calculated from the flow rate (F) and the time for dilution (T):

$$V = F \times T$$

Therefore the primary equation becomes:

$$I = C \times F \times T$$

However, with sampling along the outlet in a dynamic system, the concentration is going to be changing. It begins from zero, rises to a maximum, and then diminishes. Therefore the average concentration (C_{av}) must be used during the time of dilution, rather than using an absolute concentration. Consequently, the equation becomes:

$$I = C_{av} \times F \times T$$

$$F = \frac{I}{C_{av} \times T}$$

In a similar system, but one in which the outflow pours back into the inflow, some of the indicator will circulate back to the site of sampling before completion of the dilution process, causing a rise in the concentration (Fig. 23-3). This would definitely affect the estimation of the average concentration. However, this diminution in concentration is an exponential function of time. Therefore if this segment is plotted on a semilogarithmic scale, the expected behavior of the concentration curve can be derived by extrapolation, and the average concentration can be calculated.

The latter system simulates the heart to a great extent. If a known amount of indicator (I) is injected, the flow rate (F) or cardiac output (CO) can be estimated from the average concentration (C_{av}) and the time of dilution (T) according to the

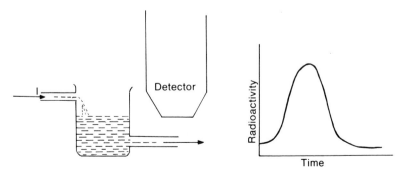

Fig. 23-2. Radionuclide dilution in a dynamic system with an inlet and an outlet.

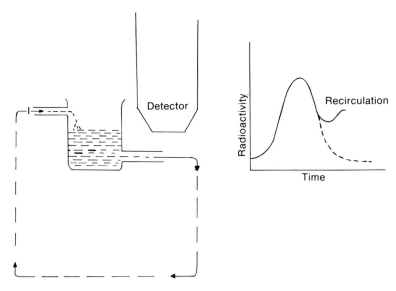

Fig. 23-3. Radionuclide dilution in a dynamic system with the outflow pouring back into the inflow.

equation just given. The indicators used are generally dyes, such as Evans blue, indigo carmine, or indocyanine green (Cardio-Green). The average concentration of the dye is obtained from serial blood samples collected at 1- to 3-second intervals by arterial puncture. To simplify matters, blood is led from an indwelling arterial needle through a constant flow cuvette with an automatic recording device to give a continuous record of the dye concentration. The concentration curve thus obtained is corrected for the effect of recirculation to determine the average dye concentration and the time of dilution, since both are needed for cardiac output determination. To obviate the need for arterial punctures, the dye concentration curve can be recorded externally by a photoelectric densitometer that measures changes in the optical density of the ear lobe after the intravenous injection of the dye. The optical density curve is treated with the application of a calibration factor relating external recording to dye concentration and corrected for the effect of recirculation.

As indicators, radionuclides have the advantage of easy and accurate quantitation even at low concentrations. In addition, gamma emitters have the unique qualification for external detection. The radionuclides used are ^{32}P-tagged red cells, ^{85}Kr, and ^{131}I-labeled human serum albumin (RISA); the latter is most commonly used. After injecting a known amount of the radionuclide, the average concentration of radioactivity during the period of observation is determined by the assay of serial arterial blood samples or from a continuous recording of radioactivity in the blood led by external tubing through a scintillation detector. This necessitates the application of a calibration factor relating the counting rate to its equivalence in concentration. This is obtained by estimating the counting rate of a known concentration of radioactivity led through the tubing.

To obviate these technical difficulties, the nuclide dilution curve is recorded by means of an external detector focused over the heart. The same principles that have been described are applicable, and the cardiac output (CO) is calculated from the following equation:

$$CO = \frac{I}{C_{av} \times T}$$

However, since the tracer concentration is not measured directly but by external monitoring, it becomes necessary to apply a factor of proportionality relating the external rate and the tracer concentration in the blood. This is achieved by recording the external counting rate (C_f) at the same time of withdrawing a venous blood sample to estimate the blood tracer concentration (C_b) by the in vitro assay of radioactivity in this sample. This proportionality factor is applied to the previous equation:

$$CO = \frac{I}{\dfrac{C_{av} \times C_b \times T}{C_f}}$$

$$= \frac{C_f \times I}{C_{av} \times T \times C_b}$$

However, the fraction $\dfrac{I}{C_b}$ represents the diluting volume of the tracer (DV), which approximates the blood volume (BV) if enough time is allowed for the tracer to attain uniform concentration and the radionuclide does not diffuse outside the vascular system. Substituting for this fraction, the equation becomes:

$$CO = \frac{C_f \times DV}{C_{av} \times T}$$

The denominator in this equation is equivalent to the area under the primary dilution curve expressed in counts. Therefore the equation will read as follows:

$$CO = \frac{C_f \times DV}{Area}$$

This area consists of the area until recirculation *(A)*, together with the extrapolated area *(B)* (Fig. 23-4). This gives the final equation:

$$CO = \frac{C_f \times DV}{(A + B)}$$

Therefore, it becomes evident that for the determination of the cardiac output, all that is needed is an estimation of the final counting rate by the external detector (C_f), the diluting volume (DV), and the total area under the primary dilution curve (A + B).

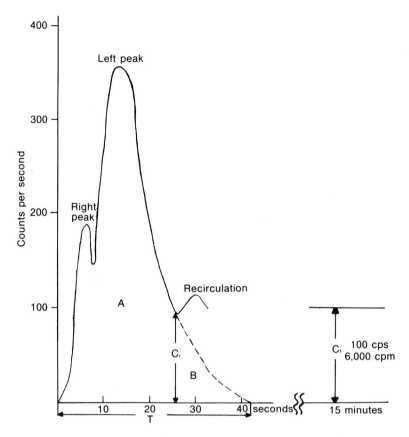

Fig. 23-4. Determination of cardiac output.

A = Area prior to recirculation
T = Time of primary circulation
C_f = Final counting rate by external monitoring
C_r = Counting rate just prior to recirculation by external counting
B = Extrapolated area

Procedure using radioiodinated human serum albumin

The patient lies comfortably in bed, and a collimated scintillation detector is placed predominantly over one side of the heart. Usually the left side is chosen, and the detector is focused over a point 4 cm (1½ inches) medial and 2 cm (1 inch) upward from the site of the maximal apical impulse. The collimator used has a straight bore, with an aperture 4 cm (1½ inches) wide; the crystal is recessed 7.5 cm (3 inches) from the surface. The information to be collected is counted through a count rate meter with a time constant of 0.5 second and is recorded on a strip-chart recorder moving at a rate of 30 cm (12 inches)per minute. After the background counting rate has been recorded, 20 to 40 μCi of radioiodinated human serum albumin in a volume not exceeding 2 ml are rapidly injected as a bolus in an antecubital vein, followed by a flushing dose of normal saline. After the passage of the radioactive bolus through the heart and the recirculation have been recorded, the time constant of the rate meter is switched to 5 to 10 seconds, and the rate of the stripchart recorder is changed to 30 cm (12 inches) per hour. After 10 to 15 minutes a venous blood sample is withdrawn from the opposite arm, and its timing is marked on the stripchart.

Radioactivity in 1 ml from the blood sample, as well as from the standard for dose calculation, is assayed in a scintillation well counter. Dividing the dose injected by the concentration of radioactivity in the blood (C_b) gives the diluting volume (DV), which, under the circumstances described, approximates the blood volume.

The final counting rate (C_f) in counts per minute is obtained from the stripchart recording at the time marked simultaneously with the blood sampling.

For calculation of the area under the primary dilution curve, the net counting rate recorded on the stripchart is replotted against time. Recirculation is identified by a sudden change in the trailing edge of the concentration curve. The count rate on the trailing edge is plotted as a function of time on semilogarithmic paper. This enables calculation of the clearance half-time ($T_{1/2}$) of RISA from the heart. By extrapolation to zero, the duration of the primary dilution curve is estimated, and the area under the curve can be completed. The whole area under the primary circulation curve is measured in square centimeters by a planimeter and is converted to its equivalent in counts by the application of the scaling factors used in plotting the data. These factors relate counts per minute per centimeter on one axis and minutes per centimeter on the other. As an alternative, the area under the primary curve until recirculation (A) is measured by planimetry, whereas the extrapolated area (B) is calculated using the following equation:

$$\text{Area B} = C_r \times T_{1/2} \times 1.443 \times \text{Scaling factor}$$

$$C_r = \text{Net counting rate at the last point before the occurrence of recirculation, as represented in centimeters in the plotted curve}$$

$$T_{1/2} = \text{Clearance half-time of RISA in seconds}$$

$$\text{Scaling factor} = \text{Factor used to relate centimeters to time in seconds}$$

If a planimeter is not available, the net counting rate as recorded on the stripchart is tabulated to give the counting rate for every 1-second interval. The area under the curve until recirculation (A) equals the sum of the products of each counting rate multiplied by the period of counting (1 second). The extrapolated area (B) is calculated from the net counting rate per second at the point prior to recirculation multiplied by 1.443 times the clearance half time ($T_{1/2}$) in seconds. The clearance half-time is obtained as usual by plotting the trailing edge of the curve on semilogarithmic paper. The whole area under the primary curve (A + B) expressed in counts is obtained by summation of area A and area B.

A much easier and more rapid method to estimate the area under the primary circulation curve is achieved through the use of a pair of printing scalers activated at 1-second intervals. The first scaler records the counting rate at increments of 1 second, whereas the second continuously integrates the isotope dilution curve. The count rate of the trailing edge of the curve as recorded by the first scaler is plotted on semilogarithmic paper against time. This yields the clearance half-time of RISA in seconds as well as the counting rate and time prior to recirculation. From these data, the extrapolated area (B) is calculated in counts as previously described. The rest of the area (A) is obtained in counts by reading the value recorded at the point prior to recirculation by the integrating scaler. The total area under the primary circulation curve expressed in counts is computed by summation of the values obtained for both areas (A and B).

Having obtained the total area under the primary circulation curve (A + B) in counts, the diluting volume (DV) in liters, and the final counting rate (C_f) as determined in counts per minute by external counting, one can then calculate the cardiac output (CO) using the following equation:

$$CO = \frac{C_f \times DV}{(A + B)}$$

To overcome the inaccuracies encountered by replotting the obtained data and the time consumed in calculations, computing techniques have been introduced for estimation of the cardiac output. The computer is programmed to recognize the final peak (left ventricular), as well as the point of recirculation of the radionuclide dilution curve, and select the optimum section of the curve between these two points to calculate the clearance half-time of RISA. Using these data, together with the information obtained from the printing scalers as previously outlined and with the diluting volume, the cardiac output is calculated.

In normal individuals, with the external radionuclide technique, the cardiac output averages 6.13 ± 0.73 L/min (mean ± 1 standard deviation), with a range of 4.93 to 7.25 L/min. The cardiac index or cardiac output/m², surface area ranges from 2.75 to 4.10 L/min/m², with a mean of 3.36 ± 0.35 L/min/m². The stroke volume or cardiac output per beat averages 92 ± 14 m/beat; the range is from 70 to 120 ml/beat. The stroke index, which represents the stroke volume/m², amounts to 50 ± 7 ml/beat/m².

Measurement of the cardiac output by the radionuclide dilution technique is safe, nontraumatic, easy to perform, and suitable for repeated determinations. It is indicated for the evaluation of cardiac cases and for the follow-up of patients submitted to cardiac surgery, as well as for those suffering from coronary disease.

CIRCULATION TIME

Circulation time represents the shortest interval between the intravascular injection of a substance and its arrival at some distant site in sufficient concentration to produce a recognizable end point.

The methods of measuring circulation time in common use depend on the application of chemicals (decholin, calcium gluconate) or volatile substances (ether) to determine the arm-to-tongue and arm-to-lung circulation times. However, these methods suffer from the disadvantage of having a subjective end point that depends on the patient's reaction and cooperation.

Radionuclides, however, produce a sharp, well-defined end point that is identifiable objectively by specialized sensitive equipment. In this connection, the most commonly used radiopharmaceutical is human serum albumin labeled with ^{131}I or with one of the short-lived radionuclides such as [99m]Tc. By use of collimated scintillation detectors connected through count rate meters to synchronized stripchart recorders, various circulation times can be measured and the velocity of flow calculated.

For the determination of the velocity of flow along the veins of the lower limbs, 10 to 20 μ Ci of RISA are injected into a vein of the dorsum of the foot. A record is obtained of the appearance of radioactivity at two points along the femoral vein by a pair of collimated scintillation detectors. From this record, the transit time of radioactivity from one detector to the other is estimated. Since the distance between the points examined is known, the velocity of the venous flow can be calculated according to the following equation:

$$\text{Velocity} = \frac{\text{Distance}}{\text{Transit time}}$$

On the arterial side, the same principle applies. The radionuclide is injected through an antecubital vein, and the velocity is calculated.

In cases of arterial obstruction, the application of a set of detectors enables identification of the site of obstruction. The detector proximal to the obstruction shows the arrival of radioactivity, whereas the distal detector does not.

Pulmonary circulation time

Measurement of the pulmonary circulation time can be achieved by the use of two synchronized sets of recording equipment. One detector is focused over the right side of the heart and the other placed over the left side. After the rapid intravenous injection of 20 μ Ci of RISA, the arrival of radioactivity in the field of each detector is recorded. The time interval between these two events roughly represents the pulmonary circulation time *(PCT)*. The same result can be obtained by means of one detector placed over the heart to record events occurring in both sides. The obtained tracing is called a *radiocardiogram* (Fig. 23-5). It is a double-peaked curve, consisting of *R* and *L* waves, which represent the right and left sides of the heart, respectively. The transitional zone between the two waves *(T)* is caused by the passage of radioactivity from the field of the detector into the lesser circulation. Thus the pulmonary circulation time can be roughly estimated by measuring the time interval between the peaks of the *R* and *L* waves. This is called the *peak-to-peak pulmonary circulation time.*

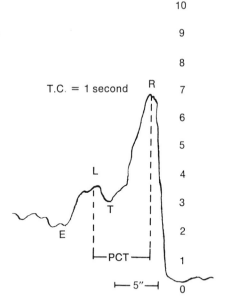

Fig. 23-5. Normal radiocardiogram. *R* represents arrival of radioactivity to the right side of the heart; *L* represents radioactivity to the left side. *T* (decrease in counting rate) is caused by passage of radioactivity from the field of the detector into the pulmonary circulation. *E* is the end of the radiocardiogram before the recirculation. The *PCT* equals the time interval between *R* and *L*. The time constant *(T.C.)* of the rate meter used in this tracing was 1 second.

In normal subjects the peak-to-peak pulmonary circulation time ranges from 2.6 to 6.1 seconds, with a mean of 4.4 ± 0.9 seconds. Diminution of the pulmonary circulation time is observed with tachycardia, severe anemia, and thyrotoxicosis. Prolongation of the pulmonary circulation time is seen with heart failure, heart block, myxedema, pulmonary hypertension, and old age.

A more accurate estimation can be obtained by correcting the peak of L for any possible lateral displacement by overlap from the terminal portion of the R wave. This is called the *corrected pulmonary circulation time.*

The most accurate of all is the *mean pulmonary circulation time* (MPCT). It was suggested that the MPCT could be estimated by measuring the time interval between the mean times for R and L waves. However, this approach led to an overestimate of the pulmonary blood volume. To circumvent this difficulty, two methods were introduced to calculate the mean pulmonary circulation time. In the midtime method the MPCT is calculated as the arithmetic average of the time of radioactivity appearance in the left heart and the time at which the left curve reaches its peak, both being measured from the time of first ejection of radioactivity from the right heart. In the left-peak method the MPCT is estimated as the time interval between the mean time of ejection of radioactivity from the right heart and the peak of the left curve.

When expressed in heart cycles instead of seconds, the mean pulmonary circulation time proved to be an objective means of assessing the impairment of the pulmonary circulation caused by left-sided heart disease. Its discriminating capacity between normal subjects and patients with left-sided heart affection appears very good.

In normal subjects the mean pulmonary circulation time averaged 6.0 ± 0.7 heart cycles (mean ± 1 SD).

Measurement of circulation times is used as an aid to proper diagnosis of cardiovascular disorders and to determine the velocity of blood flow.

RADIOCARDIOGRAPHY

Radiocardiography is the graphic recording of the precordial transit of radioactive blood through the various cardiac chambers. The radiocardiogram appears as two distinct peaks corresponding to the passage of radioactivity through the right and left cardiac chambers. From this primary indicator dilution curve together with the blood volume, the cardiac output, the pulmonary transit time, and pulmonary blood volume can be calculated. The radiopharmaceutical used should remain intravascular such as does human serum albumin labeled with either ^{131}I or [99m]Tc. Another usable radionuclide having short half-life is [113m]In, which, when injected in the blood as the chloride, combines quantitatively with transferrin and remains intravascular.

With the availability of sufficiently sensitive equipment, the precordial transit of radioactivity can be recorded at high speed using a count rate meter with a large capacity and a time constant of less than 0.1 second. Under such circumstances, the high-frequency oscillations corresponding to individual heartbeats are visualized on the downslope of the left ventricular portion of the tracing. From the magnitude of these oscillations, after background correction, it is possible to calculate the *left ventricular ejection fraction* (LVEF), which is the best estimator of the overall pump function of the heart.

Different approaches have been suggested for background correction. The first necessitates a second injection of the same radiopharmaceutical using a different collimator to eclipse the left ventricle and record the paraventricular activity or background. In contrast, the second approach requires just one injection of radionuclide through the use of a dual probe system incorporating a central collimated detector for monitoring activity in the left ventricle surrounded by a collimated annular probe to provide simultaneous monitoring of the radioactivity in the tissues providing the unwanted background. However, in both methods the precise placement of the detector over the midpoint of the left ventricle is essential and is done either by radiography or by echocardiography.

The main advantages of the probe device system are its ability to be moved to the bedside whenever needed and its relatively low cost when compared with the stationary detectors. In addition, the probe devices provide better counting statistics for calculation of the left ventricular ejection fraction, but they do not provide anatomic information. Their use in the presence of arrhythmias does not give accurate information.

In a group of normal subjects, the left ventricular ejection fraction averaged 0.64 ± 0.06 (Mean ± 1 SD), the lowest figure being 0.53.

RADIONUCLIDE ANGIOCARDIOGRAPHY

The employment of video recording devices together with the stationary scintillation detectors and concomitant use of short-lived radionuclides have enabled the development of radionuclide angiocardiographic techniques to record sequentially the passage of radioactivity through the heart and ultimately obtain a visual anatomic definition of the various cardiac chambers (Fig. 23-6). Most of the radiopharmaceuticals used are labeled with ^{99m}Tc, such as pertechnetate, human serum albumin, and autologous red cells.

The radionuclide angiocardiogram is a physiologic, safe, noninvasive procedure that is easy to perform and to repeat without undesirable side effects or discomfort to the patient. It involves much less expense than either cardiac catheterization or conventional x-ray contrast angiography.

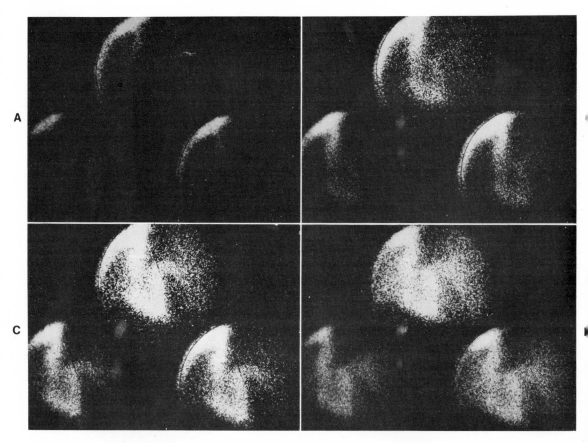

Fig. 23-6. Dynamic cardiac study following the injection of a bolus of 10 mCi pertechnetate. **A,** Bolus entering superior vena cava. **B,** Bolus has reached the level of the pulmonary outflow tract. **C** and **D,** Bolus in pulmonary vasculature

Following the intravascular injection of the radiotracer, the passage of radioactivity through the cardiopulmonary chambers is monitored by a scintillation camera, and images are sequentially recorded either directly with a rapid sequence photographic camera or on videotape for subsequent retrieval and analysis. Images of the initial-transit or first pass of radioactivity and equilibrium blood pool pictures are assessed qualitatively and/or quantitatively. Better assessment can be achieved through the use of some sort of physiologic gating to turn on the scintillation camera for a fixed time interval in relation to any specified incident in the cardiac cycle such as the R wave of the electrocardiogram for end-diastole and the second sound in the phonocardiogram for end-systole. The obtained scintigraphic data are summed over several heartbeats to produce integrated scintiphotographs representing the heart during the selected portions of the cardiac cycle.

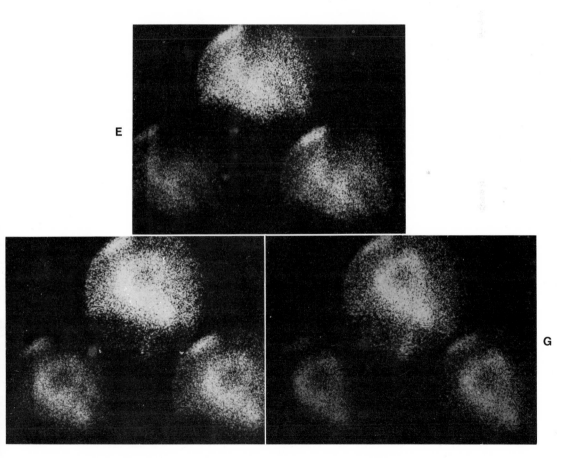

Fig. 23-6, cont'd. E, Bolus in left heart. **F,** Arch of the aorta visualized. **G,** Descending aorta visualized.

In another approach, the ungated scintillation camera data and the gating signals are recorded throughout the cardiac cycle on videotape or computer magnetic tape or disc. With the help of the computer, replaying the data provides images of selected portions of the cardiac cycle and their display either as static pictures or in the form a flicker-free movie format spanning consecutive portions of the cardiac cycle.

On a qualitative basis, the obtained scintiphotographs are used to estimate the size of the different cardiac chambers and great vessels (Fig. 23-7). In contrast to

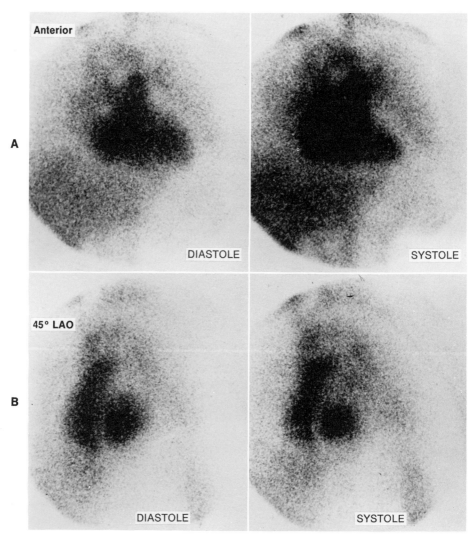

Fig. 23-7. Gated radionuclide biventriculogram in the, **A,** anterior and, **B,** 45° left anterior oblique projections at end-diastole and end-systole showing normal-size ventricles with good contractility.

radiographic ventriculography, which is used to evaluate one side of the heart at a time, radionuclide angiocardiography permits simultanous evaluation of both right and left ventricles in regard to their size (Figs. 23-8 and 23-9), as well as calculation of ejection fractions. Accordingly, this technique deserves to be called *radionuclide biventriculography*. To minimize the effect of chamber overlap, multiple views are needed. The most commonly used projections are the anterior and 45° left or 30° right anterior oblique.

In addition to assessment of chamber size, the radionuclide angiocardiogram can be utilized to detect intracardiac shunts as well as anatomic abnormalities, whether congenital or acquired. Furthermore, it has proved highly satisfactory in evaluation of ventricular wall motion.

For detection of right-to-left cardiac shunting, ^{99m}Tc albumin aggregates or microspheres are used. In the presence of shunt, the radiotracer is visualized not only in the lungs but also in other parts of the body. Another approach to this problem depends on the intravenous injection of ^{85}Kr dissolved in saline. Shunting is diagnosed if the arterial concentration of ^{85}Kr is higher than normal.

For evaluation of ventricular wall motion, imaging should be performed in

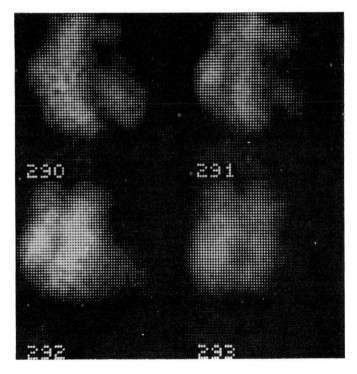

Fig. 23-8. Gated radionuclide biventriculogram in the 45° left anterior oblique projection (upper) and anterior projection (lower) in diastole (left) and systole (right) to demonstrate the enlarged right ventricle. The left ventricle is normal in size and contractility. The left ventricular ejection fraction is 0.55.

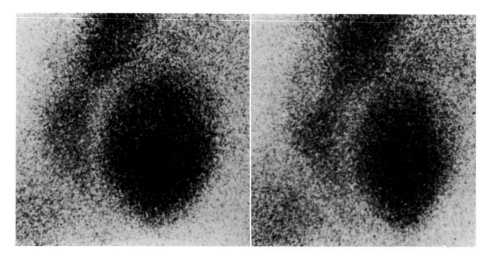

Fig. 23-9. Gated radionuclide biventriculogram in the 45° left anterior oblique view in diastole (left) and systole (right) to illustrate the enlarged left ventricle with moderate limitation in contractility.

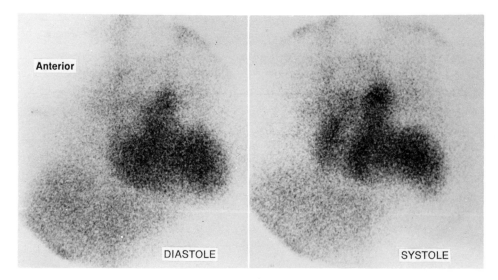

Fig. 23-10. Gated radionuclide biventriculogram in the anterior view at end-diastole and end-systole to demonstrate dyskinesia of the region of the apex of the left ventricle.

more than one projection to permit visualization of the different myocardial segments. Regions of abnormal myocardial contractility appear either as dyskinetic areas showing paradoxical bulge during systole (Fig. 23-10) or as hypokinetic regions with diminished contractility of variable degree (Fig. 23-11) up to complete akinesis.

For the quantitative analysis of the radionuclide angiocardiogram, the output

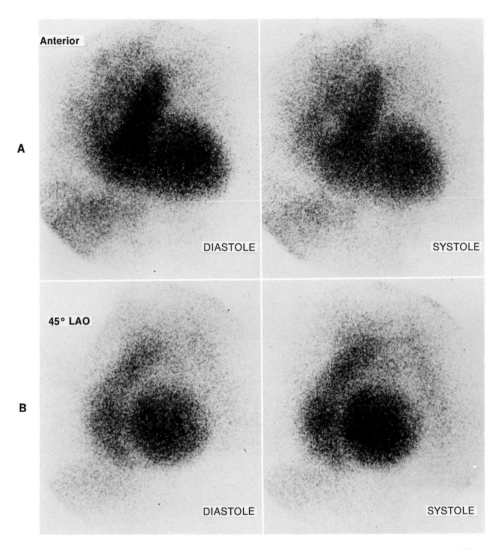

Fig. 23-11. Gated radionuclide biventriculogram in the, **A**, anterior and, **B**, 45° left anterior oblique projections at end-diastole and end-systole to demonstrate the marked limitation in contractility.

of the scintillation camera is fed into a computer system. Tracer dilution curves are determined as a function of time for each cardiac chamber or region of interest selected by light pen. In addition, signal-controlled cardiac images at end-diastole and end-systole are obtained. The ventricular ejection fraction is determined from chamber contrours either by applying the area-length formula originally developed for contrast angiography or, more accurately, by quantifying the radioactivity counting rate within a region of interest corresponding to the ventricular chamber after background correction.

$$\text{Ejection fraction} = \frac{\text{End-diastolic counts} - \text{End-systolic counts}}{\text{End-diastolic counting} - \text{Background}}$$

Sources of background counts are scattered radiation and anatomic overlap of cardiac chambers and great vessels. For correction, the counts in the incomplete ring or C-shaped area around the ventricle are normalized and subtracted from the ventricular counting rate. The background counting rates are much lower in the initial-transit recordings than at equilibrium blood pool.

Calculation of ejection fraction can be applied to both first-pass and equilibrium blood pool imaging techniques. The initial-transit technique largely eliminates the problem of chamber superimposition. However, it does not provide information regarding ventricular wall motion and requires rather a long time for image analysis. In contradistinction, the equilibrium blood pool method allows repeated imaging with the same tracer dose and permits study of wall motion. Time-activity analysis requires a relatively short time. However, the problem of chamber overlap is well manifested. In this regard, the best view to isolate the left ventricle from the other major cardiac chambers is the 45° left anterior oblique (LAO) with some degree of caudad angulation of the gamma camera.

EVALUATION OF CORONARY CIRCULATION

The main applications of radionuclides in the evaluation of coronary circulation deal with estimation of the coronary blood flow and delineation of areas of myocardial ischemia and infarction.

Determination of coronary blood flow

For estimation of the coronary blood flow, a bolus of radioactive ^{85}Kr or ^{133}Xe dissolved in saline is injected into a coronary artery and the washout of the tracer from the myocardium is followed by a precordial radiation detector. From the disappearance time constant, the flow per gram of tissue can be calculated. However, since intracoronary injection of the tracer is required, this method cannot be used for screening or for serial studies.

A different approach to this problem is based on the finding that the fraction of injected indicator taken up by the myocardium equals the fraction of cardiac output perfusing the organ.

$$\frac{\text{Coronary blood flow}}{\text{Cardiac output}} = \frac{\text{Myocardial uptake}}{\text{Injected dose}}$$

For this purpose, either radioactive potassium, thallium, or rubidium is used. In determination of the myocardial uptake by an external detector, appropriate correction for the radioactivity in the cardiac chambers has to be made. In this connection, rubidium 84 has the advantage of improved resolution based on the coincidence detection of its positron emissions.

However, both techniques enable measurement of the mean total coronary blood flow rather than evaluation of the perfusion to individual myocardial regions. Accordingly, these methods are used to assess the effects of various therapeutic measures on the total coronary blood flow.

Assessment of regional myocardial circulation

For the purpose of myocardial perfusion imaging, different isotopes of potassium, rubidium, and cesium have been used. However, when these radiopharmaceuticals are administered intravenously, their dilution into the body fluids, with resulting considerable background, together with the low myocardial uptake of the tracer, results in a poor scan image. This problem is partly solved by the intracoronary injection of a scanning agent, especially one of those with short half-lives such as ^{43}K, ^{134m}Cs, ^{129}Cs, and ^{99m}Tc-labeled albumin microspheres.

A completely different approach is offered by labeled fatty acids, which enter the cells by simple diffusion depending on the maintained concentration gradient caused by the rapid intracellular metabolism of fatty acids. In addition to being distributed in proportion to regional blood flow, labeled fatty acids are cleared from the myocardium at different rates depending on the functional status of the tissue. The main disadvantages of this radiopharmaceutical are its short half-life in the myocardium and the unavailability of sufficient commercial supplies of ^{123}I to label the fatty acids.

Out of the currently available tracers for myocardial perfusion imaging, thallium 201 appears to be the most suitable. Following its intravenous administration, the disappearance of ^{201}Tl from the blood is extremely rapid, resulting in its immediate intracellular deposition with a distribution pattern depending on the extraction rate exhibited by the different organs. Increased thallium 201 uptake is encountered in the myocardium, liver, and kidneys, especially the renal medulla, which is considered to be the critical organ. Radiothallium uptake by any organ depends mainly on the nutrient blood flow to the organ and the activity of the sodium-potassium adenosine triphosphatase transport system as well as the tissue permeability to the thallous ion.

In the heart, the concentration of radiothallium averages 2% to 5% of the administered dose. Its initial distribution parallels myocardial perfusion and simulates the distribution of potassium because of their similarity regarding the hydrated ionic radius, which is thought to be the property governing passive penetration through membranes. The myocardial extraction of this monovalent cation (thallium) is roughly 88% and is most probably caused by substitution for potassium in activation of sodium-potassium adenosine triphosphatase pump. Thallium's efflux from the myocardial cells takes place at a lower rate than potassium and consequently is a better myocardial imaging agent.

In normal persons, the concentration of ^{201}Tl is relatively uniform throughout the myocardial mass. However, because of the difference in wall thickness between the various cardiac chambers, the atria are never visualized during myocardial perfusion imaging. Similarly, because the thickness of the right ventricular myocardium is only one-third that of the left, the right ventricle is barely visualized under normal circumstances. But, if radiothallium is injected during the peak of exercise, the right ventricular myocardium becomes better visualized as a result of increased myocardial blood flow and reduction in background caused by radioactivity in the lungs and splanchnic area. In the same time, radioactivity in the left ventricular myocardium becomes more homogenous and the scan picture more sharply defined (Fig. 23-12). Exercise should be continued for about 1 minute following ^{201}Tl injection. Apart from exercise, splanchnic radioactivity can be diminished by injecting the radiothallium with the patient standing and while fasting.

Since the uptake of ^{201}Tl in the myocardial tissue corresponds to the local blood supply, an area in which the blood supply is diminished or absent will be registered as an area of reduced radioactivity (Fig. 23-13). Multiple views are needed to evaluate the different segments of the ventricular myocardium and localize areas of defective perfusion with reasonable accuracy. The interventricular

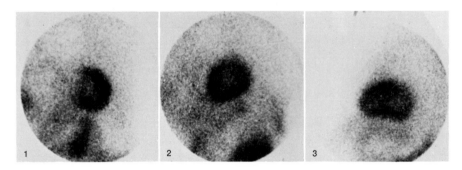

Fig. 23-12. Thallium 201 scintiscans of a subject with arteriographically normal coronary arteries. *1*, Anterior; *2*, 45° left anterior oblique; *3*, left lateral.

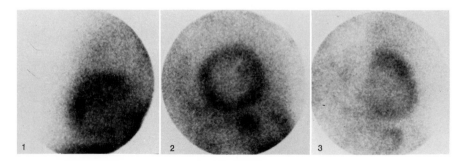

Fig. 23-13. Scintiscans with ^{201}Tl following exercise to demonstrate the left ventricular enlargement and diminished perfusion of the posterioinferior walls extending into the posterior part of the septum. *1*, Left lateral; *2*, 45° left anterior oblique; *3*, anterior.

septum and posterolateral wall are clearly visualized in the 45° left anterior oblique view. For the anterior and inferoposterior walls, the left lateral projection is the best. The anterior view is used for evaluation of the anterolateral wall. Information regarding the apex is gathered from examination of these three views. It should be noticed that radioactivity in the apical area may appear diminished even in normal subjects. However, such an area is usually small and the decrease in activity is gradual and not abrupt as is encountered with myocradial infarction.

It is advisable to start imaging within 10 minutes following the intravenous injection of 1.5- to 2.0-mCi-labeled thallium chloride; since by this time the maximal myocardial concentration of ^{201}Tl is achieved. In the meantime, the relative concentration of ^{201}Tl in the myocardium with respect to neighbouring organs such as liver and lung is optimal.

The obtained scintigraphic images are studied to determine the size and shape of each ventricle and the thickness of the myocardial muscle including the interventricular septum. Tracer distribution throughout the myocardium is examined, and areas of diminished perfusion are accurately localized.

Perfusion defects seen in images obtained with the patient at rest following ^{201}Tl injection denote areas of persistently injured myocardium produced by severe ischemia or myocardial infarction irrespective of its duration. On the other hand, areas of diminished radioactivity observed in images obtained with tracer injection during exercise and not seen in the resting scans indicate the presence of transient relative under-perfusion or ischemia. To perform such a complete study, imaging is done after ^{201}Tl injection at rest, followed few days later with another dose of tracer injected during peak exercise. In a different approach a single dose of radiothallium is injected during exercise. Myocardial perfusion images are obtained as usual. If perfusion defects are seen, scanning is repeated 3 to 4 hours later. Regions of diminished radioactivity that do not fill in with time represent prior infarction with a degree of left ventricular function impairment; whereas, transient ischemia is indicated by areas of reduced thallium activity seen on exercise that subsequently fill in with time (Fig. 23-14). This might be explained by gradual ex-

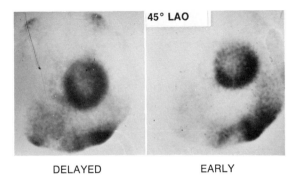

45° LAO

DELAYED   EARLY

Fig. 23-14. Thallium 201 scintiscans in the left anterior oblique projection showing an area in the septum with diminished radioactivity on exercise that filled in with time, denoting transient ischemia.

traction of the cation from the minimal concentration present in the blood pool during the 3 to 4 hours period of waiting to repeat the imaging procedure. A more objective comparison of the sequential myocardial perfusion images is achieved through profile radioactivity histograms obtained by way of computer processing of the available scintigraphic data (Fig. 23-15).

In contrast to coronary arteriography, which provides precise definition of vessel morphology, noninvasive myocardial imaging with ^{201}Tl reflects the status of the regional myocardial perfusion. With high resolution images available with the newer and more sophisticated equipment, the distribution of radioactivity throughout the myocardium is not absolutely homogenous even in normal subjects. Therefore, areas of diminished perfusion must vary by at least 25% from corresponding areas in the same projection to be considered significant.

Myocardial imaging with ^{201}Tl thallium chloride is a simple and safe technique that can be used with success for detection of fixed changes in perfusion and evaluation of perfusion reserve. It gives reasonably reproducible results and exhibits a high degree of specificity. The number of false-negative results is significant and can be partly explained by small-size lesions and those involving less than half the thickness of the myocardium. Another major contribution is the difficulty in detecting obstructive lesions involving the three major coronary arteries, leading to uniform diminution in tracer uptake throughout the ventricular myocardium. In addition to coronary artery disease, perfusion defects are encountered with infiltrative diseases of the myocardium, cardiomyopathy, and prominent abnormalities of ventricular wall motion, especially ventricular aneurysm.

A special indication for ^{201}Tl myocardial perfusion imaging is for evaluation

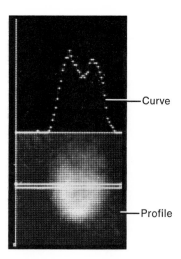

Fig. 23-15. Profile radioactivity histogram of ^{201}Tl scintiscan obtained following exercise in a normal subject.

of the effect of aortocoronary bypass graft surgery on the regional myocardial perfusion (Fig. 23-16).

Detection of acute myocardial infarction

In contrast to electrocardiography and serum enzyme tests, which yield indirect evidence of myocardial injury, radionuclides sequestered by acutely infarcted myocardium provide a direct method for detecting such an infarct and defining its size. For this purpose various radiopharmaceuticals have been used, the most important being the organomercurials and technetium chelates.

The organomercurials are represented by chlormerodrin, hydroxymercuriphthaleins, and fluoresceins. The main advantage is their fast blood clearance with rapid and large absolute uptake in the damaged myocardium. This is caused by the effect of damage on membrane permeability, permitting the influx of molecules that are ordinarily excluded and exposing the sulfhydryl groups for which mercurials have great affinity. However, these radiopharmaceuticals are difficult to prepare and their radioactive labels (197Hg and 203Hg) have poor physical decay characteristics.

Technetium chelates accumulate in areas of myocardial necrosis that still possess some residual perfusion. Their accumulation is facilitated by membrane damage, which permits the influx of the chelating agent and its binding to macromolecules to form polynuclear complexes. A more commonly used explanation is that the accumulation occurs by surface adsorption of the radiopharmaceutical to the calcium deposited in the form of apatite-like spicules or subcrystalline finely

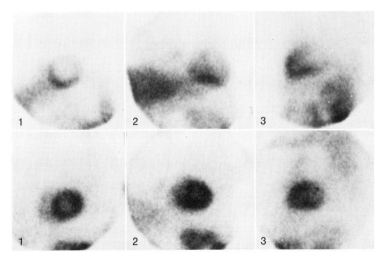

Fig. 23-16. Two sets of thallium 201 scintiscans obtained before (top) and after (bottom) aortocoronary saphenous bypass surgery to illustrate the marked improvement of the myocardial perfusion. *1*, Forty-five–degree left anterior oblique; *2*, anterior; *3*, left lateral.

granular material within the mitochondria of the irreversibly damaged myocardial cells. Another explanation suggested to account for the uptake of technetium chelates in damaged myocardium is that it occurs by transchelation of reduced technetium at the injury site by another metal with stronger affinity for the chelating agent, such as calcium.

The ^{99m}Tc-labeled complexes most commonly used as positive infarct imaging agents are tetracycline, glucoheptonate, and pyrophosphate.

Labeled tetracycline is cleared from the blood slowly and consequently necessitates a delay of 24 hours after tracer injection before imaging. However, because it accumulates only in infarcted tissue, ^{99m}Tc tetracycline can accurately define the size of acute myocardial infarction.

Glucoheptonate's rapid clearance from the body by the kidneys enables early imaging. Another advantage to its use is the absence of overlying skeletal visualization with early detection and delineation of acute infarction. However, its target-to-background ratio is low.

Of the currently available chelating agents, ^{99m}Tc stannous pyrophosphate, with its high infarct : normal myocardium concentration, is the most widely used radiopharmaceutical for acute infarct imaging. Imaging is performed 1 to 2 hours following the intravenous injection of 15 mCi of ^{99m}Tc-tagged stannous pyrophosphate. For the accurate localization of an infarct, multiple views are required, particularly the anterior, left lateral, and one or more of the left anterior oblique projections. In a good scan picture, the bones of the chest must be clearly visualized (Fig. 23-17).

To be consistently detectable by ^{99m}Tc pyrophosphate, infarcts must be at least 12 hours old and exceed 3 gm in mass. The infarct uptake of pyrophosphate reaches its maximum after 48 to 72 hours, and consequently this is the optimal time for imaging. Then the uptake fades by 6 to 7 days, to disappear by the end of 2 weeks. Occasionally the scintigrams remain persistently positive for several weeks. A possible explanation for this phenomenon is myocardial degeneration with abnormal wall motion developing into ventricular aneurysm. Other suggested causes are continued limited cell death and dystrophic calcification in the pericardium and ventricular wall.

Cardiac imaging with ^{99m}Tc stannous pyrophosphate is a simple, safe, noninvasive technique that offers high sensitivity in the detection and accurate localization of recent myocardial infarction (Fig. 23-18). This technique is particularly valuable in detecting myocardial infarction in problematic circumstances in which ordinary diagnostic methods are inconclusive, as in the presence of left bundle branch block and during the perioperative period of open heart surgery. However, the value of ^{99m}Tc pyrophosphate scintigraphy in estimating infarct size is limited, because of the increased tracer uptake in ischemic areas around the infarcted tissue.

The incidence of false-negative results, mostly caused by small infarcts, is low

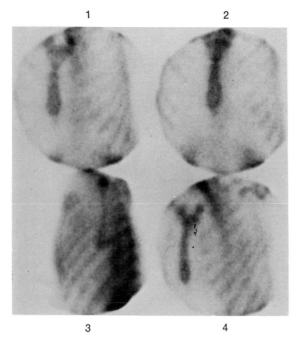

Fig. 23-17. Myocardial ⁹⁹ᵐTc pyrophosphate scintigram obtained from a normal subject in the anterior *(2)*, left lateral *(3)*, and both the 20° *(1)* and 45° *(4)* left anterior oblique projections.

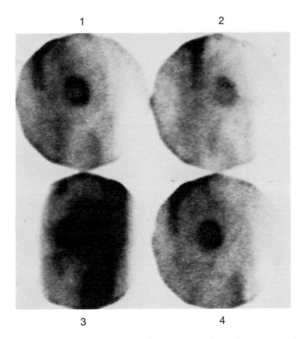

Fig. 23-18. Myocardial ⁹⁹ᵐTc pyrophosphate scintigram of a patient with an extensive transmural myocardial infarction. *1,* Twenty-degree left anterior oblique; *2,* anterior; *3,* left lateral; *4,* 45° left anterior oblique.

1   2

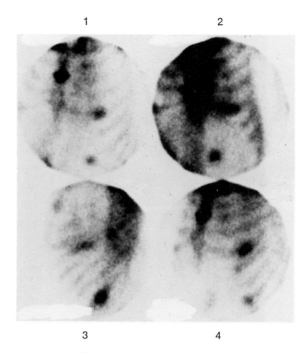

3   4

Fig. 23-19. False-positive myocardial ^{99m}Tc pyrophosphate scintiscans showing accumulation of radioactivity in the sternum, ribs, and spine. *1,* Twenty-degree left anterior oblique; *2,* anterior; *3,* left lateral; *4,* 45° left anterior oblique.

if the technical factors concerning the radiopharmaceutical and imaging procedure are well controlled. False-positive results vary between 10% and 20% according to different investigators. In this connection, breast affections in the form of tumor, inflammation, and functioning parenchyma have to be remembered. Damage of the chest wall muscles, whether following surgery or during cardioversion, is another possibility. A further cause for the extracardiac uptake of ^{99m}Tc pyrophosphate can be affection of the ribs and sternum by inflammation, neoplasm, or fracture (Fig. 23-19). In addition, false-positive scintigrams are also encountered with myocardial involvement, as in unstable angina pectoris, ventricular aneurysm, myocardiopathy, myocardial contusion, metastatic deposits, and cardiac calcifications. Lastly, a diffuse pattern of ^{99m}Tc pyrophosphate cardiac uptake is occasionally seen and represents blood pool imaging associated with delayed radionuclide clearance, which can be enhanced by reduced tissue attenuation such as that expected after left mastectomy. This problem can be easily solved by delayed imaging and comparison with the scintigrams obtained earlier.

Acute subendocardial infarction, if large enough, can be detected with reasonable accuracy by pyrophosphate scintigraphy. The radionuclide accumulation is visualized as a faint diffuse activity (Fig. 23-20) or, less frequently, as prominent localized uptake.

1   2

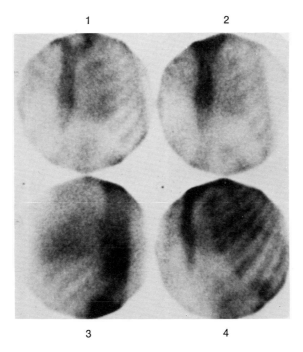

3   4

Fig. 23-20. Myocardial scintigrams to demonstrate the diffuse pattern of ^{99m}Tc pyrophosphate myocardial uptake seen in cases of myocardiopathy and subendocardial infarction. *1,* Twenty-degree left anterior oblique; *2,* anterior; *3,* left lateral; *4,* 45° left anterior oblique.

PERIPHERAL CIRCULATION

The nonradioactive techniques such as colorimetry, oscillometry, and plethysmography used to evaluate the state of the perpheral circulation are indirect and liable to technical errors and variations because of physiologic and environmental factors that are difficult to control and interpret. In contrast, procedures that employ radioactive materials directly obtain data representing the peripheral circulation (Fig. 23-21).

Although diffusion or disappearance of a freely diffusible substance injected directly into a muscle has been a satisfactory index of the vascular flow, this technique is dependent on the site, volume, and depth of injection.

A better approach depends on measurement of the uptake curves of both feet of the patient following the intravenous injection of a radionuclide. The collimated scintillation detectors used are placed in close contact with the balls of both feet. The information collected is counted by a pair of count rate meters with a time constant of 3 seconds and is recorded by a dual stripchart recorder moving at a rate of 2 cm (³/₄ inch) per minute. Labeled electrolytes were first used. However, in interpretation, the diffusion gradient of the radionuclide has to be considered, together with the degree of vascularity. Therefore, these tracers were replaced by radioactive materials that remain in the vessels and consequently reflect only the

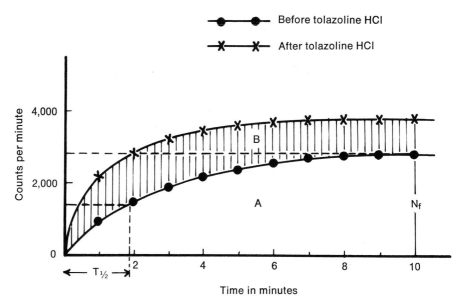

Fig. 23-21. Radioactivity build-up curve before and after the administration of tolazoline hydrochloride to demonstrate the method of calculation of the result of a test to evaluate the peripheral circulation.

A = Original build-up curve
B = Increase in build-up curve after administration of tolazoline hydrochloride
$T_{1/2}$ = Time to reach 50% of plateau activity
Time = 10 minutes
N_f = Level of activity at 10 minutes
Area = $N_f[t - (T_{1/2} \times 1.443)]$
Final result = $\dfrac{B}{A} \times 100$

intravascular radioactivity. These criteria are met by the use of labeled human serum albumin.

The test should be performed in a quiet room that is free from draft and has a relatively constant temperature. The patient is given an intravenous injection of 20 μCi of RISA, and the radioactivity build-up curves are monitored by a pair of identical, collimated scintillation detectors. The slope of the segment of the radioactivity build-up curve from the time of arrival until plateau indicates the rate of mixing of RISA with normal plasma in the capillary bed surveyed by the detector. The height of the plateau represents the size of the vascular bed in the field of the detectors. To gain more information, the ability of the vessels to dilate is tested. This is done by repetition of the test, using an exactly equal amount of RISA after the application of external heat to the legs or after an intravenous administration of a vasodilator such as 10 mg of tolazoline hydrochloride (Priscoline). External heating can be performed by applying an electric blanket to the feet for 30 minutes. If tolazoline hydrochloride is used, it is necessary to wait only 3 minutes before beginning the second test.

The result is either expressed qualitatively by visual comparison of the tracings obtained before and after the induction of vascular dilatation or quantitatively by estimating the differences between the build-up curves and expressing this difference as a percentage from the original curve $\left(\dfrac{B}{A} \times 100\right)$. The areas are either measured by planimetry or calculated according to the following equation:

$$\text{Area} = N_f \left[t - (1.443 \times T_{1/2})\right]$$

N_f = Level of activity at 10 minutes
$T_{1/2}$ = Time to reach 50% of plateau activity
t = 10 minutes (which is more than enough time to reach plateau)

Normally, under the effect of heat or tolazoline hydrochloride the vessels dilate. Consequently, the size of the vascular bed surveyed by the detector is increased, causing a higher level of plateau. Therefore in normal individuals there should be a difference between the radioactivity build-up curves recorded before and after the induction of vasodilatation. Quantitatively, the lowest figure representing the difference between the two normal tracings expressed as percentage of the original is 27%. However, it would be better to define the limits of normality by the apparatus used in each laboratory.

This test is generally used for patients who have manifestations suggestive of peripheral vascular affections, such as changes in the temperature and/or color of a limb, trophic ulcers, intermittent claudication, and absent pulse.

Another method used to study the regional blood flow in the extremities is based on quantification of the distribution of the intra-arterially injected labeled particles, with the aid of point counting or scintillation scanning.

RADIONUCLIDE VENOGRAPHY

For detection of actively forming thrombi, [125]I- or ^{131}I-labeled fibrinogen is used. Repeated point counting on successive days reveals the presence of thrombosis as evidenced by localized increase in the counting rate of at least 20% above precordial count or corresponding point on the other leg and persisting for a minimum of 24 hours. This method gives its best results in calf vein thrombosis. Its accuracy is unaffected by anticoagulant therapy. However, its accuracy diminishes as one proceeds proximally. Moreover, this test exhibits a high false-positive rate especially with recent, healed surgical incisions, hematoma, and inflammatory exudates because of their natural content of fibrin. Similarly, the test was found to be positive after contrast venography as well as in patients receiving dextran. A further disadvantage of the fibrinogen uptake test is its inability to distinguish between superficial and deep venous thrombi. Nevertheless, a negative test is strong evidence against the presence of relatively recent thrombosis.

Other much less commonly applied methods for detection of actively forming clots use labeled erythrocytes, leukocytes, platelets, or other clotting components.

For the detection of preformed deep vein thrombosis, ^{99m}Tc-labeled albumin microspheres or macroaggregates are injected into one of the veins on the dorsum of each foot, with two tourniquets placed proximally one above the ankle and the other below the knee. Scintiphotographs are taken for the calf, thigh, and pelvis to show the iliac veins and distal portion of the inferior vena cava. Evidence of abnormality may be in the form of obstruction, visualization of abnormal collateral vessels, and/or the persistence of a hot spot below the lesion or at the site of injection. It should be remembered that the finding of simple stasis in the calf region is not diagnostic.

In addition to its technical simplicity, radionuclide venography with ^{99m}Tc-labeled protein particles is highly sensitive and reliable. It enables visualization of the inferior vena cava and the iliac, femoral, and calf veins with a single injection. The procedure takes less than 30 minutes and avoids the difficulties and complications of contrast venography.

DELINEATION OF CARDIAC BLOOD POOL

If a radiopharmaceutical that remains within the cardiovascular system for a reasonable time is injected intravenously, the configuration of the cardiac blood pool can be obtained by determination of the spatial distribution of radioactivity by radionuclide scanning using a rectilinear scanner or scintillation camera (Fig. 23-6). Various radiopharmaceuticals are used, such as ^{131}I human serum albumin (150 μCi), ^{99m}Tc (5 to 10 mCi), ^{131}I cholegrafin (300 μCi), ^{99m}Tc serum albumin (2 mCi), and stabilized ^{113}In (2 mCi). Because of the better counting statistics achieved by the use of the large doses allowable with short-lived radionuclides, ^{99m}Tc and ^{113}In preparations are preferred. However, they have to be prepared and sterilized at the time of the test.

Following the intravenous injection of the radiopharmaceutical, scanning is begun from the root of the neck downward when a rectilinear scanner is used. Certain fixed reference points are marked on the scan picture to help in its accurate superimposition on the x-ray film. The suggested reference points are the suprasternal notch and the middle of the clavicles on both sides.

Since proper interpretation of the scan depends on its superimposition on a radiograph of the chest showing the exact size of the heart, the radiograph is either obtained through the anteroposterior approach at a distance of 180 cm (6 feet) or is taken in two halves to lessen the magnification of the radiographic image of the cardiac silhouette.

Normally the cardiac scan picture shows no separation from the hepatic and pulmonary blood pools and corresponds to the radiographic cardiac silhouette, which has normal dimensions. In the presence of cardiac hypertrophy or dilatation, the cardiac blood pool in the scan corresponds to the enlarged radiographic picture of the heart. With pericardial effusion, the cardiac scan measures less than 80% of the enlarged radiographic image of the heart. In addition, there is a zone of diminished radioactivity separating the cardiac from the hepatic and pulmonary blood pools. The least amount of pericardial effusion to be diagnosed by this technique is 200 ml.

By the same principles, a mediastinal shadow in which the photoscan coincides with the plain x-ray picture is diagnostic of vascular dilatation or aneurysm. On the other hand, if the shadow is caused by a mediastinal mass (glands or tumor), the cardiovascular scan is going to be smaller than the shadow observed on the x-ray film of the chest.

Cardiac photoscanning is a simple, harmless procedure that can be used to differentiate pericardial effusion from cardiac hypertrophy or dilatation or both. Furthermore, it can be applied for the differential diagnosis of cardiovascular from nonvascular shows in the mediastinum.

PLACENTAL LOCALIZATION

Because of its accuracy, safety, and relative simplicity, radionuclide placentography had gained wide acceptance over the older nonradioactive techniques. Because it is a pool of maternal blood in the gravid uterus, the placenta can be delineated by the use of radionuclides that do not leave the vascular compartment (Figs. 23-22 and 23-23). Such nuclides include ^{131}I human serum albumin (5 μCi), ^{51}Cr-tagged red cells (10 to 20 μCi), ^{99m}Tc or ^{99m}Tc-labeled serum albumin (1 mCi), and ^{113}In transferrin (1 mCi). Because of their physical characteristics, the latter two compounds are preferred. However, the excretion of ^{99m}Tc into the urinary bladder might be the cause for some confusion. The radiation dose delivered to both the mother and fetus is well below the permissible levels—much less than that received in plain radiography.

An intravenous injection of the radiopharmaceutical is given to the mother, and the placenta is localized either by point counting or by scanning with the aid of a linear scanner or the gamma camera. For point counting the abdominal surface of the uterus is divided into nine to 12 areas, and counting is done by a collimated scintillation detector. The obtained counts are expressed as percentage of the counting rate over the xiphoid.

The main indication for placental localization is to differentiate placenta previa from other causes of vaginal bleeding in the third trimester of pregnancy. An added indication is to identify the margins of the placenta to help in choosing the best site for amniocentesis.

To avoid any unnecessary exposure of the fetus to the effects of ionizing radiations, ultrasound scanning is emerging as the method of choice in placental localization. A further advantage of gray-scale ultrasonography is visualization of the

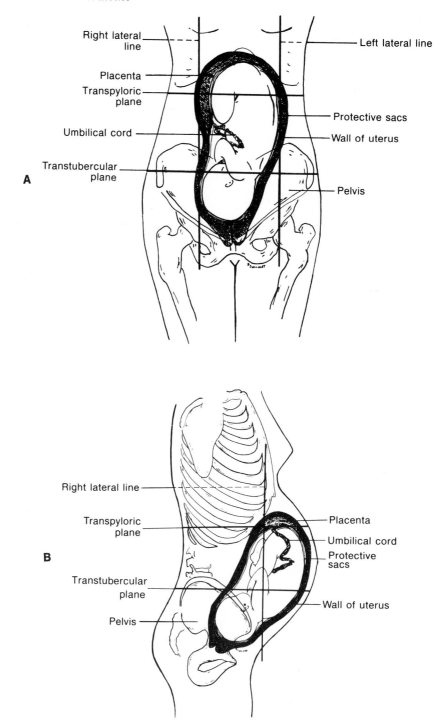

Fig. 23-22. Site of the normal placenta as seen in an anterior view (**A**) and in a lateral view (**B**).

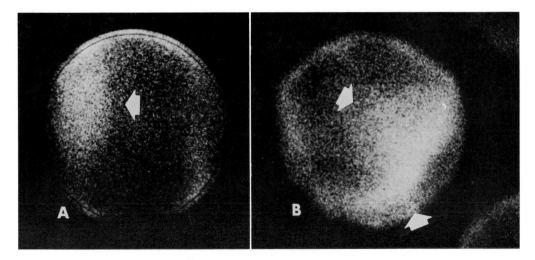

Fig. 23-23. A, Normal placental scan done shortly after the injection of 1 mCi ^{99m}Tc-labeled albumin. **B,** Abnormal placental scan. The placenta is in the lower left quadrant of the uterus covering the cervical os. (Courtesy August Miale, Jr., M.D., and Glen A. Landis, M.D., Radioisotope Unit, Georgetown University, Washington, D.C.)

inferior placental margin with its critical relationship with the presenting fetal part, cervical canal, and posterior vagina.

BIBLIOGRAPHY

Ahmad, M., Dubiel, J. P., Verdon, T. A., and Martin, R. H.: Technetium 99m pyrophosphate myocardial imaging in patients with and without left ventricular aneurysm, Circulation **53**:833-838, 1976.

Atkins, H. L., Budinger, T. F., Lebowitz, E., Ansari, A. N., Greene, M., Fairchild, R. G., and Ellis, K. J.: Thallium-201 for medical use. III. Human distribution and physical imaging properties, J. Nucl. Med. **18**:133-140, 1977.

Bailey, I. K., Griffith, L., Rouleau, J., Strauss, W., and Pitt, B.: Thallium-201 myocardial perfusion imaging at rest and during exercise. Comparative sensitivity to electrocardiography in coronary artery disease, Circulation **55**:79-87, 1977.

Berman, D. S., Amsterdam, E. A., Hines, H. H., Salel, A. F., Bailey, G. J., DeNardo, G. L., and Mason, D. T.: New approach to interpretation of technetium-99m pyrophosphate scintigraphy in detection of acute myocardial infarction. Clinical assessment of diagnostic accuracy, Am. J. Cardiol. **39**:341-346, 1977.

Berman, D. S., Salel, A. F., DeNardo, G. L., Bogren, H. G., and Mason, D. T.: Clinical assessment of left ventricular regional contraction patterns and ejection fraction by high-resolution gated scintigraphy, J. Nucl. Med. **16**:865-874, 1975.

Bradley-Moore, P. B., Lebowitz, E., Greene, M. W., Atkins, H. L., and Ansari, A. N.: Thallium-201 for medical use. II. Biologic behavior, J. Nucl. Med. **16**:156-160, 1975.

Brendt, T., Alderman, E. L., Wasnich, R., Hsich, S. C., Van Dyke, D., and Harrison, D. C.: Evaluation of portable radionuclide method for measurement of left ventricular ejection fraction and cardiac output, J. Nucl. Med. **16**:289-292, 1975.

Budinger, T. F., Yano, Y., and Hoop, B.: A comparison of ^{82}Rb and ^{13}NH$_3$ for myocardial positron scintigraphy, J. Nucl. Med. **16**:429-431, 1975.

Carr, E. A., Cafruny, E. J., and Bartlett, J. D.: Evaluation of Hg^{203} Chlormerodrin in the demonstration of human nyocardial infarcts by scanning, U. Mich. Med. Bull. **29**:27-32, 1963.

Carretta, R. F., DeNardo, S. J., deNardo, G. L., Jansholt, A., and Rose, A. W.: Early diagnosis of venous thrombosis using ^{125}I fibrinogen, J. Nucl. Med. **18**:5-9, 1977.

Cohen, W. N., and Brown, R. C.: Ultrasound, radioisotope and radiographic imaging in obstetrics.

Medcom Famous Teachings in Modern Medicine. New York 1974, Medcom.

Cook, D. J., Bailey, I., Strauss, H. W., Rouleau, J., Wagner, H. N., and Pitt, B.: Thallium-201 for myocardial imaging. I. Appearance of the normal heart, J. Nucl. Med. 17:583-589, 1976.

Davis, M. A., Holman, B. L., and Carmel, A. N.: Evaluation of radiopharmaceuticals sequestered by acutely damaged myocardium, J. Nucl. Med. 17:911-917, 1976.

Dewanjee, M. K., and Kahn, P. C.: Mechanism of localization of ^{99m}Tc-labeled pyrophosphate and tetracycline in infarcted myocardium, J. Nucl. Med. 17:639-646, 1976.

Folland, E. D., Hamilton, G. W., Larson, S. M., Kennedy, J. W., Williams, D. L., and Ritchie, J. L.: The radionuclide ejection fraction. A comparison of three radionuclide techniques with contrast angiography, J. Nucl. Med. 18:1159-1166, 1977.

Go, R.T., Doty, D. B., Chiu, C. L., and Christie, J. H.: A new method of diagnosing myocardial contusion in man by radionuclide imaging, Radiology 116:107-110, 1975.

Groch, M. W., Gottlieb, S., Mallon, S. M., and Miale, A.: A new dual-probe system for the rapid bedside assessment of left ventricular function, J. Nucl. Med. 17:930-936, 1976.

Hamilton, G. W., Trobaugh, G. B., Ritchie, J. L., Williams, D. L., Weaver, W. D., and Gould, K. L.: Myocardial imaging with intravenously injected thallium-201 in patients with suspected coronary artery disease. Analysis of technique and correlation with electrocardiographic, coronary anatomic and ventriculographic findings, Am. J. Cardiol. 39:347-354, 1977.

Hanson, R. N., Davies, M. A., and Holman, B. L.: Myocardial infarct imaging agents. III. Synthesis and evaluation of ^{203}Hg hydroxymercuriphthaleins, J. Nucl. Med. 18:1211-1214, 1977.

Hanson, R. N., Davies, M. A., and Holman, B. L.: Radiopharmaceuticals for acutely damaged myocardium. II. Synthesis and evaluation of ^{203}Hg hydroxymercurifluoresceins, J. Nucl. Med. 18:803-808, 1977.

James, A. E., Strauss, H. W., Fisher, K., Wheeless, R. C., and Longo, R.: Placental imaging with 113m-In transferrin and 99m-Tc serum albumin, Obstet. Gynecol. 37:602-611, 1971.

Janowitz, W. R., and Serafini, A. N.: Intense myocardial uptake of ^{99m}Tc-diphosphonate in a uremic patient with secondary hyperparathyroidism and pericarditis: case report, J. Nucl. Med. 17:896-898, 1976.

Jengo, J. A., Mena, I., Joe, S. H., and Criley, M.: The significance of calcific valvular heart disease in Tc-99m pyrophosphate myocardial infarct scanning: radiographic, scintigraphic and pathological correlation, J. Nucl. Med. 18:776-780, 1977.

Johnson, P. M., and King, D. L.: The placenta: evaluation by radionuclide and ultrasound, Semin. Nucl. Med. 4:75-93, 1974.

Johnston, T. B., and Whillis, J.: Gray's Anatomy, London, 1944, Longmans Green & Co.

Larson, S. M., and Nelp, W. B.: Visualization of the placenta by radioisotope photoscanning using technetium 99m labeled albumin, Am. J. Obstet. Gynecol. 93:950-956, 1965.

Lebowitz, E., Greene, M. W., Fairchild, R., Bradley-Moore, P. R., Atkins, H. L., Ansari, A. N., Richards, P., and Belgrave, E.: Thallium-201 for medical use, J. Nucl. Med. 16:151-155, 1975.

Loudon, J. R.: ^{125}I-fibrinogen uptake test, Br. Med. J. 2:793, 1976.

Lowenthal, I. S., Parisi, A. F., Tow, D. E., Barsamian, E. M., Sasahara, A. A., McCaughan, D., and Clemson, H. C.: Diagnosis of acute myocardial infarction in patients undergoing open heart surgery: a comparison of serial myocardial imaging with cardiac enzymes, electrocardiography and vectorcardiography, J. Nucl. Med. 18:770-775, 1977.

MacIntyre, W. J., Crespo, G. G., and Christie, J. H.: The use of radioiodinated (I^{131}) iodopamide for cardiovascular scanning, Am. J. Roentgenol. Radium Ther. Nucl. Med. 89:315-322, 1963.

MacIntyre, W. J., Storaasli, J. P., Krieger, H., Pritchard, W., and Friedell, H.: ^{131}I labeled serum albumin: its use in the study of cardiac output and peripheral vascular flow, Radiology 59:849-856, 1952.

McLaughlin, P. R., Martin, R. P., Doherty, P., Daspit, S., Goris, M., Haskill, W., Lewis, S., Kriss, J. P., and Harrison, D. C.: Reproducibility of thallium-201 myocardial imaging, Circulation 55:497-503, 1977.

Morris, G. K., and Mitchell, J. R. A.: Evaluation of ^{125}I fibrinogen test for venous thrombosis in patients with hip fracture. Comparison between isotope scanning and necropsy findings, Br. Med. J. 1:264-265, 1977.

Parkey, R. W., Bonte, F. J., Buja, L. M., Stokey, E. M., and Willerson, J. T.: Myocardial infarct imaging with technetium-99m phosphates, Semin. Nucl. Med. 7:15-28, 1977.

Pasquier, J., Laforte, C. D., Roux, F., Leonetti, J., Brady, A., Hegesippe, M., and Bernard, R. J.: The use of high activity ^{99m}Tc labeled red blood cells for ventricular contraction measurement with an unsophisticated cardiac synchronizer linked to a gamma camera, Eur. J. Nucl. Med. 2:13-18, 1977.

Perez, L. A.: Clinical experience: technetium 99m labeled phosphates in myocardial imaging, Clin. Nucl. Med. 1:2-9, 1976.

Pitt, B., and Strauss, H. W.: Myocardial imaging in the noninvasive evaluation of patients with suspected ischemic heart disease, Am. J. Cardiol. 37:797-806, 1976.

Poe, N. D.: Rationale and radiopharmaceuticals for myocardial imaging, Semin. Nucl. Med. 7:7-14, 1977.

Pohost, G. M., Zir, L. M., Moore, R. H., McKusick, K. A., Guiney, T. E., and Beller, G. A.: Differentiation of transiently ischemic from infarcted myocardium by serial imaging after a single dose of thallium-201, Circulation 55:294-302, 1977.

Poulouse, K. P., Kapcar, A. J., and Reba, R. C.: False positive ¹²⁵I-fibrinogen test, Angiology 27:258-261, 1976.

Prasquier, R., Taradash, M. R., Botvinick, E. H., Shames, D. M., and Parmley, W. W.: The specificity of the diffuse pattern of cardiac uptake in myocardial infarction imaging with technetium-99m stannous pyrophosphate, Circulation 55:61-66, 1977.

Prinzmetal, M., Corday, E., Bergman, H. C., Schwartz, L., and Sritzler, R. J.: Radiocardiography. A new method for studying the blood flow through the chambers of the heart in human beings, Science 108:340-341, 1948.

Razzak, M. A.: The pulmonary circulation time as measured by radiocardiography in normal individuals, J. Egypt. Med. Ass. 45:971-975, 1962.

Razzak, M. A.: Radiocardiography, J. Indian Med. Ass. 40:307-311, 1963.

Razzak, M. A.: The simultanous determination of the pulmonary and cardioportal circulation times in normal individuals by radioiodinated human serum albumin, Alex. Med. J. 9:13-16, 1963.

Razzak, M. A.: The use of a modified radioactive test for evaluating the peripheral circulation, J. Nucl. Med. 4:244-248, 1963.

Razzak, M. A.: The pulmonary circulation time and radiocardiographic pattern in bilharzial cor pulmonale, Am. J. Trop. Med. Hyg. 13:20-24, 1964.

Razzak, M. A.: Analysis of the radiocardiogram in silicosis, Nucl. Med. 4:439-444, 1965.

Razzak, M. A.: Gated radionuclide biventriculography, J. Nucl. Med. 18:1240, 1977.

Razzak, M. A., Botti, R. E., and MacIntyre, W. J.: A rapid radioisotope dilution technique for the accurate determination of the cardiac output, Nucl. Med. 7:1-7, 1968.

Razzak, M. A., Botti, R. E., MacIntyre, W. J., and Pritchard, W. H.: Consecutive determination of cardiac output and renal blood flow by external

monitoring of radioactive isotopes, J. Nucl. Med. 11:190-195, 1970.

Razzak, M. A., Hassaballa, A., and Abou-Khatwa, H.: Evaluation of the peripheral circulation in diabetics by means of a modified radioisotopic technic, Radiology 91:568-571, 1968.

Razzak, M. A., Higazi, A. M., and Guirgis, B.: Radiocardiography in rheumatic heart disease and its value in selection of cases for mitral commissurotomy, J. Nucl. Med. 5:851-863, 1964.

Razzak, M. A., and Wagner, H. N.: Cardiac photoscanning, Bull. Egypt. Soc. Cardiol. 3:44-50, 1962.

Ritchie, J. L., Hamilton, G. W., Gould, K. L., Allen, D., Kennedy, J. W., and Hammarmeister, K. E.: Myocardial imaging with indium-113m and technetium-99m macroaggregated albumin, Am. J. Cardiol. 35:380-389, 1975.

Rossman, D. J., Rouleau, J., Strauss, H. W., and Pitt, B.: Detection and size estimation of acute myocardial infarction using ⁹⁹ᵐTc-glucoheptonate, J. Nucl. Med. 16:980-985, 1975.

Ryo, U. Y., Qazi, M., Strikantaswamy, S., and Pinsky, S.: Radionuclide venography: correlation with contrast venography, J. Nucl. Med. 18:11-17, 1977.

Saperstein, L. A.: Regional blood flow by fractional distribution indicators, Am. J. Physiol. 193:161-168, 1958.

Silverstein, E. A., Turner, D. A., Fordham, E. W., and Chung-Bin, A.: Cardiac blood pool imaging over the complete cardiac cycle with a multiformat imager, J. Nucl. Med. 18:159-162, 1977.

Singh, A., and Usher, M.: Comparison of Tc-99m methylene diphosphonate with Tc-99m pyrophosphate in the detection of acute myocardial infarction: concise communication, J. Nucl. Med. 18:790-792, 1977.

Strauss, H. W., and Pitt, B.: Thallium-201 as a myocardial imaging agent, Semin. Nucl. Med. 7:49-58, 1977.

Strauss, H. W., Harrison, K., and Pitt, B.: Thallium-201 noninvasive determination of the regional distribution of cardiac output, J. Nucl. Med. 18:1167-1170, 1977.

Strauss, H. W., Harrison, K., Langan, J., Lebowitz, E., and Pitt, B.: Thallium-201 for myocardial imaging. Relation of thallium-201 to regional myocardial perfusion, Circulation 51:641-645, 1975.

Subramanian, G., McAfee, J. G., Blair, R. J., Kallfelz, F. A., and Thomas, F. D.: Technetium-99m-methylene diphosphonate. A superior agent for skeletal imaging: comparison with other technetium complexes, J. Nucl. Med. 16:744-755, 1975.

Verani, R. S., Marcus, M. L., Razzak, M. A., and Ehrhardt, J. C.: Sensitivity and specificity of thallium-201 perfusion scintigrams under exercise in the diagnosis of coronary artery disease, J. Nucl. Med. **19:**773-782, 1978.

Verani, R. S., Marcus, M. L., Spoto, G., Rossi, N. P., Ehrhardt, J. C., and Razzak, M. A.: Thallium-201 myocardial perfusion scintigrams in the evaluation of aorto-coronary saphenous bypass surgery, J. Nucl. Med. **19:**765-772, 1978.

Wackers, F. J. TH., and Dejong, R. B. J.: Myocardial imaging with thallium 201, Medicamundi **21:**103-113, 1976.

Wackers, F. J. TH., Skole, E. B., Samson, G., and Schoot, J. B.: Atlas of myocardial scintigraphy, Clin. Nucl. Med. **2:**64-74, 1977.

Wagner, H. N., McAfee, J. G., and Mozley, J. M.: Diagnosis of pericardial effusion by radioisotope scanning, Arch. Intern. Med. **108:**679-684, 1961.

Willerson, J. T., Parkey, R. W., Buja, L. M., and Bonte, F. J.: Are ^{99m}Tc-stannous pyrophosphate myocardial scintigrams clinically useful? Clin. Nucl. Med. **2:**137-145, 1977.

Willerson, J. T., Parkey, R. W., Bonte, F. J., Meyer, S. L., and Stokely, E. M.: Acute subendocardial myocardial infarction in patients. Its detection by technetium 99m-Stannous pyrophosphate myocardial scintigrams, Circulation **51:**436-441, 1975.

Zaret, B. L., and Cohen, L. S.: Radionuclides and the patient with coronary artery disease, Am. J. Cardiol. **35:**112-115, 1975.

Zweiman, F. G., Holman, B. L., O'Keefe, A., and Idoine, J.: Selective uptake of ^{99m}Tc complexes and ^{67}Ga in acutely infarcted myocardium, J. Nucl. Med. **16:**975-979, 1975.

24 Lung

ANATOMY AND PHYSIOLOGY

The main function of the lung is gaseous exchange. This exchange consists of the extraction of oxygen from atmospheric air and the disposal of gaseous waste products of the body. The diseases that affect the lung can be understood in terms of the anatomy of the airway system in which atmospheric air flow takes place and the histology of the large membrane system through which the exchange of oxygen and gaseous products takes place.

Airways

Air is carried to the lung through a system of airways that begins at the trachea and extends into alveolar units. The trachea divides into the two bronchi, which in turn divide into progressively smaller units and end at the terminal bronchioles. These bronchioles deliver air to the alveoli, the final air sacs where the exchange is made between the inspired air and the bloodstream. The airways are lined with two different types of cells, the ciliated and the goblet cells. The goblet cells produce mucus, and the ciliated cells have cilia that protect the airways. The unidirectional action of the cilia propels substances toward the mouth (Fig. 24-1).

The lung has two separate and vital functions — a ventilatory function and a respiratory function. The ventilatory function is the process of moving gas in and out of the lungs from the external environment to the alveolar wall.

The respiratory function is more complex than the ventilatory function because the transfer of gas between the alveoli and blood is an active metabolic process and is also dependent on the delivery of blood to the alveolus.

Pulmonary circulation

Approximately 90% of the blood supply of the lung is carried through the right and left pulmonary arteries, and 10% of the blood supply comes from the systemic circulation through the bronchial arteries, which come off the aorta. The pulmonary arterial system branches to the right upper lobe, to the right middle lobe and right lower lobe, and to the two major portions of the left lung (the left upper and lower lobes). The arteries then subdivide segmentally, finally to end in an arteriolar capillary unit that surrounds the alveolus.

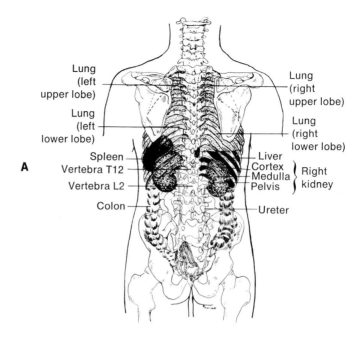

Fig. 24-1. A, Posterior anatomic relationships of large organs.

NONRADIOACTIVE METHODS OF STUDYING LUNG FUNCTION

The ventilatory function of the lung is assessed by pulmonary function studies. Volumes of air in the lung are usually studied by means of an instrument called *a spirometer*. The *residual volume*, approximately 1,200 ml of air, is the air found within the chest after a maximal expiration. A *functional residual capacity* is the resting lung volume at the end of a quiet expiration. *Tidal volume,* approximately 500 ml, is the volume of one normal breath. *Vital capacity,* approximately 4,800 ml of air, is the total volume that can be delivered after a full inspiration. *Total lung capacity,* approximately 6,000 ml, is the volume within the chest at full inspiration. *Maximal voluntary ventilation* is the greatest rate that the patient can sustain for 15 seconds and is usually expressed as amount of air exchanged per minute. With these nonradioactive studies, physicians can judge whether ventilatory impairment is obstructive or just restrictive.

The physician can also measure gas concentrations with special equipment if the patient is rebreathing in a closed system.

Tests of respiratory function usually require technical equipment and are more difficult for the physician to interpret. These studies include evaluation of the arterial and venous blood gases, both oxygen and carbon dioxide. Finally, using radiographic techniques, the radiologist may instill contrast media into the tracheobronchial system to demonstrate patency of the airway; contrast media can also be injected to visualize the major arterial system of the lung.

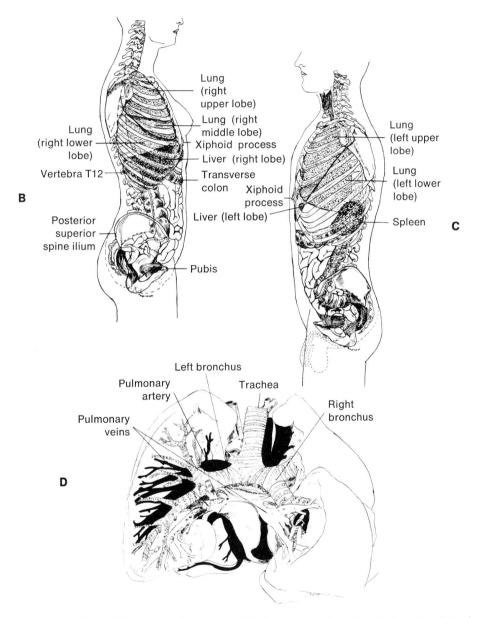

Fig. 24-1, cont'd. B, Right lateral relationships. **C,** Left lateral relationships. **D,** Posterior view of trachoebronchial tree.

NUCLEAR MEDICAL TESTS OF PULMONARY FUNCTION

Radioactive tracers have made estimation of regional pulmonary function as well as a simple estimation of pulmonary arteriolar perfusion possible.

Radioactive tests of ventilation

Radioactive aerosols may be used in the evaluation of the function of the tracheobronchial tree. Aerosol particles have varied in size from 5 to 100 μ, and various radiopharmaceuticals have been employed, including macroaggregates of albumin labeled with iodine 131 and technetium 99m. The studies are said to have accuracy in the evaluation of the patency of the tracheobronchial tree by scanning.

Respiratory ventilation has also been studied by having the patient breathe radioactive gas through a closed system. Multiple detectors or scanners qualitatively and quantitatively measure the amount of radioactivity found over areas of the lung. Oxygen 13, carbon 11, and nitrogen 13 have been used for these lung function studies. These radionuclides are primarily produced by a cyclotron. More commonly, xenon 133 is utilized to estimate both respiration and ventilation of the lung. Using a closed breathing system, the patient inspires radioactive xenon, and the radioactive gas enters various regions of the lung at a rate directly related to ventilation. This method is extended until the radioactivity reaches equilibrium. This particular equilibrium method gives an indication of alveolar ventilation. Finally, images are taken at intervals while the patient breathes room air normally and xenon is "washed out" of the lung. These washout images are indicators of the dead air spaces of the lung.

A measure of both perfusion and respiration can also be tested with radioactive xenon by placing it in solution and injecting it intravenously into the patient. The patient holds his breath during injection so that the xenon will reach the pulmonary capillary bed and diffuse into the air within the alveoli. As the patient holds his breath for 10 seconds, intrapulmonary distribution of radioactivity is determined primarily by regional pulmonary blood flow, which can be measured with external radiation detectors.

Radioactive study of lung perfusion

In recent years it has been shown that injected radioactive macroparticles lodge in the capillary bed of the lung. This has been demonstrated with the use of such materials as human albumin microspheres labeled with [99m]Tc (HAM). A direct estimation of regional perfusion can be made using external detectors. In this case, quantitative and qualitative information of perfusion can be obtained rapidly with scanners or cameras.

Human albumin microspheres labeled with [99m]Tc (HAM) can be safely administered to man. There are no hemodynamic effects from the use of the microspheres or macroaggregates, which measure approximately 40 μ in size. It has been stated that the lung contains approximately 280 billion capillary segments and in the dose of 3 mCi of macroaggregated albumin ^{131}I utilized in lung scanning, fewer than 1 million microspheres are injected. Therefore this is a relatively safe clinical procedure.

Pulmonary arterial blood flow

The major contribution of nuclear medicine to the study of lung physiology has been the evaluation of arterial blood flow. To better understand the application of this procedure the student must first know something of the normal pulmonary blood flow.

It has been shown that the regional distribution of blood flow in the lung is affected by gravity. The interalveolar structure is the same throughout the lung; however, the standing blood pressure decreases 1 ml of water per centimeter of distance from the base to the apex of the lung. Therefore, interalveolar pressure exceeds the blood pressure at the apex, alveolar blood vessels are compressed, and apical flow is minimal. When the patient is in a supine position, blood pressures become equal in the apical and basal lung regions, and the distribution of pulmonary blood flow becomes uniform. Different phases of the respiratory cycle may also influence distribution of pulmonary arterial blood flow. Therefore, the injection of the radioactive particles should take several seconds and the patient should be in a supine position. Either a scanner or a camera is used for imaging distribution of the radioactivity, and four views are usually obtained (Fig. 24-2). A note of caution should be given concerning this type of injection. The macroaggregated matter must be evenly distributed in the syringe, and blood should not be drawn back into the syringe. If a nonuniform mixture is administered or small blood clots are injected with this particular material, small areas of microembolization may be visualized.

The majority of lung tissue is posterior, therefore the best view is obtained posteriorly. Because of the focusing collimation used with rectilinear scanners, the anterior view usually does not depict the bases of the lobes, and the cardiac space will be prominent. Because the counting rate is best at the surface of the camera, it is still true that the posterior view is the best single view. Generally, however, the anterior, posterior, both lateral and posterior oblique views are obtained.

The student will recognize that emphasis is placed on complete absence or patchy absence of radioactivity in areas of the lung. Therefore, in rectilinear scanning, contrast enhancement should be minimal; otherwise, areas of poor distribution will be made absent by enhancement. As long as there is a measure of background activity on the image, minor variations in perfusion will be ascertained.

DISEASE STATES INFERRED FROM PERFUSION LUNG IMAGING
Pulmonary embolism

The search for pulmonary emboli has been one of the major uses of perfusion lung imaging. The major cause of pulmonary embolization is usually deep venous

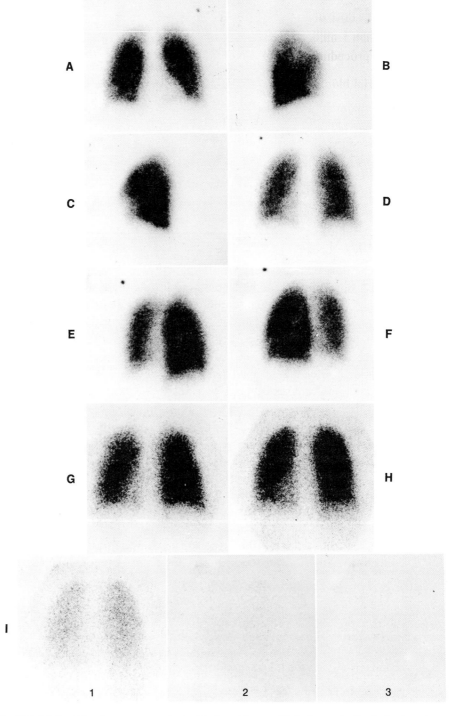

Fig. 24-2. Moderately obese young patient with short history of left chest pain. Perfusion lung images (MAA ^{99m}Tc) are within normal limits. **A,** Anterior view (slight decrease at right lateral base because of fold of fat). **B,** Right lateral view. **C,** Left lateral view. **D,** Posterior view. **E,** Right posterior oblique view. **F,** Left posterior oblique view. The ^{133}Xe ventilation study is normal. Studies were performed in posterior position. **G,** Inhalation, **H,** Equilibrium, **I,** Washout phase.

thrombophlebitis. Small fragments of the clot break loose, pass through the inferior vena cava through the right side of the heart, and lodge in the pulmonary arteriolar system. Obviously, pulmonary embolization can be caused by tumor emboli, foreign bodies, or thrombi located anywhere along the vena cava or in the right side of the heart. Pulmonary embolization may be life threatening; however, now that the diagnosis is being made with frequency, it is known that many patients who have pulmonary embolization recover without incident. The student must recognize that the signs and symptoms of this particular disease were not as well understood in the past, since the physician had no easy, direct way of estimating pulmonary perfusion. Lung scanning has given the physician a simple, nontraumatic, indirect study of pulmonary perfusion.

The signs and symptoms of pulmonary embolization listed in the medical textbooks are dramatic, but many patients with pulmonary emboli have very vague symptomatology. Frequently patients will have a fast respiratory rate and a rapid heart rate and may also have a slight fever. The patients complain of being uncomfortable and at times have slight dyspnea. However, the cardinal signs of disease, such as pain, are usually lacking in this particular disease.

A chest x-ray test in diagnosis of pulmonary embolism is only positive in 10% to 15% of patients. Usually hemorrhagic infarction is necessary before the radiograph is positive. Minor changes may be visualized that are indicative of pulmonary embolism, but these are also indicative of other disease processes. The electrocardiogram is frequently used to aid in the diagnosis of pulmonary emboli, but it is usually positive only when patients have had massive pulmonary emboli.

Chemical serum enzyme studies may be of value in the diagnosis; however, only 20% of patients with pulmonary embolization have changes in the serum enzymes associated with this diagnosis. The blood oxygen level is universally decreased in pulmonary embolization.

Finally, the radiologist may inject contrast media into the patient to visualize the pulmonary artery and its ramifications. Pulmonary arteriography, however, cannot be classed as a screening study and is usually done only when there is a real problem in interpretation of the lung image because of unexplained problems in clinical correlation or suspected underlying nonembolic lung diseases.

Lung scan. The most frequent lung perfusion findings in pulmonary embolization are lobar and segmental absences of perfusion. By planimetry it has been shown that the majority of patients with pulmonary embolization will have a decrease in or absence of perfusion of less than 20% of the total lung area.

Serial scans done on patients who have had proved pulmonary emolization have been an aid in the evaluation of the recanalization of the vessels involved in the lung (Fig 24-3). Infrequently, the lung scan will revert to normal within a very short time (within the first few days of insult). Usually, reperfusion will take place over a period of months. In older patients or those with cardiovascular conditions longer periods of time are necessary for pulmonary reperfusion. Repeated lung

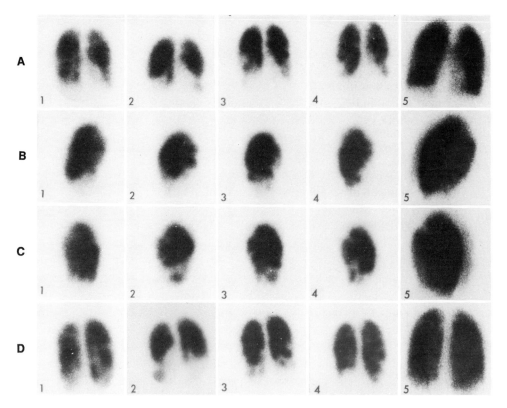

Fig. 24-3. Lung images. **A,** Anterior view. **B,** Right lateral view. **C,** Left lateral view. **D,** Posterior view. *1,* (4/2/74) Multiple segmental defects in perfusion in all lobes. Patient placed on heparin therapy. *2,* (4/9/74) Gross loss of perfusion to lower lobes with partial reperfusion of upper lobe defects. *3,* (4/16/74) Improvement in perfusion. Views on 4/22/74 *(4)* and 5/16/74 *(5)* reveal further improvement. Comment: 4/9/74 perfusion study illustrates a reperfusion "steal" phenomenon. With massive embolization in this patient, the upper lobe arterial segments were completed occluded and the lower lobe segments partially occluded. With recanalization of the upper lobe segments the lower lobe segments partially occluded were "uncovered" as perfusion shifted to the now more normally perfused upper lobes.

scans have been very helpful in following up patients who reembolized, even though they are under corrective therapy. These are the patients who are selected for surgical therapy. The primary site of the emboli is usually the deep iliac veins or the vena cava, and the surgical therapy is usually vena cava plication or ligation.

Pulmonary emphysema

The etiology of pulmonary emphysema is usually closely related to heavy smoking. In this disease the normal architecture of the tracheobronchial tree is disrupted, and bronchiolar and alveolar walls break down, resulting in large air

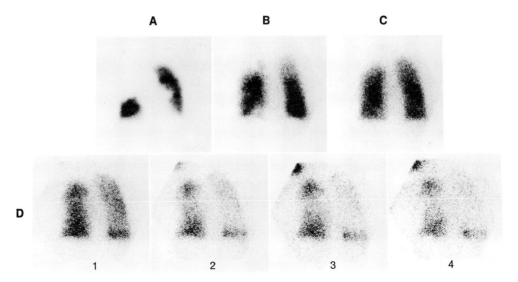

A **B** **C**

D

1 2 3 4

Fig. 24-4. Patient, 74 years of age, with moderately severe COPD (emphysema) and with an acute history of chest pain and increasing shortness of breath. **A,** Posterior perfusion (MAA ^{99m}Tc) lung image reveals absent perfusion in left upper lobe and superior left lower lobe as well as in the mediastinal region of the right lung. **B,** ^{133}Xe ventilation study (posterior position). Inhalation phase — note the ventilation of the left lung and the mediastinal portion of the right lung. **C,** ^{133}Xe equilibrium phase. Even distribution of ^{133}Xe throughout both lung fields, **D,** Washout phase. Note the delayed washout of ^{133}Xe from areas of increased dead air space (emphysema). Combined studies infer that the patient has pulmonary embolization superimposed on chronic obstructive pulmonary disease.

sacs called *blebs,* or *bullae.* These sacs do not exchange air and therefore become dead air spaces. In this group of patients, pulmonary function studies are usually abnormal. Regional vascular defects are observed by scanning in approximately 90% of the cases. The perfusion defect is usually a diffuse diminution of perfusion involving one or more areas. This perfusion defect is usually a direct effect of the distended alveoli pressing on pulmonary capillaries.

This disease could be studied by having the patient breathe a radiocolloid aerosol and imaging the normal and abnormal tracheobronchial tree. More frequently today the patient is studied with ^{133}Xe gas. The patient breathes ^{133}Xe, and the inspiratory phase and the washout phase of expiration are imaged with the scintillation camera. Thus defects of chronic bronchitis and obstructive emphysema may be inferred (Fig. 24-4).

Lung carcinoma

Lung scanning can delineate a perfusion defect caused primarily by bronchogenic carcinoma of the lung before it can be seen by standard x-ray studies (Figs. 24-5 and 24-6). These particular tumors start deep in the mediastinum and usually, by reflex action, cause a decrease in pulmonary perfusion. Since bronchogen-

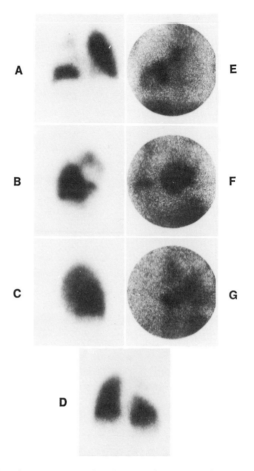

Fig. 24-5. HAM ^{99m}Tc lung images. **A,** Anterior view. **B,** Right lateral view. **C,** Left lateral view. **D,** Posterior view. Comment: almost total absence of perfusion in right upper lobe. ^{67}Ga citrate images 24 hours after administration of dose. **E,** Anterior view. **F,** Right lateral view. **G,** Posterior view. Comment: (anterior view) 6 cm concentration of gallium in right upper lobe and superior mediastinal concentration. Lateral and posterior views also reveal increased concentration in seventh dorsal vertebra. Diagnosis: bronchogenic carcinoma of right upper lobe with metastases.

ic carcinoma begins in the lumen of the bronchus, it has been found that with just a small amount of obstruction, there is a 50% decrease in perfusion in that segment of the lung. Complete absence of perfusion is the most common sign of lung carcinoma.

Inflammatory disease of the lung

In inflammatory disease of the lung the lung images are usually abnormal with areas of decreased perfusion in the regions of involvement. In acute infections of the lung the lung perfusion images may be abnormal 12 to 24 hours before the chest x-ray film becomes abnormal.

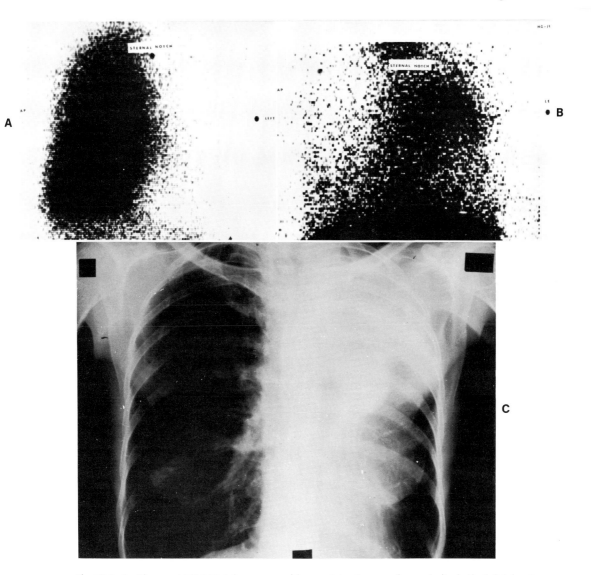

Fig. 24-6. A, Abnormal ^{131}I MAA lung scan, with complete absence of vascularity in the left lobe. **B,** [197]Hg scan revealed retention throughout the region of the left upper lobe and mediastinum. **C,** Chest x-ray film reveals large left upper lobe hilar lesion with probable secondary atelectasis. Study compatible with bronchogenic carcinoma.

Congenital and acquired heart disease

Congenital disorders of the heart will affect pulmonary circulation, and the lung scan can be informative. For example, if a single pulmonary artery has not formed, the scan will have the appearance of aplasia of the lung. When right to left side cardiac shunting is pronounced, a portion of the injected dose will often appear in other organs such as the kidney. All the rare congenital heart diseases have a bearing on pulmonary perfusion and may be studied by lung scanning. The lung scan may be of value in the diagnosis of congenital heart disease, as well as in the estimation of the amount of lung perfusion. Serial lung scans are very effective in evaluating corrective surgery.

Acquired heart diseases may be typified by mitral stenosis, which is usually a direct result of rheumatic heart disease. Patients with mitral stenosis have been found to have reversal of the gravitational perfusion of the lung. Advancing mitral stenosis will cause pulmonary venous hypertension with resultant increased blood perfusion of the apices of the lung and decreased perfusion at the bases of the lung.

Other types of heart disease, such as arteriosclerotic and hypertensive heart disease, may also change this perfusion relationship so that apical and basilar flow are almost equal.

SUMMARY

The diagnostic evaluation of pulmonary physiology has been considerably enhanced with noninvasive nuclear medicine procedures. Perfusion lung images are used routinely in the study of patients with suspected pulmonary embolization. Radioactive aerosol airway and xenon 133 ventilation images are used to visualize and quantitate the pulmonary pathophysiology caused by chronic obstructive pulmonary disease.

BIBLIOGRAPHY

Deland, F. H., and Wagner, H. N.: Atlas of nuclear medicine, Philadelphia, 1970, W. B. Saunders Co., vol. 2.

Freeman, L. M., and Blaufax, M. D.: Radionuclide studies of the lung Semin. Nucl. Med. vol. 1, no. 2, 1971.

Mandell, C. H.: Scintillation camera lung imaging — an anatomic atlas and guide, New York, 1976, Grune & Stratton, Inc.

McNeil, J.: Diagnostic strategy using ventilation — perfusion studies in patients suspect for pulmonary embolization, J. Nucl. Med. 17:613-616, 1976.

GENERAL BIBLIOGRAPHY

Ashkar, F. S., Miale, A., and Smoak, W.: A general guide to nuclear medicine, Springfield, Ill., 1975, Charles C Thomas, Publisher.

Best, C., and Taylor, N. B.: Physiological basis of medical practice, ed. 10, Baltimore, 1979, The Williams & Wilkins Co.

Blahd, W. H.: Nuclear medicine, ed. 2, New York, 1971, McGraw-Hill Book Co.

Deland, F. H., and Wagner, H. N.: Atlas of nuclear medicine, Philadelphia, 1969, W. B. Saunders Co., vol. 1.

Freeman, L. M., and Blaufax, M. D.: Physicians desk reference for radiology and nuclear medicine, Oradell, N.J., 1977-1978, Medical Economics Co.

Freeman, L. M., and Johnson, P. M.: Clinical scintillation scanning, New York, 1975, Grune & Stratton, Inc.

Grant, J. C. B., and Basmajian, J. V.: A method of anatomy, ed. 7, Baltimore, 1965, The Williams & Wilkins Co.

Gross, C. M.: Gray's anatomy of the human body, ed. 28, Philadelphia, 1966, Lea & Febiger.

Guyton, A. C.: Textbook of medical physiology, ed. 3., Philadelphia, 1966, W. B. Saunders Co.

Ham, A. W.: Histology, Philadelphia, 1957, J. B. Lippincott Co.

Holvey, D. N.: The Merck manual of diagnosis and therapy, ed. 12, Rahway, N.J., 1972, Merck Sharp & Dohme Research Lab.

Jacob, S. W., and Francone, C. A.: Structure and function in man, ed. 2, Philadelphia, 1970, W. B. Saunders Co.

Maynard, C. D.: Clinical nuclear medicine, Philadelphia, 1969, Lea & Febiger.

Powsner, E. R., and Raeside, D. E.: Diagnostic nuclear medicine, New York, 1971, Grune & Stratton, Inc.

Rhodes, B. A., editor: Quality control in nuclear medicine: radiopharmaceuticals, instrumentation, and in vitro assays, St. Louis, 1977, C. V. Mosby Co.

Shtassel, P.: Speak to me in nuclear medicine, New York, 1976, Harper & Row, Publishers.

Silver, S.: Radioactive nuclides in medicine & biology — medicine, Philadelphia, 1968, Lea & Febiger.

Wagner, H. N.: Principles of nuclear medicine, Philadelphia, 1968, W. B. Saunders Co.

Wagner, H. N.: Nuclear medicine, New York, 1975, HP Publishing, Co.

25 Urinary system

The functional portion of the urinary system is composed of two kidneys, whose primary function is to produce urine. The urine is conveyed from the kidneys by way of the ureters into the urinary bladder, where it is temporarily stored before being discharged to the outside through the urethra.

KIDNEY

The kidneys are a pair of highly vascular, retroperitoneal, elastic organs situated in the posterior part of the abdomen. They are located mainly in the lumbar regions and are embedded in a considerable mass of fatty tissue termed *renal fat* (Figs 21-1, *A* and *C*, and 24-1, *A*). Their long axes are directed downward and laterally; their upper poles are nearer to the median plane than their lower poles. The right kidney is slightly lower than the left, possibly because of its relationship to the liver. Normally the kidneys measure 11 cm (4 to 5 inches) in length, 6 cm (2.5 inches) in width, and 3 cm (1 inch) in thickness.

The outline of the kidneys can be mapped out on the patient's back within a pair of rectangles included between two horizontal lines drawn through the eleventh thoracic and third lumbar spines and two vertical lines drawn at 2.5 cm (1 inch) and 9.5 cm (4 inches) from the middle line.

In shape, each kidney resembles a bean and has an ovoid outline. The lateral border is convex; the medial border is concave in the center and convex at each end. In the central part of the medial border there is a deep vertical fissure *(hilum),* and it transmits the renal vessels and nerves, together with the funnel-shaped upper end, or pelvis, of the ureter. This hilum leads into a central recess or cavity, called the *renal sinus,* and is almost entirely filled by the *ureteral pelvis* and renal vessels. Within the sinus, the pelvis of the ureter is formed by the union of two or, less commonly, three major *calyces.* Each major calyx is formed by the union of several minor calyces that embrace the *renal papillae* and receive the urine.

The renal arteries are wide vessels that take origin from the sides of the aorta opposite the second lumbar vertebra. Before entering the kidney, each artery divides into four or five branches. Blood returns from the kidneys by way of the renal veins, which join the sides of the inferior vena cava; the left vein is longer than the right.

Structure

The kidney is enclosed by a fibrous *capsule* that is prolonged around the lips of the hilum into the renal sinus to become continuous with the outer coat of the calyces and ureteral pelvis. The kidney is made up to two main parts: an inner *medulla* and an outer *cortex*. The medulla consists of a series of conical masses (the *renal pyramids*), the bases of which face outward. They are separated by extensions from the cortex, called *cortical columns*. The apices of the pyramids converge toward the renal sinus, where they project into the interior of the calyces as small nipples, or papillae. The cortical substance is more vascular and uniformly granular. It arches over the bases of the pyramids and dips in between them.

In the renal sinus the branches of the renal artery divide into *lobar arteries,* one for each papilla. Each lobar artery divides into two *interlobar arteries* that proceed outward along the sides of the pyramids. At the junction between the medulla and cortex, the interlobar arteries divide into branches, called the *arcuate arteries,* that run at right angles to the parent stem. These give off a large number of vertically arranged branches, termed the *straight,* or *interlobular, arteries,* from which arise a number of lateral branches, called the *afferent arterioles.* Each afferent arteriole divides into about fifty capillaries that stay together to form a *glomerulus.* The blood leaves this glomerulus in a smaller *efferent arteriole* that divides to form a second capillary network around the tubules of its nephron (glomerulus and tubule). These capillaries finally converge to form *venules* that drain into the *interlobular veins.* The medulla receives its relatively scanty blood supply through branches from the efferent arterioles.

Each capillary tuft, or glomerulus, is surrounded by the expanded blind end of a renal tubule. This capsule consists of a basement membrane lined by a single layer of flattened epithelium and is called the *glomerular,* or *Bowman's, capsule.* This, together with its glomerulus, constitutes the *Malpighian,* or *renal, corpuscle.* The rest of the renal tubule runs a long tortuous course and consists of various parts, the most important of which are the *first convoluted tubule,* the *loop of Henle* (descending and ascending limbs), and the *second convoluted tubule.* This latter opens into a *collecting tubule.* The collecting tubules converge to form the *ducts of Bellini* that finally open on the summit of a papilla. The loops of Henle, the collecting tubules, and ducts of Bellini lie in the medulla; the rest of the renal tubules, as well as the renal corpuscles, are found in the cortex.

Functions

The main function of the kidney is to maintain the constancy of the osmotic pressure, volume, reaction, and composition of the extracellular fluid. This is achieved through urine secretion and elimination from the plasma of water and various nonvolatile solutes at rates and ratios that counterbalance the effects of the forces that tend to alter the composition of the internal medium. In addition, the kidney has certain functions that are unrelated to urine secretion. For example, through renin formation it may help in maintenance of normal blood pressure. Furthermore, the renal tubular epithelium carries out certain chemical transformations, including some detoxicating reactions.

Urine formation

The first step involved in the formation of urine is the maintenance of a large renal blood flow that amounts to 25% of the cardiac output (roughly 1,250 ml of blood per minute), containing approximately 700 ml of plasma. This step is followed by ultrafiltration from the plasma through the walls of the glomerular tuft of capillaries into Bowman's capsule of a large volume of fluid containing the small molecules of the plasma in unchanged concentrations. The glomerular filtrate thus formed resembles the plasma except for the absence of plasma proteins and lipids; it amounts to 120 ml/min or 170 liter/day. As it passes along the tubule, the filtrate is concentrated, and the essential substances are conserved. Most of the water is reabsorbed, so that only 1 ml/min passes into the collecting ducts to produce approximately 1.5 liters of urine per day. High threshold substances, such as glucose, sodium chloride, vitamin C, and amino acids, are nearly completely reabsorbed into the bloodstream. In contrast, only small amounts of low threshold substances such as urea, phosphates, and uric acid are reabsorbed. Practially all of substances such as creatinine and sulfates are excreted. Apart from reabsorption, the renal tubules have the power to excrete certain substances such as iodopyracet (Diodrast), organic iodine compounds, sodium para-aminohippurate, and penicillin.

After the urine is formed, it passes through the ureters into the urinary bladder, where it is temporarily stored. When empty, the urinary bladder lies in the lower and anterior part of the pelvis behind the pubic bones. As it fills, it balloons upward and rises gradually into the abdominal cavity.

DETERMINATION OF RENAL BLOOD FLOW

Radionuclide techniques used for estimation of renal blood flow in man are the inert gas washout, indicator dilution, and clearance methods.

The main advantage of the inert gas washout method is in providing information on the intrarenal distribution of the renal blood flow. However, it necessitates selective catheterization of the renal artery to enable injection of the bolus of ^{85}Kr or ^{133}Xe gas solution. After being injected, the gas diffuses rapidly into the renal tissue to reach equilibrium with the blood instantaneously. The renal radioactivity washout curve is monitored by external counting with the aid of a properly placed collimated scintillation detector. The obtained data are plotted on semilogarithmic paper and analyzed by compartmental analysis. The first, or fast, component of the washout curve represents the cortical blood flow. Using this technique, the basal renal blood flow in normal subjects with a normal sodium balance averages 4 ml/min/gm. In addition to the effect of sodium balance, another limitation to the gas washout technique is its inability to demonstrate areas that are not perfused since the slope is determined mainly by the flow in the best perfused regions.

In the indicator dilution technique, either radioiodinated human serum albumin or labeled erythrocytes are used. Catheterization of the renal artery and vein is required for injection and sampling. Therefore, the clinical application of this method has been limited.

The clearance methods are by far the most commonly used procedures for determination of the renal blood flow. According to the Fick principle, if a substance is consumed solely by one organ, the blood flow to this organ can be determined by dividing the amount consumed per unit time by the arteriovenous difference in the concentration of this material. This means that the concentration of this particular substance must be determined both in the arterial blood going to this organ and in the venous blood coming out of this organ. However, if this substance is totally consumed or excreted during a single passage through the organ, the concentration in the venous outflow will be zero. Accordingly, the arteriovenous difference is going to be equal to the arterial concentration of this material. Consequently, the blood flow to this organ can be estimated by dividing the amount consumed per unit time by the arterial concentration of this material.

In the case of the kidney, the criterion of almost complete removal from the plasma during a single passage is fulfilled by sodium para-aminohippurate (PAH). After the intravenous injection of a loading dose, PAH is administered in the form of a continuous infusion at a rate to maintain a steady blood level. So long as the PAH blood level is constant, the rate of infusion should be equal to the rate of excretion. Therefore, the renal plasma flow can be determined by dividing the amount infused or its equivalent (the amount excreted per unit time) by the plasma PAH concentration. However, maintenance of a steady blood level of PAH is not easy. Furthermore, accurate estimation of PAH urinary output per unit time necessitates the application of a urethral catheter and bladder washes.

These drawbacks were partly solved by the application of the single-injection technique with subsequent analysis of the disappearance curve of PAH from the blood. However, since the diminution in the plasma PAH concentration is not only caused by its removal by the kidneys but also by its diffusion to equilibrate in a Hippuran space, recording of the data should be extended for more than an hour to solve for the two components according to the two-compartmental system. A further disadvantage is the estimation of the rather low concentrations of PAH in the collected plasma samples.

This difficulty was overcome by the introduction of ^{131}I-tagged sodium orthoiodohippurate ([131]I Hippuran). With [131]I Hippuran the disappearance curve is recorded either by plasma sampling or by external monitoring. The obtained curve is then analyzed according to the two-compartmental system. This is both time consuming and inconvenient to the patient.

To simplify matters, a segment from the disappearance curve is selected on condition that during this period the disappearance is mainly caused by its removal by the kidney. Accordingly, the disappearance curve can be analyzed on the basis of a single-compartment system. Under such circumstances, the renal blood flow is equal to the ^{131}I Hippuran disappearance rate constant times its volume of distribution. The suggested segment is that between 8 and 18 minutes after injection. The effect of ^{131}I Hippuran diffusion on the disappearance curve during this segment is counterbalanced by the incomplete removal of ^{131}I Hippuran during its passage through the kidney. This is partly caused by the use of whole blood samples instead of plasma, taking into consideration that the intracorpuscular ^{131}I Hippuran is not as available for removal as that present in the plasma. The disappearance curve can be recorded either by serial blood sampling or by external monitoring.

Procedure

After the intravenous injection of 60 to 80 μCi of ^{131}I Hippuran, four blood samples are obtained at 3-minute intervals, starting at 9 minutes after injection. Radioactivity in 2 ml from each of these whole blood samples, as well as the standard for dose calibration, is assayed in a scintillation well counter. Radioactivity per milliliter in the serial blood samples is plotted on semilogarithmic paper as a function of time. The disappearance half-time of ^{131}I Hippuran ($T_{1/2}$) is estimated, and the disappearance rate constant (λ) is calculated: $\dfrac{0.693}{T_{1/2}}$. The volume of distribution (DV) is obtained by dividing the injected dose by the ^{131}I Hippuran concentration at zero time as derived by backward extrapolation of the exponential curve (Fig. 25-1). The renal blood flow is calculated as $\lambda \times$ DV.

By external monitoring, ^{131}I Hippuran disappearance is measured by a collimated scintillation detector placed over the manubrium sterni at the level of the second rib. Recording is performed by a rate meter and stripchart recorder or by a printing scaler. Recording is continued for about 30 minutes. Fifteen minutes after injection a blood sample is withdrawn, and the radioactivity in 2 ml from this sample is assayed. From the record curve, $T_{1/2}$ and λ are estimated. The volume of distribution is calculated as with the serial blood sampling, with the application of a calibration factor to relate the external counting rate to the level of blood radioactivity at 15 minutes. Then the renal blood flow is calculated from λ and DV (Fig. 25-2).

With these techniques, the renal blood flow in normal subjects proved to be 630 ± 70 ml/min/m^2, or $1{,}100 \pm 120$ ml/min/1.73 m^2 (mean $\pm$ 1 SD).

Having determined the renal blood flow, the relative blood flow to each individual kidney can be estimated by comparing the background-corrected, 1 to 2 minute uptake of both kidneys following the intravenous injection of ^{131}I hippurate. True blood-background correction can be obtained by estimating the uptake of a previous injection of ^{131}I human serum albumin.

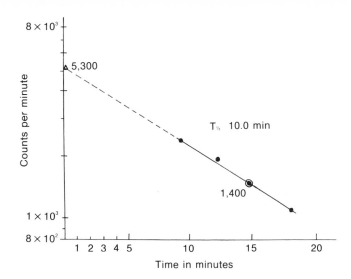

Fig. 25-1. Determination of the disappearance half-time of ^{131}I Hippuran from the circulation by serial blood sampling.

$T_{1/2}$ = 10.0 minutes
λ = 0.693 ÷ 10.0 = 0.0693 (6.93% per minute)
DV = Injected dose ÷ Intercept at zero time
   = Injected dose ÷ 5,300

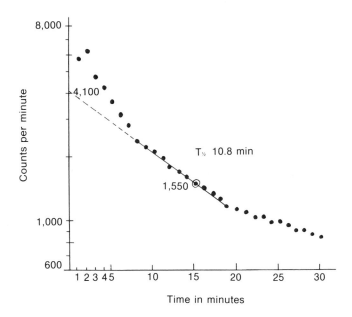

Fig. 25-2. Determination of the disappearance half-time of ^{131}I Hippuran by external monitoring.

$T_{1/2}$ = 10.8 minutes
λ = 0.693 ÷ 10.8 = 0.0642 or 6.42% per minute
External counting at 15 minutes = 1,550 cpm
Blood activity at 15 minutes (Fig. 25-1) = 1,400 cpm
Calibration factor = 1,400/1,550
Intercept at zero time = 4,100 cpm by external monitoring, which corresponds to blood activity

of $4{,}100 \times \dfrac{1{,}400}{1{,}550} = 3{,}700$ cpm

DV = Injected dose ÷ 3,700

ESTIMATION OF GLOMERULAR FILTRATION RATE

Determination of the glomerular filtration rate is based on estimation of the plasma clearance of a physiologically inert substance that is exclusively filtered by the glomeruli. This substance should not be synthesized, excreted, destroyed, or reabsorbed by the tubules.

Because of the technical difficulties encountered during the chemical determination of the test substances in plasma and urine samples, radioactively tagged compounds were introduced for determination of the glomerular filtration rate. External monitoring of these radionuclides enables recording and following the plasma radioactivity level. Accordingly, the rate of infusion of the test substance can be modified to attain a constant plasma level.

For this purpose, radioiodine-labeled inulin was used. But this compound is rather unstable, and its use has been handicapped by the presence of free radioiodine. This same disadvantage has been reported with the labeled contrast materials, which also suffer from tubular reabsorption and protein binding. In this connection, iothalamate labeled with ^{125}I is available in pure form with minimal contamination of free iodide. Its plasma binding is variable. Nevertheless, results of assessment of glomerular filtration rate with ^{125}I iothalamate are in close agreement with the inulin clearance test.

Radiocobalt-labeled vitamin B_{12} has proved to be a suitable agent for determination of the glomerular filtration rate when its protein binding is prevented by the prior administration of a large dose of stable vitamin B_{12}. Correction for the fraction that is not excreted by the kidneys should be applied. The clearance values obtained using vitamin B_{12} labeled with ^{57}Co or ^{58}Co are usually lower than those obtained by inulin clearance with a variable discrepancy between the results of these techniques.

In this connection, some chelate-forming compounds were found to be suitable for estimation of the glomerular filtration rate. These compounds have the major advantage of being extremely stable. Examples of these agents are ethylenediamine tetra-acetic acid (EDTA) labeled with ^{51}Cr and diethylenetriamine penta-acetic acid (DTPA) labeled with ^{99m}Tc, ^{113m}In, ^{58}Co, ^{169}Yb, or ^{140}La. After the intravenous injection of the calculated dose of the radionuclide, blood samples are withdrawn at 60 and 120 minutes. From the radioactivity level in these blood samples as well as in the injected dose, the glomerular filtration rate is calculated with the aid of special equations. Because of the variable percentage of ^{99m}Tc Sn-DTPA that is protein bound, the measured glomerular filtration rate is lower than that obtained with inulin.

For the determination of the glomerular filtration rate of each kidney, a method has been suggested based on the analysis of the renal time-activity curve following the intravenous administration of ^{99m}Tc DTPA and using a scintillation camera and a mini computer. Data are obtained from preselected areas representing cardiac, renal, and perirenal areas for the first 3 minutes only. The perirenal area represents the background. A blood sample is obtained to normalize the pre-cordial curve.

Similarly, individual kidney filtration fraction can be calculated through the analysis of the early segment of the kidney's time-activity curves obtained after the simultaneous administration of the tubular ^{131}I Hippuran and the glomerular ^{99m}Tc DTPA. This is based on the assumption that during the first few minutes following radionuclide injection, kidney activity is proportional to blood activity, whether tubular or glomerular, depending on the tracer used.

RADIONUCLIDE RENOGRAPHY

Although the radionuclide renogram has been in use for almost 20 years, there is no agreement regarding the radiopharmaceutical to be used, the technical details of the procedure, or the interpretation of the obtained tracing. Of the various radionuclides used, only ^{131}I sodium orthoiodohippurate and ^{197}Hg or ^{203}Hg chlormerodrin have stood the test of time. In this respect, ^{131}I Hippuran is much more widely used than labeled chlormerodrin. Hippuran is removed from the circulation partly by glomerular filtration and to a much larger extent by tubular secretion. In contrast, chlormerodrin accumulates in the proximal convoluted tubules because of their high content of sulfhydryl groups.

^{131}I Hippuran renogram

After the intravenous injection of 50 to 100 μCi of ^{131}I Hippuran with less than 1.5% free iodide, the time course of radioactivity over both kidneys is measured by a pair of well-matched collimated scintillation detectors. The information collected is counted by two rate meters with a time constant of 3 to 10 seconds; it is subsequently recorded on a dual stripchart recorder moving at a rate of 2 cm ($^{3}/_{4}$ inch) per minute over a period of 30 minutes. Recording can also be done by means of a pair of printing scalers activated at 15-second intervals. The obtained data is plotted to illustrate radioactivity as a function of time.

Although it has been shown that the shape of the renographic curve is affected to a great extent by the degree of hydration of the patient, there is disagreement as to what is the optimum state of hydration required. With hydration the tracing is more smooth, which makes calculations easier. In addition, in normal subjects the level of peak radioactivity attained by both kidneys is more or less equal, whereas in the dehydrated state the levels are not equal. Therefore it is thought that hydration is better, and this can be achieved by asking the patient to drink about 600 ml of fluids during the hour preceding the test.

In regard to the position of the patient during performance of the test, some investigators prefer the sitting position to help urine drainage by gravity. Others keep the patient supine or prone to limit movements. A combination of these benefits can be achieved by performing the renogram with the patient prone and the head of the table raised 30 degrees.

Since accurate placement of the detectors is critical, the kidneys are localized either by B-mode ultrasonography or radiography (in the same position of renography) or by moving the detectors over the patient's back after intravenous injection of 5 μCi of [125]I Hippuran or [197]Hg chlormerodrin to mark the site showing the highest counting rate.

There has been much controversy concerning the choice of collimators and depth of crystal. Wide apertures minimize the effects of errors in detector placement at the expense of including more extrarenal radioactivity. Similarly, increasing the depth of the crystal in the collimator minimizes the effect of variability in the distance at which the kidney is situated underneath the skin, but the count rate is diminished. As a compromise, a collimator with an aperature diameter of 4 cm (1.5 inch) is used, and the crystal is recessed 7 cm (3 inches) from the surface.

The obtained tracing starts with an abrupt initial rise in radioactivity because of its arrival in the field monitored by the detector. At least part of this radioactivity is extrarenal, since it can be demonstrated even after removal of the kidney. This segment is followed by a slower increase in radioactivity to reach a peak value (ascending limb). The rate of rise is affected by changes in the renal blood flow and cellular function. In addition, the rate of rise and the time necessary to reach the peak depend on the state of hydration of the patient. With hydration, the time required is shorter, and the slope of this limb is steeper. The last segment of the renogram (descending limb) represents removal of the radioactivity from underneath the detector. The rate of fall is influenced by the rate of removal of radioactivity from the renal pelvis as well as the disappearance of radioactivity from the blood. With hydration, the fall in radioactivity is initially faster and then becomes slower because of the appearance of bladder radioactivity in the field monitored by the detector (Fig. 25-3).

For the proper interpretation of the [131]I Hippuran renogram, several methods have been suggested for analysis of the obtained tracing. The easiest and quickest method is visual comparison of height and shape of the curve of both sides. However, this method of analysis cannot be applied after nephrectomy or in patients having bilateral renal affection. Therefore it was proposed that the tracings should be compared with an envelope drawn to include a group of curves from normal subjects using exactly the same procedure and equipment. However, this requires standardization of the curves to a certain height and does not allow any quantitation of the abnormality. For quantitation, various criteria were suggested, such as the time to reach peak radioactivity, the ratio of the peak values, the slope of the ascending limb, and the rate of decrease of radioactivity on the descending limb. The normal values for the suggested criteria should be determined in each laboratory using the same procedure and equipment every time.

A completely different approach in the analysis is based on the fact that [131]I Hippuran renograms represent an integrated response to changing radioactivity levels within the kidneys, as well as different levels of activity within the blood

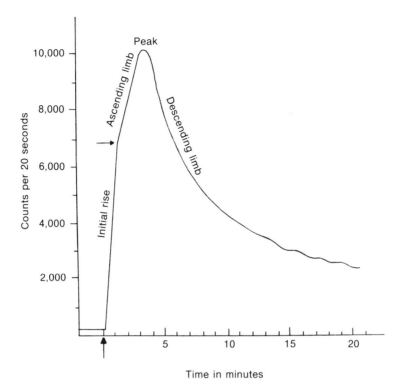

Fig. 25-3. [131]I Hippuran renogram of a normal subject after hydration with 600 ml of water.

perfusing these organs and other tissues within the area monitored by the detector. Therefore accurate correction for the external factors must be applied. This is achieved by the application of a third detector centered over the manubrium sterni and then subtraction of the obtained curve representing extrarenal radioactivity from the simultaneously recorded renograms. These mathematical manipulations are performed either manually or with the aid of a computer. The resultant curve can be called the *derived renogram* and consists of the ascending and descending limbs (Fig. 25-4). It can be analyzed by calculation of the rates of ascent and descent, respectively. A further advantage of this method of analysis is that the renal blood flow can be estimated from the tracing recorded by the sternal detector, as explained earlier (Fig. 25-2).

With the introduction of stationary detectors, errors associated with probe placement can be eliminated. Renographic and bladder activity curves can be obtained and registered on a dual-channel strip recorder attached to the output of opposite halves of the crystal or to previously chosen areas of interest. The extrarenal radioactivity contribution is reduced when each kidney is precisely defined, enabling collection of data from preselected areas of interest and subse-

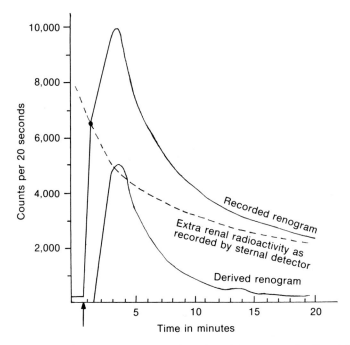

Fig. 25-4. Analysis of ^{131}I Hippuran renogram by subtraction of the extrarenal radioactivity as recorded by a sternal detector from the recorded renographic tracing.

quent analysis of the obtained data by computing techniques. However, ^{131}I is not ideal when used with the rather thin crystals of the stationary detectors, because of its relatively high-energy gamma radiation.

Clinical applications

Although renography expresses a complex function resulting from the interaction of multiple physical and physiologic factors, including geometry, background, renal hemodynamics, and various nephron mechanisms, it can provide valuable information if properly performed and interpreted. Abnormal tracings are seen with decreased kidney function or diminished blood supply or both, as well as with urinary tract obstruction whether caused by stones, tumors, or otherwise. However, it must be remembered that abnormal renogram tracings are not diagnostic of any specific disease. Thus, a cumulative type of curve can be encountered in ureteric obstruction as well as in the polyuric stage of acute renal failure. Renography has its greatest value in screening patients for a suspected abnormality when present. During pregnancy, renography is of very limited diagnostic value.

Special indications for renography include follow-up after renal artery reconstruction or kidney transplantation, in which renographic changes may precede transplant rejection. Furthermore, in rejection crisis the renal blood flow is more severely reduced than the glomerular filtration rate. Another indication is screening patients for cases of unilateral renal hypertension. An abnormal tracing on one side favors this possibility and is an indication for the application of further investigations by means of the more difficult traumatic techniques such as arteriography and differential ureteric catheterization in an effort to reach a definite diagnosis.

In doubtful cases it may be helpful to repeat the ^{131}I Hippuran renogram under restricted water intake or after loading the tubular cells with an infusion of PAH (75 mg/kg over 12 minutes). Occasionally, an antispasmodic to relieve ureteric spasm or a parasympathomimetic to correct atony of the upper urinary tract proves helpful. Further help might be obtained from radiomercury renography.

Mercury renogram

After the intravenous injection of 30 to 300 μCi of ^{197}Hg chlormerodrin, the rate of accumulation of radiomercury is measured by a pair of well-matched collimated scintillation detectors placed opposite the previously determined renal sites. The collected information is recorded by a pair of rate meters attached to a dual stripchart recorder. The result is calculated by comparison of the count rates at 30 and 60 minutes to that at 5 minutes after injection. The ratio of the rate of accumulation on the right side to that of the left is then computed. This value normally ranges from 0.85:1 to 1.05:1.

Since chlormerodrin is temporarily bound in the renal tubules, the described accumulation test is less influenced by the rate of urine flow or the state of hydration of the patient than is the case with ^{131}I Hippuran renography. Furthermore, mixing does not affect the tracing because of the slow rate of accumulation together with the long time of observation. This leaves the chlormerodrin accumulation test to be affected mainly by the renal blood flow and the renal tubular efficiency. A further advantage is the possibility of obtaining a scan picture of the kidney with the same dose of radiomercury used for the functional study. However, since the result is expressed in the form of a ratio between both sides, bilateral functional renal impairment of an equal degree would give a normal result. In addition, this test does not lead to any information about the patency of the urinary passages.

RADIONUCLIDE SCANNING OF KIDNEYS

Since chlormerodrin is extracted from the plasma by the renal tubular cells and specifically accumulated by the renal cortical tissues at a rate that greatly exceeds its excretion, this radiopharmaceutical can be used for the visualization of viable renal tissue. Usually, 300 μCi are injected intravenously, and scanning is started at least 1 hour later through the posterior approach. It must be remembered that some of the radiomercury appears in the liver (more so with depressed renal function), which could cause some confusion concerning the size of the right kidney.

To reduce the amount of radiomercury retained by the kidneys, a nonradioactive mercurial diuretic (sodium meralluride) is injected a day before the tagged chlormerodrin.

Because of the relatively high radiation dose delivered during renal scintigraphy with radiomercury, the search for better radiopharmaceuticals continues. In this respect, ^{99m}Tc iron ascorbic acid complex delivers a low radiation dose and has the other favourable characteristics of ^{99m}Tc for gamma camera scintigraphy. However, this compound is difficult to prepare and deteriorates with time; so it should be used immediately. It gives a high liver background specially with high serum creatinine levels. It is handled by both glomerular and tubular mechanisms and can be used for delayed imaging since as the compound traverses the kidney some of the ^{99m}Tc remains behind, protein bound in the tubular cells.

Another group of renal imaging agents that have become more popular are the chelate-forming compounds such as DTPA labeled with ^{113m}In or ^{99m}Tc. Since these compounds are handled solely by passive diffusion through the glomerular membrane, the obtained images could be considered as a structural representation of a physiologic function. The image quality is affected in the presence of diminished glomerular filtration, as in uremia or renal failure, with a resultant decrease in the intrarenal concentration of the radiopharmaceutical and its abnormal accumulation in the other organs, especially the liver and spleen. Immediate scans following the intravenous injection of 10 to 20 mCi of ^{99m}Tc Sn-DTPA demonstrate the perfusion pattern. Scintiphotography performed between 2 and 5 minutes after injection illustrates the kidney parenchyma before excretion of the radiotracer in the renal pelvis can obscure part of the kidney. Best images of the renal parenchyma together with the pelvic-calyceal system are obtained 10 to 15 minutes after tracer injection.

Other ^{99m}Tc-labeled compounds that have been used successfully for renal imaging include ^{99m}Tc penicillamine acetazolamide complex, labeled saccharides such as glucoheptonate, and ^{99m}Tc Sn dimercapto succinic acid.

The behaviour of ^{99m}Tc glucoheptonate simulates to a great extent the iron ascorbic acid complex, but its renal concentration is not as great. Furthermore, it delivers a lower radiation dose because of its faster blood and urinary clearance. Another advantage of ^{99m}Tc glucoheptonate is its stability, enabling its use even 5 hours after preparation. Following the intravenous injection of 15 mCi of ^{99m}Tc glucoheptonate, immediate imaging demonstrates renal perfusion (Fig. 25-5). Early sequential images illustrate the renal parenchyma followed by the pelvic-calyceal system, whereas late static scintiphotography reveals the details of the renal parenchyma alone.

Regarding ^{99m}Tc dimercapto succinic acid (DMSA), it selectively concentrates in the renal cortex and exhibits mercurial-like kinetics. Both blood clearance and urinary excretion are slow. Therefore, it enables excellent appraisal of cortical details and anatomy without interfering with activity in the pelvic-caly-

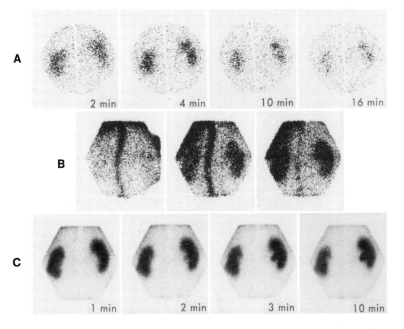

Fig. 25-5. Normal ¹³¹I Hippuran and ⁹⁹ᵐTc glucoheptonate sequential renal images. **A,** ¹³¹I Hippuran flow (2-minute sequential images; posterior position). Normal tubular function and excretion bilaterally. **B,** ⁹⁹ᵐTc glucoheptonate (4-second sequential images; posterior position). Normal perfusion bilaterally. **C,** ⁹⁹ᵐTc glucoheptonate static images (1-minute sequential images; posterior position). Sequential images reveal normal cortical volume bilaterally on 1-minute view, calyceal visualization on 2-minute view, and pelvic visualization bilaterally on 3-minute view. Ten-minute view reveals renal clearance, cortex almost completely cleared, and visualization of renal medulla and pelvis.

ceal collecting system. However, this substance must be used within 30 minutes of preparation, since it oxidizes readily. The usual dose is 1 to 5 mCi, and imaging is started immediately to evaluate the vascular supply to the kidneys. For cortical appraisal, enough time (2 hours) should elapse for the radiopharmaceutical to reach a high concentration in the renal cortex. More time is required with renal impairment, which is characterized by slow disappearance of radioactivity from the vascular compartment (Fig. 25-6).

In this connection, iodohippurate (Hippuran) tagged with ¹³¹I has been used with great success to visualize the kidneys in azotemic patients. This is based on the prolongation of the intrarenal transit time and the slow excretion of ¹³¹I Hippuran by the failing kidney, giving sufficient time for renal scintigraphy (Fig. 25-7).

Sometimes valuable information about the kidneys can be obtained indirectly during bone scintigraphy and in the course of gallium studies. During ⁹⁹ᵐTc pyrophosphate skeletal surveys, the nonvisualization of one kidney and the asymmetric or focal decreased uptake of radioactivity indicate renal abnormalities. Similarly, renal localization of ⁶⁷Ga is associated with renal pathology such as renal

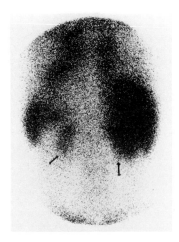

Fig. 25-6. Delayed static images following the intravenous injection of ^{99m}Tc DMSA in a patient with chronic renal failure, showing bilateral small kidneys with poor tubular function as evidenced by persistant radioactivity in the blood pool, particularly in the heart, spleen, and liver.

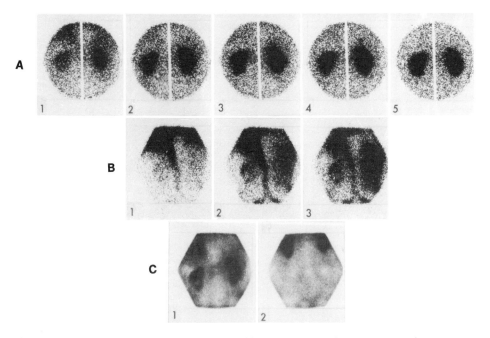

Fig. 25-7. Left renal cyst. Decreased renal function bilaterally. **A,** ^{131}I Hippuran flow (2-minute sequential images; posterior position). *1* to *4* demonstrate ill-defined decrease in concentration in lower pole of left kidney. *5,* Compared to normal tubular secretory rate, both kidneys are secreting and excreting poorly. **B,** ^{99m}Tc glucoheptonate (4-second sequential images; posterior position). *1,* Aorta; *2,* renal perfusion, avascular lesion of left kidney; *3,* relatively poor renal perfusion, since suprarenal organs have more blood flow than either kidney. **C,** ^{99m}Tc glucoheptonate static images (1-minute sequential images; posterior position). *1,* 4-minute static view: well-defined round cold lesion of left kidney; pelves have not visualized; *2,* 10-minute static view indicates poor renal function, since ureters and bladder can barely be defined.

malignancy, lymphoreticular neoplasm, leukemia, amyloidosis, and inflammatory conditions, especially renal abscess, pyelonephritis, vasculitis, and acute tubular necrosis.

Renal scanning is indicated for the accurate determination of the size, site, and shape of the kidney, together with the detection of any space-occupying lesions. The suggested reference points to be marked on the rectilinear scan picture are the midline and the last rib and iliac crest on both sides. Normally the renal picture measures 12 by 6 cm or 5 by 2.5 inches.

Scanning is diagnostic of morphology and not pathology. A space-occupying lesion in a scan picture might be caused by a tumor, cyst, abscess, or infarct (Figs. 25-7 and 25-8). Ultrasonography can accurately differentiate cysts from other space-occupying lesions.

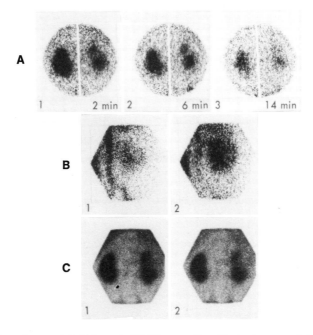

Fig. 25-8. Renal carcinoma, right kidney. **A,** [131]I Hippuran flow (2-minute sequential images; posterior position). *1,* 2-minute view: right kidney, decreased concentration in medial and superior portion; left kidney normal; *2,* 6-minute view: normal secretion and excretion of left kidney and functional portion of right kidney; *3,* 14-minute view: normal secretion and excretion of left kidney and functional portion of right kidney. **B,** [99m]Tc glucoheptonate (4-second sequential images; posterior position). NOTE: camera was centered over the abnormal right kidney. *1,* Right kidney: normal arterial perfusion in lower pole, uneven and abnormal perfusion in medial and superior pole; *2,* capillary/venous phase revealing perfusion of a nonfunctional space-occupying lesion in the medial superior right kidney. **C,** [99m]Tc glucoheptonate static images (1-minute sequential images; posterior position). *1,* 2-minute static image: normal left renal cortical volume, pelvis, and ureter; right kidney, large, nonfunctional space-occupying lesion in superior medial right kidney; normal inferior cortical function, pelvis, and ureter; *2,* 6-minute static image: cortical excretion with visualization of the left renal medulla and functional remnants of the right kidney.

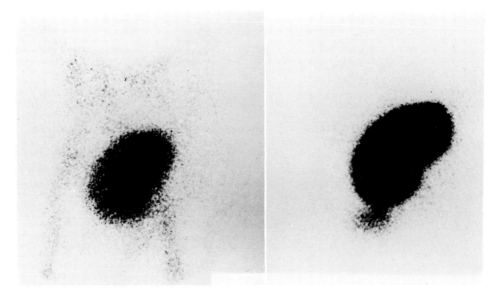

Fig. 25-9. ^{99m}Tc DMSA sequential renal scans obtained immediately (left) and at 3 hours (right) following tracer injection to evaluate renal transplant. Scans show normal perfusion and tubular function.

A special indication for radionuclide scanning of the kidneys is the detection of tumors that do not cause distortion of the calyceal system and consequently would be missed by intravenous pyelography. Another indication for renal scanning is the investigation of patients who are allergic to iodine-containing contrast media. In addition, in the presence of moderate renal failure, scanning usually succeeds in visualization of the kidneys when pyelography fails. Another method that can be used to delineate the size and configuration of the nonfunctioning kidney is B-mode ultrasound.

Stationary detectors are becoming more and more popular in the field of renal scintigraphy, particularly since they provide added information about kidney function. Sequential scintigraphy with ^{131}I Hippuran, ^{99m}Tc Sn-DTPA, ^{99m}Tc glucoheptonate, and ^{99m}Tc DMSA has proved very helpful in the diagnosis of various renal disorders, including the evaluation of renal transplants (Fig. 25-9).

The transplanted kidney is subjected to a variety of immunologic, vascular, and obstructive processes that are not easy to detect early by conventional diagnostic techniques. Renal arteriography and biopsy can establish the diagnosis, but they cannot be performed serially. In contrast, radionuclide techniques are easy to perform and to repeat without risk to the patient. In addition, they can provide valuable diagnostic information.

Since fibrin is deposited in the vascular and interstitial tissues of renal transplants undergoing rejection, labeled fibrinogen has been used for the diagnosis of this complication by external counting as well as by determination of clearance

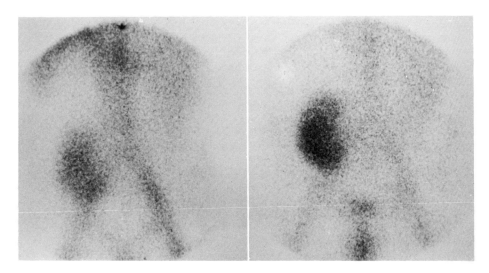

Fig. 25-10. Sequential renal scans obtained at 10 minutes and 3 hours after ⁹⁹ᵐTc DMSA injection. The transplant has poor perfusion and markedly diminished tubular function.

rate or imaging. However, optimal imaging is delayed for 24 hours and the obtained pictures are poor in quality. False-positive results are encountered with wound hematoma, perirenal hemorrhage, and urinary leakage. On the other hand, false-negative results have been reported with chronic rejection.

Another radiopharmaceutical that has been used with success to detect transplant rejection is ⁹⁹ᵐTc sulfur colloid, which appears to accumulate in areas of intravascular thrombosis in acutely and chronically rejecting renal transplants. No accumulation of the radiocolloid is seen in normal-functioning renal transplants. On the other hand, acute and chronic rejection, with evidence of residual function and preserved blood supply, show radiocolloid accumulation in the graft. False-negative results are seen with necrotic transplants and cases treated with high doses of heparin, as well as in end-stage chronic rejection with absent vascularity. False-positive results are sometimes observed with acute tubular necrosis, especially when there is history of previous rejection episodes.

Similarly, renal transplants undergoing rejection accumulate ⁶⁷Ga citrate. However, the detection procedure takes a longer time and is technically more complicated than that used with ⁹⁹ᵐTc sulfur colloid.

Added evidence for rejection can be obtained from diminution of the renal blood flow as determined by external monitoring of ¹³¹I Hippuran clearance. This is further supported by sequential scanning that shows diminished uptake in the early phase, with delay in the intrarenal transport and evacuation of the radio-Hippuran. Another advantage to the use of ¹³¹I Hippuran is the ability to detect posttransplant urinary extravasation and to evaluate urinary tract patency. This information can be similarly obtained with ⁹⁹ᵐTc Sn-DTPA.

To demonstrate patency of the arterial tree and evaluate renal perfusion, sequential scintiphotography is performed immediately following the intravenous injection of ^{99m}Tc pertechnetate, ^{99m}Tc DTPA, or ^{99m}Tc DMSA (Fig. 25-10). Information obtained from scans performed later depends on the radiopharmaceutical used. With rejection, the transplant appears enlarged as a result of edema. An area of diminished or absent uptake can be explained by infarction. Multiple small defects and diminished radioactivity uptake are seen with advanced graft rejection and acute tubular necrosis.

BIBLIOGRAPHY

Arnold, R. W., Subramanian, G., McAfee, J. G., Blair, R. J., and Thomas, F. D.: Comparison of ^{99m}Tc complexes for renal imaging, J. Nucl. Med. **16:**357-367, 1975.

Assailly, J., Pavel, D. G., Bader, C., Chanard, J., Ryerson, T. W., Cotard, J., and Funk-Brentano, J.: Noninvasive experimental determination of the individual kidney filtration fraction by means of a dual tracer technique, J. Nucl. Med. **18:**684-691, 1977.

Blau, M., McAfee, J. G., Rohri, R. H., Synder, W. S., and Smith, E. M.: Summary of current radiation dose estimates to human from ^{197}Hg and ^{203}Hg labeled chlormerodrin, J. Nucl. Med. **16:**1095-1098, 1975.

Blaufox, M. D., Potchen, E. J., and Merrill, J. P.: Measurement of effective renal plasma flow in man by external counting methods, J. Nucl. Med. **8:**77-85, 1967.

Burke, G., and Halko, A.: Dynamic clinical studies with radioisotopes and the scintillation camera: sodium iodohippurate I^{131} renography employing electronic crystal splitting, Am. J. Roentgenol. Radium Ther. Nucl. Med. **100:**792-800, 1967.

Burke, G., Halko, A., and Coe, F. L.: Dynamic clinical studies with radioisotopes and the scintillation camera. I. Sodium iodohippurate I^{131} renography, J.A.M.A. **197:**15-24, 1966.

Cantalamessa, L., Giustina, G., and Valentini, F.: The renal accumulation test with ^{203}Hg neohydrin in the diagnosis of unilateral nephropathies, Minerva Nucl. **10:**447-451, 1966.

Cohen, M. B., Pearman, R. O., Mims, M. M., and Blahd, W.: Radioisotope photoscanning of the kidneys in urologic disease, J. Urol. **89:**360-365, 1963.

Dabaj, E., Menges, H., and Pritchard, W. H.: Determination of renal blood flow by single injection of hippuran-I^{131} in man, Am. Heart J. **71:**79-83, 1966.

Frankel, R. S., Richman, S. D., Levenson, S. M., and Jochnston, G. S.: Renal localisation of gallium-67 citrate, Radiology **114:**393-397, 1975.

Freeman, L. M., and Blaufox, M. D.: Radionuclide studies of the genitourinary system, New York, 1974-1975, Grune & Stratton, Inc.

Funk-Brentano, J. L., Lellouch, J., and Leski, M.: Nouvelle methode de mesure de la filtration glomerulaire sans prelevement d'urine. Mesure de la clearance du DTPA Lanthane-140 par enregistrement de la decroissance par detection externe, Rev. Fr. Etudes Clin. Biol. **12:**790-798, 1967.

Ganong, W. F.: Review of medical physiology, Los Altos, California, 1967, Lange Medical Publications.

George, E. A., Codd, J. E., Newton, W. T., Haibach, H., and Donati, R. M.: Comparative evaluation of renal transplant rejection with radioiodinated fibrinogen, ^{99m}Tc sulfur colloid and ^{67}Ga citrate, J. Nucl. Med. **17:**175-180, 1976.

Gott, F. S., Pritchard, W. H., Young, W. R., and MacIntyre, W. J.: Renal blood flow measurement from the disappearance of intravenously injected Hippuran ^{131}I, J. Nucl. Med. **3:**480-485, 1962.

Handmaker, H., Young, B. W., and Lowenstein, J. M.: Clinical experience with ^{99m}Tc-DMSA (dimercaptosuccinic acid), a new renal-imaging agent, J. Nucl. Med. **16:**28-32, 1975.

Johnson, D. E., Taplin, G. V., Dore, E. K., and Hayashi, J.: The radioisotope renocystogram, J. Nucl. Med. **2:**8-23, 1961.

Johnston, T. B., and Whillis, J.: Gray's anatomy, London, New York and Toronto, 1944, Longmans, Green & Co.

Koplowitz, J. M., Mitchell, J. F., and Blahd, W. H.: The radioisotope renogram. A comparison of qualitative and quantitative interpretation, J. A. M. A. **192:**1032-1034, 1965.

Kristiansen, J. H., Hammelloff, K. E., Fredridsen, P. B., and Svendsen, V.: The diagnosis of urinary extravasation using gamma camera scintigraphy, Scand. J. Urol. Nephrol. **11:**69-72, 1977.

Kumar, B., and Coleman, R. E.: Significance of delayed ^{67}Ga localization in the kidneys, J. Nucl. Med. **17:**872-875, 1976.

Maher, F. T.: Evaluation of renal and urinary tract

abnormalities noted on scintiscans. A retrospective study of 1711 radioisotope skeletal surveys performed in an 18-month period, Mayo Clin. Proc. **50:**370-378, 1975.

McAfee, J. G., and Wagner, H. N.: Visualization of renal parenchyma by scintiscanning with ²⁰³Hg Neohydrin, Radiology **75:**820-821, 1960.

Nielsen, S. P., Moller, M. L., and Trap-Jensen, J.: ⁹⁹ᵐTc-DTPA scintillation camera renography: a new method for estimation of single-kidney function, J. Nucl. Med. **18:**112-117, 1977.

Pedersen, F., and Poulsen, P. E.: Hippuran I¹³¹ renography and clearance measurements used for determination of the individual kidney function, J. Urol. **97:**180-183, 1967.

Philips, J. F., Neiman, H. L., and Brown, T. L.: Ultrasound diagnosis of post-transplant lymphocele, Am. J. Roentgenol. Radium Ther. Nucl. Med. **126:** 1194-1196, 1976.

Razzak, M. A.: Radionuclide evaluation of crossed renal ectopia, Strahlentherapie **147:**258-262, 1974.

Razzak, M. A., Botti, R. E., and MacIntyre, W. J.: Interrelationship between hydration, urine flow, renal blood flow and the radiohippuran renogram, J. Nucl. Med. **10:**672-675, 1969.

Razzak, M. A., Botti, R. E., and MacIntyre, W. J.: Analysis of radiohippuran renogram by subtraction of extrarenal radioactivity, J. Urol. **115:**494-496, 1976.

Razzak, M. A., Botti, R. E., MacIntyre, W. J., and Pritchard, W. H.: External monitoring of ¹³¹I-Hippuran disappearance as a measure for renal blood flow, Int. J. Appl. Radiat. Isot. **18:**825-828, 1967.

Razzak, M. A., Botti, R. E., MacIntyre, W. J., and Pritchard, W. H.: Determination of renal blood flow by external monitoring of radiohippuran disappearance, J. Urol. **100:**209-214, 1968.

Razzak, M. A., Botti, R. E., MacIntyre, W. J., and Pritchard, W. H.: Consecutive determination of cardiac output and renal blood flow by external

monitoring of radioactive isotopes, J. Nucl. Med. **11:**190-195, 1970.

Razzak, M. A., Hassaballa, A. M., and Naguib, M.: Estimation of renal blood flow in dogs by rate of disappearance of Hippuran I¹³¹ from the vascular system, J. Urol. **94:**475-478, 1965.

Reba, R. C., Wagner, H. N., and McAfee, J. G.: Measurement of Hg²⁰³ chlormerodrin accumulation by the kidneys for detection of unilateral renal disease, Radiology **79:**134-135, 1962.

Selkurt, E. E.: The renal circulation. In Hamilton, W., and Dow, P., editors: Handbook of physiology. Circulation, vol. II, Baltimore, 1965, The Williams & Wilkins Co.

Shames, D. M., and Korobkin, M.: A simple technique for measuring relative renal blood flow, J. Nucl. Med. **17:**876-879, 1976.

Sodee, B. D.: The screening of renal hypertension utilizing the mercury-197 chlormerodrin uptake study and scan, J. Urol. **94:**313-319, 1965.

Texter, J. H.: Scintigraphy in early diagnosis of urine leakage following renal transplantation, J. Urol. **116:**547-549, 1976.

Vieras, F., and Boyd, C. M.: Diagnostic value of renal imaging incidental to bone scintigraphy with ⁹⁹ᵐTc-phosphate compounds, J. Nucl. Med. **16:**1109-1114, 1975.

Wagoner, R. D., Tauxe, W. N., Maher, F. T., and Hunt, J. C.: Measurement of effective renal plasma flow with sodium iodohippurate I¹³¹. J. A. M. A. **187:**811-813, 1964.

Winston, M. A., Halpern, S. E., Weiss, E. R., Emdow, J. S., and Blahd, W. H.: A critical evaluation of ⁹⁹ᵐTc-Fe ascorbic acid complex as a renal scanning agent, J. Nucl. Med. **12:**171-175, 1971.

Woodruff, M. W., Kibler, R. S., Bender, M. A., and Blau, M.: Hg-203 Neohydrin photoscan as an adjuvant to diagnosis of renal disease, J. Urol. **89:**746-752, 1963.

26 Radiopharmaceutical tumor localization

Cancer has been found to be an extremely pleomorphic disease without a single characteristic that is common to all neoplastic processes. There are many sensitive imaging procedures that detect pathophysiologic change in the regions surrounding neoplasms, such as bone scanning with ^{99m}Tc phosphates and liver imaging with ^{99m}Tc colloids. However, the radiopharmaceuticals used to measure tumor concentration are dependent, for their increased concentration, on factors that differ between various cancers and that are frequently held in common with inflammatory disease states.

FACTORS INVOLVED IN TUMOR LOCALIZATION

Vascularity. In the brain the "blood-brain" barrier is the physiochemical phenomenon that allows only those nutrients needed by the brain cell to cross from the brain capillary into the cell space. In neoplastic change, this regulatory mechanism is lost and any chemical crosses into the cell to be held by the cell or in the false extracellular space created. Thus many radiopharmaceuticals have been found efficacious for brain tumor localization.

Neovascularity. After tissue injury the body responds by forming new capillaries that are advanced into the region of imaging. These new capillaries are like systemic capillaries and will allow the protein-bound or nonprotein-bound radiopharmaceutical to "leak" into the region of injury. Thus nonspecific injury (infection, infarction) as well as tumor regions will be visualized by imaging procedures.

Increased metabolic rate. Some tumors have an increased metabolic rate and increased DNA formation. These tumors will usually have an increase in blood flow (perfusion). Thus these tumors have been more successfully imaged by protein precursors (Se 75 methionine) and blood protein-carried radiopharmaceuticals (^{197}Hg Cl, ^{197}Hg chlormerodrin, ^{67}Ga citrate).

Immune factor. The immune mechanism of the body does respond to cancer; therefore, radionuclide labeling of specific tumor antibodies has been shown to be successful in imaging tumors. These studies are in the clinical experimental state at the present time.

GALLIUM 67 IN TUMOR LOCALIZATION

In today's practice, ^{67}Ga citrate is the primary "tumor localizing" radiopharmaceutical. ^{67}Ga is carried in the blood stream by the plasma transferrin and has

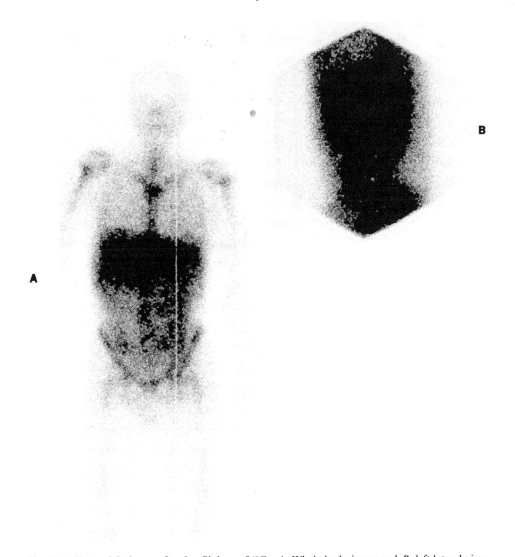

Fig. 26-1. Forty-eight hours after 5-mCi dose of ^{67}Ga. **A,** Whole-body image and, **B,** left lateral view. Patient developed a fever of unknown origin with elevated white blood count 10 days after partial gastrectomy. The ^{67}Ga images are abnormal, revealing an abscess in the mid infradiaphragmatic region posterior to the left lobe of the liver.

been found to be concentrated by the lysosomes of cells. Specifically why the lysosomes of tumors have an avidity for gallium is still being studied. White blood cells have a high concentration of lysosomes, and this partially explains why gallium is also concentrated in and around regions of inflammation and abscess formation.

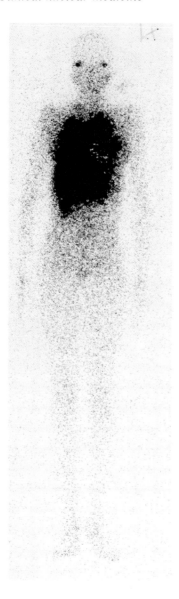

Fig. 26-2. Ninety-six hours after 5-mCi dose of ^{67}Ga. Young female patient with fever and an abnormal chest x ray. ^{67}Ga images are abnormal and reveal marked concentration of nuclide in the perihilar and lung regions, in the liver, and in the region of the lacrimal glands in this patient with sarcoidosis, a benign granulomatous disease process.

^{67}Ga whole-body imaging has been particularly useful in staging patients with Hodgkin's disease, non-Hodgkin's lymphoma, and bronchogenic carcinoma. Abscesses, osteomyelitis, and acute tissue inflammatory conditions are a few of the nonmalignant disease states localized by ^{67}Ga whole-body imaging.

It should be stressed that ^{67}Ga localization is nonspecific and that malignant and nonmalignant disease may be found in the same patient. Finally, histologically similar malignant lesions may have markedly different ^{67}Ga concentrations without obvious reasons.

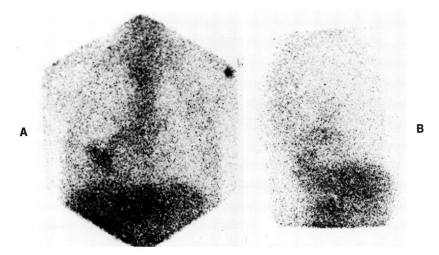

Fig. 26-3. Forty-eight hours after 5-mCi dose of ⁶⁷Ga. **A,** Anterior view and, **B,** right lateral view (sitting). Abnormal ⁶⁷Ga images of the thorax; 5 × 3 cm concentration of nuclide in right lower lobe and linear extension to the right hilum in a bronchogenic carcinoma with right perihilar metastatic disease.

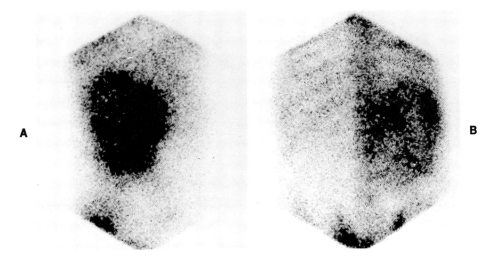

Fig. 26-4. Forty-eight hours after 3-mCi dose of ⁶⁷Ga. **A,** Anterior and, **B,** posterior abdominal images in a patient who had undergone right nephrectomy 2 years prior to study. ⁹⁹ᵐTc sulfur colloid images revealed compression of the liver anteriorly by a posterior mass lesion. Gallium images reveal uneven increased concentration of gallium in a 20 × 30 cm residual mass of renal cell carcinoma. Areas of decreased concentration approximate areas of tumor necrosis.

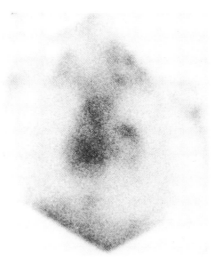

Fig. 26-5. Seventy-two hours after 9-mCi dose of [67]Ga. Abnormal ^{67}Ga concentration in cervical, supraclavicular, mediastinal, and perihilar lymph nodes in Hodgkin's disease.

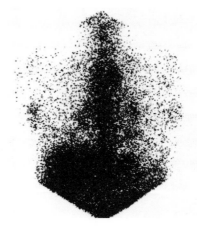

Fig. 26-6. Forty-eight hours after 5-mCi dose of [67]Ga. Abnormal ^{67}Ga concentration in axillary and perihilar nodes in a patient with lymphoma.

SUMMARY

There are several mechanisms that form the basis for tumor localization, which include abnormal capillary and cell permeability and enhanced metabolic incorporation of "tumor-localizing" radiopharmaceuticals into tumors. The tumor-localizing radiopharmaceutical sensitivity is excellent in some tumor systems, but their nonspecificity demands close correlation with the patient's clinical signs and symptoms, as well as with all other related diagnostic studies.

BIBLIOGRAPHY

Asckar, F.: Practical nuclear medicine, New York, 1974, Medcom Press.

Cross, M., and others: New techniques in tumor localization and radioimmunoassay, New York, 1974, John Wiley & Sons, Inc.

Greenlaw, R. H., and others: ^{67}Ga-citrate imaging in untreated malignant lymphoma: preliminary report of cooperative group, J. Nucl. Med. **15:**404-407, 1974.

Johnson, G., and Jones, A.: Atlas of gallium 67 scintigraphy, New York, 1973, Plenum Publishing Corporation.

Johnson, G. S., and others: The gallium-67 scan in clinical assessment of cancer, J. Surg. Oncol. **5:** 529-538, 1973.

Johnston, G., and others: ^{67}Ga-citrate imaging in untreated Hodgkin's disease: preliminary report of cooperative group, J. Nucl. Med. **15:**399-403, 1974.

Sauerbrunn, B. J. L., and others: Ga-67 citrate imaging in tumors of the genito-urinary tract: report of cooperative study, J. Nucl. Med. **19:**470-475, 1978.

Subramanian, G., and others, editors: Radiopharmaceuticals, New York, 1975, The Society of Nuclear Medicine.

Tsan, M.: Studies on gallium accumulation in inflammatory lesions. III. Roles of polymorphonuclear leukocytes and bacteria, J. Nucl. Med. **19:**492-495, 1978.

27 Technetium 99m biorouting

William Miller, B.S.

Nuclear medicine testing in most instances involves the internal administration of radioactive substances to the patient. Once administered, the radioactive substance is distributed within the body according to its physical-chemical properties. This distribution can be defined simply as the *biorouting* of the administered substance.

To gain information useful in diagnosing disease there must be a clear understanding of the normal biorouting of a radiosubstance. It is the observation of a body's irregular handling of this agent that enables the physician to suggest the presence of disease. Furthermore, if certain patterns are noted in the abnormal biorouting and the patient's history and other clinical findings are correlated, invaluable assistance may be rendered in establishing the exact nature of the disorder.

The purpose of this chapter is to introduce the student to a variety of radioagents containing technetium 99m. Chemical, physical, and physiologic factors that govern their biorouting will be discussed. Finally, the individual compounds will be discussed and their normal biorouting described.

RADIOPHARMACEUTICALS

Radiopharmaceuticals can be defined as atoms or molecules consisting of or containing as part of their structure radioactive atoms. These substances have been processed in such a manner so as to ensure safe use in humans. In the preparation of these radiopharmaceuticals due consideration must be given to sterility, pyrogenicity, toxicity, and the presence of contaminants, both stable and radiochemical. In addition, consideration must be given to problems specific to certain radiopharmaceuticals. Particulate sizing, colloid stability, and presence or absence of carrier are but a few. Last, clinical usefulness demands that radiopharmaceuticals be prepared and packaged in such a fashion that they are not unwieldy to use.

PERTECHNETATE

Sodium pertechnetate ($Na^{99m}TcO_4$), procured either prepackaged or from a $^{99}Mo/^{99m}Tc$ generator system, is chemically a salt. When this salt is placed in water, a solution is formed in which two ions are produced.

$$Na^{99m}TcO_4 \rightarrow Na^+ \text{ and } ^{99m}TcO_4^-$$

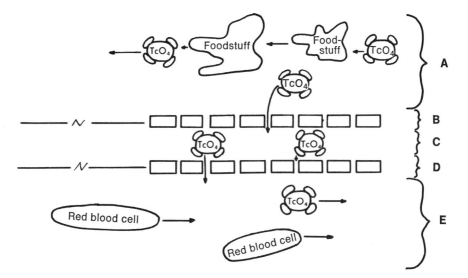

Fig. 27-1. *A* represents the gut contents compartment. *B* represents the layer of cells in intimate contact with the gut contents. *C* represents the interstitial spaces separated from the gut contents by layer *B*. *D* represents the single layer of endothelial cells that line the intrinsic walls and are common to the entire vascular compartment. *E* represents the vascular compartment or the compartment in which the formed elements of the bloodstream are confined.

The sodium cations present are required only for electrical neutrality purposes. Any positive ion can serve the same role. When introduced into the body, the positive ion does not follow the biopathway of the negative ion.

The pertechnetate anion (TcO^-_4) may be administered either orally or intravenously. If given orally in solution form, the ion will quickly pass from the digestive tract to the bloodstream by simple diffusion. The diffusionary movement to the bloodstream requires only that the gut content concentration be higher than that of the bloodstream.

Movement from the gut contents to the bloodstream requires passage through several layers separating the various fluid compartments of the body. To illustrate this movement, a simple schematic diagram is provided showing the structures involved in the passage of materials from the gut contents to the capillary vessel serving that tissue part (Fig. 27-1).

The passage from the gut contents *(A)* through the cell layer *(B)* can be by one of two processes: simple diffusion or passive transport, in which the substance in question flows between the cells of the layer, or a process of active transport in which the substance passes into the cells of layer *B* and is discharged into compartment *C*. Substances arriving in the interstitial fluids *(C)* can then move through the endothelial layer *(D)*, which is the capillary membrane, by similar processes to become bloodborne in compartment *E*.

The passage of pertechnetate ion from gut contents to blood is by simple diffusion. Its absorption begins in the stomach and is essentially completed early in its passage through the small intestine. Gut contents at the time of oral administration govern the rate of absorption to the bloodstream. A normal fasting patient will achieve maximum blood levels within 30 minutes after oral dosing.

Because of uncertain absorption rates and the resulting variation in blood levels among patients, the intravenous administration of pertechnetate is the method of choice. In this way 100% of the dose is bloodborne immediately. This choice of route also allows for the observation of the initial vascular distribution of the agent seconds after administration and forms the basis for the new common flow studies.

If blood samples were collected from a patient every minute for several hours after dosing and the samples counted in a well counter, there would be a fall in activity per sample not explained by decay. By plotting activity per sample versus time, one would achieve a multiphasic curve as illustrated in Fig. 27-2.

The overall loss of pertechnetate from the vascular compartment can be explained as the product of many physiologic factors acting independently but simultaneously, resulting in what is known as a disappearance curve. Each physiologic factor contributes to this vascular loss for a different reason and in a different way.

Immediately after injection, pertechnetate ions are partly bound to serum proteins. This binding is reversible but initially accounts for as much as 70% to 80% of the injected dose. Capillary membrane cells lining the vascular compartment are held together by a cellular "glue" that is somewhat porous.

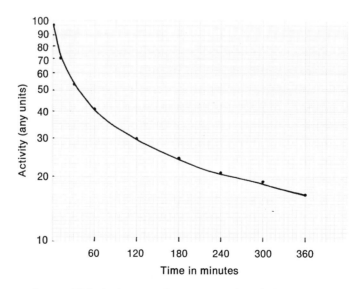

Fig. 27-2. Biologic clearance of pertechnetate from the bloodstream.

These pores readily allow by simple diffusion the passage of molecules whose molecular weights (mol wt) are less than 50,000 to 70,000. Molecules larger than these can pass, but it must be by active transport, a much slower process. Pertechnetate-binding serum proteins in general are of a high molecular weight. Because their weights exceed 70,000, they and the pertechnetate they carry are confined to circulate in the vascular compartment.

The unbound pertechnetate ions are small (165 mol wt). They are not confined to the vascular compartment but rapidly escape through the capillary membranes to the interstitial fluids.

At the same time that the free ions are leaving the vascular compartment, it follows that the concentration of these ions in this compartment is falling. As the free ion concentration falls, the protein-bound ion percentage in the vascular fluid is increasing. This is not to say that the total pertechnetate bound to protein is increasing but rather that the percentage of the total radioions present in the vascular compartment that are bound is increasing. This then requires a shift in the equilibrium of this situation favoring release of protein-bound pertechnetate. As these newly freed ions become available, they, too, can escape the vascular compartment into the interstitial fluid. Thus, there is a mechanism that will allow for complete escape from the vascular compartment of the pertechnetate ions injected. The rate of this escape is ultimately governed by the concentration of the radioion in the interstitial spaces.

Since the interstitial fluid volume is three to four times larger than the vascular volume, as much as 75% of the free ions leave the vascular compartment by simple diffusion. Equilibrium, or equal concentration of free ions in the vascular compartment and the interstitial fluids, is achieved in as short a time as 2 to 3 minutes. This, then, is the first factor in explaining the initial rapid loss of pertechnetate from the vascular compartment.

Pertechnetate ions arriving in the interstitial fluids can be removed from this fluid compartment in significant quantities by only a few organ systems: the stomach, thyroid, salivary glands, bowel (both small and large), to some extent sweat glands, mucous membrane tissue, choroid plexus of brain, and, last very important, kidney. All other organ systems essentially exclude pertechnetate from their intracellular fluids, including the brain. The organs just listed provide the second major reason for the loss of pertechnetate from the vascular compartment.

Stomach

The affinity of the stomach for pertechnetate is caused by its similarity to chloride. Both ions are negative one anions. The parietal acid-producing cells of the stomach produce carbon dioxide by normal metabolic pathways. This CO_2 is converted to carbonic acid by enzymatic activity. Following on p. 548 is a summary of reactions occurring in the stomach producing pertechnic acid.

$$CO_2 + H_2O \xrightarrow{\text{enzymes}} H_2CO_3$$

$$H_2CO_3 \xrightarrow{\text{dissociates}} H^+ + HCO_3^-$$

$$(H^+ + HCO_3^-) + (TcO_4^-) \xrightarrow{\text{exchange}} (H^+ + TcO_4^-) + (HCO_3^-)$$

$$H^+ + TcO_4^- \xrightarrow[\text{stomach contents as}]{\text{secreted to}} \text{pertechnic acid}$$

Carbonic acid is passed to ducts carrying these secretions to the stomach contents. Here the carbonic acid dissociates into hydrogen ions and bicarbonate. The bicarbonate exchanges with pertechnetate (both are negative one anions), with the former taking the place of the pertechnetate in the interstitial fluids of the stomach. The hydrogen along with pertechnetate is secreted into the stomach contents as pertechnic acid in the same fashion as is hydrochloric acid. Thus intravenously administered pertechnetate will accumulate quickly in the stomach wall and contents shortly after administration. Within 30 minutes after administration the stomach, because of its size, will yield the highest external counting rate. Pertechnetate so secreted into the stomach contents is readily reabsorbed, thus producing an internal cycle.

Salivary glands

Salivary gland accumulation again is produced by the similarity of pertechnetate ions to other anions of similar charge. Saliva is produced in large amounts and contains considerable salts, including negative anions. Pertechnetate escaping the vascular compartments to the salivary gland interstitial fluid will be taken up by these cells and secreted into the salivary ducts as a constituent of saliva. Although initially secreted saliva is isotonic to blood (and therefore contains an equal salt concentration to that of the plasma from which it arises), it paradoxically is rendered hypotonic by fluid-secreting cells lining the ducts carrying the saliva from the glands to the mouth. This would lead one to conclude that the overall concentration of pertechnetate in the gland is lower than that of the blood perfusing it. One might further conclude that the salivary glands should appear as an area of poor uptake on imaging rather than an area of increased uptake. This latter conclusion is false, however. If one considers the salivary glands as a four-compartment system (that is, vascular, interstitial, cellular, and secretion-collecting) and compares this to other tissues not exhibiting a secretory function such as muscle, the reason the salivary glands reveal themselves as "hot" in an imaging procedure can be explained. Muscle tissue and its interstitial fluid surrounding the salivary glands can only achieve a concentration as high as the vascular supply servicing it. Salivary gland cells, on the other hand, permit the entry of pertechnetate anions and in doing so have a concentration as high as the blood and interstitial fluid supply in their vicinity. This anion is then secreted into ducts leaving the salivary gland cells. The fluid in the duct also has a concentration of the anion as high as cells from which it arose. In a gram of salivary tissue, therefore, there are four fluid compartments all containing pertechnetate, whereas in a gram of muscle tissue only two compartments contain the anion. Thus the salivary glands are easily visualized in a sea of muscle.

Classically, the time of imaging is chosen when the target-to-nontarget ratio is the highest (hopefully). The accumulation of pertechnetate in the salivary glands appears to reach its maximum in less than 10 minutes after dosing. It is at this point that the highest target-to-nontarget ratio is achieved. To wait for vascular clearance is futile because there is an outflux from the gland of the radionuclide that follows the decrease in vascular pertechnetate. Thus, although the ratio remains the same, the count rate differential closes with time. In addition, there is a gradual loss of overall count rate caused by decay, which will ultimately result in a lengthened time required to perform the imaging procedure. This is a disadvantage in most cases.

Some clinicians prescribe atropine as an adjunct to salivary gland imaging. Atropine interferes with the discharge of saliva from the gland by blocking the nervous stimulation. Thus saliva formed within the gland is retained. This, according to some, should increase the target-to-nontarget ratio. However, the enrichment of salivary gland tissue with pertechnetate depends on the block of two avenues of escape. The release to the oral cavity of the saliva is successfully blocked by atropine, but "obstructed" pertechnetate will return to the vascular compartment by diffusion as the concentration in the blood falls. Atropine is not recommended by all. There may be another and more significant merit to the use of atropine in that the oral cavity contamination buildup of pertechnetate that may obscure the image is avoided.

Secreted saliva that finds its way to the oral cavity is swallowed passing to the stomach, providing the patient does not permit its loss. The pertechnetate is in effect recycled at this point. It might be pointed out that the unconscious patient may drool on the pillowslip or other bedding. This wetness will contain activity that can cause artifacts in subsequent imaging procedures.

Thyroid

An organ that has been successfully studied in so many ways with the iodine radionuclides can also be looked at in a much more limited fashion with the pertechnetate ion. The avidity of the thyroid for iodide ions is well known. Iodide is trapped, oxidized, converted to the positive ionic species, and coupled to the organic molecule thyronine to produce thyroid hormone. Only the first step in this sequence can be duplicated with pertechnetate.

Pertechnetate ions are rapidly trapped on arrival at the surface of the acinar cells of the thyroid. This trapping is against a concentration gradient and therefore is a form of active transport. The end result is that the gland will have a higher concentration of pertechnetate than the blood supply servicing the organ.

The mechanism of the trap for iodide is not clear, much less the mechanism for the entrapment of pertechnetate. A reasonable hypothesis has been proposed that in two ways supports an explanation for the similarity of the trap between the two ions. First, the iodide ion has a negative one charge. So does the pertechnetate ion. This is apparently partly responsible for the failure of the thyroid to distinguish between the two ions. In addition, other negative one anions are also trapped (for example, perchlorate, ClO_4^-, and iodate, IO_3^-). The whole story does not stop here, however, because there are some negative one ions that are not so avidly accumulated, such as fluoride (F^-) or chloride (Cl^-). A review of an $^{18}F^-$ bone scan will fail to reveal the high degree of thyroid uptake normally seen in an iodide or pertechnetate scan.

In an attempt to clarify the picture, the second part of the hypothesis takes into consideration the molecular weight of the ions exhibiting a negative one charge. In examining the list of these ions one finds that among the halogens only iodide (I^-) and astatine* (At^-) are significantly trapped. In addition, certain combinations of atoms with overall negative one charges are also trapped, including perchlorate (ClO_4^-), iodate (IO_3^-), and pertechnetate (TcO_4^-). Those halogens that are trapped and the combination ions just listed have two properties in common. All are negative one anions, and each has an ionic weight of about 100 or more. It is interesting to note that halogen ions (F^-, Cl^-, Br^-) and combination ions (NO_3^-, HCO_3^-) with weights less than 100 are not significantly trapped.

It appears therefore that at least two conditions must be met before the thyroid will take up a substance: negative one charge and ionic weight of more than 100. Obviously many other molecules also fill these qualifications; therefore, other properties probably should be considered such as molecular configuration and ionic volume.

After trapping, the second step in the iodide conversion to the hormonal state requires its oxidation to I^0. This involves the removal of an electron, that is, $I^- \rightarrow I^0 + 1$ electron. At this point in biorouting, iodide and pertechnetate (along with other oxygen-carrying trap competitors) enter dissimilar pathways. Iodide can be oxidized. Pertechnetate, perchlorate, and others cannot. Thus pertechnetate is accumulated by the thyroid but cannot be further processed. It is instead released from the gland as the pertechnetate (TcO_4^-) ion.

After an intravenous injection of pertechnetate the vascular levels fall rapidly, during which time the thyroid accumulates a portion of the radionuclide. The high efficiency of the trap mechanism yields a thyroid concentration that rises normally to a level approximately ten times that of the surrounding vasculature. Since the gland is not able to organify the pertechnetate, the trapped ion escapes and diffuses back to the bloodstream. The ten-to-one ratio is maintained for some time as blood levels fall, with thyroid activity falling proportionately.

---

*Astatine is the heaviest of the Group VII elements. It exhibits properties similar to those of others in this group. Its atomic number is 85, and its average weight is 210. All known forms are radioactive.

Normally accumulation of pertechnetate in the gland is positive throughout the first 10 to 15 minutes after dosing even though blood levels are falling rapidly. It should be remembered that the reason the blood levels are falling is because organs such as the thyroid are taking it up. These levels plateau for the next 30 to 45 minutes, during which time blood levels continue to fall, that is, the percentage of the administered dose in the gland remains relatively stable. After 1 hour or so the maximum thyroid-to-blood ratio has been achieved, and a further drop in blood activity results in a proportionate drop in thyroid activity. Total clearance of pertechnetate follows total clearance of the ion from the vascular compartment. Fig. 27-3 may be helpful in clarifying what is happening in the thyroid during the first few hours after dosing.

The optimum time for imaging, then, is sometime after 30 to 40 minutes following dosing. To wait longer would serve no purpose because the best target-to-nontarget ratio has already been reached by this time. Further delay would only result in loss of count rate as a result of decay and biologic clearance.

Small and large bowel

Twenty-four hours after dosing, the organ system exhibiting the highest concentration of pertechnetate is the large bowel. To follow the biorouting of pertechnetate an understanding of the secretory and absorption function of the bowel in this regard is necessary.

Pertechnetate is found in the stomach contents after either its oral or intrave-

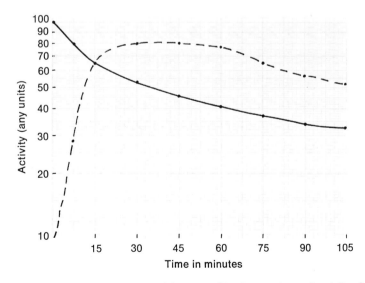

Fig. 27-3. Comparison of thyroid (- - · - -) activity versus bloodstream (———) activity after the intravenous injection of pertechnetate. Maximum target-to-nontarget ratios are obtained between 30 to 60 minutes after injection of the dose.

nous injection. The reader is requested to review the role of the stomach in the secretion of pertechnetate from the vascular volume to the stomach contents.

Pertechnetate in the stomach and the upper reaches of the small bowel will be absorbed by diffusion only so long as blood levels are lower. When blood levels reach a concentration equal to that of the bowel contents, the absorption of pertechnetate ceases. Because vascular-bound pertechnetate is removed by other organs handling anions, it would appear that absorption would continue indefinitely, cycling back through the stomach as acid and from swallowed saliva. The gut content, however, becomes more and more dilute as it passes from the proximal to the distal small bowel because the secretion of fluids exceeds the absorbed volume. Thus pertechnetate becomes less likely to be absorbed by the diffusion process the longer it remains in the gut content because it is being diluted by the secreted hypotonic fluids.

The ever-more-dilute phenomenon ceases with passage to the large bowel. At this point the very liquid chyme begins a process of drying out until by the time the material reaches the descending colon it has attained the semisolid consistency of feces. During this process most of the water and salts to be conserved by the body are being reabsorbed. At the same time some pertechnetate is included in those salts that are reabsorbed. As the chyme becomes a solid, however, the remaining pertechnetate is trapped and eventually retained for passage in the stools. This pertechnetate remaining in the fecal mass is partly responsible for the large bowel activity observed on abdominal images acquired many hours after dosing.

A second explanation for the activity remaining in bowel, not as part of its contents but rather as part of the gut wall, rests in the active absorption and secretion processes. The active transport of salts in the gut is well recognized. Water carrying many mineral ions is secreted and absorbed by this process. No doubt pertechnetate is also handled in this fashion. Since active transport requires the attachment of the absorbed substance to an intracellular carrier that will transport the substance from the cell membrane facing one compartment through the cell cytoplasm to the membrane facing the appropriate compartments for release, it allows for a higher cellular concentration than is present in the surrounding fluids. The intestinal mucosa, one of the cellular compartments permitting the entry of pertechnetate, thus retains a portion of the activity when the blood levels have fallen. For this reason, cleaning of the bowel prior to abdominal imaging is not a totally satisfactory method of removing all bowel activity.

Since so much of the administered pertechnetate is involved with the gastrointestinal tract, it is not surprising to note the high degree of excretion by the fecal route. Estimations have shown that about 30% to 40% of an administered dose of pertechnetate will be passed in the stools in the first 48 to 72 hours after dosing. Trace amounts totaling an additional 5% to 10% are added in the succeeding 2 weeks; however, physical decay of technetium 99m does not allow detection after the initial 72 hours.

Choroid plexus

The choroid plexus is composed of a layer of cells found on the interior surfaces of the ventricles of the brain. The function of these cells is to produce the cerebrospinal fluid (CSF) by extracting the required materials from the vascular compartment and secreting it into the CSF spaces. This fluid then bathes the brain tissue and serves among other purposes as a protective layer between the brain substance and the skull.

The CSF is continuously produced by the choroid but is not absorbed by the same tissue. Instead it flows throughout the many channels of the brain and finally reaches the arachnoidal granulations over the cerebrum where the fluid empties into the venous sinuses.

The composition of the CSF is similar to that of plasma. It contains among others electrolytes and certain protein materials but no formed elements. The mechanics of the production of CSF by the choroid layer is thought to be primarily one of exuding fluid from the vascular arteriole capillary of the choroid to the CSF space. This should mean that the plasma and CSF composition is the same with regard to electrolytes. It has been found, however, that this is not the case. Pertechnetate will be caught in the choroid cells but not be transferred to the CSF. This apparent filtering of pertechnetate ions by the choroid cells may be responsible for the increased activity seen in this area during imaging. Clearance of pertechnetate from the choroid requires a drop in blood concentration of the ion whereby it will wash out by a diffusionary process. In any event the accumulation of the radioion above that of the surrounding tissue is reached shortly after dosing and the ratio remains in favor of choroid throughout the succeeding hours as vascular levels fall.

Although the uptake of pertechnetate by the choroid plexus of the brain is an extremely small fraction of the administered dose, the presence of this minute amount has caused great concern among clinicians interpreting brain images. The problem is compounded by the fact that the uptake is variable between patients. In some patients the choroid plexus visualizes, whereas in equal numbers the area does not visualize.

So bothersome is this accumulation of pertechnetate that a great deal of effort has been spent toward the development of blocking agents that would prevent this uptake. To date two agents have found their way into common usage as an adjunct to pertechnetate brain imaging.

Lugol's solution, a combination of elemental iodine and potassium iodide, has been used with very limited success. Orally administered, Lugol's solution prevents accumulation of pertechnetate in the choroid plexus apparently by a flooding mechanism whereby stable iodide ions simply dilute the pool of negative one ions available for uptake by this tissue. Unfortunately, clinical use resulted in successful blockage of perhaps only half of those whose choroid would have visualized without the solution. To compound the problems with use of Lugol's solution, the agent has a bad taste, has to be administered sometime prior to the injection of pertechnetate, and cannot be given to those patients sensitive to iodine or who are unable to take medications orally.

The use of Lugol's solution has given way to potassium perchlorate. This agent administered orally in doses of 200 to 1,000 mg has been shown to be more effective but still does not result in a 100% block of all choroid plexus uptakes. On the negative side, perchlorate must be administered orally before pertechnetate dosing, is barely soluble in water (about 7 mg/ml at 20°C), and is contraindicated in patients with gastric or duodenal disorders.

The solution to the choroid uptake problem lies with the introduction of chelated forms of technetium. In this chemical form the agent no longer accumulates in the choroid plexus because its negative one charge is altered. The chelated forms of technetium will be discussed on p. 562.

Brain

In a discussion of biorouting of pertechnetate the omission of a section on the brain would be a major oversight because of the very prevalent practice of using this agent for brain imaging purposes. The fact is that brain tissue, with the exception of the choroid plexus, has no effect on the biodistribution of the pertechnetate ion. Indeed brain tissue substance for the most part rejects the entry of the pertechnetate ion into its intracellular compartment.

The unique structural arrangement of brain tissue provides a compact assembly of cells with little if any interstitial space. This clustered arrangement, together with capillaries that have far less permeability than capillaries elsewhere in the body, produces a barrier between the vascular compartment and the brain intracellular compartment commonly referred to as the *blood-brain barrier.*

Since the blood-brain barrier rejects the entry of pertechnetate into the brain substance, in the normal patient an image of the brain will reveal only the vascular structures. A disruption of the barrier from nearly any cause will allow for infiltration by diffusion of the pertechnetate ion from the high concentration in the vascular compartment to the abnormal areas not protected by the "barrier." Thus immediately after injection and mixing, all vascular compartment fluids should have the same concentration. Any area exhibiting a high vascular content, such as the heart, placenta, nasal sinuses, or venous sinuses of brain, will be revealed as an area of increased activity over the surrounding tissue. Hypervascular lesions of the brain are often visualized seconds to minutes after injection.

Other lesions not well perfused or where perfusion is absent will accumulate pertechnetate by a slower process, requiring in some cases hours. When blood levels fall, the activity in the lesion remains for some time, producing a favorable target-to-nontarget ratio.

Clearance of pertechnetate from the brain directly follows vascular clearance. Clearance from abnormal areas follows vascular clearance but at a reduced rate.

Sweat glands

The sweat glands are an organ system that can influence the biorouting of pertechnetate. A brief discussion on the mechanics of skin water loss is necessary to understand how the sweat glands can participate in this role.

Water is lost from the body through the skin by two methods: insensible and sensible perspiration. The former involves mere evaporation. Sensible perspiration, on the other hand, requires secretion of fluid by the sweat glands through ducts to the surface of the body. Perspiration contains essentially the same electrolytes as are found in the balance of the body's extracellular fluid. Since salts are part of the sweat, pertechnetate will be included in the materials that are secreted to the surface of the skin.

If active perspiration is not underway, the amount of pertechnetate lost in this fashion is negligible. If, however, a patient is actively sweating a normal composition fluid, he can lose a fraction of an administered dose in this manner. The total amount lost in the perspiration depends to a great degree on the electrolyte composition of the extracellular fluid and the amount of sweat being secreted. Therefore, skin deposition as a transferable liquid or as a removable dry salt will vary greatly among patients.

When sodium ^{131}I iodide, a similarly biorouted radionuclide, is administered in therapeutic amounts, linen contamination by perspiration is a factor that must be dealt with. This contamination resulted in procedures for monitoring bed garments, pillowslips, and so on and possible storage for decay of these articles prior to laundering. Although pertechnetate given in equal activities to ^{131}I is just as likely to contaminate bedding, equal concern has not been thought warranted, probably because of its shorter half-life. The fact remains that ^{99m}Tc can be lost in the perspiration. Technologists handling patients and their bedding do acumulate activity on their fingers. This activity can easily be transferred to glassware and test tubes. An exterior surface-contaminated test tube in a low counting Schilling procedure can add significantly to the urine count, producing a false-negative result. Some care should be exercised to avoid these types of pitfalls.

Kidney

The role of the kidney in biorouting of the pertechnetate ion cannot be underestimated. The kidney plays the most significant role in the removal of vascular-bound pertechnetate because the ions it removes are not made available again to the vascular compartment. This is not the case with the two or three other systems that influence vascular pertechnetate, the stomach, thyroid, and salivary glands.

Blood arriving at the kidney passes through the renal artery of the afferent arteriole. The afferent arteriole enters the glomerulus, which is composed of about 50 parallel capillaries encased in a structure known as Bowman's capsule. During this passage through the glomerulus, the blood is reduced in volume by about 10%.

This reduction is at the expense of the liquid fraction of the blood and not the formed elements. Included in this fraction, which is now known as the glomerular filtrate, is a wide variety of dissolved salts, glucose, amino acids, and fats and a limited amount of some small proteins. Dissolved substances that are vascular bound and larger than 50,000 to 70,000 molecular weight cannot be filtered and exit the glomerulus by means of an outbound vessel known as the *efferent arteriole*. Of course, all undissolved substances are much too large to be filtered and therefore remain vascular. In addition, a very large number of soluble protein molecules and substances that are complexed to protein molecules and whose aggregate molecular weight exceeds 70,000 are also confined to the vascular compartment. The biorouting of pertechnetate is greatly influenced by these parameters.

After arrival in the bloodstream, pertechnetate is in significant quantity bound to plasma proteins. These bound ions enter the glomerulus and exit by the efferent arterioles to the peritubular vessels that finally coalesce to form the renal vein.

The free pertechnetate ions that enter the glomerulus are filtered and pass into the tubules that eventually condense to form the ureter. Once in the ureter these ions are for all practical purposes lost to the body although they will be temporarily stored in the bladder before being discharged in the urine. The blood leaving by the renal vein will have a pertechnetate bound-to-free ratio greater than that on entry through the renal artery. This cannot remain, because, when there is an excess bound pertechnetate in the blood, a portion will disassociate to become free. There is then a reestablishment of the same bound-to-free ration that existed at the time the blood entered the renal artery. The only difference is that the total pertechnetate entering the kidney is reduced by 10% on its exit because of that lost to the glomerular filtrate.

Considering that 25% of the cardiac output flows through the kidneys and that 10% of the blood is cleared to pertechnetate by glomerular filtration, a bit of mathematical liberty will produce a half-time clearance of the entire bloodstream in about 30 minutes. This is, of course, after the initial loss during the first hour in which equilibrium with the extracellular compartment is reached. In addition, the other organs removing pertechnetate from the vascular compartment will also have reached their peak concentration and will be taking up the ion at the same rate they are discharging it.

The 30-minute half-time clearance just calculated in no way agrees with the actual measured vascular clearance half-time. Commencing at 1 hour after dose, biologic half-times on the order of 2 to 3 hours would be much more realistic. A better explanation than just glomerular filtration as the mechanism for vascular clearance is in order.

The answer apparently lies in the reabsorption phenomena that occurs between the kidney tubule fluid and the efferent arteriole and peritubular capillary fluids. The normal function of the kidney includes the salvaging of 99% of the fluid filtered by the glomerulus. To do this, substances to be conserved must either diffuse from the tubules to the bloodstream or be actively reabsorbed by the tubule cells. Unwanted substances pass on to form the urine.

Pertechnetate ions that are filtered from the plasma by the glomerulus are present in the filtrate in the same concentration as the plasma from which it came. Because the fluid leaving the glomerulus by the efferent arteriole is reduced in volume, the bound-to-free ion ratio is upset, but the remaining free ion concentration is to this point the same as that in the glomerular filtrate. As the vascular fluid moves through the efferent arteriole to the peritubular capillaries, the volume is increased by the reabsorption process. This process probably does not include the active transport of pertechnetate, but this is conjecture. In any event, as the vascular volume increases, the concentration of free pertechnetate falls. At the same time the tubular volume (which is going on to become the urine) is decreasing. The pertechnetate concentration in the tubules is therefore increasing. Now, because the tubular fluid pertechnetate concentration exceeds the vascular pertechnetate concentration, diffusion of the radioion begins its trek across the tubule membrane to the fascular compartment. Thus the pertechnetate is conserved, and the longer blood half-time disappearance is reasonable.

Fifty percent of an administered dose of sodium pertechnetate will be removed from the body by the urinary tract in the first 24 hours. The temporary storage of this ion in the bladder cannot be overlooked when this organ becomes part of a pelvic or lower abdominal view. A thyroid uptake with pertechnetate always requires a blood background to be subtracted from the neck count. The thigh is often chosen, and care must be exercised not to include the bladder in the field of view.

By using long-lived ^{95}Tc pertechnetate it has been shown that 100% of a dose will be excreted within 2 weeks. The urinary route accounted for half and the fecal route a bit less than half. Traces were lost through perspiration and skin sloughing.

TECHNETIUM SULFUR COLLOID

Sodium thiosulfate, when boiled in the presence of acid, will precipitate colloidal sulfur. The reaction is as follows:

$$8Na_2S_2O_3 + H^+ \xrightarrow[\text{heat}]{} 8Na_2SO_3 + S_8 \downarrow + H^+$$

When sodium pertechnetate is included in the reaction, the technetium combines with sulfur as follows:

$$2TcO_4^- + 7S + 16H^+ \rightarrow Tc_2S_7 + 8H_2O$$

Since the pertechnetate used in the reaction is carrier-free, the amount of technetium sulfide produced is insufficient to produce even one particle. The latter reaction therefore is assumed, but support is given from studies using rhenium, an element similar to technetium, in which Re_2S_7 was formed.

Since the technetium sulfide is produced in the presence of precipitating elemental sulfur, it has been proposed that the tracer is incorporated as a part of the colloidal sulfur particle. Properly synthesized, the reaction will allow incorporation of more than 95% of the technetium in the particulate structure and less than 5% remaining as free pertechnetate.

Technetium sulfur colloid is commercially available as the prepackaged agent, or it may be synthesized on site using kits containing all the ingredients except the pertechnetate. The procedure involves mixing pertechnetate, the thiosulfate, and an acid in a vial. The vial is then heated in a boiling water bath for about 10 minutes. After cooling, a buffer is added to bring the solution to a pH suitable for injection.

An important material present in all sulfur colloid preparations is gelatin. The purpose of this agent is to stabilize the colloidal particles formed. The gelatin coats the particles and since the substance absorbs water on its surface, the individual particles are kept separate by layers of water. It is important to note that the more gelatin used, the smaller the mean particle size. This can have some influence on the biorouting of the colloid.

Technetium sulfur colloid preparations contain particles whose diameters range in size from as low as 0.1 m μ to as large as 1 μ. The amount of gelatin used, the heating time, and the presence of contaminants such as aluminum cations (possibly from the generator column) will affect the particle size distribution. Compared to colloidal gold, the agent formerly used because of its colloidal properties, the size range of sulfur colloid is wide, that is, 0.1 m μ to 1 μ for sulfur colloid versus 3 to 20 m μ for gold. This difference has resulted in a significantly altered biodistribution with the technetium compound versus that of gold colloid. Variations in the particle size range between sulfur colloid preparations will also affect its biorouting after administration.

Technetium sulfur colloid injected into the vascular compartment will be confined to this volume because of its size. The colloidal particles, although smaller than some formed blood elements such as red cells, are much larger than any molecule able to escape the vascular compartment. The colloid particles as foreign bodies will be removed from the vascular compartments by the organ systems housing the protective cells of the reticuloendothelial system (RES). The RES system is composed primarily of the Kupffer cells lining the sinousoids of the liver (75% to 80%) and found to a lesser extent in the spleen, with the remainder mostly in the bone marrow. The exact mechanism whereby the liver removes colloid particles from the vascular compartment has been assumed to the phagocytosis by the Kupffer cells. This concept has been challenged recently in comparative autoradiographic studies done in animals between the clearance of gold colloid and technetium sulfur colloid. The gold was shown to be incorporated into the Kupffer cells, whereas the sulfur colloid particle was not. Other factors appear to be involved. In any event the circulating technetium sulfur colloid will be cleared to organ systems housing RES cells. Whether the RES cells are the only cells responsible for this clearance will have to be settled by further investigation.

The clearance of technetium sulfur colloid is very rapid with a half-time on the order of 2 to 5 minutes. Maximum organ concentrations will be achieved in about 10 minutes, at which time circulating radiocolloid will be reduced to zero.

The entire RES cannot be looked on as being equally efficient in the removal of foreign particles from the bloodstream. The spleen, for example, tends to favor the accumulation of the larger particles. This is not to say that the spleen is unable to remove small particles but rather that it is more efficient at removing large particles. The marrow, on the other hand, favors removal of small particles. There is some difference in the normal distribution of the particles after the colloid has been cleared from the bloodstream, depending on the particle size distribution. The particle size distribution can be altered by several preparation variables as already mentioned. Fig. 27-4 may assist in this concept.

If the mean particle size is reduced, the uptake to spleen will be less, and more will go to the marrow. If the mean size is increased, the uptake to spleen will be increased. If the particles are too large ($>1.0\ \mu$), the agent will be trapped in the lung capillaries on its first transit from the heart. It is worthy to note that normal-

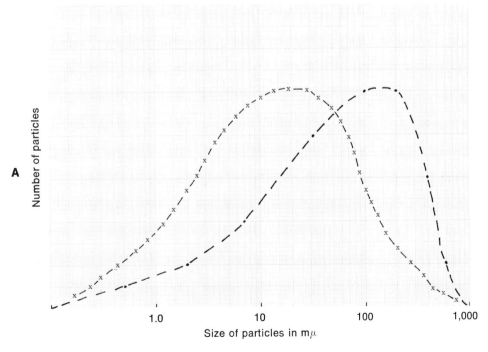

Fig. 27-4. A, Effects of heating and the amount of gelatin present on the size of the technetium sulfur colloid particle formed. - · - - -, Average heating with optimum gelatin produces a particle size distribution with a mean of 100 to 200 mμ. - x - x - x, Prolonged heating or added gelatin or both produce a particle size distribution with a mean of 10 to 30 mμ.   *Continued.*

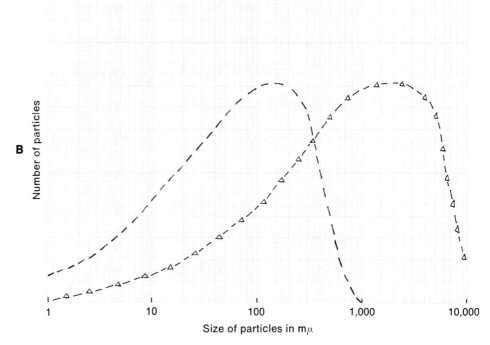

Fig. 27-4, cont'd. B, Effects of aluminum contaminant on the size of the technetium sulfur colloid particles formed. - - - -, Sulfur colloid preparations with minimal or no aluminum contaminant produce particle size distributions with a mean of 100 to 200 mμ. - - $\triangle$ - $\triangle$, Sulfur colloid preparations with an excess aluminum contamination produce a particle size distribution with a mean size greater than 1,000 mμ. Settling of the undisturbed preparation will be noted, and, if used, a large number of the particles will lodge in the lung.

size particles will often be seen in the lung field when liver disease or infection has caused an increase in circulatory macrophages. These bodies will engulf the particles and be retained in the lung bed because of increased size. For these reasons it is important that good quality control measures be instituted to ensure that a product of uniform size is produced batch after batch.

Distribution of technetium sulfur colloid is dependent on blood flow to RES organs and the functional ability of these organs to remove foreign particles. Any disease state that destroys or alters either blood flow or function will alter the distribution of the cleared colloid. If the disease process is in the early stages, shunting of the activity away from the diseased organ will result in an increased uptake in the remaining RES-bearing organs. This of course will cause an increase in activity in the normal portion of the RES at the expense of the diseased portion. If the disease process has progressed, the blood clearance time may be extended greatly.

Technetium sulfur colloid trapped by RES-bearing organs will remain indefinitely. Because of the short half-life of ^{99m}Tc, extended testing is impossible. Indications are, however, that the colloid is not biodegradable and therefore does remain indefinitely.

A word of caution should be mentioned at this point. Although the literature indicates that the biologic half-life of technetium sulfur colloid is infinity, one must not be fooled into thinking urine and stools will be devoid of activity when conducting tests involving these specimens. It must be remembered that only about 95% of the pertechnetate in the sulfur colloid preparation is so incorporated in the particles. About 5% remains as pertechnetate; of this, surely, there are in solution a sizable number of soluble Tc_2S_7 molecules small enough to enter the glomerular filtrate. The pertechnetate, of course, enters a biopathway of its own that includes excretion by the urinary and fecal routes.

TECHNETIUM MACROAGGREGATED ALBUMIN

Human albumin extracted from blood sera is a soluble protein. This material, however, can be rendered insoluble if merely heated in its water solution with either a little acid or base added. If the conditions of heating are proper and the solution is stirred at the appropriate rate, the precipitating protein will form independent aggregates with dimensions on the order of 10 to 100 μ. Commercial preparations of this product actually have a tighter range of particles than this, made possible by rigid production and separation techniques. A more accurate description of the product would include a particular size range of 20 to 50 μ for 90% of the preparation.

If stannous chloride with tin in the +2 valence state is mixed with the macroaggregated albumin and a solution of sodium pertechnetate is then added, a reaction will occur in which the macroaggregated albumin will be tagged with ^{99m}Tc. The exact chemical mechanism has yet to be elucidated. It is thought, however, that the albumin contains at least 2 oxygen atoms oriented in such a fashion as to allow binding by the stannous ion. Once bound to the albumin, the tin atom has available additional binding sites that will couple with pertechnetate, probably through one or more of the oxygens joined to the technetium atom. In any event the tag of albumin through tin is quite stable of physiologic pH.

All easily accessible veins lead to the right side of the heart. In going from the site of injection to the heart the vessel diameter enlarges. From the right side of the heart the blood is pumped to the lung through the pulmonary artery. At this time the vessel diameter reduces at each branch until, at the alveoli level, the vessels are at precapillary size, 10 to 20 μ.

Aggregates of albumin tagged with ^{99m}Tc will be swept along by blood flow to the heart and thence to the lungs, at which time vessel diameter will be too small for passage. The particles will then be trapped in the lung tissue.

There is no physiologic or chemical property of lung tissue that produces this localization as is seen in pertechnetate thyroid images. It is mere vessel blockage with harmless particles that obstruct only an insignificant fraction of the precapillary vessels of the lung. An intra-arterial injection serving any organ would serve the same purpose and allow for visualization of its arterial capillary bed.

Distribution of the particles in the lung will be strictly in accordance to blood flow. Areas well perfused will deposit large numbers of aggregates, whereas areas of poor or absent perfusion will receive few or no particles. If a major supply vessel is occluded, then all downstream vessels and the areas of the lung they serve will be devoid of trapped particles. This initial distribution and subsequent imaging procedure then allow the interpretation of perfusion defects in the lung.

Since albumin is a physiologic substance (even aggregated), it is not surprising to find that biorouting does not stop here as it does with technetium sulfur colloid. Clearance of the tagged macroaggregates from the lung requires three processes. First, bloodstream enzymes begin immediately to dissolve the particles. This dissolution process commences on the outer surface, thus shrinking the particle. It is somewhat analogous to the melting of an ice cube. Second, respiratory motion continually causes the lung tissue to expand and contract. This motion also elongates and compresses the particles. Third, there is a constant blood pressure being delivered in a rhythmic fashion. These three forces eventually push the particles through the lung capillary bed to the pulmonary vein and out to the systemic circulation. Estimates on clearance rates have been varied with reports of biologic half-times of 3 to 9 hours.

Particles so removed from the lung are now in the colloidal size range. Being "foreign" particles, the tagged aggregates are removed by the RES, primarily the liver. It is known that the albumin will be fully digested by this system, with the end products recycled. The fate of the technetium-tin complex is unknown because of its short physical half-life. Again the reader is cautioned to exercise care when required to do dual studies involving the assessment of the activity in the urine or stools of a patient who has recently undergone a lung imaging procedure. Although the tag to albumin aggregates is again about 95%, this does leave a quantity of free technetium to follow the path of its own biorouting.

TECHNETIUM DTPA

Diethylenetriamine penta-acetic acid (DTPA) is an organic molecule and one of a unique class of similar compounds exhibiting the property of being able to bind certain metals. Molecules of this class are referred to as chelating agents. The word *chelate* is derived from a Greek word meaning a claw or grasp. Chelating molecules accomplish the binding of metals generally by donating unused electrons to the metal atom from either nitrogen or oxygen without actually giving them up. In this way certain metallic cations in solution will attach themselves to the organic molecule and on introduction to the human body will be swept along the biopathway of the chelate rather than as the free cation.

Many substances in the body perform this same type of task. In most cases, however, the body's chelating substances are large proteins, and in general they and their bound substances are confined to the vascular pool.

The value of DTPA (Fig. 27-5) rests with the fact that it is a small molecule (less than 500 mol wt), is soluble, and is stable at physiologic pH. Metallic cations when attached to DTPA do not alter the biorouting of the parent molecule.

Two metals are currently used as instruments to effect the binding of technetium to DTPA — iron and tin. When ferrous iron (Fe^{++}) is mixed with pertechnetate, a complex is formed that binds to DTPA, producing a single molecule of technetium iron DTPA. To maintain the iron in the Fe^{++} state a reducing agent such as ascorbic acid is required. Therefore a fraction of the end product ends up as a technetium iron ascorbate. These two products exhibit somewhat different bioroutes, which will be explained shortly.

When a stannous (Sn^{++}) ion is mixed with pertechnetate again a complex is formed that will join DTPA to form a technetium stannous DTPA. Since the stannous ion can be produced in the lyophilized (freeze-dried) state and is stable in the absence of oxidizers, the reagents can be mixed and packaged without ascorbate. The addition of pertechnetate then produces a pure product. Regardless of whether iron or tin is used, much less than 10% of the technetium added to the reaction is left as free pertechnetate ion. With tin, however, only one product is produced, whereas with iron around 10% of the technetium added tags ascorbate and not DTPA.

When ^{99m}Tc DTPA with either tin or iron is introduced to the vascular compartment, a rapid equilibrium within the extracellular compartment is established. DTPA, being small, can freely diffuse across the capillary membrane. Since the molecule is unneeded by any cell of the body and is rejected even by the liver, it would remain circulating for an indefinite time if it were not for the glomerulus of the kidney. DTPA and its tag that escape the vascular compartment by the

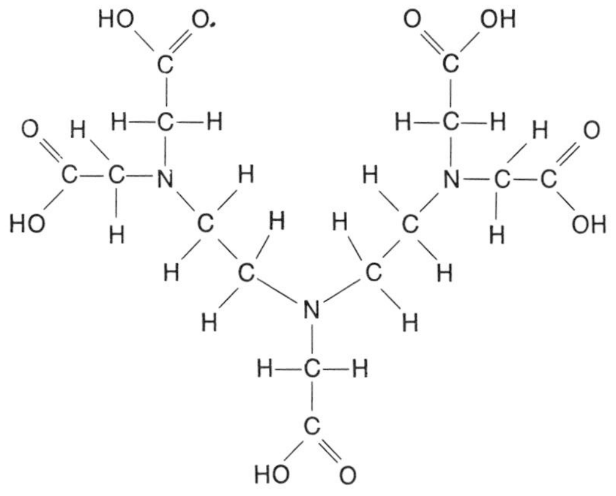

Fig. 27-5. Diethylenetriamine penta-acetic acid (DTPA).

glomerular filtrate will not be reabsorbed by the tubules. This failure to reabsorb takes both mechanisms, diffusion and active transport, into consideration. The molecules will not diffuse back to the vascular compartment as does pertechnetate nor will the tubule cells actively absorb DTPA as they do glucose and so many other substances.

The initial disappearance curve for ^{99m}Tc DTPA tin or iron is similar to that of pertechnetate. Within 5 minutes after injection and surely by 10 minutes, when mixing is assured, the concentration of the agent is uniformly distributed throughout the extracellular compartment. At this point further bloodstream clearance is produced exclusively by the action of the glomerulus. Since the extracellular compartment is three to four times larger than the vascular compartment, the time required to clear the bloodstream to half its original levels is on the order of several hours. During this time the kidney tubular system carrying the cleared chelate to the ureters has a significantly higher activity than the surrounding tissue.

When using the DTPA iron complex product, the presence of the ^{99m}Tc iron ascorbate should be recalled. This agent, which is approximately 10% of the ad-

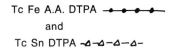

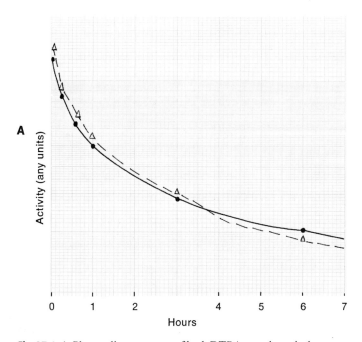

Fig. 27-6. **A,** Plasma disappearance of both DTPA complexes is the same.

ministered dose, is also cleared by the kidney. Although the mechanism is not clear, there is a tubular retention of this agent. The retention appears to involve the tagging of the iron to transferrin or transferrin-like molecules in the tubular cells. This, of course, carries with it the technetium.

The ultimate fate of this kidney binding is unknown; however, it does allow for imaging of the organ at much later times than with the tin complex, which exhibits an in-and-out biorouting. A whole-body disappearance curve for the ^{99m}Tc DTPA tin and iron products is shown in Fig. 27-6.

Imaging of the kidney can be performed with both agents almost immediately after injection. Indeed, if using enough of the DTPA complex to yield a high enough count rate, one can observe the function of the kidney through serial images. Seconds after injection the radioagent may be observed perfusing the kidney by the renal artery input. The agent will immediately begin clearing to the tubular system and only minutes later will arrive in the collecting tubules and calyxes. By about 5 minutes after dosing, the ureters draining the complex to the bladder will be visualized.

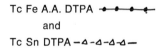

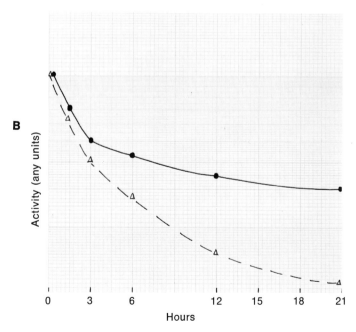

Fig. 27-6, cont'd. B, The whole-body retention of the iron-containing agent is higher, however. The retained substance is localized entirely in the kidney and is thought to be the technetium iron ascorbate component of this complex.

The bladder will act as a temporary storage compartment until the patient voids. Patients should be encouraged to void within the hour after the imaging procedure is complete to reduce the bladder radiation dose. Fecal or other routes of elimination are unknown. We have not had any experience with stool sample counting after dosing with ^{99m}Tc DTPA (Sn or Fe) but would strongly suspect contamination to be there.

Brain imaging with the tagged DTPA complexes is successful for the same reason it is successful with pertechnetate. Initially, high concentrations of both agents will infiltrate areas of the brain not protected by a blood-brain barrier and will be left behind when the bloodstream clears to the agent. The advantage of using the DTPA complex over pertechnetate rests with the increased clearance rate of the former, resulting in a high target-to-nontarget ratio at an earlier time after dosing.

TECHNETIUM PHOSPHATES AND DIPHOSPHONATES

A revolution in bone imaging has been made possible through the development of two classes of ^{99m}Tc-labeled compounds. For many years it was known that phosphate labeled with ^{32}P would localize preferentially around skeletal lesions. The unavailability of a suitable gamma-emitting nuclide of either phosphorous or oxygen made the use of these nuclides clinically impractical. The discovery of a method by which technetium can be made to bind to phosphate or diphosphonate has made possible further progress along these lines.

Until recently bone imaging agents had developed through the use of radionuclides whose properties were similar to calcium or the hydroxy grouping of which bone mineral is composed in part. ^{47}Ca, two strontium nuclides, and ^{18}F were tried and used with limited success. ^{18}F as the fluoride ion that will enter bone mineral content in exchange for the hydroxy (OH^-) group was the most successful, but because of a half-life a bit too short (110 minutes) and an energy too high (511 kev), it has been abandoned by most for the technetium compounds. Tagging of technetium to either phosphate or diphosphonate is accomplished through the use of a metal intermediary as was the case with the DTPA compounds. The stannous ion again appears to be the most successful metal used. Tagging under the proper circumstances can be virtually 100%. Difficulties in the preparation of these compounds generally result from failure to maintain tin in the +2 valence state. Conversion of tin from the +2 to the +4 state will occur in the presence of almost any oxidant.

Any oxidizing agent present in the generator eluent or the pertechnetate supply will produce this adverse effect. Oxygen dissolved in water or moisture will also produce a stannic (+4) ion. For this reason the radiopharmaceutical companies provide these agents in a lyophilized form within nitrogen-purged vials.

The technologist tagging the bone agent by the use of these kits would be well advised to avoid the introduction of air into these vials. Failure to maintain the tin as the stannous ion will result in a significant fraction of the activity remaining as free pertechnetate.

Although the chemical structure of technetium stannous polyphosphate, pyrophosphate, or diphosphonate is somewhat in doubt, the diagram shown in Fig. 27-7 represents the general consensus of opinion.

To appreciate the mechanism whereby the polyphosphates and diphosphonates are able to assist in the revelation of bone defects, a brief description of the anatomy and physiology of bone is necessary.

True osseous tissue, as distinguished from bone marrow, is made up of two major components: an organic matrix and a complex of mineral salts. The organic matrix consists of protein, 95% of which is fibrous collagen. The balance of the protein is referred to as a ground substance composed of several identifiable proteins with a consistency ranging from that of interstitial fluid to that of a semisolid gel.

Intermixed in the organic matrix are a large number of mineral crystals composed of positive calcium, magnesium, sodium, and hydrogen ions and negative phosphate, carbonate, and hydroxide ions. These ions are arranged in a complex crystalline structure that closely resembles that of the apatite minerals such as $CaCO_3 \cdot 3Ca_3(PO_4)_2$. The carbonate apatite mineral $CaCO_3 \cdot 3Ca_3(PO_4)_2$ is preferably written $Ca_{10}(PO_4)_6CO_3$, since x-ray diagrams of it are quite distinct from those of $CaCO_3$ and $Ca_3(PO_4)_2$. This is also true for bone mineral in that x-ray diffraction techniques do not identify patterns of $CaCO_3$ and $Ca_3(PO_4)_2$ as such but arrangement in the crystalline order characteristic of the apatite minerals.

Also intermixed in the organic matrix of bone are the osteoblasts, dormant bone cells that when triggered become osteocytes. Osteocytes are active bone-forming cells. Bone forming means that the cells are laying down the minerals resulting in the actual crystalline structure of bone. It is at this point that the radiobone agents, when introduced to the vascular system, will be incorporated in the mineral being deposited. The technetium-labeled phosphates have also been shown to have selective binding affinity by immature collagen.

The triggering of the osteocytes is a poorly understood phenomenon. It ap-

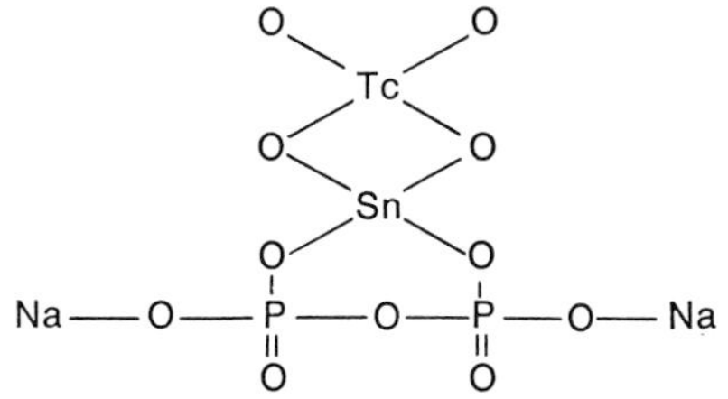

Fig. 27-7. Proposed structure of technetium stannous bone imaging agents. The compound illustrated is that of pyrophosphate. The polyphosphates are longer chains of that shown. The structure of the diphosphonates is similar to that described except that the central oxygen between the two phosphorus atoms is replaced by a carbon atom.

pears, however, to be in some way related to blood flow. When blood flow is generous to a certain area of bone, the osteocytic activity increases and bone mineral deposition is positive. Bone growth thus results. When the blood flow to the osteocytes becomes impaired, the activity of these cells diminishes. This process of building continues to some point where there is no longer a net increase in bone mineral deposition and osteocytic activity is limited to wear and tear repair. At this time the deposition of new mineral salts is offset by a reabsorptive mechanism whereby deposited salts are solubilized and returned to the vascular compartment. Thus there is a mineral turnover but no net gain in either direction.

Blood flow to both newly forming bone and injured bone is increased over that to stable or mature bone. Apparently in the process of reaching maturity or full repair the blood flow is gradually reduced by the accumulation of deposited minerals. The reduction in blood flow results in less osteocytic activity.

Bone-seeking radiominerals will then be deposited in or around bone defects according to two parameters: perfusion and osteocytic activity. In areas such as these the increased activity deposited will result in an increased count rate over that recorded from normal bone.

After intravenous injection the technetium tin—tagged phosphates and diphosphonates will be distributed throughout the extracellular spaces with a mixing time not much greater than 10 minutes. Loose binding to protein to the extent of 80% of the injected dose delays mixing and clearance somewhat.

Blood clearance of the technetium bone seekers is effected primarily by bone and kidney. The blood clearance rate is markedly influenced by the degree of renal function. When kidney function is poor, the half-time clearance may be delayed several hours more than normal. Clearance by kidney appears to be by glomerular filtration. Filtered phosphates, however, are reabsorbed by the tubules. Diphosphonates also are reabsorbed but apparently a bit less efficiently. This is probably because of the dissimilarity in chemical structure of the two classes of compounds. It may also explain why the clearance of diphosphonates is a bit faster than that of the phosphates.

The increased accumulation in bone will be positive for about 1 hour, at which time approximately 50% of the injected dose will be localized in bone. The amount in bone remains at this level for several hours with no additional accumulation or washout.

The remaining 50% of the dose, however, is cleared by the kidney with a half-time of about 4 hours. Urinary clearance of 15% by 1 hour growing to 28% by 4 hours has been reported. This means that the remaining activity in the extracellular (vascular and interstitial) spaces will fall from 35% at 1 hour to 22% at 4 hours after dose. Since the bone concentration remains the same, the target (bone)-to-nontarget (background) ratio improves with the passage of time.

Since vascular clearance of the 50% not bound to bone is quite slow, the optimum time for imaging has been the subject of debate. Target-to-nontarget ratios improve for many hours after injection. Recent reports indicate that the best ratios occur at as long as 12 hours after injection; however, most clinicians are imaging at 2 to 3 hours after injection. Hydration of the patient is indicated to produce a urine flow. Voiding is recommended prior to imaging the pelvic region because of the bladder accumulation influence.

Excretion of the technetium bone agents by other routes is not well documented with regard to quantity. Since phosphate is a normal constituent of most all body fluids, it would seem reasonable to assume that contamination of all fluids would occur. Any fluid loss would then be accompanied by a corresponding loss of activity. The bulk of the excretion of these bone agents is by the kidney. Of the 50% of the dose not bound to bone, the urinary clearance route accounts for about 95% in less than 24 hours. Release of the 50% deposited in bone is considerably slower, and physical decay does not allow for quantitation much beyond 48 to 72 hours. Experiments in animals have shown that deposited phosphate (^{32}P) disappears with a biologic half-time of 38 to 40 days.

BIBLIOGRAPHY

Adams, E. H.: Sulfur colloid flocculation due to acid leached aluminum, J. Nucl. Med. **13:**707, 1972.

Aronson, R. S.: Source of contaminants in technetium generators, J. Nucl. Med. **12:**271, 1971.

Arras, J. M., and Schadt, W. W.: Determination of radiochemical contamination on columns of Tc-99m generators, J. Nucl. Med. **11:**620, 1970.

Bardfield, P. A., and Rubin, S.: Comparative study of instant technetium from various commercial suppliers, J. Nucl. Med. **14:**880, 1973.

Berger, A., Elenbogen, G. D., and Guris, L. G.: Pyrogens, Adv. Chem. Ser. **16:**168, 1956.

Boyd, G. E.: Recent developments in generators of Tc-99m, radiopharmaceuticals and labelled compounds, vol. 1, Vienna, 1973, IAEA, pp. 3-25.

Briner, W. H.: Sterile kits for the preparation of radiopharmaceuticals: some basic quality control considerations. In Subramanian, G., and others, editors: Radiopharmaceuticals, New York, 1975, Society of Nuclear Medicine, pp. 246-253.

Briner, W. H., and Harris, C. C.: Radionuclide contamination of eluates from fission product molybdenum-technetium generators, J. Nucl. Med. **15:**466, 1974.

Brucer, M.: 118 medical radioisotope cows, Isot. Radiat. Tech. **3:**1, 1965.

Brucer, M.: A herd of radioisotope cows. In Vignettes in nuclear medicine, No. 3, St. Louis, Mallinckrodt Inc., 1966.

Brucer M.: A tracer has no pharmacology. In Vignettes in nuclear medicine, No. 24, St. Louis, Mallinckrodt Inc., 1967.

Callahan, R. J.: Technetium-99m human serum albumin: evaluation of a commercially produced kit, J. Nucl. Med. **17:**47, 1976.

Chen, M., Rhodes, B. A., Larson, S. M., and others: Sterility testing of radiopharmaceuticals, J. Nucl. Med. **15:**1142-1144, 1974.

Code of federal regulations, Title 10, chapter 1, part 20.205, Washington D.C., 1973, United States Government Printing Office.

David, G. S.: Quality of radioiodine. Science **184:**1381, 1974.

Eckelman, W., Atkins, H. L., Richards, P., and others: Visualization of the human spleen with Tc-99m-labeled red blood cells, J. Nucl. Med. **12:**310, 1971.

Gerlit, J. B.: Some chemical properties of technetium, Proceedings of the International Conference on Peaceful Uses of Atomic Energy **7:**145, 1956.

Haney, T. A.: Physical and biological properties of a Tc-99m-sulfur colloid preparation containing disodium edetate, J. Nucl. Med. **12:**64, 1971.

Harper, P. V.: Technetium-99m as a scanning agent, Radiology **85:**101, 1965.

Krogsgaard, O. W.: Radiochemical purity of various Tc-99m labelled bone scanning agents, Eur. J. Nucl. Med. **1:**15, 1976.

Krogsgaard, O. W.: Technetium-99m sulfur colloid: in vitro studies of various commercial kits, Eur. J. Nucl. Med. **1:**31, 1976.

Lathrop, K. A.: Preparation and control of Tc-99m radiopharmaceuticals; proceedings of a panel on radiopharmaceuticals from generator produced radionuclides, STI-PUB-294, Vienna, 1971, IAEA, pp. 39-52.

Physicians' desk reference for radiology and nuclear

medicine, ed. 30, Oradell, N.J., 1976, Medical Economics Co., pp. 92-94.

Spatz, D. D.: Reverse osmosis: the mechanism and application to dialysis, Med. Instrum. **8**:209, 1974.

Stern, H. S.: Preparation, distribution and utilization of technetium-99m sulfur colloid, J. Nucl. Med. **7:** 655, 1966.

Walker, H. G.: Effect of Tc-99m on bone scan agents in subsequent pertechnetate brain scans, J. Nucl. Med. **16:**579, 1975.

Zimmer, A. M., and Holmes, R. A.: Radiochemical purity and stability of commercial Tc-99m-Sn-diphosphate kits using a new chromatography technique, J. Nucl. Med. **16:**584, 1975.

28 Computed tomography

Ronald J. Ross, M.D.

Computed tomography is the newest diagnostic modality utilizing ionizing radiation. The theoretic principles for computed tomography were formulated many years ago. G. N. Hounsfield, a British engineer, developed the proper technical apparatus in 1971. J. Ambrose utilized this equipment in clinical experiments. The advent of computed tomography (CT) has revolutionized diagnostic imaging in radiology and has been compared in importance to Roentgen's discovery of the x-ray in 1895.

Since technical improvements have occurred rapidly and the equipment is costly ($500,000 and up), there are now rigid governmental controls that will limit the establishment of further CT facilities. There are approximately 950 CT scanners and 15,000 radioisotope scanners or cameras in the United States. Thus many hospitals will not have CT facilities in the near future and will have to refer their in-hospital patients to existing CT facilities in their area.

Computed tomography utilizes an x-ray–emitting source, sensitive detectors that receive the transmitted x-ray beam, advanced data processing computers that evaluate the information from the detectors, and various recording devices to display the final results.

The patient is properly positioned for the CT examination of the part of the body of interest (Fig. 28-1). The x-ray source rotates around the structure to be examined and emits very finely collimated x-ray beams. These x-ray beams (photons) are partially absorbed as they pass through the body structures. The altered beams pass into a detector system. This information passes from the detector system to the computer, which evaluates, computes, and reconstructs the results into a picture on a television screen (Fig. 28-2). The CT unit can evaluate various thicknesses of body structures, for example, 5 mm, 1.3 cm, and 2.6 cm. After each rotation around the patient, the conveyer table advances a determined distance and another complete rotation occurs until the entire structure has been evaluated in a series of thin slices (tomographic sections). The brain is evaluated with 8 to 10 slices. Hundreds of thousands of equations are solved by the computer during each examination.

Various systems are used, including rotating sources, rotating detectors, and fixed detectors. Depending on the equipment, the radiation dosage varies but usu-

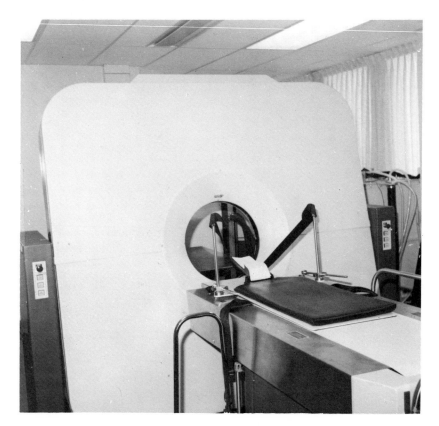

Fig. 28-1. CT gantry and patient table. Patient's head or body passes into circular opening in the center of the gantry. (From Young, W. S.: CT in a private practice radiology office, Radiology – Nuclear Medicine Magazine 8(2):11, 1978.)

ally is the same or less than the radiation doses for comparable routine radiographic examinations. The total time of the examination and recording of the information varies depending upon the equipment and the part of the body examined. The brain can be examined in times ranging from 3 to 15 minutes. Examinations of the abdomen and various intra-abdominal structures take longer. Some CT scanners can only perform examinations of the head, while the head and whole-body scanners can examine all parts of the body.

The computers utilize various mathematic procedures, and the reproduced images of the results of these computations are demonstrated on the television screen in black and white or color. The resultant television images are recorded on various formats including x-ray film, 70- to 100-mm film and Polaroid film (Fig. 28-3). The images are also stored on magnetic tape and can be recalled at any time.

Every structure in the patient's body can be examined with CT. However, an estimated 90% of all CT examinations now being performed are of the brain.

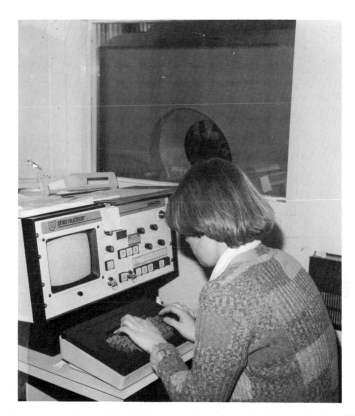

Fig. 28-2. Technician control panel. Technician control panel entering information into CT system and monitoring CT examination in progress on television screen. The patient is observed passing through the gantry during the examination. (From Young, W. S.: CT in a private practice radiology office, Radiology – Nuclear Medicine Magazine 8(2):11, 1978.)

Since the brain is encased by the bony calvarium, it was formerly only accessible by special radiologic procedures such as angiography, pneumoencephalography, and ventriculography. Radioisotope brain scanning is still the most frequently utilized diagnostic procedure for the evaluation of the brain.

The CT unit has the ability to accurately differentiate tissues and structures of all densities utilizing absorption coefficients and attenuation values. The gross normal anatomy of the brain is demonstrated and pathologic variations are detected (Fig. 28-4). The bony calvarial structures can be evaluated (Fig. 28-5). Brain parenchyma is differentiated from the cerebrospinal fluid-filled ventricular system. CT demonstrates areas of brain abnormalities resulting from ischemic or hemorrhagic infarctions, tumors (Fig. 28-6), calcification, structural abnormalities (Fig. 28-7), aneurysms, hematomas (Fig. 28-8), and hemorrhages. CT has the ability to evaluate the brain for atrophy (Fig. 28-9), communicating (Fig. 28-10) or obstructing hydrocephalus (Fig. 28-11), and postoperative and postirradiation changes.

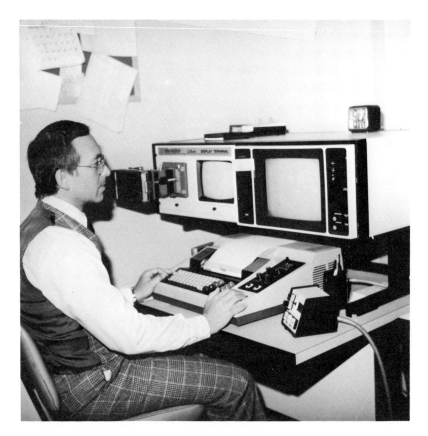

Fig. 28-3. Physician control panel. Physician monitor and control television screens (CRT, cathode ray tube) and keyboard controls. Polaroid reproductions and film hard copies are reproduced from magnetic tape images displayed on CRT. (From Young, W. S.: CT in a private practice radiology office, Radiology – Nuclear Medicine Magazine **8**(2):11, 1978.)

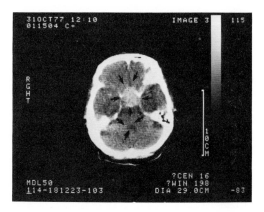

Fig. 28-4. Pituitary tumor in enlarged sella turcica. Contrast enhancing pituitary tumor in an enlarged sella turcica. The normal fourth ventricle is delineated in the posterior fossa.

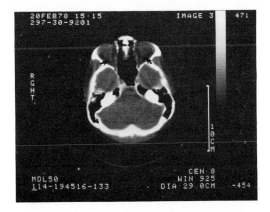

Fig. 28-5. Optic nerves and bony structures. Optic nerves passing to the optic globes and bony structures at this level are delineated.

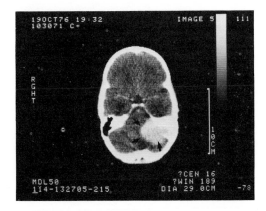

Fig. 28-6. Posterior fossa – cerebellar tumor. Large contrast-enhanced astrocytoma in posterior fossa – left cerebellar hemisphere adjacent to petrous ridge.

A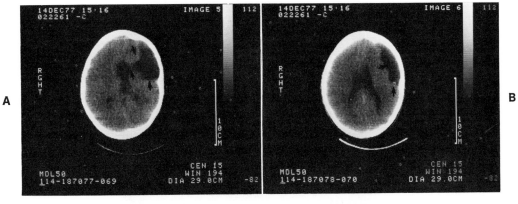B

Fig. 28-7. Porencephaly. **A,** Large area of porencephaly communicating with left frontal horn. **B,** Higher level scan shows continuation of porencephaly 1.3 cm cranially into left frontotemporal region. Bodies and occipital horns of lateral ventricles demonstrated.

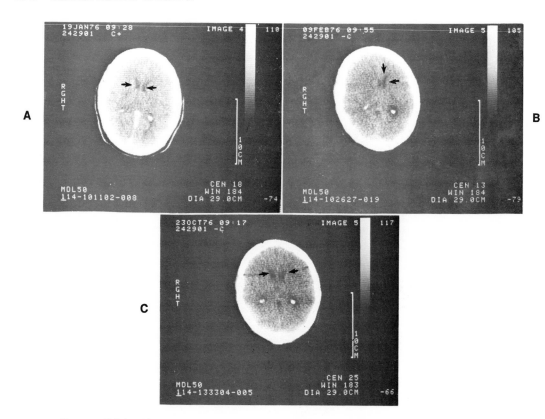

Fig. 28-8. Subdural hematoma. **A,** Normal brain scan with frontal horns in normal position. **B,** Following minor head trauma, brain scan now shows compression of right frontal horn and displacement of right and left frontal horns to left side. Acute subdural hematoma was found at surgery 6 hours after scan. **C,** Progress brain scan again shows normal position of frontal horns.

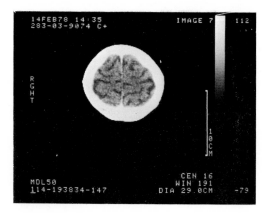

Fig. 28-9. Peripheral cortical atrophy. Deepened convexity sulci indicating moderate peripheral cortical atrophy.

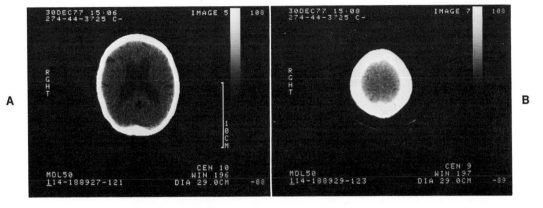

Fig. 28-10. Communicating hydrocephalus. **A,** Large dilated lateral ventricles with no obstructing lesion in a 69-year-old female. **B,** Same patient with section at convexity of brain demonstrating no deepening of sulci as is usually present in elderly people. Thus **A** and **B** indicate communicating (normal pressure) hydrocephalus.

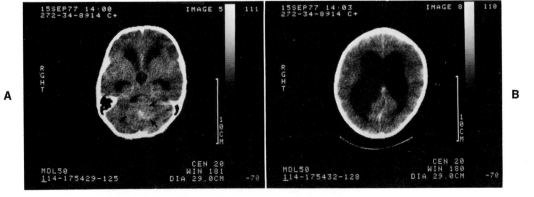

Fig. 28-11. Obstructive hydrocephalus – posterior fossa lesion. **A,** Obstructive hydrocephalus with dilation of entire ventricular system secondary to posterior fossa tumor; **B,** 4 cm cranially is massive dilation of lateral ventricles.

Although CT is considered to be a noninvasive procedure, intravenous contrast material is frequently injected into an arm vein prior to CT scanning of the brain. The circulating contrast material enhances certain normal and abnormal structures in the brain and aids in differential diagnosis (Fig. 28-12). Approximately 25% of CT scans are performed without the injection of contrast material. Fifty percent of the CT scans are performed following the injection of contrast material, and 25% of the CT scans are performed initially without contrast material and subsequently with contrast material.

Although CT is a major technologic advance available for diagnostic purposes in evaluating the brain, it does not eliminate other diagnostic procedures such as radioisotope scanning and angiography (Fig. 28-13). Most pathologic processes

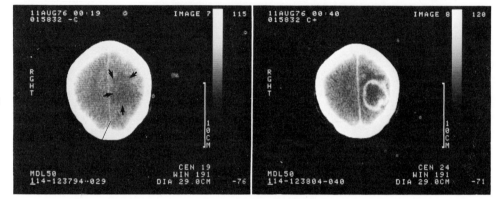

Fig. 28-12 Glioma without and with contrast enhancement. **A,** Poorly demarcated large area of decreased density in left parietal lobe. No contrast material injected (−C). **B,** Following the intravenous injection of contrast material, contrast-enhanced glioma with surrounding edema and central necrosis is delineated.

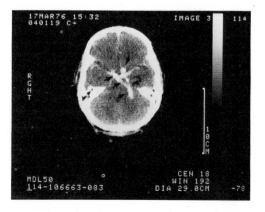

Fig. 28-13. Contrast-filled vessels of circle of Willis and ectatic basilar artery demonstrated on CT scan and corroborated by cerebral angiography.

and structural abnormalities of the brain are accurately and expeditiously diagnosed with CT. However, a CT scan of the brain may be negative in various pathologic entities, such as some acute ischemic cerebral infarctions and a few brain tumors in their early phases (Fig. 28-14). Also, current CT methods cannot evaluate cerebral blood flow abnormalities in occlusive vascular disease or the

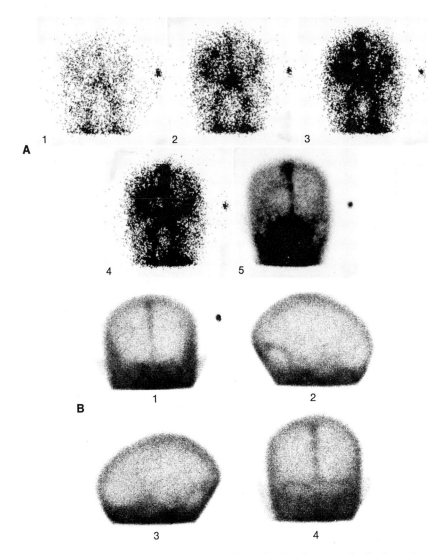

Fig. 28-14. Astrocytoma. **A,** January 1977. Dynamic cerebral perfusion study. In the early arterial phase (*1* and *2*) there is increased perfusion in the right frontal parietal region that persists throughout the capillary *(3)* and venous phase (*4* and *5*). **B,** January 1977. Two hours after dose static images reveal an irregular slightly increased concentration of nuclide in the right frontal region. Five-hour residual images revealed no further concentration of nuclide in the abnormal region. Study compatible with an AVM (arteriovenous malformation) or low grade glioma. *Continued.*

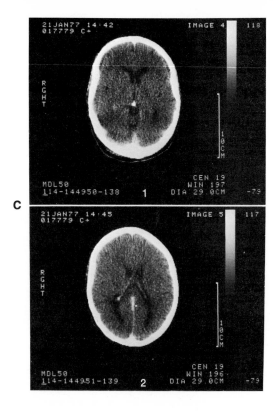

C

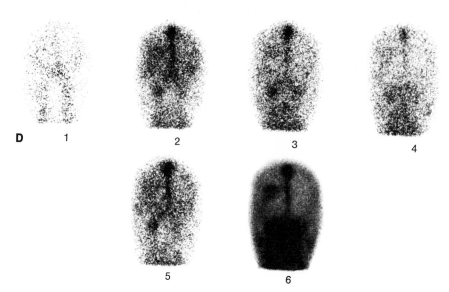

D

Fig. 28-14, cont'd. C, *1* and *2*, January 1977. CT scan of brain with contrast injection was normal. **D,** *1* to *6*, May 1977. Dynamic cerebral perfusion study reveals an increase in size in the lesion in the right frontal region and an increase in perfusion as well as early concentration of nuclide.

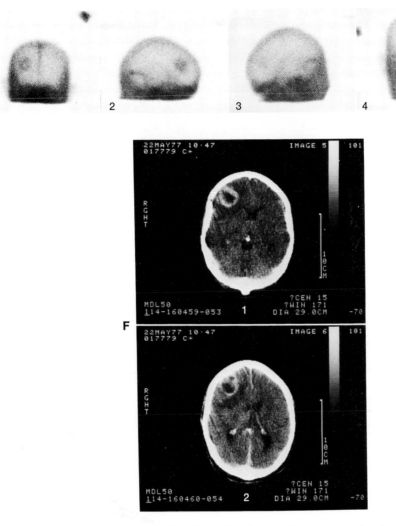

Fig. 28-14, cont'd. E, May 1977. Two hours after dose, static images reveal an irregular 4-cm lesion in the right frontal region. The lesion has a doughnut configuration as seen in central necrosis. **F,** *1* and *2*, May 1977. CT scan of brain. Contrast is enhancing mass lesion in right frontal lobe (with contrast injection). Pathologic diagnosis: astrocytoma Gd II.

smaller cerebral aneurysms. Thus, if clinical symptomatology warrants further investigation, a negative CT examination of the brain does not rule out the possibility that further diagnostic studies should be performed, such as a radioisotope brain scan or cerebral angiography or both.

CT scanning can be used to evaluate structures other than the brain, some of which are difficult to assess by other diagnostic modalities. These include the

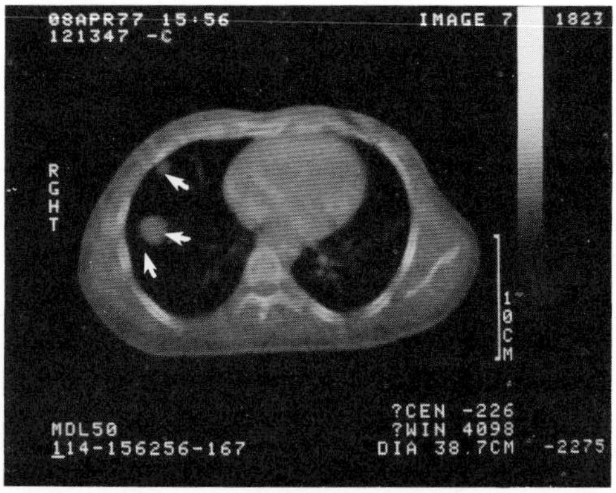

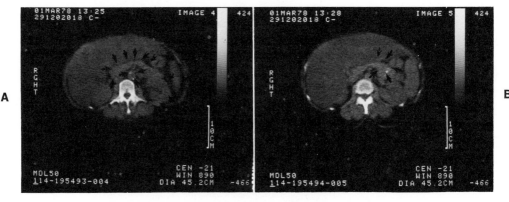

Fig. 28-15. Lung parenchymal and pleural lesions in right lung.

Fig. 28-16. Normal pancreas. A, Normal head and body of pancreas anterior to partially calcified aorta and vertebral body. The liver is enlarged. Mid portion of left kidney and lower portion of spleen delineated. B, Same patient 1.3 cm cranially. Tail of pancreas has small calcifications. Mid portion of spleen and kidney delineated.

mediastinum, the pleura (Fig. 28-15), the pancreas (Fig. 28-16), the liver and biliary ductal system (Fig. 28-17), and the pelvic viscera. Bone and soft tissues can be evaluated, and the extent of lesions in these regions can be determined (Fig. 28-18). Since CT is a three-dimensional approach to diagnosis, lesions can be very accurately localized and measured. This is of great benefit for medical, surgical, and radiotherapy treatment.

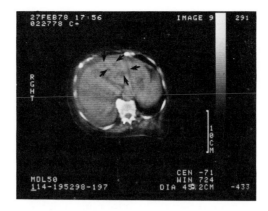

Fig. 28-17. Liver and biliary ductal system. Dilated bile ducts and enlarged liver in a patient with a hepatoma of the right lobe of the liver and obstructive jaundice.

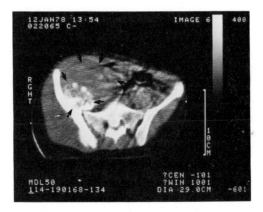

Fig. 28-18. Chondrosarcoma of iliac bone. Large chondrosarcoma arising from right iliac bone and protruding into true pelvis. Calcified and soft-tissue portions delineated.

BIBLIOGRAPHY

Abrams, H. L., and McNeil, B.: Medical implications of computed tomography, N. Engl. J. Med. **298**(5): 255-261, and **298**(6): 310-318, 1978.

Gambarelli, J., Guerinel, G., Chevrot, L., and Mattel, N.: Computed axial tomography, Heidelberg, 1977, Springer-Verlag.

Gonzalez, C., Grossman, C., and Palacios, E.: Computed brain and orbital tomography, New York, 1976, John Wiley & Sons, Inc.

Lanksch, W., and Kazner, E.: Cranial computerized tomography, Heidelberg, 1976, Springer-Verlag.

New, P., and Scott, W.: Computed tomography of the brain and orbit, Baltimore, 1975, The Williams & Wilkins Co.

Ramsey, R.: Computed tomography of the brain, Philadelphia, 1977, W. B. Saunders Co.

Ross, R.: Computed tomography in a private practice office, Radiology **127**(3):693-696, 1978.

29 Ultrasound imaging

Diagnostic ultrasound has become the most promising noninvasive medical modality to complement the anatomic physiologic information obtained with nuclear medicine procedures. In nuclear medicine imaging, radiation dosages to the patient have been reduced to the minimum as compared to radiologic procedures. However, diagnostic ultrasound has proved to be innocuous in terms of physical or genetic damage.

PRINCIPLES OF ULTRASOUND

Ultrasound refers to sound waves at frequencies that are inaudible to the human ear. For diagnostic purposes, frequencies in the 1 to 10 MHz range are employed. Resolution is dependent on the wavelength (λ), which is related to the frequency (F) and velocity (C) of the ultrasound beam. Therefore $F \times \lambda = C$. Thus the wavelength varies inversely with the frequency, and better resolution can be obtained with higher frequencies. Tissue attenuation increases with frequency, thus limiting the depth visualized at higher frequencies.

Production

Ultrasound is created by the piezoelectric effect. An electric potential is placed across the piezoelectric material, which responds by undergoing mechanical deformation, producing a short series of compressions and rarefactions that are transmitted into the surrounding medium (tissue). The transducer is then used as an ultrasound receiver converting reflected acoustic energy into signals that may be displayed. The transducer acts as a sender of ultrasound energy 0.1% of the time and a receiver 99.9% of the time, thus explaining the safety of ultrasound resulting from the very short pulses of energy emitted.

Reflection

Specular reflectors. As the ultrasound beam passes through tissue and reaches an interface with a medium of different acoustic properties, the reflected beam will be of large amplitude and its reflection will equal its angle of incidence, much like light reflected from a mirror. When the angle approaches 0°, the reflected beam will be received by the transducer. When the densities of two media differ drastically, as do air and tissue, there is close to 100% reflection at the interface. Velocity of sound density and the bulk modulus of an organ are also related to the sound reflected. It is thus postulated that the display of the organs is dependent on the collagen-supporting structures (bulk moduli 10,000 times greater than surrounding soft tissues) in blood vessels, bile ducts, and organs. Thus replacement or displacement of the supporting structures would be displayed as an abnormal anatomic defect.

Backscattered echoes. Backscattered echoes are the low-amplitude echoes returned in the same plane of the incident beam. These low level echoes, which may be displayed by gray-scale ultrasonography, have added greatly to the visual perception of the tissue background in an organ.

GRAY-SCALE ULTRASONOGRAPHY

Gray-scale ultrasonography allows the operator to preferentially amplify the low-level echoes (backscatter echoes) and compress the high-level echoes (specular echoes) so that the consistency of tissue (collagen) may be displayed as well as the contour of the organ. Progress in gray-scale instrumentation and research on the higher frequency-focused transducers made useful by instrumentation advances have shown gray-scale ultrasonography images to have greater solid organ and vascular information than the more costly CT radiologic scanning images. Real-time ultrasound imaging utilizing phased array transducers, a parabolic mirror, or a rotating transducer has proved of great aid in vascular visualization and in screening abdominal and pelvic anatomy.

LIVER

Ultrasonically the normal liver has a uniform echo pattern, a well-defined contour, and normal caliber vessels and biliary tree (common bile duct and gailblad-der). In its examination multiple transverse and longitudinal plane images are done while the patient holds inspiration. Primary and secondary liver tumors, cysts, abscesses, and gallbladder calculi have characteristic echo patterns (Figs. 29-1 to 29-3). The majority of metastatic disease sites usually have decreased echogenicity as compared to normal liver tissue. The resolution of gray-scale ultrasound imaging is greater than the nuclear image when both are performed with technical expertise. However, ultrasound, as practiced today, still is hampered by technical and interpreter vagaries that prompt most clinicians to screen patients with suspected metastatic disease with both modalities. While the nuclear image reveals a space-occupying lesion, ultrasound can characterize the nature of the lesion into malignant, abscess, inflammation, or cyst by its ultrasonic properties.

PANCREAS

In approximately 80% to 90% of patients studied the gray-scale ultrasonogram can demonstrate the normal or abnormal pancreas (Figs. 29-4 and 29-5). While in many instances ultrasound cannot differentiate malignancy from inflammatory

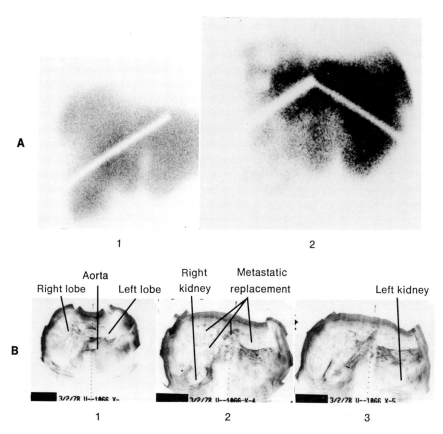

Fig. 29-1. A, Anterior liver images performed with [99mTc] sulfur colloid. Images done February 1976, *1,* and March 1978, *2,* demonstrate progression of the disease with replacement of normal liver tissue. **B,** Ultrasound study (5-MHz transducer). Three sagittal abdominal ultrasound views: *1,* xiphoid, *2,* xiphoid minus 4 cm, and *3,* xiphoid minus 5 cm. There is an uneven echo pattern throughout entire liver with loss of normal architecture and multiple sonolucent areas of malignancy. Diagnosis: hepatoma.

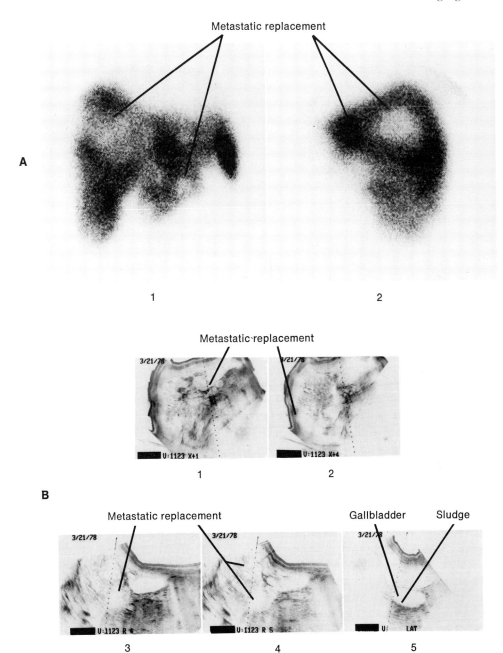

Fig. 29-2. A, Liver images performed with ^{99m}Tc sulfur colloid. *1,* Anterior view; *2,* right lateral view. There are multiple sites of metastatic disease throughout the liver. **B,** Ultrasound study (5-MHz transducer). Sagittal body section, *1,* xiphoid plus 1 cm and *2,* xiphoid plus 4 cm. Grossly abnormal liver architecture. Note the metastatic lesions on the periphery of the left lobe. *3* and *4* are longitudinal sections of the right upper quadrant. Multiple sonolucent metastatic lesions are present throughout the right lobe. *5,* Lateral sector image demonstrating the cystic gallbladder with fine dependent echogenicity of debris. Diagnosis: metastatic lung carcinoma.

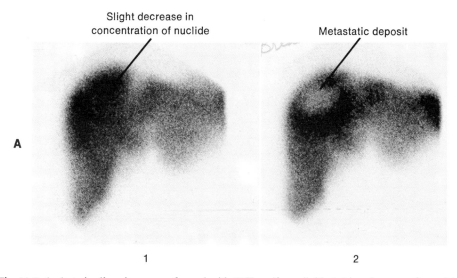

Slight decrease in concentration of nuclide

Metastatic deposit

A

1

2

Fig. 29-3. A, Anterior liver images performed with ^{99m}Tc sulfur colloid. *1,* Liver image performed in 1977 reveals a minimal ill-defined decreased concentration of nuclide in superior right lobe. *2,* Liver image performed 1 year later reveals a space-occupying lesion in the superior right lobe measuring approximately 7 cm. **B,** Ultrasound study (5-MHz transducer). *1,* Sagittal section of the body 2 cm below the xiphoid. *2* to *5,* Longitudinal section of the right upper quadrant. Ultrasound study reveals a 5-cm echogenic focus surrounded by 2-cm rim of sonolucency. In the center of the lesion there is an area of central necrosis. Note the resolution of the surrounding vascular structures, the kidney, and the normal liver parenchyma.

disease, ultrasound has become the screening technique of choice in studying patients with suspected pancreatic disease. (CT visualization of the pancreas is also useful with approximately the same sensitivity and specificity as ultrasound. However, the CT image is vastly improved if there are peripancreatic fatty deposits.) The pancreatic image with ^{75}Se selenomethionine has slightly better sensitivity; however, its specificity suffers primarily because of differing technical approaches and interpretor experience. The pancreatic nuclear image is usually reserved for those patients whose pancreases are not visualized by ultrasound or CT imaging.

ABDOMINAL VASCULAR ANATOMY

Gray-scale ultrasonography, whether sectional or real time, is of primary importance in the identification of normal and abnormal intra-abdominal vessel anatomy. The larger vascular structures are identified (aorta, superior mesenteric artery, inferior vena cava, superior mesenteric vein, and portal vein) (Figs. 29-6 and 29-7).

PELVIS

As a result of its lack of potentially harmful effects, ultrasound is ideally suited for the study of pregnancy and fetal development. Because of their position be-

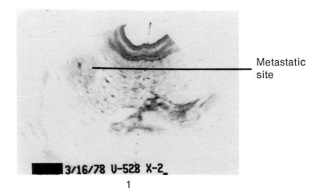

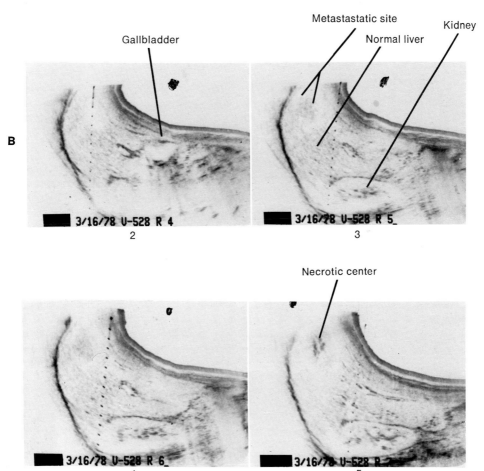

Fig. 29-3, cont. For legend see opposite page.

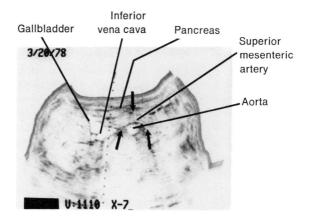

Fig. 29-4. Sagittal ultrasound (5-MHz transducer with extended gray scale) study 7 cm below the xiphoid revealing the pancreas and its relationship to the surrounding structures. The aorta and superior mesenteric artery are directly posterior to the body of the pancreas and the pancreatic head is anterior to the inferior vena cava. The normal pancreas is slightly more echogenic than the hepatic tissue.

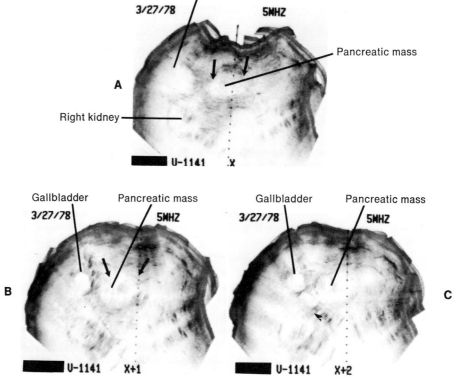

Fig. 29-5. Sagittal abdominal sections at the xiphoid, **A,** and 1 cm, **B,** and 2 cm, **C,** above the xiphoid reveal a large complex mass involving the entire pancreas. The poor detail behind the pancreatic mass is caused by sound absorption by the solid pancreatic carcinoma.

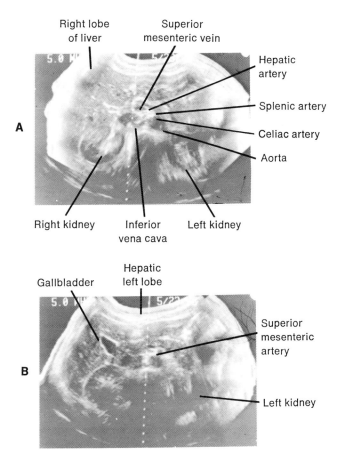

Right lobe of liver
Superior mesenteric vein
Hepatic artery
Splenic artery
Celiac artery
Aorta
A
Right kidney
Inferior vena cava
Left kidney

Hepatic left lobe
Gallbladder
Superior mesenteric artery
B
Left kidney

Fig. 29-6. Normal abdominal vascular study. **A,** X-3. Sagittal section 3 cm below the xiphoid reveals normal cross section of aorta at level of celiac artery. The splenic artery, hepatic artery, aorta, inferior vena cava, and the superior mesenteric vein are demonstrated. **B,** X-4. Note the cross section of the take-off from the aorta anteriorly of the superior mesenteric artery. *Continued.*

hind a full bladder, the pelvic organs may also be imaged, showing much detail, with relative ease. The anatomic detail of ultrasound imaging has caused it to largely replace radionuclide and x-ray studies in the pregnant female (Fig. 29-8).

SUMMARY

The growth of the anatomic imaging field of gray-scale ultrasonography is a mirror image of the growth of physiologic nuclear medicine. Their combined information has added greatly to the precise patient diagnostic information obtainable today on a noninvasive, nontraumatic basis. Ultrasound information is limited by attenuation of the ultrasound beam by bone and gas, therefore hampering the

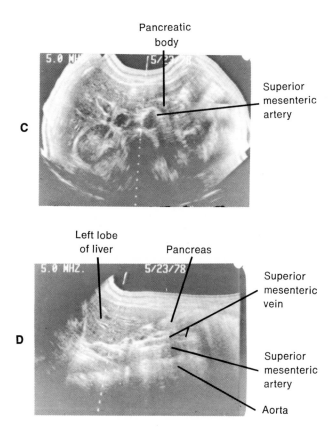

Fig. 29-6, cont'd. C, X-5. Cross section of the superior mesenteric artery anterior to the aorta. The body of the pancreas is anterior to the superior mesenteric artery. **D,** L-1. Longitudinal section 1 cm to the left of the midline demonstrates the normal aorta and the superior mesenteric artery and vein. The pancreas lies directly above the superior mesenteric vein.

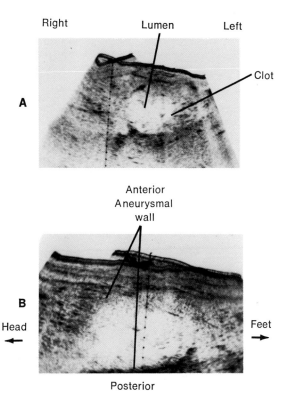

Fig. 29-7. A, Sagittal section of the abdomen 1 cm below the umbilicus reveals an aortic aneurysm. Note the round, 3.5-cm aortic "lumen" that is sonolucent with the surrounding tissue, which has fine texture echogenicity and a few harsh echoes. This tissue is intra-aneurysmal clot. **B,** Longitudinal section reveals a very large aneurysm filled with echogenic clot. Note the increased sound transmission through the aneurysm with resultant dense echo pattern behind the aneurysm.

Placenta

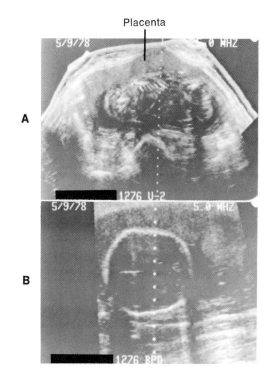

Fig. 29-8. A, Longitudinal section 2 cm to the right of the midline reveals the fine echogenicity of the anterofundal placenta and the fetal parts posterior to the placenta. Note the sound shielding posterior to the baby. **B,** A view of the fetal biparietal diameter, which is an excellent method of assessing the gestational age of the fetus. The biparietal diameter is 60 mm (1-cm electronic marker is placed on film), which is the equivalent of a 25-week gestation.

evaluation of structures underlying the ribs, lung, and intestinal gas. Ultrasound evaluation also needs a skilled operator, good quality control, and good interpretative skills. However, the future is bright for advances in ultrasound with application of automation, data processing, and computerization that have been applied to nuclear medicine imaging and CT imaging.

BIBLIOGRAPHY

DiMagno, E., and others: A prospective comparison of current diagnostic tests for pancreatic cancer, N. Engl. J. Med. **297**(14):737-742, October, 1977.

Jaffe, C., and Simonds, B.: Computed tomography and ultrasound of the abdomen: diagnostic implications of the imaging process, Appl. Radiol. **7**:81-84, 1978.

Tayler, K.: Atlas of grey scale ultrasonography, New York, 1978, Churchill Livingstone.

30 Radioimmunoassay

Rama Narra, Ph.D.
William Miller, B.S.

A significant contribution of immunology to modern clinical medicine has been the development of radioimmunoassay procedures for the determination of serum concentrations of certain physiologically important substances that cannot be easily detected or measured by standard laboratory techniques.

Before the advent of radioimmunoassay the assay of polypeptide hormones was mostly considered a research topic, and their assessment was made indirectly. The earliest method of measuring peptide hormones in plasma depended on bioassay. This was performed by comparing the hormonal effect produced by an unknown in a laboratory animal with that produced by a known standardized preparation of the hormone. Several bioassays have been developed. However, they are generally lacking either in sensitivity or specificity. To improve both sensitivity and specificity it became necessary to concentrate the hormone in question from a large volume of animal plasma. This animal preparation, as well as the processing of the material for use, was time consuming and tedious. Although these methods yielded much physiologic information in the past, the technical requirements and poor reproducibility restricted the clinical use of bioassays to relatively few laboratories.

The direct chemical assay of peptide hormones has likewise been fraught with problems. The chemical assay of thyroidal and steroidal hormones is possible because they possess distinctive chemical groupings. In addition, their concentrations in plasma are *three* to *five* orders of magnitude higher than those of the peptide hormones present with them. Unlike thyroidal and steroidal hormones, peptide hormone analysis has escaped accurate assay because there are ve:y few uniquely reacting groups that can be used to identify the hormone in the presence of other peptides. Even when specific reaction sites do exist on the peptide hormone in question, they are not readily distinguishable from the remainder of the plasma proteins, which are present at a *millionfold* to *billionfold* higher concentration.

Immunologic reactions, because of their characteristic "lock and key" mechanism, exhibit high specificity and sensitivity. These methods have demonstrated the capability of measuring 10^{-9} to 10^{-12} molar concentrations of peptide hor-

Fig. 30-1. Clinical radioimmunoassay.

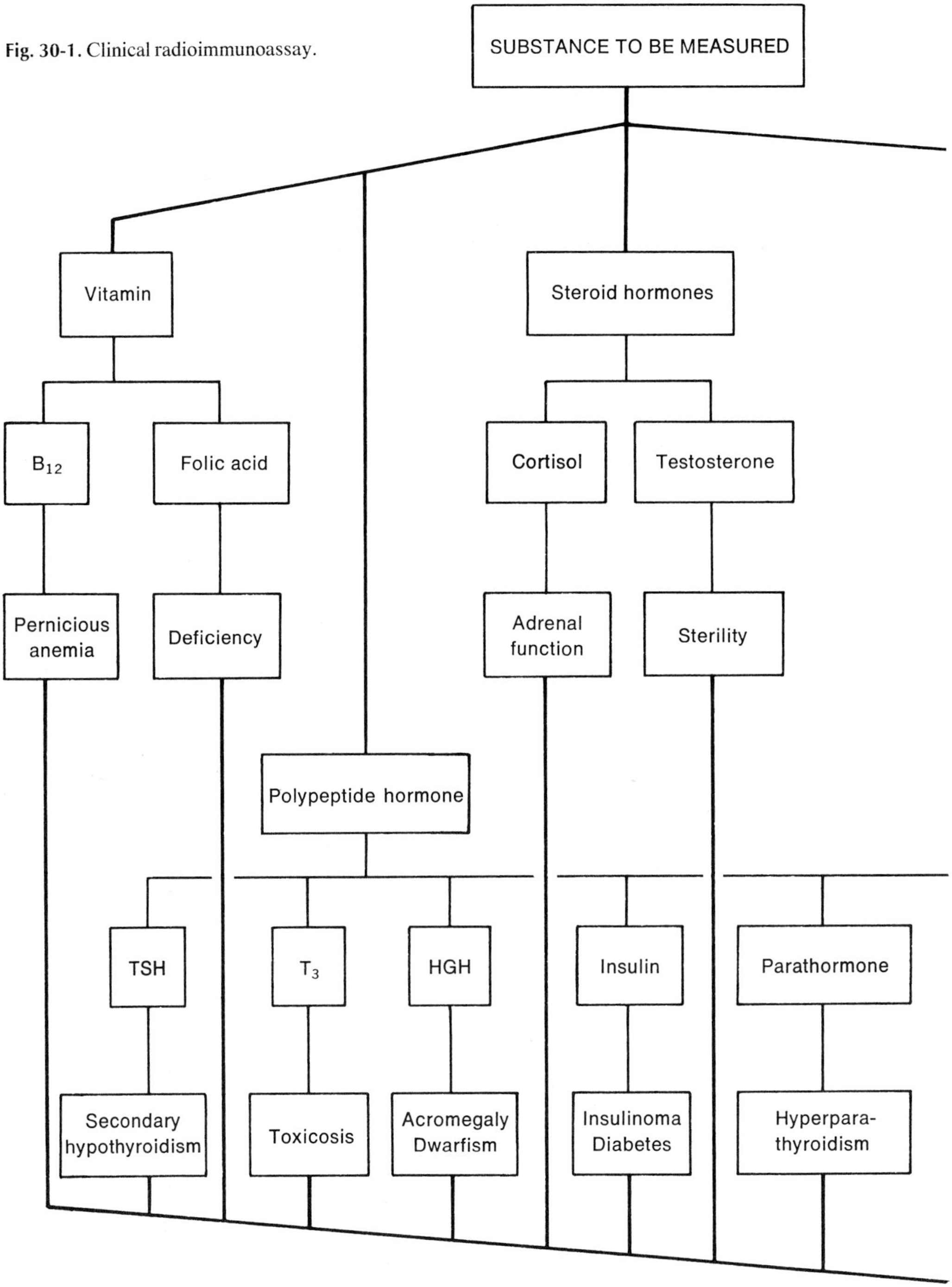

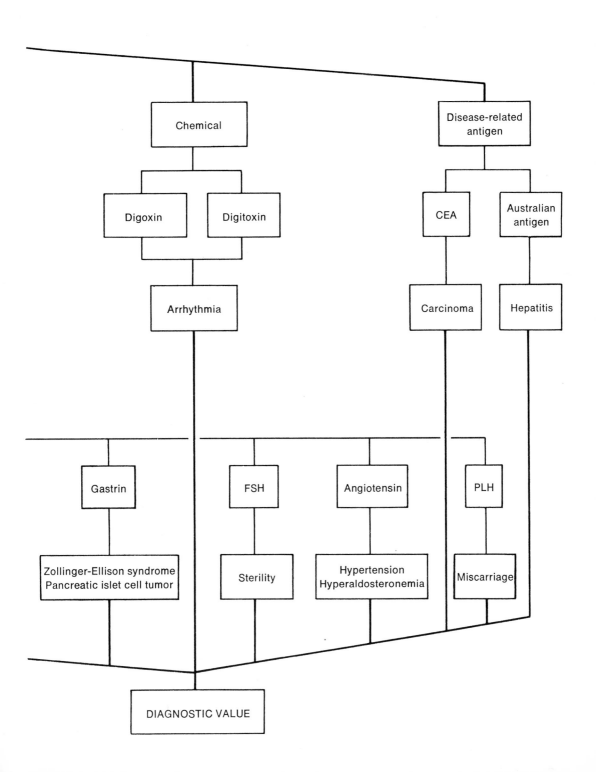

mones. Radial immunodiffusion and radioimmunoassay are two widely employed immunochemical methods used for the determination of serum concentrations of physiologically important substances.

In radial immunodiffusion, the measurement is accomplished by comparing the visible precipitate between the test protein in the plasma and its corresponding antibody with the visible precipitate formed with a known amount of the protein and its antibody. Theoretically, radial immunodiffusion methods can be used to determine the serum concentrations of any serum protein for which a specific antibody can be prepared. However, since they involve the formation of the visible precipitate between the test protein and its specific antibody, they cannot be used for the detection of antigens whose serum concentration is too low to form a visible precipitate or whose molecular size is too small to form a precipitable complex when bound to its corresponding antibody.

Radioimmunoassay methods possess the unique advantages of being sensitive, specific, and precise and therefore have gained the widest acceptance. The radioimmunoassay technique, as the name implies, achieves sensitivity through the use of radionuclides and specificity that is uniquely associated with immunochemical reactions. The two profound observations by Yalow and Berson,[1] that insulin-treated diabetics develop antibodies that could bind ^{131}I-labeled insulin and that the percentage of the labeled insulin bound to the antibody decreases progressively with the addition of increasing amounts of unlabeled insulin to the incubating mixture, form the basis for the development of radioimmunoassay. These investigators first published their classic paper on the assay of plasma insulin in humans by immunologic methods in 1960.[1] Since then, this technique has been extended to the measurement of most of the peptide hormones and a great variety of biologically active compounds and drugs. The high sensitivity attained in these procedures has undoubtedly increased the diagnostic accuracy in conditions associated with these hormones and drugs. Fig. 30-1 illustrates the broad scope of substances, conditions, and involved organs that may be measured and evaluated by modern radioimmunoassay techniques. Because of its widespread application in the biomedical field, it is important to know the basic principles, requirements, and, finally, the criteria necessary to have a valid radioimmunoassay.

TERMINOLOGY

It is important to define a number of words peculiar to the field of radioimmunoassay before proceeding with the text. Following is a radioimmunoassay glossary:

accuracy* The extent to which a given measurement agrees with its actual value.

adjuvant A substance that increases the formation and persistence of antibodies when injected together with antigens.

Freund's adjuvant In the incomplete form consists of a mixture of neutral detergent and mineral oil; the complete form also contains killed mycobacteria.

affinity Related to the energy of reaction and most often used synonymously with *avidity*. The simple difference between these two terms

---
*For footnote see opposite page.

is that avidity specifically refers to the quality of the antibody, whereas affinity reflects the quality of the antigen. Both avidity and affinity effect the overall binding in antigen/antibody complex formation.

antibody (Ab) A substance produced in response to an antigen that reacts specifically with that antigen.

antigen (Ag) Any substance that can induce the formation of antibodies and that reacts specifically with the antibodies formed.

antigen/antibody complex The product of the joining of an antigen to an antibody. The complex has both chemical and physical properties different from either the antigen or the antibody.

antigenicity The ability of a substance to induce the immune response. Antigenicity of a substance depends both on its molecular size and chemical composition. Certain substances, because of their small molecular size (for example, digoxin, angiotensin I, angiotensin II, triiodothyronine), will be able to induce the immune response only when they are coupled to larger molecules.

avidity Represents the energy of binding between an antibody and its specific antigen.

buffer(s) or **buffer solution** The ability of a system to resist changes in pH on the addition of acid or base or on diluting it with the solvent. pH may be defined as the negative logarithm of the hydrogen ion concentration. Mathematically it is written as $pH = -\log [H^+]$. A weak acid or weak base in the presence of one of its salts forms a buffer solution. Examples of typical buffer systems include the following: acetic acid (CH_3COOH) and sodium acetate (CH_3COONa), sodium dihydrogen phosphate (NaH_2Po_4) and disodium hydrogen phosphate (Na_2HPo_4), and ammonium hydroxide (NH_4OH) and ammonium chloride (NH_4Cl).

concentration The amount of a substance in weight or moles present in unit volume of a solution.

molar concentration Concentration expressed as moles per liter or millimoles per milliliter ($1mM = 0.001 mol$). A *mole* is Avogadro's number (6.023×10^{23}) of molecules of a substance or mass numerically equal to the molecular weight. It is usually expressed as the gram molecular weight.

cross-reactivity Closely resembles specificity. Reactions where antibodies react with two or more antigens of similar structure are known as cross-reactions. Cross-reactivity can occur between different hormones from the same species. For example, there is partial or complete cross-reactivity between FSH, LH, and TSH and HGH and HPL.

hapten Any substance unable to induce antibody formation by itself but able to incite antibody formation with antigenic specificity when joined to a large protein molecule.

hormones Substances secreted by the endocrine, or ductless, glands that influence the activity of the various organs of the body and thus regulate the metabolic processes. Chemically these represent a diverse group of compounds and can be divided into three classes: (1) Polypeptide or protein hormones: the hormones secret-

---

*Accuracy and precision: Accuracy refers to the extent to which a given measurement agrees with its actual value. Precision is concerned with the reproducibility of a certain measurement. These two terms can best be understood with reference to a particular example. Suppose that a serum sample having a known concentration of digoxin, 1.85 ng/ml (nanograms, or ng = 10^{-9} grams), was supplied to four different laboratories for digoxin assay. Each laboratory performed four measurements, and the following results were reported.

Serum sample	Digoxin concentration (ng/ml)			
	Lab A	*Lab B*	*Lab C*	*Lab D*
1	1.52	1.65	1.43	1.72
2	1.47	2.00	1.77	1.87
3	1.57	2.15	1.90	1.80
4	1.59	1.70	1.35	1.95
Avg ± SD	1.54 ± 0.08	1.88 ± 0.25	1.61 ± 0.26	1.82 ± 0.09

Inference: Lab A, precise but not accurate; Lab B, accurate but not precise; Lab C, not precise, not accurate; Lab D, precise and accurate.

ed by pituitary, parathyroid, and pancreas (for example, thyrotropin, TSH, growth hormone, HGH, follicle-stimulating hormone, FSH, parathormone, calcitonin, and insulin). The molecular weights of these hormones range from approximately 1,000 to 30,000 or more. (2) Steroid hormones: the hormones produced by the adrenal cortex and gonads (for example, aldosterone, corticosterone, testosterone, progesterone, and estrogens). (3) Simple hormones: hormones produced by adrenal medulla and thyroid. These are neither protein nor steroid but simple amino acid derivatives (for example, epinephrine, triiodothyronine [T_3], and thyroxine [T_4].

immunogen See *antigen.*

immunogenicity See *antigenicity.*

immunoreactivity Reaction that takes place between an antigen and its antibody.

precision* Concerned with the reproducibility of a certain measurement.

sensitivity Minimum amount of hormone that can

be measured without introducing significant error. In addition, it can be used to indicate the slope of a dose-response curve.

species specificity Situation in which the same antigen from two different animal species exhibits different reactivity toward an antibody. Hormones exhibit species specificity to a high degree. When assaying these hormones, it is often necessary to use the same antigen for the preparation of tracer and standards and the production of antibodies. In these cases, of course, all the antiserum must be obtained from the same species.

specificity Implies that an antibody can only react with the antigen responsible for its formation. However, certain antibodies are nonspecific and react with a variety of antigens from the same animal species, providing they are similar in their structure.

titer Optimal or final concentration of the antibody present in the assay system.

THEORY

The radioimmunoassay technique is based on the isotope dilution principle, along with the use of a specific antibody to bind a portion of a substance to be measured. If an antigen (for example, a hormone) is mixed with a specific antibody to that substance, an interaction will occur, forming an antigen/antibody complex that is chemically different from either the antigen or the antibody. If there is insufficient antibody to complex all the antigen present, mixing of the anti-

---

*Accuracy and precision: Accuracy refers to the extent to which a given measurement agrees with its actual value. Precision is concerned with the reproducibility of a certain measurement. These two terms can best be understood with reference to a particular example. Suppose that a serum sample having a known concentration of digoxin, 1.85 ng/ml (nanograms, or ng = 10^{-9} grams), was supplied to four different laboratories for digoxin assay. Each laboratory performed four measurements, and the following results were reported.

Serum sample	Digoxin concentration (ng/ml)			
	Lab A	*Lab B*	*Lab C*	*Lab D*
1	1.52	1.65	1.43	1.72
2	1.47	2.00	1.77	1.87
3	1.57	2.15	1.90	1.80
4	1.59	1.70	1.35	1.95
Avg ± SD	1.54 ± 0.08	1.88 ± 0.25	1.61 ± 0.26	1.82 ± 0.09

Inference: Lab A, precise but not accurate; Lab B, accurate but not precise; Lab C, not precise, not accurate; Lab D, precise and accurate.

body with a known amount of isotopically labeled antigen along with an unknown amount of labeled antigen allows quantitation of the unlabeled antigen. The following diagram and example may help illustrate the point:

If:

Antigen + Antibody → Complex + Leftover antigen

And:

Antigen* + Antibody → Complex* + Leftover antigen

Then:

Antigen + Antigen* + Antibody → Complex* + Complex +

Leftover antigen + Leftover antigen*

If the amount of antigen* present is fixed, then by competitive binding the amount of antigen/antibody complex* formed will be *inversely* dependent on the amount of unlabeled antigen present. Another way of explaining this is that the leftover labeled antigen remaining will be in *direct* proportion to the unlabeled antigen present in the reaction mixture.

Example. Suppose 1 mg of the hormone insulin is mixed with 1 mg of insulin labeled with ^{125}I, and this mixture is treated with enough antibody to complex only a total of 1 mg of the hormone. Then, by competitive binding, 0.5 mg of labeled complex will be formed, along with 0.5 mg of unlabeled complex. If, however, 3 mg of the hormone insulin is mixed with 1 mg of the insulin labeled with ^{125}I and again the mixture is treated with only enough antibody to complex a total of 1 mg of the hormone, then, by competitive binding, 0.25 mg of the labeled complex will form along with 0.75 mg of the unlabeled complex. Thus increasing the amount of unlabeled hormone in the reaction mixture decreases the amount of labeled complex formed and vice versa. At the same time one should recognize that by increasing the amount of unlabeled hormone, the amount of labeled hormone remaining uncomplexed also increases.

• • •

Prior to testing unknowns it is necessary to prepare a series of solutions of increasing antigen concentration. These solutions of known antigen concentration are referred to as *standard solutions*. To these solutions is added a fixed amount of labeled antigen and antibody *insufficient* to bind all the antigen present. The complex is permitted to form, and the bound antigen is separated from the free antigen. By relating the count from the separated complex to the control, one can establish a standard curve as illustrated in Fig. 30-2. From this standard curve, unknown samples run concurrently can be quantified.

---

*Labeled with radioactive tracer.

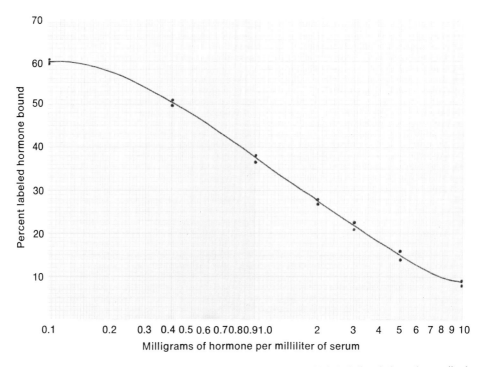

Fig. 30-2. Typical standard curve as constructed with percentage of labeled digoxin bound to antibody versus ng/ml digoxin contained per standard tube. (From Sodee, D. B., and Early, P. J.: Technology and interpretation of nuclear medicine procedures, ed. 2, St. Louis, 1975, The C. V. Mosby Co.)

STANDARD CURVE

A plot of the distribution of radioactivity as a function of the amount of unlabeled antigen present is known as a *standard*, or *dose-response, curve*. Standard curves are plotted in a variety of different ways. The most commonly used response curves are the bound-free (B/F) ratio, free-bound (F/B) ratio, or fraction-bound (b) ratio and occasionally b/b_0, in which b_0 corresponds to the percent bound in the absence of unlabeled antigen. The dose can be plotted on either the arithmetic or logarithmic scale. Some typical dose-response curves are presented in Fig. 30-3.

To obtain response curves that are essentially linear over a large part of the antigen concentration, the logit function defined as follows has been used:

$$\text{logit (y)} = \ln \frac{y}{1 - y}$$

Where:

$$y = \text{either } B/B_0 \text{ or } (B/F)/(B_0/F_0)$$

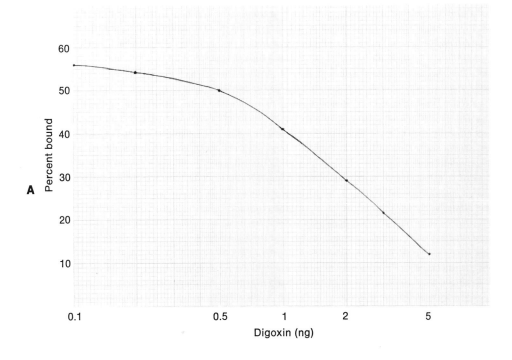

A

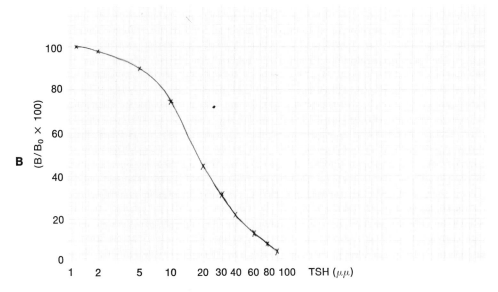

B

Fig. 30-3. Experimental dose-response curves. **A,** Digoxin radioimmunoassay standard curve, obtained with Schwarz/Mann Digoxin (^{125}I) radioimmunoassay kit. **B,** TSH radioimmunoassay standard curve, with reagents prepared in the laboratory. Antigen and antiserum were obtained from NPA (National Pituitary Agency, National Institute of Arthritis and Metabolic Diseases). (Double antibody separation technique.)   *Continued.*

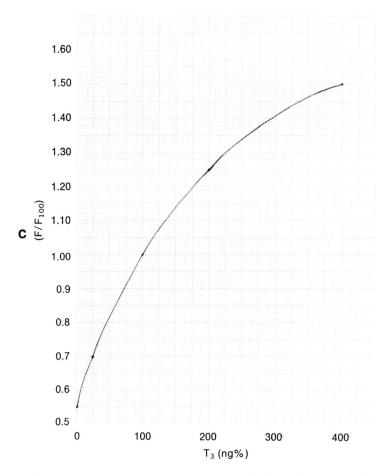

Fig. 30-3, cont'd. C, T_3 radioimmunoassay standard curve, obtained with Nuclear Diagnostics T3 RIA-STAT kit. Note that the dose-response curve is different in each case.

When logit (y) is plotted against the log concentration of the antigen, a linear dose-response curve results for most of the assay systems.[2, 3] Dose-response curves that are essentially linear can also be obtained by plotting $F/B - F_0/B_0$ against the antigen concentration on a log-log graph. Computer programs are now available to analyze the data and present the assay results, together with the associated error.

KINETICS

A knowledge of the basic kinetics involved in the antigen/antibody reaction is necessary for a clear understanding of radioimmunoassay test principles. We shall begin with the simplest possible system with the following assumption: that the antigen and antibody are univalent. This means that one antigen can react with one and only one molecule of antibody. This assumption seems very unrealistic because it has been established that antibodies are bivalent and antigens are multivalent. However, with this assumption for the sake of simplicity, the reaction between antigen and antibody can be represented as follows:

$$Ag + Ab \underset{K_2}{\overset{K_1}{\rightleftharpoons}} Ag \cdot Ab \qquad (30\text{-}1)$$

Where:

K_1 = Rate constant for association
K_2 = Rate constant for dissociation

According to the law of mass action, the equilibrium constant or the affinity constant K then becomes:

$$K = \frac{K_1}{K_2} = \frac{(AgAb)}{(Ag)(Ab)} \qquad (30\text{-}2)$$

Where:

(Ag) = Molar concentration of free antigen
(Ab) = Molar concentration of free antibody
$(AgAb)$ = Molar concentration of antigen-antibody complex

At equilibrium the ratio of bound antigen (B) to free antigen (F) is given as follows:

$$\frac{B}{F} = \frac{(AgAb)}{(Ag)} \qquad (30\text{-}3)$$

It is clear from formulas 30-2 and 30-3 that

$$\frac{B}{F} = K \cdot (Ab) \qquad (30\text{-}4)$$

and, expanding,

$$\frac{B}{F} = K\left[(Ab_0) - B\right] \qquad (30\text{-}5)$$

Where:

(Ab_0) = Initial concentration of antibody

If we represent the fraction of the bound antigen component by b, we can write the following:

$$B = b (Ag_0)$$

Where:

(Ag_0) = Initial or total antigen concentration

Therefore, from formulas 30-5 and 30-6 it can be concluded that B/F decreases as $b (Ag_0)$ increases.

However, since b cannot exceed 1, the reduction in B cannot be noticeable if (Ag_0) is much less than (Ab_0). Therefore, to be able to detect a hormone of concentration (H), it is essential that (Ab_0) be a value not much higher than (H).

From formula 30-5 it can be seen that there is a linear relationship between the B/F ratio and the concentration of the bound antigen (B). A graphic representation of formula 30-5 — a plot of the B/F ratio versus bound antigen (B) — is known as the *Scatchard plot*. The Scatchard plot can be used to estimate the affinity constant (K) and the total concentration of the antibody binding sites (Ab_0) from the experimental results. The slope of the straight line in the Scatchard plot corresponds to $-K$, and the intercept on the horizontal axis corresponds to (Ab_0). The effect of the antibody concentration and the equilibrium constant value on the sensitivity of the assay will be considered in detail later in the chapter.

REQUIREMENTS

Radioimmunoassay involves three components: pure antigen, radiolabeled antigen, and antiserum (antibody). Also, a suitable separation technique is essential to estimate the distribution of radioactivity in the free and bound fractions. In summary, the essential requirements for any radioimmunoassay can be listed as follows:
1. A highly purified preparation of the antigen
2. Radiolabeled antigen
3. Antiserum with good binding affinity
4. A method for the separation of antigen-antibody complex from the free antigen

The sensitivity of an assay depends to a large extent on the quality of these components and choice of a particular separation technique. Various considerations involved in the preparation of these substances and the methods of separation will be discussed briefly.

Pure antigen

The preparation of standards and tracer and the production of antibodies depends on the availability of pure antigen. Several procedures, such as electrophoresis, chromatoelectrophoresis, gel filtration, ion exchange chromatography, and precipitation by salt and organic solvents, are available for the extraction and purification of hormones from biologic samples. A pure synthetic preparation, if available, can be substituted for the natural preparation. A number of hormones produced synthetically are now available with a purity to match the best materials isolated from natural sources.

In any case, before the antigen, either synthetic or natural, can be used as a standard, the specificity between this antigen and the antigen in the test sample toward the antibody binding sites must be clearly established.

Radiolabeled antigens

A radiolabeled antigen possessing an unimpaired reactivity with an antibody is one of the essential components of any radioimmunoassay test. The sensitivity of an assay is dependent on two factors relating to the antigen. First, the labeled antigen should react with the antibody in the same fashion as does the unlabeled antigen. If a portion of the labeled antigen fails to react with the antibody, then an increased amount of antibody will be required to allow formation of sufficient labeled complex to provide a suitable counting rate. This added antibody, however, will bind a proportionally larger amount of the unlabeled antigen present. As described earlier, the steepest portion of any standard curve will occur where equal numbers of labeled and unlabeled antigen are present for binding by the limited amount of antibody. All ratios either greater or less will fall on a less steep portion of the curve, thus the sensitivity will be reduced. Second, for similar reasons the specific activity of the labeled antigen should be great enough to provide suitable counting rates. If the specific activity is low, then the quantity of labeled antigen present must be high. If the labeled antigen quantity is high, then the antibody quantity must also be high for the same reasons and with the same results just described.

Extremely high specific activities can also present problems. Damage during preparation and self-irradiation during storage can introduce a wide variety of both radioactive and chemical contaminants. Thus it is necessary to make a reasonable compromise between too low a specific activity, with its associated loss of sensitivity, and too high a specific activity, with its molecular damage resulting in a loss of specificity.

Antigen labels

The choice of a radionuclide for labeling purposes is dictated mostly by the availability of a suitable procedure to tag the antigen under study. Radionuclide half-life, specific activity available, and cost are other items that must be considered. ^{3}H and ^{14}C find application in steroid analyses, in which it is convenient to tag these radionuclides into the ring portions of the molecule. The inherent disadvantage in using these isotopes arises from their long half-life and pure beta-emissions. ^{57}Co has found application only in the vitamin B$_2$ radioimmunoassay. ^{75}Se is also used in limited applications.

The most widely used radionuclides in the radioimmunoassay of peptide hormones, viral antigens, and drugs are the isotopes of iodine, ^{125}I and ^{131}I. The incorporation of iodine into polypeptides and proteins that contain tyrosine residues can be easily achieved. For compounds that do not possess tyrosine groups, it might be necessary to attach a tyrosine or a peptide containing tyrosine to achieve iodination. The main advantage of these isotopes is that they can be obtained in higher specific activities than can be found with either ^{3}H or ^{14}C.

¹²⁵I has become the isotope of choice for most compounds in radioimmunoassay. The reasons for preferring ^{125}I over ^{131}I are many:

1. The isotopic abundance of ^{125}I as supplied by many commercial firms is over 96%, whereas the isotopic abundance of a ^{131}I preparation is about 15% to 20%. In other words, when ^{131}I is used for radioiodination, on the average 4 to 6 atoms of nonradioactive [127]I are present for every [131]I. This situation might well result in reducing the immunoreactivity of the labeled antigen.
2. The counting efficiency for ^{125}I is much higher than that for ^{131}I because of the higher energy of the latter.
3. The longer half-life of [125]I (60 days) compared with that of [131]I (8.08 days) prolongs the shelf life of a particular preparation.
4. The handling of ^{125}I presents a lesser health physics problem than the handling of [131]I.

Radioiodination of the antigen

To have a radioimmunoassay test with good sensitivity, the radioiodine-labeled compound used must have a specific activity of 100 to 300 mCi/mg. The early investigators, Yalow and Berson[1] and Samols and Willliams,[4] were successful in preparing substances with such specific activities. However, because of the poor reaction yields, their methods required very high starting activities.

The most commonly used radioiodination technique is the one developed by Hunter and Greenwood,[5] popularly known as the *chloramine-T method*. The procedure is easy and consists simply of adding the protein and the chloramine-T to a solution of sodium iodide (Na[125]I). The mechanism of the reaction is not clearly understood, but it is believed that the chloramine-T forms hypochlorites in water and thus acts as a mild oxidizing agent. The oxidative process is essential in producing the radioiodide ion with a positive charge for substitution onto the tyrosine fraction of the protein molecule.

The amount of chloramine-T required is dictated by the quantity and nature of the protein that is being iodinated. If excess quantity of the oxidizing agent is used, the protein might be damaged. Thus, to prevent such damage, it is advisable to limit both the reaction time and the amount of the oxidizing agent. Hunter and Greenwood reported that one molecule of chloramine-T is required for every one of iodide, when the protein concentration is high and the molar ratio of iodide to protein is maintained high. At lower concentrations of iodide, relatively more chloramine-T is required. Maximum yields were realized by Hunter and Greenwood using as many as 100 molecules of chloramine-T for every iodide at very low concentrations of iodide.

The effect of pH on the iodination of proteins was studied by several workers, and it was shown that there is a fairly sharp pH optimum at a pH of 7.5 for most of the proteins.

For routine iodinations the following procedure is usually adopted:

[125]I, approximately 1 mCi (0.5 to 2 mCi)	10 μl
Sodium phosphate, pH 7.5, 0.5M	10 μl
Hormone, 5 μg (2.5 to 5 μg) in 0.01M phosphate buffer	10 μl
Chloramine-T, 50 μg (30 μg) in 0.01M phosphate buffer	10 μl
Reaction volume	40 μl

These reagents are added rapidly, and the reaction mixture is kept under gentle agitation for about 30 to 45 seconds. At the end of this period 50 mg of reducing agent, sodium bisulfite, in 50 μl of 0.01M buffer is added. This reduces the unreacted iodine back to iodide and brings the reaction to an end. The amount of bisulfite needed is simply the chemical equivalent of the amount of chloramine-T added. It is important to keep the reaction volumes to a practical minimum because the percentage incorporation of iodine is markedly dependent on the concentration of the protein. Separation of the labeled antigen from the unreacted radioiodide, reactants, and damaged proteins is achieved immediately after iodination.

Several techniques, such as adsorption chromatography, thin-layer chromatography, ion-exchange chromatography, electrophoresis, chromatoelectrophoresis, and gel filtration are available for the purification of tagged antigens.

Gel filtration employing Sephadex or Bio-Gel provides a quick and satisfactory separation in most cases. Column preparation is an important part of the purification of the labeled antigens. The selection of the proper type of gel and its packing in the column are points to consider. Often the column must be pretreated with protein such as albumin to saturate the adsorption sites on the gel to reduce nonspecific binding.

An example of the purification of a labeled antigen (^{125}I-labeled TSH) with Sephadex G-75 is shown in the elution pattern illustrated in Fig. 30-4.

The specific activity (expressed as mCi/mg or μCi/μg) and the iodination yields can be estimated by measuring the activity found in various stages during radiolabeling. A comparison of the total activity in the various labeled fractions with the initial starting activity gives the percent recovery (r). The ratio of the activity in the hormone peaks to the total activity recovered represents the iodination yield. Knowing the percent recovery (r), amount of hormone (H) initially used, and radioactivity present in the hormone peak (A$_h$), the specific activity is estimated as follows:

$$\text{Specific activity} = \frac{A_h \text{ (mCi)}}{r \times H \text{ (mg)}}$$

The estimation of yield following iodination is sometimes obtained by precipitating a sample of the reaction mixture with 10% trichloroacetic acid. The ratio of the radioactivity present in the precipitate to the total radioactivity in the sample gives the iodination yield. This ratio is usually known as the TCA factor. When

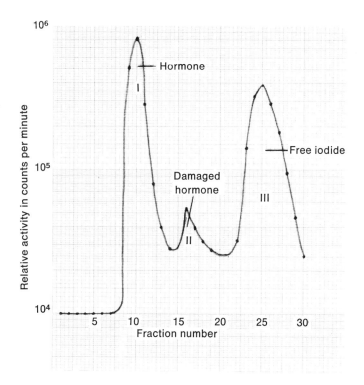

Fig. 30-4. Elution pattern from Sephadex G-75 of the reaction mixture after iodination of TSH. Iodination was carried out by the chloramine-T method. The reaction mixture containing labeled hormone, damaged hormone, and free iodide was loaded on the column. By use of a suitable buffer, the column was eluted and separate fractions collected and counted. Counts versus fraction were plotted on graph paper. The fractions corresponding to those producing the first peak contained the pure hormone; those producing the second and third peaks contained damaged hormone and free iodide, respectively.

the amount of hormone and the radioactivity used in iodination are kept constant, the TCA factor indicates changes in the specific activity of the labeled hormone.

The immunoreactivity of the labeled antigen can be assessed by obtaining a set of antiserum titration curves. For this purpose the radiolabeled antigen alone (for one curve) and then the radiolabeled antigen diluted with the unlabeled antigen (for another curve) are incubated with the antiserum at different dilutions. The antigen concentration is maintained in both cases. Almost identical antiserum curves establish the fact that the iodination process has not caused any damage to the antigen.

ANTISERUM (ANTIBODY)

Antibodies are a group of serum proteins that are also known as *gamma globulins*, or *immunoglobulins*. Antiserum with appropriate *titer*, *specificity*, and *affinity* is one of the basic requirements for the development of a particular radioimmunoassay. It is appropriate to discuss briefly the production, quality assessment, and storage of antiserum.

Production

Production of antiserum involves rather a complex procedure and is characterized more an an art than a science. Antibodies are relatively easily raised against protein compounds of molecular weight in excess of 4,000 to 6,000. For smaller proteins and nonimmunogenic substances such as thyroid and steroid hormones, cyclic nucleotides, and drugs, it is necessary to conjugate the compound to a larger polypeptide or a protein such as albumir., thyroblogulin, or polylysine prior to immunization. It is customary to couple the hapten in such a way as to expose any functional groups characteristic of the molecule, so that the likelihood of production of specific antibodies is enhanced. A variety of chemical procedures are available for the covalent linkage of small molecules to larger molecules.[6-8]

The quality of antiserum prepared against an antigenic hormone depends on several factors, such as the following:
1. Molecular size and chemical composition
2. Timing of injections and bleeding
3. Adjuvant and total dose of immunogen
4. Route of administration
5. Choice of animal species

The general method of inducing antibody formation is to inject into a number of animals the pure antigen mixed with Freund's adjuvant. Based on the view that impurities may have an adjuvant effect, some investigators prefer to immunize with relatively impure material, rather than a highly purified or synthetic equivalent. The selection of animal species (rabbit, guinea pig, sheep, goat, chicken, or monkey) depends on the volume of antisera desired. More important, however, the antigen for which antibodies are desired must be antigenic (foreign) to the animal selected, otherwise antibodies will not form. The techniques for antigenic injections vary according to routes of administration, dose, and frequency. The available evidence suggests that the various routes of administration may be ranked in decreasing order of effectiveness as follows: into the lymph nodes, intraarticular (usually into the knee joint), intradermal, intramuscular, intraperitoneal, subcutaneous, and, finally, intravenous. As with other variables, the sensible course is to select a route of injection to begin with and change to another route later if unsuccessful. In general, 0.2 to 2 mg of the antigenic preparation is injected as a suspension, although in certain cases it may be necessary to use larger quantities. In other cases as little as 20 to 100 μg of the immunogen is sufficient. Antibody response is virtually independent of immunogen dosage over a wide range, once a certain minimum quantity injected is exceeded. Antibody levels rise relatively slowly after a primary injection, reaching a peak about 6 weeks later. Usually, booster doses are not given earlier than 4 weeks after the first injection and repeated once each month thereafter. Antibody levels rise to a maximum about 10 days after each booster injection, and the bleeding of the animals is performed around this period.

Assessment

The assessment of antiserum includes a measurement of titer, effective avidity, and specificity.

Titer. The estimation of titer value of the antiserum is normally obtained from the antiserum titration curves, provided that a labeled antigen of known purity is available. Constant amounts of the labeled antigen are incubated with different dilutions of antiserum, and the distribution of radioactivity between the antibody-bound (B) and free (F) fractions is determined after separation. A plot of B/F or percent bound versus antiserum dilution is known as the antiserum titration, or dilution, curve. The titration curve will indicate the working dilution at which the antiserum should be used. Normally the dilution is chosen so that 40% to 60% of the labeled antigen is bound in the absence of unlabeled antigen. Use of an excess of antibody results in loss of sensitivity, since all the binding sites must be occupied before the unlabeled material being assayed can compete with labeled antigen.

Avidity. Avidity describes the binding affinity and chemical attraction of ligand and binding agent, therefore describing the stability of the resultant complex in terms of binding energy.

Specificity. As mentioned earlier, radioimmunoassay is based on the competition between labeled and unlabeled antigens for a limited number of specific antibody bindings sites. Anything that competes for such sites or in any other way inhibits the binding of labeled antigen by the antibody will influence the measurement. Nonimmunologic factors such as pH, osmolality, high concentration of proteins in plasma, and presence of absorbents like charcoal or Fuller's earth in the incubation mixture can easily affect the assay. Competition for binding sites, other than by the antigen under test, can result when the incubation mixture contains the following:

1. Biologically inactive fragments of the antigen
2. Fragments of the antigen containing only part of the antigenic determinant
3. Other compounds containing structural groups that are identical with or closely related to the antigen

Specificity of the antiserum is assessed by introducing known likely competitors into the reaction mixtures containing the antibody and observing the extent to which they displace the labeled antigen. Even when a particular antiserum is seen to be of poor specificity, it is sometimes possible to obliterate nonspecific antibodies in the antiserum by deliberately introducing large amounts of cross-reacting antigen into the system, thus leaving only antibodies specific to the test antigen to participate in the assay.

Final tests of specificity of the antiserum in the actual assay system as a whole must be carried out on the unknown samples by the preparation of sample dilution curves and the comparison of their slopes with that obtained using the purified standard. Additional checks of assay specificity can be carried out by assaying unknowns with different antibody concentrations. The measurements in all such cases must be identical to establish the validity of assay.

Storage

Antiserum is a precious material in radioimmunoassay technology, and as such every effort should be made to preserve this material in its highest quality. The best way of storing antiserum is in lyophilized (freeze-dried) form. There have been reports indicating that the freeze-dried antiserum suffers a loss of 20% to 30% in its original titer value. Nevertheless, once it has been freeze dried, the titer value remains absolutely constant. Freeze drying whole serum is considered better than freeze drying the antibody extracts. The next alternative is to store the serum at 0° C. It is desirable to freeze even the diluted antiserum, until there is substantial evidence to indicate that the antiserum at the working dilutions does not show any loss of activity after being kept at 4° C for a prolonged period. In all these instances repeated freezing and thawing is to be avoided. Another most promising method for preserving antibodies is the use of insoluble solid polymers. To accomplish this, a coupling between the antibodes and solid bodies such as cyanogen bromide, activated Sephadex, or polyacrylamide gel particles is performed. In this form the antibodies will be preserved for an indefinite length of time. These methods not only help solve the storage problems and improve the stability of antibodies but also provide an easy means for separation of the *bound* labeled antigen from the *free*.

SEPARATION TECHNIQUES

The last and very important requirement for a good radioimmunoassay test is a reliable technique for clean and rapid separation of the antigen-antibody complex from the free antigen. An ideal separation must meet the following requirements:
1. Give a clean separation of the free and bound fractions
2. Be reproducible
3. Be independent of nonspecific factors
4. Be able to handle large volumes of the incubate
5. Be simple and inexpensive

A great variety of methods have been developed and used successfully. However, there is no single system that is universally applicable for all tests and that satisfies even the majority of the requirements just cited. Each separation technique has its particular advantages and disadvantages. Some of the well-adapted methods are discussed here under the following categories: (1) electrophoresis and chromatoelectrophoresis, (2) gel filtration, (3) solid-phase adsorption of antigen, (4) solid-phase adsorption of antibody, (5) immunoprecipitation using a second antibody, and (6) fractional precipitation using neutral salts or organic solvents.

Electrophoresis

Simple electrophoresis is based on the unequal migration of bound and free fractions in the presence of an electric field. Neither component can have appreciable affinity for the support medium. The disadvantage with this method is that separation is not complete and the time required is rather long, sometimes extending into several hours.

Chromatoelectrophoresis

Chromatoelectrophoresis is an improvement over simple electrophoresis. This method combines the principles of separation by electrophoresis as well as separation by paper chromatography. Paper strips that have a high affinity for free antigen are suitable for this technique. Free antigen binds firmly at the point of application, whereas the complex AgAb is displaced primarily by the hydrodynamic flow. The application of an electric field accelerates the flow and sharpens the resolution. The time required for this type of separation is around 30 minutes. After the separation is completed, the strips are dried and the radioactivity counted using a strip counter.

Chromatoelectrophoresis is a highly reliable method, providing excellent separation of the free and bound fractions. Hormone damaged in iodination of incubation will usually not bind to the paper and can easily be recognized on the strip as a separation component. However, there are certain practical disadvantages that make this method unsuitable for routine radioimmunoassay procedure. The sensitivity of these assays is very much restricted because the amount of material that can be applied onto the paper is limited. The separation is laborious and time consuming (although short compared to simple electrophoresis) and often demands a cold room. High specific activities of the labeled antigen are required for accurate counting. Strip counters add to the expense.

Gel filtration

Gel filtration is also based on unequal migration of bound and free fractions. Because of the difference in their size, free and antibody-bound antigens will migrate through cross-linked dextrans (Sephadex) at different rates, thus providing a clean separation. Although theoretically very attractive, this method is not convenient because the preparation of individual columns demands meticulous care and consumes a great deal of time. Also, the collection of eluates from the columns requires constant technician attention or expensive automatic fraction collectors.

Solid-phase absorption of antigen

Separations by solid-phase precipitation are based on the ability of certain absorbing substances such as charcoal, talc, Florisil, and certain resins to bind most peptide hormones and steroids instantaneously. These methods are very popular because of their simplicity, economy, speed, and reproducibility. Ideally the absorbent should not possess any affinity for the antigen-antibody complex. However, all the adsorbents just mentioned show some affinity for the complexes, which can be reduced by prior treatment of the adsorbent. Too low a concentration of plasma protein will cause some of the antibody to be adsorbed, whereas an excess of plasma proteins often leads to decreased adsorption of the antigen. Thus a balanced proportion of these proteins and the adsorbent becomes a primary requisite for a good separation.

Many radioimmunoassays utilize charcoal coated with dextrans of molecular weights from 10,000 to 250,000, depending on the size of the hormone to be assayed. The dextrans coat the surface of the activated charcoal and act as a sieve. Larger molecules such as antigen-antibody complexes cannot penetrate the dextran coating and get into the interstices of the charcoal and thus cannot be adsorbed. In contrast, the smaller molecules like free antigen can penetrate into the interstices, where they can be taken up by a large internal adsorbing area of the activated charcoal. Simply by adding a suitable amount of the dextran-coated charcoal at the end of the incubation period to the reagent mixture containing antibody, labeled antigen, and unlabeled antigen, it is possible to remove all the free antigen from the solution. After centrifugation, all the radioactivity present in the supernatant represents antibody bound to antigen. At the same time the unbound antigen appears in the charcoal precipitate. The radioactivity present in either one or both of the fractions can be counted, and the B/F ratio or the percent bound can be calculated.

The adsorption methods for the separation of the free from the bound clearly reveal the relative ratio of bound-to-free labeled hormone, but in no case can it be assumed that they give an absolute separation. There have been many reports indicating that the supernatant fraction, following the dextran-coated charcoal (DCC) separation, contains labeled hormone. Chromatoelectrophoresis was used in all these cases to establish the presence of the undamaged hormone in the supernatant. An incomplete separation of the free tracer from other fractions does not necessarily invalidate the assay results, as long as the relative changes in the B/F ratio in the standards and the unknowns are fully appreciated.

Solid-phase antibody systems

Antigens and antibodies can be coupled chemically to an insoluble matrix with the retention of immunologic reactivity. These solid-phase antibody techniques utilize antibodies covalently linked to insoluable polymers, covalently cross-linked to one another, or physically adsorbed to a plastic. In this system the antibody-bound antigen always presents in the solid phase, whereas the unbound antigen remains in the solution. In this way separation can be accomplished by simple decantation or centrifugation. Binding of the antigen in most cases is rapid and virtually irreversible. To obtain a reliable radioimmunoassay, it is essential that the immunoadsorbents retain their immunoreactivity for long periods during dry storage. At the same time it is necessary that the same amount of immunoadsorbent be found in each tube. There are different forms of solid-phase system. Examples are fine particles, thin discs, and plastic tubes. This separation technique was originally developed and extensively applied by Catt and associates,[9, 10] and by Wide and Porath.[11] For a detailed account of activation of the polymers, coupling of the antibodies, and optimization of the assay, the reader is advised to refer to the article by Wide and Porath. In its simplest form a radioimmunoassay test using the solid-phase coupled antibodies is in no way different from that using simple antibodies. The amount of labeled antigen and coupled antibodies is chosen in such a way that there will be about 30% to 40% binding of the labeled antigen to the antibodies within a reasonable length of time. It is desirable to keep the reagent mixture under constant agitation during incubation. At the end of incubation the bound and free components are separated by simple centrifugation or decanting or both. A simple washing with a suitable buffer solution will be sufficient in the case of antibody-coated plastic tubes.

Double antibody method

The separation of the antigen and antigen-antibody complex by precipitating with a second antibody was reported first by Utiger and associates.[12] In this method the second antibody used to precipitate the bound component is produced against the gamma globulin of the species used to raise the antihormone serum. The original complex AgAb normally appears as a soluble component and cannot be precipitated by centrifugation even at very high g values. On the other hand, the complex formed after the addition of the second antibody becomes large enough so that it can be separated by centrifugation and decanting. The flow chart for the simple and most widely used method is shown on the opposite page.

The reaction mixture containing Ag, Ag*, and the first antibody Ab_1 is incubated long enough for the primary reaction to attain equilibrium. The second antibody is added in excess and incubated for a further period to get 100% binding of the complex, after which the tubes are centrifuged. The supernatant containing the free hormone fraction is then decanted, and the tubes containing the doubly bound hormone as a precipitate are used to estimate the bound activity. When carried out in this way, there will always appear a considerable nonspecific trapping of the free hormone in the precipitate. However, a wash with a proper diluent

---

*Antigen labeled with radiotracer.

RIA sequence with double antibody separation

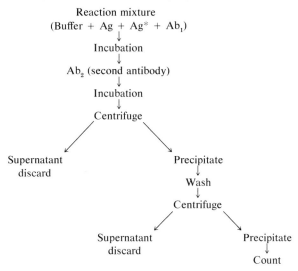

and a repeat centrifugation followed by decanting would reduce the portion of free hormone appearing in the bound component to less than 2%.

The advantages of this method include the following: (1) there is a clean separation of the bound from the free, (2) large volumes of the incubating mixture can be handled, and (3) it can be used practically for any radioimmunoassay. The disadvantages include cost of the second antibody and increase in error because of added handling.

Because of the large amount of precipitating antiserum required to achieve 100% binding of the primary complex in a reasonable length of time, the second antibody is usually produced in larger animals (sheep, goat, donkey) against the gamma globulin of the animal used to induce the first antibody. Rabbits are generally the animals of choice for raising antibodies against most peptide hormones. Since the second antibody is produced against the rabbit gamma globulin, it is called *antirabbit gamma globulin* (anti-RGG). In addition, the speed of precipitation depends on the concentration of the antibody; therefore, it must invariably be concentrated either by salt precipitation or simple DEAE chromatography before it is used in an assay.

Inhibition of the precipitation by the second antibody can be affected by a number of constituents of plasma or serum and may give rise to falsely elevated values in any assay. However, plasma may actually increase the efficiency of precipitation in double antibody separation systems.[13] The promotor of immunopre-

---

*Antigen labeled with radiotracer.

cipitin in human serum has not been clearly identified. However, the effect of serum proteins can be markedly reduced by using the precipitating serum at its optimal dilution. If the problem persists, further improvement can be expected by the use of a diluent containing polyvinyl pyrrolidone (PVP) at a final concentration of 4% in the incubating mixture. In certain cases, when all these efforts fail, it may be necessary to equalize the concentration of plasma throughout all the assay tubes, including those containing the standards.

The second antibody may cross-react with the human gamma globulin. Although the cross-reaction is slight, sometimes it is desirable to balance these effects by the addition of increasing quantities of nonimmune rabbit serum.

Recognition of immunologic damage to labeled hormone during iodination and incubation is difficult to detect with the double antibody method. In general, the double antibody method presents incubation damage as a diminished percentage of bound hormone and will be interpreted as real hormone. The quality of labeled hormone is critical for the successful use of the double antibody technique. To make sure that the quality of the labeled hormone is satisfactory, the purification of the labeled hormone just before introducing it into an assay system is suggested as an additional procedural step.

Fractional precipitation

Fractional precipitation is based on the nonspecific precipitation of antigen-antibody complex under conditions that leave the labeled antigen in solution. Neutral salts such as sodium sulfite and ammonium sulfate and organic solvents such as ethanol have been tried by various investigators. Mostly because significant free antigen is trapped in the precipitate, this method has not gained any practical importance in routine assays.

PROCEDURE

A major step in making radioimmunoassay work is the reagent preparation and optimizing the working concentration of these reagents. Once this is achieved, the rest of the procedure is quite simple. However, there are a number of quality control checks required to establish the validity of an assay.

The general procedure consists of adding suitable quantities of standards, unknowns, labeled antigen, and antibodies to a buffer solution and allowing the reaction to reach equilibrium. Most of the competitive binding assays are of equilibrium type, in which all the reagents are added at the same time and the reaction is allowed to proceed until equilibrium is established. In some cases it might be necessary to add the tracer at a late stage to improve the sensitivity. This type is known as the sequential saturation analysis. At the end of the incubation period the free and bound fractions are separated using a suitable technique. The distribution of radioactivity in each sample is determined by counting either *free* or *bound* or *both* with the use of suitable counting equipment. The estimation of antigen concentration is made by comparing the inhibition observed in the unknown with that produced by standard solutions of known antigen concentration. For this purpose the dose-response curves are plotted using the data from the standard tubes, and the antigen concentration present is read directly from the graph.

All the radioimmunoassay procedures must be thoroughly checked for any nonspecific interactions and identity between the standards and unknowns established before they can be routinely adopted. Immunologic identity between the unknown samples and the standards can be examined by using multiple dilutions of an unknown sample in an assay. These dilutions can be compared with the curve prepared from the standards. A close parallellism between these will establish immunologic identity.

Another important factor to be examined is *reproducibility*. This reveals to what extent the reagents are stable. A control sample must be included each time an assay is performed. The estimated values from different assays must lie within 10% of the average.

Although attractive and finding increasing acceptance, radioimmunoassay is not without problems. The problems mainly arise from instability of the reagents, lack of reference standards, physiologic factors, and methodologic differences. As these problems are overcome, reliable assays of minute quantities of serum-borne substances will be practical in all laboratories.

REFERENCES

1. Yalow, R. S., and Berson, S. A.: Immunoassay of endogenous plasma insulin in man, J. Clin. Invest. **39**:1157, 1960.
2. Rodbard, D., Rayford, P. L., Cooper, J. A., and Ross, G. T.: Statistical quality control of radioimmunoassays, J. Clin. Endocrinol. **28**:1412, 1968.
3. Rodbard, D., Bridson, W., and Rayford, P. L.: Rapid calculation of radioimmunoassay results, J. Lab. Clin. Med. **74**:770, 1969.
4. Samols, E., and Williams, H. S.: Trace labelling of insulin with iodine, Nature **190**:1211, 1961.
5. Hunter, W. M., and Greenwood, F. C.: Preparation of iodine-131 labelled human growth hormone of high specific activity, Nature **194**:495, 1962.
6. Deodhar, S.: Immunologic production of angiotensin. I. Preparation of angiotensin protein complex antigen, J. Exp. Med **111**:419, 1960.
7. Goodfriend, T. L., Levine, L., and Fasman, G. D.: Antibodies to bradykinin and angiotensin, a use of carbodiimides in immunology, Science **144**:1344, 1964.
8. Abraham, G. E., and Grover, P. K.: Covalent linkage of hormonal haptens to protein carriers for use in radioimmunoassay. In Odell, W. D., and Daughaday, W. H., editors: Principles of competitive protein-binding assays, Philadelphia, 1971, J. B. Lippincott Co.
9. Catt, K., Niall, H. D., and Treager, G. W.: Solid-phase radioimmunoassay of human growth hormone, J. Lab. Clin. Med. **70**:820, 1967.
10. Catt, K. J., Niall, H. D., and Treager, G. W.: A disc method for solid phase radioimmunoassay of proteins, Aust. J. Exp. Biol. Med. Sci. **45**:703, 1967.
11. Wide, L., and Porath, J.: Radioimmunoassay of proteins with the use of Sephadex-coupled antibodies, Biochem. Biophys. Acta **130**:257, 1966.
12. Utiger, R. F., Parker, M. L., and Daughaday, W. H.: Studies on human growth hormone: a radioimmunoassay for human growth hormone, J. Clin. Invest. **41**:254, 1962.
13. Burr, I. M., Grant, D. B., Sizonenko, P. C., Kaplan, S. L., and Grumbach, M. M.: Some critical factors in double antibody radioimmunoassay systems utilizing sheep anti-rabbit precipitating sera for measurement of human serum LH, FSH and HGH, J. Clin. Endocrinol. **29**:948, 1969.

BIBLIOGRAPHY

Berson, S. A., and Yalow, R. S.: Assay of plasma insulin in human subjects by immunological methods, Nature **184:**1648, 1959.

Collip, J. B., and Anderson, E. M.: The production of serum inhibitory to the thyrotropic hormone, Lancet **226:**76, 1934.

Ekins, R. P.: The estimation of thyroxine in human plasma by an electrophoretic technic, Clin. Chim. Acta **5:**453, 1960.

Ekins, R. P.: Radioimmunoassay, protein-binding assay and other saturation assay technics, Year Book of Nuclear Medicine, Chicago, 1973, Year Book Medical Publishers, Inc.

Hunter, W. M.: The preparation and assessment of iodinated antigens. In Kirkham, K. E., and Hunter, W. M., editors: Radioimmunoassay methods, Baltimore, 1971, The Williams & Wilkins Co.

In vitro procedures with radioisotopes in medicine, Vienna, 1970, International Atomic Energy Agency.

Odell, W. D., and Daughaday, W. H., editors: Principles of competitive protein-binding assays, Philadelphia, 1971, J. B. Lippincott Co.

Radioisotopes in medicine: in vitro studies, Conf. 671111, Oak Ridge, Tenn., 1968, U. S. Atomic Energy Commission.

Smith, T. W., Butler, V. P., and Haber, E.: Determination of therapeutic and toxic serum concentrations by radioimmunoassay, N. Engl. J. Med. **281:**1212, 1969.

31 Radionuclide therapy

James H. Larose, M.D., M.M.Sc.

TREATMENT OF HYPERTHYROIDISM
Graves' disease

Graves' disease is an autoimmune condition of the thyroid manifest by thyrotoxicosis, a diffusely enlarged gland, and a probable (80% if the gamma globulin fraction is concentrated) positive long-acting thyroid stimulator (LATS) titer. Therapy is designed to temporarily suppress secretion of thyroid hormone into plasma. If successful, the derangement driving the thyroid into uncontrolled secretory activity seems to abate and in months or years the gland is able to reestablish a normal homeostatic relationship with the pituitary and to supply the body with physiologic amounts of thyroid hormone.

Nonradioactive *iodine* immediately inhibits the release of thyroid hormone from the gland. Unfortunately, its effectiveness in controlling thyrotoxicosis is only partial and frequently not sustained. It is also used preoperatively to decrease the vascularity of the thyroid gland. *Propylthiouracil* (PTU) inhibits the synthesis of thyroid hormone but does not affect the storage or release of preformed thyroid hormone. This explains the delayed onset of clinical change in many cases. Prolonged remission has been reported in 45% to 72% of patients who received long-term therapy (follow-up period of 4 years or more). *Methimazole* (Tapazole) is at least ten times more potent than PTU and therefore is given in proportionately lower doses. Neither drug has an overwhelming advantage over the other. *Guanethidine* (Ismelin) and *reserpine* are useful adjuncts in thyrotoxicosis and thyrotoxic crisis. They do not affect the hyperactivity of the thyroid gland but do decrease the accompanying increased adrenergic activity. This action relieves tachycardia, palpitation, and hypertension and may help prevent cardiac decompensation. Similarly, *propranolol* (Inderal), by virtue of its ability to completely block beta-adrenergic receptors, also has been advocated as an adjunct in the treatment of thyrotoxicosis. One advantage of this regimen is the prompt symptomatic improvement in all patients.

Radioiodine (^{131}I) is an acceptable method of treatment in practically all adults with Graves' disease except those who are pregnant or lactating. Since the average range of the beta particles in tissue is 0.5 mm, there is no significant extrathyroidal radiation. There are only two reports of possible injury to parathyroid glands or other perithyroidal tissues. Salivary gland amylase has been noted to be depressed temporarily after radioiodine therapy. This can be substantially reduced by administering 0.4 mg atropine along with the radioiodine dose to decrease iodine accumulation in the salivary glands. It is probably safe to treat females during or shortly after their menstrual periods. The radioiodine dose can be delivered either in one dose or in small doses at short intervals. The administration of 2 mCi every few weeks until clinical cure is to be frowned on for the following reasons:

1. The radioiodine dose is not fully delivered to the thyroid in the first few weeks, and it is a bad policy to retreat before the total effect of the first dose has been evaluated.
2. Subsequent doses of radioiodine are always less effective because of the decreased uptake.

The preferred method of treatment is with a single dose and is frequently designed to deliver 80 to 100 μCi per gm of thyroid tissue to the gland at 24 hours.[1]

$$D\ (\mu Ci) = \frac{(80\ \mu Ci/gm)\ (gram\ weight\ of\ gland)}{24\text{-}hr\ radioiodine\ uptake\ as\ fraction}$$

$$D\ (\mu Ci) = \frac{80\ \mu Ci/gm \times 45\ gm\ estimated\ gland}{0.45}$$

$$Dose = 8,000\ \mu Ci$$

If the glands are greater than 50 gm, then the dose for that part of the gland over 50 gm should be cut to 40 μCi/gm. Some practitioners prefer to deliver 3.2 mCi to the gland, which is essentially the same technique just mentioned except that all glands are assumed to be approximately 40 gm. Reevaluation should take place in 2 to 3 months after the first dose, and the decision to retreat should be a clinical and not a laboratory decision.

Toxic nodular goiter

There is no uniform agreement about the role of radioiodine therapy in *toxic nodular goiter*. Dose calculations are less accurate here than for Graves' disease because (1) the iodine uptake is irregularly distributed, and many of the nodules will receive little or no radiation because of a low uptake: (2) there is difficulty in estimating the gland size because of the irregularity and frequent retrotracheal and substernal extensions; and (3) relapses are more likely to occur in this disease. Hamburger and co-workers[2] suggest treating "small glands" with 8 mCi retained in the gland and the largest glands with up to 20 mCi retention, with administered doses of 20 to 50 mCi.

Thyrocardiac symptoms are particularly troublesome in Plummer's disease, *true autonomous toxic nodular goiter*. An initial retained dose of 20 mCi has been suggested by Skillern and co-workers.[3] Myxedema is seldom seen after radioiodine therapy because the normal suppressed gland gets little radiation.

Euthyroid heart disease

Radioiodine is used intermittently in the treatment of *euthyroid heart disease.* It was shown in the early 1930s that relief of angina pectoris could be obtained in thyrotoxic patients by surgical thyroidectomy. Surgery and later antithyroid drugs were shown to alleviate both congestive failure and angina in patients with euthyroid status. Blumgart and associates[4, 5] introduced radioiodine therapy to produce a relative hypothyrodism in an attempt to decrease the work on the heart. They also showed in five autopsy cases that the incidence of atheroma was not increased in these patients, followed up from 1 to 11 years. Supraventricular tachyrhythmias are also successfully treated with this technique.[6] The atrium appears hypersensitive to thyroid hormone or an imbalance in the free-to-bound thyroid ratios as can be produced by decreased TBG levels. This mode of therapy fell into disuse with the introduction of propranolol, a beta adrenergic blocking agent. Currently, only an occasional patient breaks out of control with propranolol and is referred for radioiodine therapy.

• • •

The *Cooperative Thyrotoxicosis Therapy Follow-up Study* of over 36,000 treated hyperthyroid patients[7] showed an age-adjusted leukemia incidence of 11 per 100,000 patient years for radioiodine-treated patients and 14 per 100,000 patient years in patients treated with surgical thyroidectomy. Radiododine therapy delivered about 13 to 14 rads to the total body in these cases. This finding is consistent with the two other existing dose-effect studies of radiation leukemogenesis in human adults (that is, the atomic bomb survivors and ankylosing spondylitis studies). All three studies fail to demonstrate induction of leukemia at low total-body doses of irradiation.

Lima and his group[8] have just reported the fourth case of thyroid cancer after iodine 131 therapy of hyperthyroidism. This was a follicular carcinoma that was found 4 years after the start of therapy. All four cases were in females and developed 2 to 10 years after the beginning of therapy.

THYROID CARCINOMA

Thyroid carcinoma is a relatively rare disease, occuring with an incidence of 3.9 cases per 100,000 population per year in the United States. This is an increase from the incidence reported by the Second National Cancer Survey in 1947, when the occurrence rate was 2.4 per 100,000 population. This is at least partially a result of radiation-induced carcinoma.

For several decades, beginning in the 1920s, radiation therapy was considered good medical practice and very effective treatment for patients with such conditions as enlargement of the thymus gland, hypertrophy of tonsils and adenoids, deafness caused by hypertrophied lymphoid tissue around the eustachian tubes, cervical adenitis, hemangiomas of the head and neck, tinea capitus, and acne.

A linkage of thyroid tumors with prior irradiation was not recognized until these tumors began to be diagnosed with increasing frequency in individuals more than 5 years after their initial treatments.

It is now recognized that the effect of these treatments continues into adult life, and intervals of more than 35 years between irradiation and diagnosis have now been recorded.[9]

The majority of thyroid carcinomas are likely to be fully removable by surgery, which further reduces the frequency that they will be seen by the nuclear medic. These carcinomas are very frequently well differentiated, which has led to confusion and the introduction of self-contradicting terms such as "benign metastasizing thyroid" and "lateral aberrant thyroid." The thyroid is an embryologically midline organ, and it is the general consensus currently that any lateral tissue is a metastasis. Fortunately, radioiodine has been found to concentrate in over 50% of the carcinomas and probably in about 80% of all adenocarcinomas of the thyroid, provided that tests are made at times up to 4 months or more after total ablation of all normal thyroid tissue. Not just the follicular but also the papillary carcinomas have been shown to accumulate radioiodine. The undifferentiated, medullary, and Hürthle cell carcinomas rarely concentrate efficiently, nor do they respond to radioiodine therapy. A few adenocarcinomas have been shown to be autonomous, that is, to concentrate radioiodine in the presence of normal functioning thyroid tissue. Usually uptake develops only after removal or ablation of all normal thyroid tissue. Radioiodine therapy should be attempted no matter what the uptake or histopathology shows, since radiosensitivity does not correlate with iodine uptake, a biopsy showing an undifferentiated carcinoma may be incomplete, and a treatable adenocarcinoma may also be present.

When a histologically differentiated tumor is found by biopsy or at operation, it is now common surgical practice to attempt a total thyroidectomy as well as a total removal of recognizable thyroid tissue, since any intrathyroidal or multicentric tumor development is thereby dealt with and since radioiodine uptake is accelerated in any tumor tissue that remains. Some clinics prefer a hemithyroidectomy followed by radioiodine ablation (80 to 100 mCi) of the remaining normal functioning thyroid tissue to reduce the indicence of hypoparathyrodism. After removal of the normal thyroid tissue, Pochin[10] prefers to treat thyroid adeniocarcinomas with repeated doses of 150 mCi[131]I. He typically uses 3 to 7 therapeutic doses given over a course of 2 to 5 years before all clinical and counting evidence of remaining tumor tissue is abolished. Quantitative information can probably best be obtained by determination of the percentage of the administered dose that is organically bound in plasma taken 6 days after the dose is given. This protein-bound iodine concentration appears in the absence of normal thyroid tissue to parallel the remaining amount of functioning tumor tissue and the process of its destruction during treatment, in the same way as do the more direct measures of tumor uptake. It has the added merits of summing the activity of all functioning tumor deposits, however disseminated, and of distinguishing between apparent retention produced by physiologic sites of iodine concentration and organic synthesis occurring in tumor tissue. If normal thyroid tissue has been ablated, remaining tumor activity is likely if the protein-bound (PB)[131]I exceeds 0.006% per liter and certainly if it exceeds 0.010% per liter, but is unlikely with values below 0.003% per liter. Counting urinary radioiodine for 7 days is not a feasible method of determining retention.

Marrow depression is found to be uncommon on normal dosage regimens except when bone metastases are present. In these cases longer intervals between doses, at least after the first few doses, are desirable.

Patients are treated with replacement doses of thyroxine during the 3, 6, or 12 months between radioiodine doses. This is discontinued 4 weeks before each dose (2 weeks if the patient is maintained on triiodothyronine) and resumed 2 days after it. Tracer doses of 1 to 5 mCi are given, occasionally, with TSH, to exclude recurrence with the scanning or counting techniques. Care must be taken to use TSH only occasionally, since this material is extracted from bovine pituitary. Repeated doses have been known to occasionally cause sloughing at the injection site.

A retrospective study of 33 children and adolescents treated with large doses of ^{131}I for thyroid cancer has shown no subsequent detrimental effect on their fertility or birth histories.[11]

Another retrospective study has suggested that the prevalence of breast cancer is higher in women receiving thyroid hormone therapy than those who do not receive this therapy. Several prospective studies are currently trying to clarify some of the incompletely documented aspects of this study.[12]

POLYCYTHEMIA VERA

Polycythemia vera is a chronic hematologic disorder characterized by increased proliferative activity of erythroid, myeloid, megakaryocytic, and fibroblastic cell lines. The early and erythrocytotic phase often progresses through a phase of myelofibrosis with myeloid metaplasia (MMM), which is also called the *spent phase* and is marked by anemia, a leukoerythrobastic blood picture, and hepatosplenomegaly. This eventually progresses to an accelerated malignant phase indistinguishable from acute myeloblastic leukemia (AML). An elevated hematocrit, hemoglobin, or RBC count does not suffice for a diagnosis of true erythrocytosis. An absolute increase in the red cell mass can be determined only by direct measurement using ^{51}Cr- (or ^{32}P-) labeled autologous erythrocytes. The presence of a compensatory erythrocytosis resulting from tissue hypoxia must be ruled out by the demonstration of a normal arterial O_2 concentration in the absence of an abnormal hemoglobin with increased O_2 affinity or diminished O_2-carrying capacity. The presence of erythropoietin-secreting tumors must be ruled out. Once these possibilities have been eliminated, confirmatory evidence of a panmyelosis must be obtained, including the finding of splenomegaly or two or more of the following: leukocytosis greater than 12,000, thrombocytosis greater than 400,000, elevated leukocyte alkaline phosphates, or elevated serum unsaturated B_{12} binding capacity.[13]

After confirmation of the disease process, 3 to 5 mCi of radiophosphate are injected intravenously. Patients are reevaluated at 10 to 12 weeks, and this dose is repeated if the patient's clinical status and laboratory data so indicate. This period of time is necessary because the circulating red cells normally disappear from the circulation so slowly that a significant change could not be expected at an earlier time. A single course of therapy may induce a remission lasting several years. The ^{32}P dose probably should not exceed 6 mCi during any 6-month period. Treatment with ^{32}P should preferably not be used if the platelet count is less than 15,000, the reticulocyte count less than 0.2%, or the blood cell count less than 3,000. In 1969 Lawrence's group[14] reviewed their 181 patients treated with ^{32}P and observed to termination. Fourteen percent developed an acute myelogenous leukemia-like state, and 25% developed significant splenic myeloid metaplasia. These investigators believe that the increased incidence of both acute leukemia and splenic myeloid metaplasia was a result of prolonged survival, since these patients were younger at the time of diagnosis and survived longer than those ^{32}P-treated patients who died of causes other than myeloid metaplasia or acute leukemia. The massive retrospective survey of Modan and Lilienfeld[15] noted an 11% incidence of acute leukemia in ^{32}P-treated patients and an 8.9% incidence in x-irradiated subjects. The significance of the less than 1% incidence of acute leukemia in the nonirradiated treated group is subject to the limitations they so ably discuss— improper diagnostic criteria, lack of selection of comparable cases, differences in quality of medical care, and frequency in duration in follow-up visits. No one has yet proved the speculation that the risk of acute leukemia is increased in irradiated patients. A *Polycythemia Vera Cooperative Study* is currently in progress under the sponsorship of the National Cancer Institute. Spiers and co-workers[16] have calculated the total absorbed dose to marrow in trabecular bone at 24 rads per mCi of phosphorus 32 injected.

INTRACAVITARY USE OF RADIOACTIVE COLLOIDS

The control of recurrent effusions in the pleural and periotoneal cavities that result from a malignant disease presents a serious and difficult problem. Not only is the repeated drainage of these cavities an uncomfortable procedure for the patient, but also usually it has to be repeated at frequent intervals with resulting loss of vital body proteins. Crystalloid solutions are not suitable for this purpose because they are absorbed into the bloodstream, thus subjecting the patient to significant total body radiation. Colloids introduced into the cavity are first engulfed by the floating macrophages and then fixed by the tissue macrophages lining the wall of the serous cavity. Some of the material reaches the local lymph nodes to be deposited there.

Colloidal gold 198 was initially chosen because it had both beta and gamma radiation. The beta radiation provided the therapy, and the gamma radiation allowed determination of the spatial distribution of the radiocolloid. The difficulty with the gold colloid is the exposure risk to the personnel administering this material. The mechanism of action of the radiocolloids is fibrosis of the mesothelium and small blood vessels and a direct action on the free tumor cells in the fluid and the tumor seedings along the pleura.

Colloidal chromic phosphate ($Cr^{32}PO_4$) has been used extensively in recurrent neoplastic effusions with a response rate of over 50% in several series. Radiophosphorus is preferred over radiogold because it is less expensive, has a longer physical half-life, and is a pure beta emitter. Radiogold (^{198}Au) has fallen into disuse because of cost, its short half-life, and FDA regulations that demand that a patient remain in the hospital until the dose in the body has decayed to not more than 30 mCi. (This applies to both living and deceased patients.) Yttrium 90 has been used in doses of 10 to 30 mCi intrapleurally. There is still some difficulty in obtaining a stable colloidal suspension of the yttrium chloride.

Intraperitoneal use of these three radionuclides is essentially the same as intrapleural except that the average dose may be up to twice that used in the pleura. Intrapericardial instillation with 5 mCi of ^{32}P has been used for treatment of recurrent malignant pericardial effusion.

METASTATIC BONE DISEASE

In clinical practice, breast, prostate, bronchial, renal, and thyroid carcinomas account for most of the metastatic bone disease seen. Thyroid carcinoma has been discussed previously. The Maxfields[17] attempted to increase localization of ^{32}P in and around tumors by pretreatment with aqueous testosterone in doses of 100 mg parenterally for 5 days prior to and after therapy with ^{32}P. Autoradiographs of vertebrae showed that there was a 20:1 tumor-to-nontumor ratio produced with this technique. Patients are selected because of (1) relapsed intractable pain after castration and prolonged estrogen therapy, (2) rapid deterioration of the patient's condition as a result of the disease, (3) the need for frequent and high doses of narcotics for relief of pain, and (4) the radiographic evidence of bony metastases. Testosterone has been shown to stimulate the formation of new bone and therefore increase the demand for phosphorus. The differential uptake between tumor and nontumor allows desirable doses to be delivered to the area of the tumor without dangerous levels to the normal tissues, which include the marrow. A partial reason for a lack of marrow depression could be the stimulating effect of testosterone on the marrow proper. On a microscopic level it has been shown that the ^{32}P is taken up in the new bone rather than in the adjacent tumor tissue. This technique has no appreciable effect on soft tissue metastases.

An alternate method of therapy has recently been proposed by Tong,[18] who objects to the testosterone techniques because they reactivate prostate metastases and often intensify the existent bone pain. He injects 100 units of fresh parathyroid extract intramuscularly three times a day for 7 days and forces fluids to prevent any possible renal precipitation of calcium salts. Parathormone acts predominately on the bone and renal tubules. It mobilizes calcium and phosphates out of bone, producing hypercalcemia and hypercalciuria. Simultaneously it lowers the renal tubular threshold for phosphates, causing hypophosphatemia. A rebound occurs 24 hours after withdrawal of parathormone and demonstrates a reverse action. Increased deposition of calcium phosphate in bone associated with a diminished output of calcium and phosphates in the urine takes place. Radiophosphorus in the form of sodium phosphate given at this time will be maximally absorbed. Tong gives three consecutive daily doses (3 mCi, 2 mCi, and 2 mCi). In the second and third weeks 2 mCi are given twice weekly, and in the next 3 weeks 1 mCi is given twice weekly. Vitamin D and calcium gluconate are administered orally during and after the course of radiophosphorus to accelerate deposition of the radiosotope in the unsaturated bone. Intractable bone pain was alleviated in all of his cases which has also been our experience. Pain relief usually occurs 2 to 3 weeks after therapy.

POSTOPERATIVE IRRADIATION OF PTERYGIUM

Surgical ablation is essential in the treatment of pterygium, irrespective of whether the lesion is primary or recurrent after previous treatment. However, an overall 20% to 30% recurrence rate follows surgery alone. To reduce this rate of recurrence, prophylactic postoperative irradiation has been advocated and proved successful in many centers. If beta radiation of low-tissue penetration is used, the dose to the lens is very low and the incidence of radiation cataract is correspondingly reduced to negligible proportions. A series of 1,300 pterygia were reported by van den Brenk,[19] who used a flat, circular ^{90}Sr applicator to the limbus over the bare area produced at surgery. The pterygium received either 800 or 1,000 rads surface dose of beta radiation, respectively, on postoperative days 0,7, and 14. The recurrence rate was reduced to less than 2% as compared to the 25% recurrence rate with 2 doses of 900 rads. Doses of 3 × 1,000 rads often caused a diffuse erythematous reaction at the site or irradiation with some edema and formation of a fibrinous exudate, but this reaction invariably resolved within 1 to 2 weeks of the first dose. Scleral or corneal damage or both occurred in only five cases. No cases of cataract formation were seen.

INTRAVASCULAR PARTICULATE RADIONUCLIDE THERAPY

Local irradiation of tumor tissue has been accomplished by intravascular injection of radionuclide-labeled particles into the vessel supplying the tumor. Yttrium 90 appears to be the most popular radionuclide for this use because it is a pure beta emitter. It has been tagged to microspheres or used as yttrium oxide that has been sieved so that the particle distribution ranges from 50 to 100 μ. This will produce a temporary, diffuse, homogeneous field of radiation within a selected region of the body without resulting in embolic ischemic necrosis. Injection of the radiopharmaceutical is usually preceded by radiopaque angiography so that the catheter can be selectively placed in the vessel that feeds the lesion. This technique has been used only in terminal cases, and in Nolan and Grady's series[20] the median survival was only 4 months. There appears to be continuing modification in techniques and dosage, and this procedure will probably remain experimental until these problems can be more accurately resolved.

Intra-arterial phosphorus 32 radiocolloid has been injected into celiac and superior mesenteric arteries to give prophylactic homogeneous internal hepatic radiotherapy. This is done following placement of the catheter at angiography and obviates having to surgically enter the peritoneum. This enteric intra-arterial injection gives a more homogeneous radiation since there is no streamlining as is seen with injection into the portal vein. It also causes less bone marrow and spleen irradiation than a straight intravenous injection would. This technique has been used prophylactically in patients operated on "for cure" for colon and rectal cancer, since as many as 60% of these patients will have microscopic hepatic metastases at the time of their surgery.[21]

INTRA-ARTICULAR THERAPY

Early clinical studies have shown significant improvement in many patients with chronic effusions associated with rheumatoid arthritis who were treated with intra-artericular injections of yttrium 90. Muller and associates[22] have chosen ^{90}Y because of its short, 2.7-day half-life and primary beta particle radiation that gives a depth penetration of 4 to 5 mm. They use ^{90}Y bound to amorphous silicate particles that are about 100 mm in size and that will be phagocytized rapidly by the synovial cells. A range of 3 to 6 mCi of ^{90}Y was injected into a series of 40 joints. There was complete elimination of effusion in 43% of joints. Skin necrosis occurred in only one case. Statistically significant improvement was noted in pain at rest, pain on motion, pain on starting motion, swelling, and elevated joint temperature. Concurrent oral corticosteroid therapy had no essential influence on the results.

REFERENCES

1. Silver, S.: Radioactive nuclides in medicine and biology, Philadelphia, 1968, Lea & Febiger, p. 168.
2. Hamburger, J. I., Kadian, G., and Rossin, H. W.: Why not radioactive iodine therapy for toxic nodular goiter? Arch. Intern. Med. **119:**75, 1967.
3. Skillern, P. G., McCullagh, E. P., and Clamen, M.: Radioiodine in diagnosis and therapy of hyperthyroidism, Arch. Intern. Med. **110:**888, 1962.
4. Blumgart, H. L., Freedberg, A. S., and Kurland, G. S.: Hypothyroidism produced by radioactive iodine (^{131}I) in treatment of euthyroid patients with angina pectoris and congestive heart failure: early results in various types of cardiovascular diseases and associated pathologic states, Circulation **1:**1105, 1950.
5. Blumgart, H. L., Freedberg, A. S., and Kurland, G. S.: Treatment of incapacitated euthyroid cardiac patients with radioactive iodine; summary of results in treatment of 1070 patients with angina pectoris or congestive heart failure, J.A.M.A. **157:**1, 1955.
6. Corday, E., Gold, H., and Jaffe, H. L.: Radioiodine treatment of paroxysmal supraventricular

tachycardia in the euthyroid patient, Circulation **17:**900, 1958.

7. Tompkins, E.: Late effects of radioiodine therapy. In Medical radionuclides: radiation dose and effects, AEC Symposium Series **20:**431, 1970.

8. Lima, J. B., Catz, B., and Perzik, S. L.: Thyroid cancer following ^{131}I therapy of hyperthyroidism, J. Nucl. Med. **11:**46, 1970.

9. United States Department of Health, Education & Welfare: Information for physicians — irradiation related thyroid cancer, DHEW publication, no. (NIH) **77:**1120.

10. Pochin, E. E.: Radioiodine therapy of thyroid cancer, Semin. Nucl. Med. **1:**503, 1971.

11. Sarkar, S., Beierwaltes, W. H., Gill, S. P., and Cowley, B. J.: subsequent fertility and birth histories of children and adolescents treated with ^{131}I for thyroid cancer, J. Nucl. Med. **17:**460-464, 1976.

12. Gorman, C.A., Becker, D. V., Greenspan, F. S., and others Breast cancer and thyroid therapy — statement by the American Thyroid Association, J.A.M.A. **237:**1459-1460, 1977.

13. Krauss, S., and Wasserman, L. R.: Leukemia in patients with polycythemia vera treated with radioisotopes. In Medical radionuclides; radiation dose and effects, AEC Symposium Series **20:**441, 1970.

14. Lawrence, J. H., Winchell, H. S., and Donald, W. G.: Leukemia in polycythemia vera: relationship to splenic myeloid metaplasia and therapeutic radiation dose, Ann. Intern. Med. **70:**763, 1969.

15. Modan, B., and Lilienfeld, A. M.: Polycythemia vera and leukemia — the role of radiation treatment, a study of 1222 patients, Medicine **44:**305, 1965.

16. Spires, F. W., Beddow, A. H., King, S. D., and others: The absorbed dose to bone marrow in the treatment of polycythemia by ^{32}P, Br. J. Radiol. **49:**133-140, 1976.

17. Maxfield, J. R., Jr., Maxfield, J. J. G., and Maxfield, W. S.: Use of radioactive phosphorus and testosterone in metastatic bone lesions from breast and prostate, South. Med. J. **51:**320, 1958.

18. Tong, E. C. K.: The treatment of bone metastases with parathormone followed by radiophosphorus, Am. J. Roentgenol. **99:**422, 1967.

19. van den Brenk, H. A. S.: Results of prophylactic postoperative irradiation in 1,300 cases of pterygium, Am. J. Roentgenol. **103:**723, 1968.

20. Nolan, T. R., and Grady, E. D.: Intravascular particulate radioisotope therapy: clinical observations of 76 patients with advanced cancer treated with 90 yttrium particles, Am. Surg. **35:**181, 1969.

21. Grady, E. D., Nolan, T. R., Crumbley, A. J., Larose, J. H., and Cheek, W. V.: Internal hepatic radiotherapy. II. Intra-arterial radiocolloid therapy for hepatic tumors, Am J. Roentgenol. Radium Ther. Nucl. Med. **124:**596-599, 1975.

22. Muller, W., Pavelka, K., and Fridrich, R.: Treatment of chronic arterial effusions with 90-Yttrium (^{90}Y), Scand. J. Rheumatol. **4:**216-220, 1975.

Glossary

aberrant Deviated from normal structure.

ablation Removal.

absorption The process by which radiation imparts some or all of its energy to any material through which it passes. (See *Compton effect, photoelectric effect,* and *pair production.*)

absorption coefficient Fractional decrease in the intensity of a beam of radiation per unit thickness (linear absorption coefficient), per unit mass (mass absorption coefficient), or per atom (atomic absorption coefficient) of absorber.

acinus Saccular terminal division of a compound gland having a narrow lumen, as contrasted with an alveolus. Several acini combine to form a lobule.

activation analysis A method of chemical analysis especially for small traces of material, based on the detection of characteristic radionuclides following nuclear bombardment.

activity See *radioactivity.*

acute exposure Term used to denote radiation exposure of short duration.

adenopathy Any disease of the glands, especially lymph glands.

adrenergic Activated or transmitted by epinephrine. A term applied to those nerve fibers that liberate sympathin at a synapse when a nerve impulse passes (that is, the sympathetic fibers).

agglutination Mass formed by the joining together or aggregation of suspended particles.

akinesis Absence of motor function or activity.

allergy Altered reaction capacity to a specified substance; acquired sensitivities to drugs and biologic substances.

alpha particle A helium nucleus, consisting of 2 protons and 2 neutrons; it has a double positive charge and possesses a mass of 4.00278 atomic mass units (amu).

alveolus Designates a small saclike dilation; an air cell of the lung.

amplification As related to radiation detection instruments, the process (either gas or electronic or both) by which ionization effects are magnified to a degree suitable for measurement.

anemia Deficiency of blood as a whole or deficiency of hemoglobin or in the number of red blood cells.

angstrom unit (Å) 10^{-8} cm. Used to measure the wavelength of electromagnetic radiations.

anion Negatively charged ion.

ankylosis Abnormal immobility and consolidation of a joint.

annihilation radiation The photons produced when an electron and a positron unite and then cease to exist. The annihilation of a positron-electron pair results in the production of 2 photons; each has an energy of 0.51 mev.

anode A positive electrode; the electrode to which negative ions (anions) are attracted.

anoxia Oxygen deficiency; a condition that results from a dminished supply of oxygen to the tissues.

antecubital vein Vein located in front of the elbow in each arm.

antibiotic A substance of biologic origin that inhibits the growth of or kills microorganisms. Common examples are penicillin, streptomycin, and aureomycin.

anticoincidence circuit A circuit with two input terminals that delivers an output pulse if one input terminal receives a pulse but not if both input terminals receive a pulse simultaneously or within a predetermined time interval. A principle used in pulse height analysis.

aplasia Developmental defect or congenital absence of a part.

arrhythmia Absence of rhythm.

arteriogram Radiographic study of an artery following injection of contrast media.

arteriosclerosis Hardening of the arteries.

atheroma Arteriosclerosis with marked degenerative changes.

atom The smallest particle of an element that is capable of entering into a chemical reaction.

atomic mass unit (amu) Unit of mass equal to $1/12$ the arbitrary mass assigned to carbon 12. One amu is equivalent to 931.2 mev of energy.

atomic number Symbol: Z. The number of protons in the nucleus; therefore, the number of positive

631

charges in the nucleus. The atomic number also reflects the number of electrons outside the nucleus of a neutral atom.

atomic weight The relative weight of the atom of an element compared with the weight of one atom of oxygen taken as 16.

atrophy Size reduction of an organ, cell or tissue.

attenuation The process by which radiation is reduced in intensity when passing through some material. This is a combination of absorption and scattering processes.

autoimmune Immunity directed against the body's own tissue.

autologous A part of, or derived from, an organism.

autonomous Self-governing, independent function.

autoradiograph The record of radiation from radioactive material in an object that is made by placing its surface in close proximity to a photographic emulsion.

avalanche The multiplicative process in which a single charged particle accelerated by a strong electric field produces additional charged particles through collision with neutral gas molecules.

average life (mean life) The average of the individual lives of all the atoms of a particular radioative substance. This average is 1.443 times the radioactive half-life of the substance.

avidity An intense eagerness for.

Avogadro's number The number of molecules in a gram molecular weight of any substance (6.03 × 10^{23} molecules); also, the number of atoms in a gram atomic weight of any element.

background radiation Radiation caused by cosmic rays, radioactive materials in the vicinity, and a slight radioactive contamination of the materials of which the instrument is made.

backscattering The process of scattering or deflecting into the sensitive volume of a measuring instrument radiations that originally had no motion in that direction. The process is dependent on the nature of the mounting material, the nature of the sample, the type and energy of the radiations, and the particular geometric arrangement.

barrier Shields of radiation-absorbing material, such as lead and concrete.

benign Not malignant.

beta particle A charged particle emitted from the nucleus of an atom. Its mass and charge are equal in magnitude to those of the electron.

betatron A device for accelerating electrons by means of magnetic induction.

binary scaler A scaler in which the scaling factor is 2 per stage. (See *scaler*.)

binding energy The energy represented by the difference in mass between the actual mass of the nucleus and the sum of the component parts.

biologic half-life The time required for the body to eliminate one half of an administered dose of any substance by regular processes of elimination. This time is approximately the same for both stable and radioactive isotopes of a particular element.

bleb A bubble (culla) or vesicle filled with fluid or air.

blood pigments Pigments normally found in blood, such as hemoglobin and bilirubin.

bone marrow The soft material that fills the cavity in most bones and manufactures most of the formed elements of the blood.

Bremsstrahlung The secondary photon radiation produced by the deceleration of charged particles as they pass through matter.

cancer Popular terminology for any malignant neoplasm.

capillary Small, hairlike vessel connecting arterioles and venules.

carcinogenic Cancer-producing.

carcinoma Malignant epithelial tumor.

carrier (1) A quantity of an element that may be mixed with its radioisotopes to give enough of a quantity to facilitate chemical operations. (2) A substance that, when associated with a trace of another substance, will carry the trace with it through a chemical or physical process.

carrier-free An adjective applied to radioisotopes undiluted with stable isotope carrier.

catabolism Destructive phase of metabolism in which complex compounds are broken down by the cells of the body often with the liberation of energy; the opposite of anabolism.

cataract A clouding of the lens of the eye that obstructs the passage of light.

cathode A negative electrode; the electrode that attracts positive ions.

cation A positively charged ion.

cell Fundamental unit of structure and function in living organisms.

chain reaction Any chemical or nuclear process in which some of the products of the process, including energy, are instrumental in the continuation or magnification of the process.

characteristic radiation Radiation originating from an atom after the removal of an electron or excitation of the nucleus.

chronic exposure The term used to denote radiation exposure of long duration.

cirrhosis Chronic, progressive disease of the liver, essentially inflammatory, characterized by proliferation of connective tissue, degeneration of parenchymal cells, and distortion of architectural pattern.

The liver may be either enlarged or reduced in size.

clot retraction Contraction or shrinkage of a blood clot resulting in the extrusion of serum.

cloud chamber A device for observing the paths of ionizing particles that is based on the principle that supersaturated vapor condenses readily on ions.

coagulation Formation of a coagulum or clot, as in blood or milk.

coincidence The occurrence of one or more ionizing events in one or more detectors simultaneously or within an assignable time interval.

coincidence circuit A circuit with two input terminals that delivers an output pulse only when both input terminals receive pulses simultaneously or within a predetermined time interval. A principle used in the detection of positron emitters.

collimator A device for confining the elements of a beam within an assigned solid angle.

Compton effect Absorption effect observed for x- and gamma radiation in which the incident photon interacts with an orbital electron on the absorber atom to produce a recoil electron and a photon of energy less than the incident photon.

congenital Existing at birth.

conservation of mass-energy Energy and mass are interchangeable, as evidenced by the equation $E = mc^2$, where E is energy, m is mass, and c is velocity of light.

contamination, radioactive Deposition of radioactive material in any place where its presence may be harmful. The harm may be in invalidating the experiment or procedure or in actually being a source of danger to personnel.

corpuscle (1) Encapsulated sensory nerve end-organ. (2) Old term for cell, especially a blood cell.

cosmic rays Radiation, both particulate and electromagnetic, that originates outside the earth's atmosphere.

count (radiation measurements) External indication of a device designed to enumerate ionizing events. It may refer to a single detected event or to the total number that is registered in a given period of time.

count rate meter A device that gives a continuous indication of the average rate of ionizing events.

cumulative dose (radiation) Total dose resulting from repeated exposures. This may be radiation to the same region or to the whole body.

curie That quantitiy of a radioactive material having associated with it 3.7×10^{10} disintegrations per second.

cyclotron A device for accelerating charged particles in a spiral fashion to high energies by means of an alternating electric field between electrodes placed in a constant magnetic field.

cytoplasm Protoplasm of a cell other than that of the nucleus, as opposed to nucleoplasm.

daughter A synonym for a product of decay.

decade scaler A scaler that has a power of 10 for a scaling factor.

decay, radioactive The disintegration of the nucleus of an unstable atom by the spontaneous emission of charged particles and/or photons.

decay constant The fraction of the number of atoms of a radionuclide that decay in unit time.

decay curve A curve showing the relative amount of radioactive substance remaining after any given time.

densitometer An instrument utilizing the photoelectric principle to determine the degree of darkening of developed photographic film.

density A term used to denote the degree of darkening of photographic film.

desquamation A shedding of the superficial epithelium, renal tubules, mucous membranes, and skin.

detoxify Process, usually consisting of a series of reactions, by which a substance foreign to the body is changed to a compound or compounds more readily excreted.

deuterium ($^2_1$H) A heavy isotope of hydrogen having 1 protron and 1 neutron in the nucleus. It is sometimes called "heavy hydrogen."

deuteron The nucleus of a deuterium atom, containing 1 proton, 1 neutron, and no orbital electrons.

diastole A period of relaxation and dilation of a heart chamber during which it fills with blood.

disintegration, nuclear Spontaneous nuclear transformation (radioactivity) characterized by the emission of energy and/or mass from the nucleus.

disintegration constant The fraction of the number of atoms of a radionuclide that decay per unit time.

dose (dosage) According to current usage, the radiation delivered to the whole body or to a specified area or volume.

dose rate Radiation dose delivered in unit of time.

dose rate meter Any instrument that measures dose rate.

dosimeter An instrument used to detect and measure an accumulated dose of radiation. In common usage, it is a pencil-size ionization chamber, with or without a built-in, self-reading electrometer used for personnel monitoring.

dot scan A display, on paper, of equidense dots in a manner that reproduces the spatial distribution of radioactivity in the area desired to be visualized.

dyskinesis Impairment of motor function or activity.

dyspnea Labored or difficult breathing.

ectopic Away from normal position.

effective half-life The time required for a radionuclide introduced into a biologic system to be reduced to one half as a result of the combined action of radioactive decay and biologic elimination.

efficiency (of counters) A measure of the probability that a count will be recorded when radiation is "seen" by a detector.

ejection fraction Percent of difference between ventricular systolic and diastolic volume.

electrode Either terminal of an electric source.

electrolyte Substance that in solution is capable of conducting an electric current and is decomposed by it.

electron A negatively charged particle that is a constituent of every neutral atom. A unit of negative electricity equal to 4.80×10^{-10} electrostatic units. It has a mass of 0.000549 atomic mass units (amu).

electron capture A method of radioactive decay involving the capture of an orbital electron by its nucleus.

electron volt (ev) The amount of energy gained by an electron as it passes through a potential difference of 1 volt.

electrophoresis Migration of charged colloidal particles through the medium in which they are dispersed when placed under the influence of an applied electric potential.

electroscope An instrument for detecting electric charges by the deflection of charged bodies.

element A pure substance consisting of atoms of the same atomic number.

elution Process of extraction of the adsorbed substance from the solid adsorbing medium in chromatography.

embolus Any foreign matter, as a blood clot or air bubble, brought by the blood through a larger vessel and forced into a smaller one obstructing circulation.

emphysema Overdistension of the air spaces (alveoli) in the lungs.

endocrine Internal secretion; pertaining to ductless glands that secrete substances directly into the bloodstream.

endogenous Produced within or as a result of internal causes; applied to the formation of cells or of spores within the parent cell.

endothelium Mesodermally derived, simple, squamous epithelium lining any closed cavity in the body.

energy The capacity to do work. Potential energy is the energy inherent in mass because of its position with reference to other masses. Kinetic energy is the energy possessed by mass because of its motion.

enriched material Material in which the relative amount of one or more forms of an element has been increased.

enzyme Substance formed by living cells, having the capacity to facilitate a chemical reaction.

epidermis The outer layer of the skin.

epilation The temporary or permanent loss of hair.

epithelium The cells lining all canals and surfaces having communication with external air; cells specialized for secretion in certain glands.

erg The unit of work done by a force of 1 dyne acting through a distance of 1 cm. The unit of energy that can exert a force of 1 dyne through a distance of 1 cm.

erythema Redness of the skin produced by congestion of the capillaries, which may result from a variety of causes, the etiology or a special type of lesion often being indicated by a modifying term.

erythematous Of the nature of erythema (red).

erythrocyte Red blood corpuscle. A small, circular disc, with both faces concave, containing hemoglobin that carries oxygen to the body tissues.

erythrocytosis Increased erythrocyte count of more than two standard deviations above mean normal as determined by use of the same method on blood of healthy persons of the patient's age and sex and associated with increased total blood volume.

erythroid Of a red color; reddish; pertaining to red cell series.

erythropoietin Factor elaborated by the kidney (juxtaglomerular cells) that stimulates red cell production.

etiology The study of the causes of disease and mode of operation.

exocrine Pertaining to glands that deliver their secretion or excretion to an epithelial surface, either directly or by means of ducts.

exophthalmos Protrusion of eyeball from the orbit.

extracellular Occurring outside the cell.

exudation Passage of various constituents of blood through the walls of vessels into adjacent tissues or spaces in inflammation.

fibroblast Stellate or spindle-shaped cell with a large, oval, flattened nucleus and a thin layer of cytoplasm found in fibrous tissue.

film badge Photographic film used for the approximate measurement of radiation exposure for personnel monitoring purposes.

fission The splitting of a nucleus into two or more parts with the subsequent release of enormous amounts of energy.

fission products The elements resulting from fission.

flat-field collimator A collimator constructed so as to permit a broad area to be visualized by a radiation detector. It is usually made of lead with a single aperture that is either cylindrical or slightly conical in shape.

focused collimator A collimator constructed so as to permit only a restricted area to be visualized at one time. It is usually made of lead with holes arranged in a honeycomb fashion and converging at some point distant to the face of the collimator.

follicle A small secretory or excretory sac or gland.

fusion The act of combining two or more nuclei into one nucleus.

gamma globulin Globulins of plasma that in neutral or alkaline solutions have the slowest electrophoretic mobility. Most antibodies are gamma globulins.

gamma ray A short wavelength, electromagnetic radiation of nuclear origin with a range of wavelengths from 10^{-9} to 10^{-12} cm, emitted from the nucleus.

gas amplification The release of additional ions from neutral atoms caused by collisions of electrons that are set free in response to the paths of ionizing radiation and that have acquired high energies as a result of an increased electrical field. A phenomenon seen in proportional counters.

gas-flow counter A radiation detector in which an appropriate atmosphere is maintained in the counter tube by allowing a suitable gas to flow slowly through the sensitive volume.

Geiger region An ionization radiation detector whose operating voltage interval in which the charge collected per ionizing event is essentially independent of the number of primary ions produced in the initial ionizing event.

Geiger threshold The minimum voltage at which a Geiger-Mueller tube operates in the Geiger region.

Geiger-Mueller (G-M) counter tube A highly sensitive gas-filled, radiation-measuring device that operates at voltages in the region of avalanche ionization.

genetic effect of radiation Inheritable changes (mutations) produced by the absorption of ionizing radiations.

germ cells (genetic cells) The cells of an organism whose function is to reproduce its kind. These cells are characteristically haploid.

globulin Class of proteins characterized by being insoluble in water but soluble in saline solutions.

glycogen A carbohydrate formed by and largely stored in the liver.

half-value layer (half-thickness) The thickness of any material required to reduce the intensity of an x-ray or gamma-ray beam to half its original value.

Hashimoto's struma Diffuse enlargement of the thyroid characterized by atrophy of the thyroid parenchyma, fibrosis, and excessive formation of lymphoid tissue.

hematopoiesis Formation of blood cells.

hematuria Urine containing blood.

hemolysis Destruction of red cells and the resultant escape of hemoglobin.

hydrocephalus Increased volume of cerebrospinal fluid within the skull.

hypertonic Above normal tension or strength.

hypertrophy Increase in size.

hypochondrium Upper lateral area of abdomen below the rib cage.

hypokinesis Decreased motor function or activity.

hypotonic Below normal tension or strength.

hypoxia Oxygen want or deficiency; any state wherein a physiologically inadequate amount of oxygen is available to or utilized by tissue without respect to cause or degree.

induced radioactivity That activity produced in a substance after bombardment with neutrons or other particles.

inert Lacking activity.

infarct An area of dead tissue produced by interference with blood flow.

integrating circuit An electronic circuit that records, at any time, an average value for the number of ionization events occurring per unit time, or an electrical circuit that records the total number of ions collected in a given time.

internal conversion A method of radioactive decay in which the gamma rays from excited nuclei cause the ejection of orbital electrons from the atom.

interstitial (1) Situated between important parts; occupying the interspaces or interstices of a part. (2) Pertaining to the finest connective tissue of organs.

intrathecal Within a sheath, particularly within the meninges into the subarachnoid space.

intrinsic factor Substance produced by the stomach that combines with extrinsic factor (vitamin B_{12}) to yield an antianemic factor.

ion An atomic particle; an atom or chemical radical bearing an electric charge that is either positive or negative.

ion pair Two particles of opposite charge; usually refers to the electron and positive atomic or molecular residue resulting after the interaction of radiation with the orbital electrons of atoms.

ionization The process or the result of any process by which a neutral atom or molecule acquires a charge, either positive or negative.

ionization chamber An instrument designed to measure the quantity of ionizing radiation in terms of the charge of electricity associated with ions that are produced within a defined volume.

ionization potential The potential necessary to separate one electron from an atom, resulting in the formation of an ion pair.

ionizing energy The average energy lost by ionizing

radiation for the production of an ion pair in air — about 34 electron volts (ev).

ionizing event Any process whereby an ion or group of ions is produced.

ionizing radiation Any electromagnetic or particulate radiation capable of direct or indirect ion production in its passage through matter.

irradiation Any exposure of matter to radiation.

ischemia Local deficiency of blood supply associated with obstruction or functional constriction.

isobar One of two or more different nuclides having the same mass number.

isocount curves Curves showing the distribution of radiation in a medium by means of lines or surfaces drawn through points receiving equal doses.

isomer One of several nuclides having the same number of neutrons and protons, but capable of existing for a measurable time in different energy states. Usually, the isomer of higher energy decays to one with lower energy by the process of isomeric transition.

isomeric transition (IT) The process by which a nuclide decays to an isomeric nuclide of lower energy state. Isomeric transitions proceed by gamma ray and/or internal conversion electron emission.

isoresponse curves See *isocount curves.*

isotone One of several nuclides having the same number of neutrons in their nuclei.

isotope One of several different nuclides having the same number of protons in their nuclei and therefore the same atomic number. However, they differ in the number of neutrons and hence in the mass number. Isotopes have almost identical chemical properties.

jaundice Yellowness of skin, secretions, and mucous membranes because of bile pigments in the blood.

K capture A colloquialism for K electron capture; also loosely used to designate any orbital electron capture process.

kev One thousand electron volts (10^3 ev).

kinetic Pertaining to motion; producing motion.

labeled compound A compound consisting, in part, of labeled molecules. By observations of radioactivity or isotopic composition, this compound or its fragments can be followed through various physical, chemical, or biologic processes.

labeled molecule A molecule containing one or more atoms distinguished by unnatural isotopic composition (with radioactive or stable isotopes).

lamella Thin leaf or plate, as of bone.

LD$_{50}$ (lethal dose) The dose of radiation that causes mortality in 50% of a species.

lead equivalent The thickness of lead that results in the same reduction in radiation dose rate under specified conditions as the material in question.

ligation Tying off, especially arteries, veins, or ducts.

line space The distance between lines of dots on a dot or photo scan; usually expressed in centimeters.

linear absorption coefficient An expression of the fraction of a beam of radiation absorbed in unit thickness of material.

linear accelerator A device for accelerating charged particles, using alternate electrodes and gaps arranged in a straight line. These electrodes and gaps are so proportioned that when their potentials are varied in the proper amplitude and frequency, particles passing through them receive successive increments of energy.

linear amplifier A pulse amplifier in which the output pulse height has been amplified to a height that is proportional to the input pulse height.

lobule Small lobe or a subdivision of a lobe.

lysis Dissolution, setting free, releasing, or destruction-decomposition.

macrophage Phagocytic cell (not a leukocyte) belonging to the reticuloendothelial system. It has the capacity for storing certain aniline dyes in its cytoplasm in the form of granules.

mass absorption coefficient The linear absorption coefficient per centimeter divided by the density of the absorber in grams per cubic centimeter.

mass defect The difference between the mass of the nucleus as a whole and the sum of the nuclear components weighed separately.

mass number Symbol: A. The number of nucleons in the nucleus of an atom.

matrix Basic material from which a thing develops.

maturation Process of coming to full development.

maximum permissible dose (MPD) The maximum dose of radiation permitted for persons working with ionizing radiation. MPD for whole body = $5(N-18)$ rems; N=age.

median lethal dose (MLD/30) The dose of radiation required to kill 50% of the individuals in a large group of animals or organisms within 30 days.

medulla The middle; the marrow.

megakaryocyte Giant cell of the bone marrow containing a large, irregularly lobulated nucleus; the progenitor of blood platelets.

megaly Denoting great size.

metabolism The sum of all the physical and chemical processes by which a living substance is produced and maintained and by which energy is made available for the uses of the organism.

metaplasia Change in the type of adult cells in a tissue to a form that is not normal for that tissue.

metastable state An excited state of a nucleus that returns to its ground state by the emission of a gamma ray. Ground state is not achieved immediately, but over a measurable half-life.

metastatic Pertaining to the spread of malignant cells.

mev One million electron volts (10^6 ev).

microcurie (μCi) 3.7×10^4 disintegrations per second (one millionth of a curie).

micromicrocurie (Picocurie) ($\mu\mu$ Ci) 3.7×10^{-2} disintegrations per second (one millionth of a microcurie).

millicurie (mCi) 3.7×10^7 disintegrations per second (one thousandth of a curie).

millimicrocurie (Nanocurie) (mμCi) 37 disintegrations per second (one thousandth of a microcurie).

milliroentgen (mr) One thousandth of a roentgen.

mitral stenosis Diseased valve causing obstruction of the flow of blood through left atrioventricular opening.

molecule The ultimate unit of a compound that can exist by itself and retain all the properties of the original substance.

monitoring The periodic or continuous determination of the amount of ionizing radiation or radioactive contamination present in an occupied region.

area monitoring Routine monitoring of the level of radiation or of radioactive contamination of any particular area, building, or room.

personnel monitoring Monitoring of any part of an individual such as breath, excretions, or clothing.

monoenergetic radiation Radiation of a given type in which all photons or particles have the same energy.

morphogenesis Structural changes during development of an organism.

mutation A change in the characteristics of any organism as a result of an alteration of the usual hereditary pattern.

myelofibrosis Replacement of the bone marrow by fibrous tissue occurring in association with a myeloproliferative disorder or another unrelated condition.

myeloid Pertaining to, derived from, or resembling bone marrow.

myxedema Swelling associated with hypothyroidism. A sallow, puffy appearance, particularly in hands and face, is characteristic.

necrosis Decay or death of tissue as a result of loss of blood supply.

negatron (β^-) A particle having a mass and charge equal to that of an electron, but originating from the nucleus. Its mass is 0.000548 amu. This term is not used in the United States.

neoplasia New growth, usually applied to a tumor.

nephritis Inflammation of the kidneys.

neutrino A neutral particle of very small mass (approaches zero rest mass) emitted during various processes of decay.

neutron An elementary, electrically neutral nuclear particle with a mass approximately the same as that of a proton. Its mass is 1.00898 atomic mass units (amu).

nuclear reactor An apparatus in which the nuclear fission reaction may be self-sustaining.

nucleon A common term for a constituent particle of the nucleus; usually applies to protons and neutrons.

nucleus (of an atom) That part of an atom in which most of the mass and the total positive electric charge are concentrated.

nuclide A general term referring to any nucleus (stable or radioactive) plus its orbital electrons.

occult Hidden; concealed; not evident as occult blood — the blood in excrement or secretion not clearly evident to the naked eye.

operating voltage The voltage across the electrodes in the detecting chamber required for proper detection of an ionizing event.

osmotic pressure Pressure developed when a solution and its solvent component are separated by a membrane permeable to the solvent only or when two solutions of different concentration of the same solute are similarly separated.

ossification Method by which fibrous tissue or cartilage is converted into bone or a bony substance.

osteoblast Cell arising from a fibroblast that, as it matures, plays a role in the production of bone.

osteoid Resembling bone. Also the organic matrix of bone; young uncalcified bone.

osteon Basic unit of structure of compact bone: haversian canal and its concentrically arranged lamellae (four to 20, each 3 to 7μ thick) in a single (haversian) system. Such units are directed mainly in the long axis of the bone.

osteoprogenitor cells Forefather or ancestor of cells of the bone marrow.

pair production An absorption process for x- and gamma radiation in which the incident photon is annihilated in the vicinity of the nucleus of the absorbing atom, with subsequent release of a positron and a beta particle. This reaction cannot occur for incident radiation energies of less than 1.02 mev.

pancreozymin Crude extract of the intestinal mucosa that stimulates the secretion of pancreatic enzymes.

panmyelosis Multiplication of all the elements of the bone marrow.

parent A radionuclide that yields another nuclide on disintegration. The latter (the daughter) may be radioactive or stable.

patency Open.

pernicious anemia Anemia that results from defects of the bone marrow, such as hypoplasia, euplasia, and degenerative changes. It is caused by a deficiency of red cells, hemoglobin, and granular cells and a predominance of lymphocytes.

phagocytosis Ingestion of foreign or other particles, principally bacteria, by certain cells.

photoelectric effect A process by which a photon ejects an electron from an atom and thereby is totally absorbed.

photographic dosimetry The determination of the accumulative radiation dosage by use of photographic film.

photomultiplier tube A tube in which small electron currents are amplified by a cascade process employing secondary emission.

photon A quantity of electromagnetic energy.

photo scan A display on x-ray film of variable density dots in a manner that reproduces the spatial distribution of radioactivity in the area desired to be visualized.

physical half-life (T_p or $T_{1/2}$) The time required for a source of radioactivity to lose 50% of its activity by decay.

piezeoelectric effect Charges of electricity developed when pressure is applied to certain crystals.

pile See *nuclear reactor*.

pinocytosis Absorption of liquids by cells.

Planck's constant A natural constant of proportionality (h) relating the frequency of a quantum of energy to the total energy of the quantum; equivalent to 6.61×10^{-7} erg-sec.

planimetry The measurement of level surfaces; plane geometry.

plateau As applied to radiation detector chambers, the level portion of the voltage curve where changes in operating voltage introduce minimum changes in the counting rate.

pleomorphic Widely different forms of the same species.

plication Designated a fold or ridge.

positron A particle having a mass equal to the electron and having an equal but opposite charge. Its mass is 0.000548 atomic mass units (amu).

precordium Area of the chest overlying the heart.

progenitor To bring forth.

prone Lying with face downward.

proportional counter A gas-filled radiation detector in which the pulse produced is proportional to the number of ions formed in the gas by the primary ionizing particle.

proportional region The voltage range in which the gas amplifcation is greater than 1 and in which the charge collected is proportional to the initial ionizing event.

proteolysis Enzymatic or hydrolytic conversion of proteins into simple substances.

proton An elementary nuclear particle with a positive electric charge equal numerically to the charge of the electron and having a mass of 1.00759 atomic mass units (amu).

pterygium Anything like a wing; disease of the eye in which a membrane grows over it from the inner corner.

ptosis (ptotic) Falling down of an organ; prolapse; abnormal position.

pulse height analyzer Any circuit designed to select and pass voltage pulses in a certain range of amplitudes.

pyknosis Thickening; especially degeneration of a cell in which the nucleus decreases in size and the chromatin condenses.

quantum See *photon*.

quenching The process of inhibiting discharge in a counter tube that uses gas amplification.

quenching gas A polyatomic gas used in Geiger-Mueller counters to quench or extinguish avalanche ionization.

radiation absorbed dose (rad) A measure of the amount of energy imparted to matter by ionizing radiation per unit mass of irradiated material at the place of interest; equivalent to 100 ergs of absorbed energy per gram of irradiated material.

radioactive half-life See *physical half-life*.

radioactivity The process whereby certain nuclides undergo spontaneous disintegration in which energy is liberated, generally resulting in the formation of new nuclides. The process is accompanied by the emission of one or more types of radiation, such as alpha and beta particles and gamma radiation.

radioresistance The relative resistance of cells, tissues, organs, or entire organisms to the injurious action of radiation.

radiosensitivity The relative susceptibility of cells, tissues, organs, entire organisms, or any substances to the injurious action of radiation. Radioresistance and radiosusceptibility are at present employed in a qualitative or comparative sense, rather than in a quantitative or absolute one.

read-out A method of presenting a total count or rate of detected radiation events.

relative biologic effectiveness (RBE) The ratio of x- or gamma ray dose to the dose that is required to produce the same biologic effect by the radiation in question.

relativistic mass The increased mass associated with a particle when its velocity is increased. The increase in mass becomes appreciable only at velocities approaching the velocity of light (3×10^{10} cm/sec).

resolving time, counter The minimum time interval between two distinct ionization events that will permit both to be counted.

roentgen The quantity of x- or gamma radiation such that the associated corpuscular emission per 0.001293 gram of air produces, in air, ions carrying 1 electrostatic unit of electrical charge, either positive or negative.

roentgen equivalent, man (rem) A unit of human biologic dose as a result of exposure to one or many types of ionizing radiation. It is equal to the absorbed dose in rads times the RBE of the particular type of radiation being absorbed

scaler An electronic device that produces an output voltage pulse whenever a prescribed number of input pulses has been received.

scanner A device used to display a two-dimensional portrayal of the variations of concentration of radioactivity in any volume of material.

scan speed The rate of travel of the scanner detector as it traverses the area being visualized.

scattering The change of direction of particles or photons as a result of a collision or interaction.

scintillation counter The combination of phosphor, photomultiplier tube, and associated circuits for counting light emissions produced in the phosphors by ionizing radiation.

secondary radiation Radiation originating as the result of interactions of other radiation in matter. It may be either electromagnetic or particulate in nature.

secretin Hormone produced in the epithelial cells of the duodenum by the contact of acid. It is absorbed from the cells by the blood and excites the pancreas to activity; it has been isolated as secretin picrotonate.

self-absorption The absorption of radiation by the matter in which the radioactive atoms are located; in particular, the absorption of radiation within the sample being assayed.

sequestration Separation.

shunting Alternate way, bypass.

somatic (1) Pertaining to the body. (2) Pertaining to the framework of the boedy and not to the viscera, such as the somatic musculature (the muscles of the body wall or somatopleure) as distinguished from the splanchnic musculature (the splanchnopleure).

somatic cells Body cells, usually having two sets of chromosomes. Germ cells have only one set.

specific activity (1) Of a compound: fatal radioactivity per gram of compound; (2) of an element: total radioactivity per gram of element; (3) of an isotope: total radioactivity per gram of radiosotope.

specific gravity Measured mass of a substance with that of an equal volume of another taken as a standard. For gases, hydrogen of air may be the standard; for liquids and solids, distilled water at a specified temperature is the standard.

spectrometer A device used to count an emission of radiation of a specific energy or range of energies to the exclusion of all other energies.

spondylitis Inflammation of the spine with pathologic changes in the vertebrae and intravertebral joints.

spurious count The count caused by any agency other than the radiation desired to be detected.

stable isotope An isotope of an element that is not radioactive.

steatorrhea (1) Increased flow of the secretion of the sebaceous follicles. (2) Fatty stools.

stray radiation Radiation serving no useful purpose.

supine Lying on back with face upward.

synchrotron A device for accelerating particles, ordinarily electrons, in a circular orbit with frequency-modulated electric fields combined with an increasing magnetic field applied in synchronism with the orbital motion.

systole Contraction of the heart chambers.

tachycardia Excessive rapidity of the heart's action.

tagged compound See *labeled compound.*

teledeltos paper A black paperlike material with a white chalklike overlay. The overlay is burned away by the passage of a current pulse through a stylus to a metal back-plate on which the teledeltos paper is mounted. The result is a black dot on a white field.

threshold (1) Lower limit of stimulus capable of producing an impression on consciousness or of evoking a response in an irritable tissue. (2) Entrance of a canal.

thrombocytosis Condition marked by the presence of a large number of blood platelets in the blood.

thrombosis Formation of a clot of blood.

thyrotoxicosis Hyperthyroidism of any type

titer The amount of a substance (standard) needed to react with a volume of another substance.

tracer, isotopic The isotope or nonnatural mixture of isotopes of an element that may be incorporated into a sample to make possible observation of the course of that element through a chemical, biologic, or physical process.

transferrin Siderophilin; a pseudoglobulin of blood, having molecular weight of about 90,000. It is capable of combining with 2 atoms of ferric iron to form a compound that serves as a transport form of iron in blood.

tritium (^{3}H or ^{3}T) An isotope of hydrogen having a mass number of 3 (1 proton, 2 neutrons).

vagus nerve Parasympathetic pneumogastric nerve; the tenth cranial nerve, composed of both motor and sensory fibers. It has a wide distribution in the neck, thorax, and abdomen and sends important branches to the heart, lungs, stomach, and so on.

vascular Pertaining to, consisting of, or provided with vessels.

viscus Any one of the organs enclosed within one of the four great cavities; the cranium, thorax, abdomen, or pelvis, especially an organ within the abdominal cavity.

vitamin B$_{12}$ Essential vitamin needed for the normal maturation of cells of the erythrocytic series and for normal neurologic function. When given parenterally, it corrects both the hematologic and neurologic symptoms of pernicious anemia.

wavelength The distance between the same point on two subsequent electronmagnetic waves.

window A term that describes the upper and lower limits of energy of radiation accepted for counting by a spectrometer; also termed window width.

x rays Penetrating electromagnetic radiations having wavelengths much shorter than those of visible light.

zymogen Inactive precursor of an enzyme that, on reaction with an appropriate kinase or other chemical agent, liberates the enzyme in active form.

PREFIXES

A prefix consists of one or two syllables placed before a word to modify the meaning. These syllables are often prepositions or adverbs.

a, an	Without, negative
ab	From, away from
ad	Adherence, increase, near, toward
ante, antero	Before, forward, front
anti	Against
auto, aut	Self
bi, bis	Twice, double
cata	Lower, down, negative
co, com, con	Together, with
contra	Against, counter, opposite
de	Down from
di	Double, twice
dia	Through, apart
dis	Apart, away from
dys	Painful, difficult
ec	Out of
ecto	Outside
em, en	In, into
end, endo	Within
entero	Intenstine
epi	Upon, at, in addition to
ex, exo	Out, away from, over, outside
gastro	Stomach
hemi	Half
hemo	Blood
hyper	Above, excessive, beyond
hypo	Decreased, under
infra	Beneath, below
inter	Among, between
intra, intro	Into, within
macro	Large
micro	Small
multi	Many
myo	Muscle
neuro	Nerve
ortho	Straight, normal
pan	All, every
para	Around, beside, by, beyond, abnormal, near
patho	Disease
per	Through
peri	Around
poly	Many
post	After, behind
pre	Before, in front of
pro	In front of, forward
pseudo	False
py	Pus
re	Again, back
retro	Back, backward
semi	Half
steno	Narrow, contracted
sub	Under, below, beneath
super, supra	Above, beyond, superior
sym, syn	With, along, together, beside
tendo	Tendon
trans	Across, over, through
tri	Three
ultra	Excess, beyond

SUFFIXES

A suffix is a syllable or syllables added to the end of a word or root to modify its meaning.

algia	Pain
dynia	Pain
ectomy	Surgical removal of
genic	Origin, producing
genous	Kind
gram	Picture, tracing
lysis	Dissolution, breaking down
oid	Resembling, like
ology	Science of, study of
oscopy	Diagnostic examination
ostomy	Opening
otomy	Incision
penia	Lack, decrease
plegia	Paralysis
trophy	Nutrition
uria	Urine

DIAGNOSTIC SUFFIXES OR COMBINING FORMS

cele	Hernia, tumor
ectasis	Expansion, dilation
emia	Blood
iasis	Condition, presence of
itis	Inflammation
malacia	Softening
megaly	Enlargement
oma	Tumor
osis	Condition, disease
pathy	Disease
ptosis	Falling
rrhexis	Rupture

POSITION OR DIRECTION

anterior or ventral	Front of
posterior or dorsal	Back of
superior or upper	Situated above
inferior or lower	Situated beneath
cranial, craniad, cephalic	Nearest or toward the head
caudal, caudad	Away from the head, inferior in position
medial	Middle, internal
lateral	Side, to the side
proximal	Near the source or attachment
distal	Away from the source

APPENDIXES

A Physical data for radionuclides used in nuclear medicine

Element	Chemical symbol (X)	Atomic number (Z)	Mass number (A)	Half-life	Radiation	Principal gamma energy (mev)
Arsenic	As	33	74	17.9d	EC, β^+, β^-, γ	0.596
Calcium	Ca	20	47	4.5d	β^-, γ	1.308
Carbon	C	6	11	20.3m	β^+	None
			14	5730y	β^-	None
Cesium (^{137m}Ba)	Cs	55	137	30y	β^-, γ	0.662
Chromium	Cr	24	51	27.8d	EC, γ	0.320
Cobalt	Co	27	57	270d	EC	0.122
			58	71.3d	EC, β^+, γ	0.810
			60	5.26y	β^-, γ	1.17, 1.33
Gallium	Ga	31	67	78h	EC, γ	0.091, 0.093 (38%) 0.184(24%) 0.300(16%) 0.394(4%)
Gold	Au	79	198	2.7d	β^-, γ	0.412

Element	Symbol		Mass No.	Half-life	Decay	Energy (MeV)
Iodine	I	53	123	13h	EC, γ	0.159
			125	60d	EC, γ	0.035γ(7%) 0.027x(1.15%) 0.031x(25%)
			131	8.06d	β⁻, γ	0.364
Iron	Fe	26	59	45d	β⁻, γ	1.17, 1.33
Indium	In	49	111	2.8d	EC, γ	0.173(89%) 0.247(94%)
Krypton	Kr	36	79	1.45d	EC, γ	0.398, 0.606
Mercury	Hg	80	197	2.7d	EC, γ	0.077
			203	46.9d	β⁻, γ	0.279
Molybdenum	Mo	42	99	2.78d	β⁻, γ	0.740
Oxygen	O	8	15	2.1m	β⁺	None
Phosphorus	P	15	32	14.3d	β⁻	None
Rubidium	Rb	37	86	18.7d	β⁻, γ	1.078
Selenium	Se	34	75	120d	EC, γ	0.265
Strontium	Sr	38	85	64d	EC, γ	0.514
			87m	2.83h	IT, γ	0.388
			90	27.7y	β⁻	None
Technetium	Tc	43	99m	6h	IT, γ	0.140
Thallium	Tl	81	201	73h	EC, γ, x	0.135γ(3%) 0.167γ(10%) 0.068 – 0.080x(94.5%)
Tin	Sn	50	113	115d	EC, γ	0.255
Tritium	H	1	3	12.26y	β⁻	None
Xenon	Xe	54	127	36.4d	EC, γ	0.172(22%) 0.203(65%) 0.375(20%)
			133	5.31d	β⁻, γ	0.08
Ytterbium	Yb	70	169	32d	EC, γ	0.177(22%) 0.198(35%)

B Universal decay table

Activity remaining for t ÷ $T_{1/2}$ from 0 to 1.00

	.000	.001	.002	.003	.004	.005	.006	.007	.008	.009
	1.00000	.99931	.99861	.99792	.99723	.99654	.99585	.99516	.99447	.99378
.01	.99309	.99240	.99172	.99103	.99034	.98966	.98897	.98829	.98760	.98692
.02	.98623	.98555	.98487	.98418	.98350	.98282	.98214	.98146	.98078	.98010
.03	.97942	.97874	.97806	.97739	.97671	.97603	.97536	.97468	.97400	.97333
.04	.97265	.97198	.97131	.97063	.96996	.96929	.96862	.96795	.96728	.96661
.05	.96594	.96527	.96460	.96393	.96326	.96259	.96193	.96126	.96059	.95993
.06	.95926	.95860	.95794	.95727	.95661	.95595	.95528	.95462	.95396	.95330
.07	.95264	.95198	.95132	.95066	.95000	.94934	.94868	.94803	.94737	.94671
.08	.94606	.94540	.94475	.94409	.94344	.94278	.94213	.94148	.94083	.94017
.09	.93952	.93887	.93822	.93757	.93692	.93627	.93562	.93498	.93433	.93368
.10	.93303	.93239	.93174	.93109	.93045	.92980	.92916	.92852	.92787	.92723
.11	.92659	.92595	.92530	.92466	.92402	.92338	.92274	.92210	.92146	.92083
.12	.92019	.91955	.91891	.91828	.91764	.91700	.91637	.91573	.91510	.91447
.13	.91383	.91320	.91257	.91193	.91130	.91067	.91004	.90941	.90878	.90815
.14	.90752	.90689	.90626	.90563	.90501	.90438	.90375	.90313	.90250	.90188
.15	.90125	.90063	.90000	.89938	.89876	.89813	.89751	.89689	.89627	.89565
.16	.89503	.89440	.89379	.89317	.89255	.89193	.89131	.89069	.89008	.88946
.17	.88884	.88823	.88761	.88700	.88638	.88577	.88515	.88454	.88393	.88332
.18	.88270	.88209	.88148	.88087	.88026	.87965	.87904	.87843	.87782	.87721
.19	.87661	.87600	.87539	.87478	.87418	.87357	.87297	.87236	.87176	.87115
.20	.87055	.86995	.86934	.86874	.86814	.86754	.86694	.86634	.86574	.86514
.21	.86454	.86394	.86334	.86274	.86214	.86155	.86095	.86035	.85976	.85916
.22	.85857	.85797	.85738	.85678	.85619	.85559	.85500	.85441	.85382	.85323
.23	.85263	.85204	.85145	.85086	.85027	.84968	.84910	.84851	.84792	.84733
.24	.84675	.84616	.84557	.84499	.84440	.84382	.84323	.84265	.84206	.84148
.25	.84090	.84031	.83973	.83915	.83857	.83799	.83741	.83683	.83625	.83567
.26	.83509	.83451	.83393	.83335	.83278	.83220	.83162	.83105	.83047	.82989
.27	.82932	.82874	.82817	.82760	.82702	.82645	.82588	.82531	.82473	.82416
.28	.82359	.82302	.82245	.82188	.82131	.82074	.82017	.81960	.81904	.81847
.29	.81790	.81734	.81677	.81620	.81564	.81507	.81451	.81394	.81338	.81282

	0	1	2	3	4	5	6	7	8	9
.30	.80720	.80776	.80832	.80888	.80944	.81000	.81057	.81113	.81169	.81225
.31	.80163	.80218	.80274	.80329	.80385	.80441	.80497	.80552	.80608	.80664
.32	.79609	.79664	.79719	.79775	.79830	.79885	.79941	.79996	.80051	.80107
.33	.79059	.79114	.79169	.79223	.79278	.79333	.79388	.79443	.79499	.79554
.34	.78513	.78567	.78622	.78676	.78731	.78785	.78840	.78895	.78949	.79004
.35	.77970	.78025	.78079	.78133	.78187	.78241	.78295	.78350	.78404	.78458
.36	.77432	.77486	.77539	.77593	.77647	.77701	.77755	.77809	.77862	.77916
.37	.76897	.76950	.77004	.77057	.77111	.77164	.77218	.77271	.77325	.77378
.38	.76366	.76419	.76472	.76525	.76578	.76631	.76684	.76737	.76791	.76844
.39	.75838	.75891	.75944	.75996	.76049	.76102	.76154	.76207	.76260	.76313
.40	.75315	.75367	.75419	.75471	.75524	.75576	.75628	.75681	.75733	.75786
.41	.74794	.74846	.74898	.74950	.75002	.75054	.75106	.75158	.75210	.75262
.42	.74278	.74329	.74381	.74432	.74484	.74536	.74587	.74639	.74691	.74742
.43	.73765	.73816	.73867	.73918	.73969	.74021	.74072	.74123	.74175	.74226
.44	.73255	.73306	.73357	.73408	.73458	.73509	.73560	.73611	.73662	.73713
.45	.72749	.72799	.72850	.72900	.72951	.73002	.73052	.73103	.73154	.73204
.46	.72247	.72297	.72347	.72397	.72447	.72497	.72548	.72598	.72648	.72699
.47	.71747	.71797	.71847	.71897	.71947	.71997	.72047	.72096	.72146	.72196
.48	.71252	.71301	.71351	.71400	.71450	.71499	.71549	.71598	.71648	.71698
.49	.70760	.70809	.70858	.70907	.70956	.71005	.71055	.71104	.71153	.71203
.50	.70271	.70320	.70368	.70417	.70466	.70515	.70564	.70613	.70662	.70711
.51	.69786	.69834	.69882	.69931	.69979	.70028	.70076	.70125	.70174	.70222
.52	.69304	.69352	.69400	.69448	.69496	.69544	.69592	.69641	.69689	.69737
.53	.68825	.68873	.68920	.68968	.69016	.69064	.69112	.69160	.69208	.69255
.54	.68349	.68397	.68444	.68492	.68539	.68587	.68634	.68682	.68729	.68777
.55	.67877	.67924	.67971	.68019	.68066	.68113	.68160	.68207	.68255	.68302
.56	.67408	.67455	.67502	.67549	.67596	.67642	.67689	.67736	.67783	.67830
.57	.66943	.66989	.67036	.67082	.67129	.67175	.67222	.67268	.67315	.67362
.58	.66480	.66526	.66573	.66619	.66665	.66711	.66757	.66804	.66850	.66896
.59	.66021	.66067	.66113	.66159	.66204	.66250	.66296	.66342	.66388	.66434
.60	.65565	.65611	.65656	.65702	.65747	.65793	.65838	.65884	.65930	.65975
.61	.65112	.65157	.65203	.65248	.65293	.65338	.65384	.65429	.65474	.65520
.62	.64662	.64707	.64752	.64797	.64842	.64887	.64932	.64977	.65022	.65067
.63	.64216	.64260	.64305	.64349	.64394	.64439	.64483	.64528	.64573	.64618
.64	.63772	.63816	.63861	.63905	.63949	.63994	.64038	.64082	.64127	.64171
.65	.63332	.63376	.63420	.63464	.63508	.63552	.63596	.63640	.63684	.63728
.66	.62894	.62938	.62982	.63025	.63069	.63113	.63156	.63200	.63244	.63288

Continued.

Activity remaining for t ÷ T₁/₂ from 0 to 1.00

	.000	.001	.002	.003	.004	.005	.006	.007	.008	.009
.67	.62851	.62807	.62764	.62720	.62677	.62633	.62590	.62546	.62503	.62460
.68	.62417	.62373	.62330	.62287	.62244	.62201	.62157	.62114	.62071	.62028
.69	.61985	.61942	.61900	.61857	.61814	.61771	.61728	.61685	.61643	.61600
.70	.61557	.61515	.61472	.61429	.61387	.61344	.61302	.61259	.61217	.61174
.71	.61132	.61090	.61047	.61005	.60963	.60921	.60878	.60836	.60794	.60752
.72	.60710	.60668	.60626	.60584	.60542	.60500	.60458	.60416	.60374	.60332
.73	.60290	.60249	.60207	.60165	.60123	.60082	.60040	.59999	.59957	.59915
.74	.59874	.59832	.59791	.59750	.59708	.59667	.59625	.59584	.59543	.59502
.75	.59460	.59419	.59378	.59337	.59296	.59255	.59214	.59173	.59132	.59091
.76	.59050	.59009	.58968	.58927	.58886	.58845	.58805	.58764	.58723	.58682
.77	.58642	.58601	.58561	.58520	.58479	.58439	.58398	.58358	.58317	.58277
.78	.58237	.58196	.58156	.58116	.58075	.58035	.57995	.57955	.57915	.57875
.79	.57834	.57794	.57754	.57714	.57674	.57634	.57594	.57554	.57515	.57475
.80	.57435	.57395	.57355	.57316	.57276	.57236	.57197	.57157	.57117	.57078
.81	.57038	.56999	.56959	.56920	.56880	.56841	.56801	.56762	.56723	.56683
.82	.56644	.56605	.56566	.56527	.56487	.56448	.56409	.56370	.56331	.56292
.83	.56253	.56214	.56175	.56136	.56097	.56058	.56019	.55981	.55942	.55903
.84	.55864	.55826	.55787	.55748	.55710	.55671	.55632	.55594	.55555	.55517
.85	.55478	.55440	.55402	.55363	.55325	.55287	.55248	.55210	.55172	.55133
.86	.55095	.55057	.55019	.54981	.54943	.54905	.54867	.54829	.54791	.54753
.87	.54715	.54677	.54639	.54601	.54563	.54525	.54488	.54450	.54412	.54374
.88	.54337	.54299	.54261	.54224	.54186	.54149	.54111	.54074	.54036	.53999
.89	.53961	.53924	.53887	.53849	.53812	.53775	.53737	.53700	.53663	.53626
.90	.53589	.53552	.53514	.53477	.53440	.53403	.53366	.53329	.53292	.53255
.91	.53218	.53182	.53145	.53108	.53071	.53034	.52998	.52961	.52924	.52888
.92	.52851	.52814	.52778	.52741	.52705	.52668	.52632	.52595	.52559	.52522
.93	.52486	.52449	.52413	.52377	.52340	.52304	.52268	.52232	.52196	.52159
.94	.52123	.52087	.52051	.52015	.51979	.51943	.51907	.51871	.51835	.51799
.95	.51763	.51727	.51692	.51656	.51620	.51584	.51548	.51513	.51477	.51441
.96	.51406	.51370	.51334	.51299	.51263	.51228	.51192	.51157	.51121	.51086
.97	.51051	.51015	.50980	.50945	.50909	.50874	.50839	.50803	.50768	.50733
.98	.50698	.50663	.50628	.50593	.50558	.50523	.50488	.50453	.50418	.50383
.99	.50348	.50313	.50278	.50243	.50208	.50174	.50139	.50104	.50069	.50035
1.00	.50000									

The accompanying table can be used to determine the fraction of activity remaining of any radionuclide, from 0.001 half-life to 1.00 half-life.

To use the table:

1. Divide elapsed time by the known physical half-life of the radionuclide under consideration (t ÷ $T_{1/2}$). NOTE: The same time unit must be used in each instance.
2. Use this answer (to three significant figures) in locating the percent of original activity remaining. The first two significant figures are listed on the vertical column at the left of the table; the third significant figure is listed on the horizontal across the top of the table.
3. Multiply original activity by this percentage figure to obtain amount remaining.

Example: What is the strength of a 10 mCi ^{131}I source after 2 days?

1. t ÷ $T_{1/2}$ = 2 ÷ 8.1 = 0.247.
2. Fraction remaining from decay table = 0.84265.
3. 10 mCi × 0.84265 = 8.43 mCi.

C Table of atomic mass units

Symbol	Element	Atomic mass units (amu)
e	Electron	0.000549
n	Neutron	1.008665
p	Proton	1.007277
$^{1}_{1}H$	Hydrogen	1.007825
$^{2}_{1}H$	Deuterium	2.014102
$^{3}_{1}H$	Tritium	3.016050
$^{3}_{2}He$		3.016030
$^{4}_{2}He$	Isotopes of	4.002603
$^{5}_{2}He$	helium	5.012297
$^{6}_{2}He$		6.018893
$^{10}_{6}C$		10.016810
$^{11}_{6}C$		11.011432
$^{12}_{6}C$	Isotopes of	12.000000
$^{13}_{6}C$	carbon	13.003354
$^{14}_{6}C$		14.003242
$^{15}_{6}C$		15.010600
$^{12}_{5}B$		12.014354
$^{12}_{6}C$	Isobars of mass 12	12.000000
$^{12}_{7}N$		12.018641
$^{16}_{8}O$	Oxygen	15.994915
$^{32}_{15}P$	Isobars of mass 32	31.973910
$^{32}_{16}S$		31.972074

D Four-place logarithms*

N	0	1	2	3	4	5	6	7	8	9
10	0000	0043	0086	0128	0170	0212	0253	0294	0334	0374
11	0414	0453	0492	0531	0569	0607	0645	0682	0719	0755
12	0792	0828	0864	0899	0934	0969	1004	1038	1072	1106
13	1139	1173	1206	1239	1271	1303	1335	1367	1399	1430
14	1461	1492	1523	1553	1584	1614	1644	1673	1703	1732
15	1761	1790	1818	1847	1875	1903	1931	1959	1987	2014
16	2041	2068	2095	2122	2148	2175	2201	2227	2253	2279
17	2304	2330	2355	2380	2405	2430	2455	2480	2504	2529
18	2553	2577	2601	2625	2648	2672	2695	2718	2742	2765
19	2788	2810	2833	2856	2878	2900	2923	2945	2967	2989
20	3010	3032	3054	3075	3096	3118	3139	3160	3181	3201
21	3222	3243	3263	3284	3304	3324	3345	3365	3385	3404
22	3424	3444	3464	3483	3502	3522	3541	3560	3579	3598
23	3617	3636	3655	3674	3692	3711	3729	3747	3766	3784
24	3802	3820	3838	3856	3874	3892	3909	3927	3945	3962
25	3979	3997	4014	4031	4048	4065	4082	4099	4116	4133
26	4150	4166	4183	4200	4216	4232	4249	4265	4281	4298
27	4314	4330	4346	4362	4378	4393	4409	4425	4440	4456
28	4472	4487	4502	4518	4533	4548	4564	4579	4594	4609
29	4624	4639	4654	4669	4683	4698	4713	4728	4742	4757
30	4771	4786	4800	4814	4829	4843	4857	4871	4886	4900
31	4914	4928	4942	4955	4969	4983	4997	5011	5024	5038
32	5051	5065	5079	5092	5105	5119	5132	5145	5159	5172
33	5185	5198	5211	5224	5237	5250	5263	5276	5289	5302
34	5315	5328	5340	5353	5366	5378	5391	5403	5416	5428
35	5441	5453	5465	5478	5490	5502	5514	5527	5539	5551
36	5563	5575	5587	5599	5611	5623	5635	5647	5658	5670
37	5682	5694	5705	5717	5729	5740	5752	5763	5775	5786
38	5798	5809	5821	5832	5843	5855	5866	5877	5888	5899
39	5911	5922	5933	5944	5955	5966	5977	5988	5999	6010
40	6021	6031	6042	6053	6064	6075	6085	6096	6107	6117
41	6128	6138	6149	6160	6170	6180	6191	6201	6212	6222

Continued.

*Modified from Quimby, E. H., and Feitelberg, S.: Radioactive isotopes in medicine and biology, Philadelphia, 1963, Lea & Febiger.

N	0	1	2	3	4	5	6	7	8	9
42	6232	6243	6253	6263	6274	6284	6294	6304	6314	6325
43	6335	6345	6355	6365	6375	6385	6395	6405	6415	6425
44	6435	6444	6454	6464	6474	6484	6493	6503	6513	6522
45	6532	6542	6551	6561	6571	6580	6590	6599	6609	6618
46	6628	6637	6646	6656	6665	6675	6684	6693	6702	6712
47	6721	6730	6739	6749	6758	6767	6776	6785	6794	6803
48	6812	6821	6830	6839	6848	6857	6866	6875	6884	6893
49	6902	6911	6920	6928	6937	6946	6955	6964	6972	6981
50	6990	6998	7007	7016	7024	7033	7042	7050	7059	7067
51	7076	7084	7093	7101	7110	7118	7126	7135	7143	7152
52	7160	7168	7177	7185	7193	7202	7210	7218	7226	7235
53	7243	7251	7259	7267	7275	7284	7292	7300	7308	7316
54	7324	7332	7340	7348	7356	7364	7372	7380	7388	7396
55	7404	7412	7419	7427	7435	7443	7451	7459	7466	7474
56	7482	7490	7497	7505	7513	7520	7528	7536	7543	7551
57	7559	7566	7574	7582	7589	7597	7604	7612	7619	7627
58	7634	7642	7649	7657	7664	7672	7679	7686	7694	7701
59	7709	7716	7723	7731	7738	7745	7752	7760	7767	7774
60	7782	7789	7796	7803	7810	7818	7825	7832	7839	7846
61	7853	7860	7868	7875	7882	7889	7896	7903	7910	7917
62	7924	7931	7938	7945	7952	7959	7966	7973	7980	7987
63	7993	8000	8007	8014	8021	8028	8035	8041	8048	8055
64	8062	8069	8075	8082	8089	8096	8102	8109	8116	8122
65	8129	8136	8142	8149	8156	8162	8169	8176	8182	8189
66	8195	8202	8209	8215	8222	8228	8235	8241	8248	8254
67	8261	8267	8274	8280	8287	8293	8299	8306	8312	8319
68	8325	8331	8338	8344	8351	8357	8363	8370	8376	8382
69	8388	8395	8401	8407	8414	8420	8426	8432	8439	8445
70	8451	8457	8463	8470	8476	8482	8488	8494	8500	8506
71	8513	8519	8525	8531	8537	8543	8549	8555	8561	8567
72	8573	8579	8585	8591	8597	8603	8609	8615	8621	8627
73	8633	8639	8645	8651	8657	8663	8669	8675	8681	8686
74	8692	8698	8704	8710	8716	8722	8727	8733	8739	8745
75	8751	8756	8762	8768	8774	8779	8785	8791	8797	8802
76	8808	8814	8820	8825	8831	8837	8842	8848	8854	8859
77	8865	8871	8876	8882	8887	8893	8899	8904	8910	8915
78	8921	8927	8932	8938	8943	8949	8954	8960	8965	8971
79	8976	8982	8987	8993	8998	9004	9009	9015	9020	9025
80	9031	9036	9042	9047	9053	9058	9063	9069	9074	9079
81	9085	9090	9096	9101	9106	9112	9117	9122	9128	9133
82	9138	9143	9149	9154	9159	9165	9170	9175	9180	9186
83	9191	9196	9201	9206	9212	9217	9222	9227	9232	9238
84	9243	9248	9253	9258	9263	9269	9274	9279	9284	9289

N	0	1	2	3	4	5	6	7	8	9
85	9294	9299	9304	9309	9315	9320	9325	9330	9335	9340
86	9345	9350	9355	9360	9365	9370	9375	9380	9385	9390
87	9395	9400	9405	9410	9415	9420	9425	9430	9435	9440
88	9445	9450	9455	9460	9465	9469	9474	9479	9484	9489
89	9494	9499	9504	9509	9513	9518	9523	9528	9533	9538
90	9542	9547	9552	9557	9562	9566	9571	9576	9581	9586
91	9590	9595	9600	9605	9609	9614	9619	9624	9628	9633
92	9638	9643	9647	9652	9657	9661	9666	9671	9675	9680
93	9685	9689	9694	9699	9703	9708	9713	9717	9722	9727
94	9731	9736	9741	9745	9750	9754	9759	9763	9768	9773
95	9777	9782	9786	9791	9795	9800	9805	9809	9814	9818
96	9823	9827	9832	9836	9841	9845	9850	9854	9859	9863
97	9868	9872	9877	9881	9886	9890	9894	9899	9903	9908
98	9912	9917	9921	9926	9930	9934	9939	9943	9948	9952
99	9956	9961	9965	9969	9974	9978	9983	9987	9991	9996

E Exponentials*

X	e^{-x}	X	e^{-x}	X	e^{-x}
0.00	1.000	0.40	0.670	1.0	0.368
0.01	0.990	0.41	0.664	1.1	0.333
0.02	0.980	0.42	0.657	1.2	0.301
0.03	0.970	0.43	0.651	1.3	0.273
0.04	0.961	0.44	0.644	1.4	0.247
0.05	0.951	0.45	0.638	1.5	0.223
0.06	0.942	0.46	0.631	1.6	0.202
0.07	0.932	0.47	0.625	1.7	0.183
0.08	0.923	0.48	0.619	1.8	0.165
0.09	0.914	0.49	0.613	1.9	0.150
0.10	0.905	0.50	0.607	2.0	0.135
0.11	0.896	0.52	0.595	2.1	0.122
0.12	0.887	0.54	0.583	2.2	0.111
0.13	0.878	0.56	0.571	2.3	0.100
0.14	0.869	0.58	0.560	2.4	0.0907
0.15	0.861	0.60	0.549	2.5	0.0821
0.16	0.852	0.62	0.538	2.6	0.0743
0.17	0.844	0.64	0.527	2.7	0.0672
0.18	0.835	0.66	0.517	2.8	0.0608
0.19	0.827	0.68	0.507	2.9	0.0550
0.20	0.819	0.70	0.497	3.0	0.0498
0.21	0.811	0.72	0.487	3.2	0.0408
0.22	0.803	0.74	0.477	3.4	0.0334
0.23	0.795	0.76	0.468	3.6	0.0273
0.24	0.787	0.78	0.458	3.8	0.0224
0.25	0.779	0.80	0.449	4.0	0.0183
0.26	0.771	0.82	0.440	4.2	0.0150
0.27	0.763	0.84	0.432	4.4	0.0123
0.28	0.756	0.86	0.423	4.6	0.0101
0.29	0.748	0.88	0.415	4.8	0.0082
0.30	0.741	0.90	0.407	5.0	0.0067
0.31	0.733	0.92	0.399	5.5	0.0041
0.32	0.726	0.94	0.391	6.0	0.0025
0.33	0.719	0.96	0.383	6.5	0.0015
0.34	0.712	0.98	0.375	7.0	0.0009
0.35	0.705			7.5	0.0006
0.36	0.698			8.0	0.0003
0.37	0.691			8.5	0.0002
0.38	0.684			9.0	0.0001
0.39	0.677				

*Courtesy Editors of Handbook of chemistry and physics, Chemical Rubber Co.

F Data for decay of radionuclides used in nuclear medicine*

Radionuclide	$T_{1/2}$	$\bar{E}_\beta(mev)$	Principal photon energies (mev)	Fractional emission (n_i)	$\Delta_i\left(\dfrac{g \cdot rad}{\mu Ci \cdot hr}\right)$
^{18}F	110m	0.250	–	–	0.5157
			0.511	1.94	2.1115
^{24}Na	15h	0.555	–	–	1.180
			1.37	0.999	2.915
			2.75	0.999	5.861
^{32}P	14.3d	0.695	–	–	1.4799
^{51}Cr	27.8d	0.005	–	–	0.011
			0.320	0.102	0.0694
^{59}Fe	45d	0.117	–	–	0.255
			0.142	0.0096	0.003
			0.19	0.029	0.012
			0.033	0.002	0.002
			1.10	0.56	1.299
			1.29	0.44	1.214
^{60}Co	5.26y	0.093	–	–	0.202
			1.17	0.99	2.494
			1.33	0.99	2.838
^{67}Ga	78h	–	–	–	0.0685
			0.0933	0.3797	0.0754
			0.1845	0.2388	0.0939
			0.2090	0.0247	0.0110
			0.3002	0.1613	0.1031
			0.3936	0.0429	0.0359
			0.0086 (x ray)	0.3075	0.0056
^{75}Se	120d	–	–	–	0.0316
			0.1986	0.0135	0.0057
			0.2646	0.5710	0.3218
			0.2795	0.2388	0.1421
			0.3038	0.0123	0.0080
			0.4005	0.1164	0.0993

Continued.

---

*Data derived primarily from MIRD Supplement No. 2, pamphlet 4, March, 1969, and MIRD Supplement No. 4, pamphlet 6, March, 1970, New York, Society of Nuclear Medicine.

Radionuclide	$T_{1/2}$	$\overline{E}_\beta$(mev)	Principal photon energies (mev)	Fractional emission (n_i)	Δ_i $\left(\dfrac{g \cdot rad}{\mu Ci \cdot hr}\right)$
^{99m}Tc	6h	0.014	—	—	0.0371
			0.018 (x ray)	0.044	0.0017
			0.021 (x ray)	0.011	0.0004
			0.140	0.879	0.2630
^{113}In	1.7h	0.133	—	—	0.277
			0.392	0.621	0.518
			0.024 (x ray)	0.124	0.0064
^{123}I	13h	0.026	—	—	0.0602
			0.027 (x ray)	0.71	0.0415
			0.159	0.84	0.2831
			0.53	0.01	0.0118
^{125}I	60d	0.014	—	—	0.0463
			0.027 (x ray)	1.152	0.0671
			0.031 (x ray)	0.248	0.0163
			0.035	0.07	0.0050
^{131}I	8.06d	0.188	—	—	0.4135
			0.080	0.026	0.004
			0.284	0.058	0.035
			0.364	0.820	0.637
			0.6367	0.065	0.0886
			0.723	0.017	0.027
^{133}Xe	5.31d	0.110	—	—	0.299
			0.031 (x ray)	0.387	0.025
			0.081	0.36	0.062
^{137}Cs(^{137m}Ba)	30y	0.226	—	—	0.5367
			0.032 (x ray)	0.059	0.0039
			0.66	0.898	1.266

G

Relationships between "special" units and the SI units

Quantity	Dimensions	Previous SI unit	New SI unit; name (abbreviation)	Relationships with special unit
Activity	s^{-1}	s^{-1}	becquerel (Bq)	1 Ci $= 3.7 \times 10^{10}$ Bq 1 Bq $\simeq 2.703 \times 10^{-11}$ Ci
Exposures	$s \cdot A \cdot kg^{-1}$	$C \cdot kg^{-1}$	—*	1 R $= 2.58 \times 10^{-4}$ C/kg 1 C/kg $= 3.876 \times 10^{3}$ R
Absorbed dose	$N \cdot m \cdot kg^{-1}$	$J \cdot kg^{-1}$	gray (Gy)	1 rad $= 10^{-2}$ Gy 1 Gy $= 100$ rad
Dose equivalent	$N \cdot m \cdot kg^{-1}$	$J \cdot kg^{-1}$	—†	1 rem $= 10^{-2}$ J/kg 1 J/kg $= 100$ rem

*No name proposed; it is anticipated that this unit will eventually disappear.
†The question of a separate name for this SI unit is subject to further discussion: See also Dose Equivalent, Supplement to ICRU Report 19(1973).

Conversion factors for units of activity (A) and absorbed dose (D)

Activity (A)

1 picocurie	(1 pCi)	$= 10^{-12}$ Ci	$=$ 37 millibecquerels	(37 mBq)
1 nanocurie	(1 nCi)	$= 10^{-9}$ Ci	$=$ 37 becquerels	(37 Bq)
1 microcurie	(1 μCi)	$= 10^{-6}$ Ci	$=$ 37 kilobecquerels	(37 kBq)
1 millicurie	(1 mCi)	$= 10^{-3}$ Ci	$=$ 37 megabecquerels	(37 MBq)
1 curie	(1 Ci)	$=$ 1 Ci	$=$ 37 gigabecquerels	(37 GBq)
1 kilocurie	(1 kCi)	$= 10^{3}$ Ci	$=$ 37 terabecquerels	(37 TBq)
1 megacurie	(1 MCi)	$= 10^{6}$ Ci	$=$ 37 petabecquerels	(37 PBq)
1 gigacurie	(1 GCi)	$= 10^{9}$ Ci	$=$ 37 exabecquerels	(37 EBq)
1 becquerel	(1 Bq)	$=$ 1 Bq	$=$ 27.03 picocuries	(27.03 pCi)
1 kilobecquerel	(1 kBq)	$= 10^{3}$ Bq	$=$ 27.03 nanocuries	(27.03 nCi)
1 megabecquerel	(1 MBq)	$= 10^{6}$ Bq	$=$ 27.03 microcuries	(27.03 μCi)
1 gigabecquerel	(1 GBq)	$= 10^{9}$ Bq	$=$ 27.03 millicuries	(27.03 mCi)
1 terabecquerel	(1 TBq)	$= 10^{12}$ Bq	$=$ 27.03 curies	(27.03 Ci)
1 petabecquerel	(1 PBq)	$= 10^{15}$ Bq	$=$ 27.03 kilocuries	(27.03 kCi)
1 exabecquerel	(1 EBq)	$= 10^{18}$ Bq	$=$ 27.03 megacuries	(27.03 MCi)

Continued.

Absorbed dose (D)

1 millirad	(1 mrad)	= 10^{-3} rad	= 10 micrograys	(10 μGy)
1 rad	(1 rad)	= 1 rad	= 10 milligrays	(10 mGy)
1 kilorad	(1 krad)	= 10^3 rad	= 10 grays	(10 Gy)
1 megarad	(1 Mrad)	= 10^6 rad	= 10 kilograys	(10 kGy)
1 microgray	(1 μGy)	= 10^{-6} Gy	= 100 microrads	(100 μrad)
1 milligray	(1 mGy)	= 10^{-3} Gy	= 100 millirads	(100 mrad)
1 gray	(1 Gy)	= 1 Gy	= 100 rads	(100 rad)
1 kilogray	(1 kGy)	= 10^3 Gy	= 100 kilorads	(100 krad)

Index

A

Abdomen
  blood vessels in, 588, 591, 592, 593
  landmarks in, 343-344
  transverse sections through, 440, 441
Abscesses
  gallium 67 citrate imaging and, 539, 540
  hepatic, 539, 585
  renal, 533
  splenic, 369
Absorbed fraction of energy, 128-137, 140
  bone and, 133-134
  calculations in, 130-131
  embryo and, 138-139
  liver and, 130-133, 134, 140
  problem in, 131-133
  "S" tables in, 135-139
  spleen and, 133
  uterus and, 134-135
Absorbed radiation dose, average, 127
Absorption in counting and imaging, 252-253
Acceleration, 44, 47
Accelerators, 85-86
Access time, 233
Accidents in surgery or autopsy, 323; *see also* Safety
ACD; *see* Acid citrate dextrose
Acid citrate dextrose, 349, 356, 365, 367-368
Acinar cells, 458
Acini, 458
ACTH; *see* Adrenocorticotropic hormone
Actinium series, 32
Activated charcoal traps, 307, 309
Activation, neutron, 5, 80-84
Activators, 278
Activity
  on hand, 302
  specific; *see* Specific activity
Acute radiation syndrome, 158-159, 160
Acute somatic effects, 158-162
ADC converters, 219-221
Addition
  binary system and, 229
  static studies and, 240
Address wires, 234
Address word, 229
Adenomas of thyroid, 403
Adjuvant, 598
Adrenocortical hormone, 377
Adrenocorticotropic hormone, 396

Adsorption methods, 615
Aerosols, radioactive, 508, 513
Afferent arterioles, 519, 555
Affinity, 598-599
Age, 155
Aging, early, 163
Air, absorption and, 252
Airways, 505
ALARA; *see* As low as reasonably achievable
Albumin, 345
  excessive loss of, 435-436
  macroaggregates of, labeled
    with iodine 131, 508, 515
    with technetium 99m, 508, 510, 513, 561-562
  radiochromium serum, 437
  radioiodinated serum
    brain and, 415-416, 424, 427
    cardiac blood pool and, 498
    cardiac output and, 472, 474-476
    cerebrospinal fluid and, 424
    circulation time and, 477
    denatured, liver and, 442, 444, 447, 452
    hematology and, 347, 348, 351
    kidneys and, 521
    peripheral circulation and, 496
    placental localization and, 499
    protein absorption and, 433
    protein loss and, 436
    radiocardiography and, 479
  technetium 99m serum
    angiocardiography and, 480, 483
    cardiac blood pool and, 498
    cerebrospinal fluid and, 424
    circulation time and, 477
    coronary circulation and, 487
    hematology and, 348
    macroaggregates of, 508, 510, 513, 561-562
    microspheres of, 483, 487, 498, 508-509, 514
    placental localization and, 499, 501
    radiocardiography and, 479
    venography and, 498
    thyroid function and, 392
Alpha emitters, pure, 34
  decay schemes of, 65
Alpha particles, 27
  decay methods of, 35-37, 65, 67, 68
  emissions of, 33, 34
    reaction of, 37
  intensity of, 121